Routledge Revivals

Selected Genetic Papers of J.B.S. Haldane

First published in 1990, this is a compilation of several important papers that have contributed to the foundation of population genetics, evolutionary biology and human genetics. The collection includes Haldane's first paper in genetics, which was published in 1915, reporting the first case of linkage in a mammal, and - fifty years later, in 1965 - his last paper in genetics on selection for a single pair of allelomorphs with complete replacement. Haldane's Rule, the only idea named after him, was published in 1922 and is still valid today. Other papers, which include many Haldane firsts, such as the first estimation of a human mutation rate, first human gene map, first papers in population genetics, first estimate of the probability of fixation of a new mutation, and first measurement of mutation impact on a population, leading to the "genetic load" concept, are included. The volume also includes a paper presenting an ancient logical system for interpreting scientific results.

Selected Genetic Papers of J.B.S. Haldane

Edited with an Introduction by
Krishna R. Dronamraju

Foreword by
James F. Crow

Routledge
Taylor & Francis Group

First published in 1990
by Garland Publishing, Inc.

This edition first published in 2014 by Routledge
2 Park Square, Milton Park, Abingdon, Oxon, OX14 4RN
and by Routledge
711 Third Avenue, New York, NY 10017
Routledge is an imprint of the Taylor & Francis Group, an informa business

Publisher's Note
The publisher has gone to great lengths to ensure the quality of this reprint but points out that some imperfections in the original copies may be apparent.

Disclaimer
The publisher has made every effort to trace copyright holders and welcomes correspondence from those they have been unable to contact.

A Library of Congress record exists under LC control number: 90014125

ISBN 13: 978-1-138-78337-9 (hbk)
ISBN 13: 978-1-315-76869-4 (ebk)
ISBN 13: 978-1-138-78343-0 (pbk)

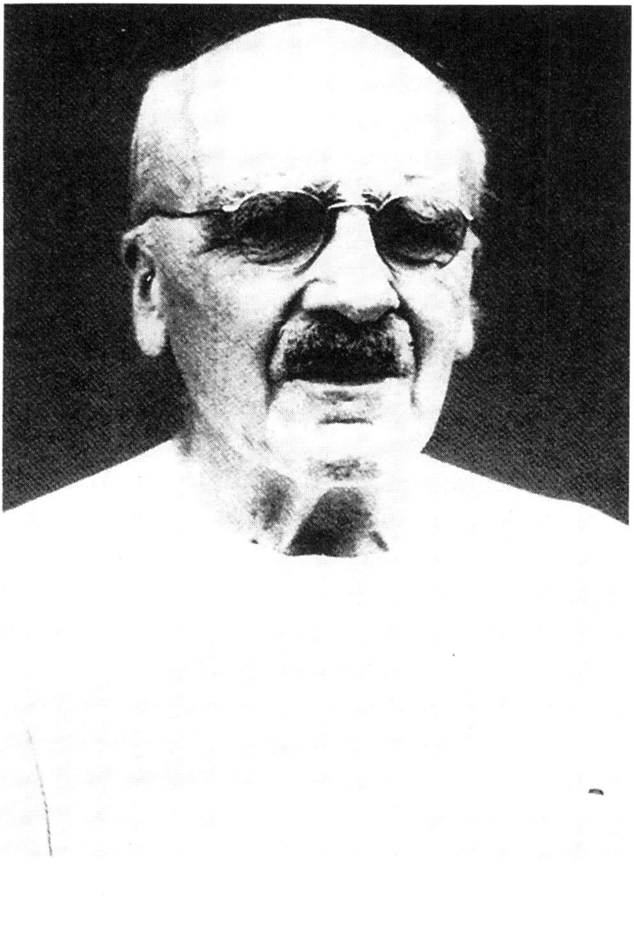

Haldane in India in 1961, Research Professor at the Indian Statistical Institute, Calcutta.

Selected Genetic Papers of

J.B.S. Haldane

Edited with an introduction by
Krishna R. Dronamraju

Foreword by
James F. Crow

Garland Publishing, Inc.
New York & London
1990

The editor and publisher are grateful to the University of Chicago Press for permission to reprint The *Effect of Variation on Fitness* and *A Defense of Beanbag Genetics;* and to Macmillan Magazines, Ltd. for permission to reprint *The Theory of Natural Selection Today and The Genetics of Cancer.*

Library of Congress Cataloging-in-Publication Data

Haldane, J.B.S. (John Burdon Sanderson), 1892–1964.
Selected genetic papers of J.B.S. Haldane / edited with an introduction by Krishna R. Dronamraju ; foreword by James F. Crow.
p. cm.
Includes bibliographical references.

ISBN 0-8240-0473-6 (alk. paper)

1. Genetics. 2. Human genetics. 3. Evolution. 4. Haldane, J.B.S. (John Burdon Sanderson), 1892–1964. I. Dronamraju, Krishna R. II. Title.
[DNLM: 1. Haldane, J.B.S. (John Burdon Sanderson), 1892–1964. 2. Genetics—collected works. QH 431 H158s]
QH438.H35 1990 575.1—dc20
DNLM/DLC for Library of Congress 90-14125

Printed on acid-free, 250-year-life paper.
Manufactured in the United States of America.

Design by Julie Threlkeld

Contents

Statement by Joshua Lederberg ix
Foreword by James F. Crow xi
Acknowledgements xiii
Introduction by Krishna R. Dronamraju xv

Perspectives in Biology

A Defense of Beanbag Genetics. 1
Perpectives in Biology & Medicine, 7: 343–359, 1964.
An Autobiography in Brief. 19
Illustrated Weekly of India, Bombay, 1961.
The Theory of Evolution, Before and After Bateson. 25
Journal of Genetics, 56:1–17, 1958.
The Theory of Natural Selection Today. 43
Nature, 183: 710–713, 1959.

Selection

A Mathematical Theory of Natural and Artificial Selection. Part I. 57
Transactions of the Cambridge Philosophical Society, 23: 19–41, 1924.
A Mathematical Theory of Natural and Artificial Selection. Part IV. 81
Proceedings of the Cambridge Philosophical Society, 23: 607–615, 1927a.
A Mathematical Theory of Natural and Artificial Selection, Part V.
Selection and Mutation. 90
Proceedings of the Cambridge Philosophical Society, 23: 838–844, 1927b.
A Note on Fisher's Theory of the Origin of Dominance, and on a Correlation
Between Dominance and Linkage. 97
American Naturalist, 64: 87–90, 1930.
A Mathematical Theory of Natural Selection. Part VIII.
Metastable Populations. 101
Proceedings of the Cambridge Philosophical Society, 27: 137–142, 1931.
The Time of Action of Genes, and Its Bearing on
Some Evolutionary Problems. 107
American Naturalist, 66: 5–24, 1932.
Suggestions as to Quantitative Measurement of Rates of Evolution. 127
Evolution, 3: 51–56, 1949.
The Measurement of Natural Selection. 133
Caryologia (suppl.), 6: 480–487, 1954.
The Theory of Selection for Melanism in Lepidoptera. 141
Proceedings of the Royal Society, B, 145: 303–308, 1956.
The Conflict Between Inbreeding and Selection, I. Self-Fertilization. 147
Journal of Genetics, 54: 56–63, 1956.
The Cost of Natural Selection 155
Journal of Genetics, 55: 511–524, 1957.

(with S.D. Jayaker) Polymorphism Due to Selection Depending on the Composition of a Population. 169
Journal of Genetics, 58: 318–323, 1963.
(with S.D. Jayakar) Selection for a Single Pair of Allelomorphs with Complete Replacement. 175
Journal of Genetics, 59: 81–87, 1965.

Mutation and Human Genetics

A Method for Investigating Recessive Characters in Man. 185
Journal of Genetics, 25: 251–255, 1932. .
The Part Played by Recurrent Mutation in Evolution. 191
American Naturalist, 67: 5–19, 1933.
The Rate of Spontaneous Mutation of a Human Gene. 207
Journal of Genetics, 31: 317–326, 1935.
The Effect of Variation on Fitness. 217
American Naturalist, 71: 337–349, 1937.
(with J. Bell) The Linkage Between the Genes for Colour-Blindness and Haemophilia in Man. 231
Proceedings of the Royal Society of London, B, 123: 119–150, 1937.
The Relative Importance of Principal and Modifying Genes in Determining Some Human Diseases. 263
Journal of Genetics, 41: 149–157, 1941.
Selection against Heterozygosis in Man. 273
Annual of Eugenics, 11: 333–340, 1942.
The Interaction of Nature and Nurture. 281
Annual of Eugenics, 13: 197–205, 1946.
The Mutation Rate of the Gene for Haemophilia, and Its Segregation Ratios in Males and Females. 291
Annual of Eugenics, 13, 262–271, 1947.
The Formal Genetics of Man. 301
Proceedings of the Royal Society, B, 135: 147–170, 1948.
Disease and Evolution. 325
La ricerca scientifica, supplemento, 19: 2–11, 1949.
The Association of Characters as a Result of Inbreeding and Linkage. 335
Annual of Eugenics, 15: 15–23, 1949.
Parental and Fraternal Correlations for Fitness. 345
Annual of Eugenics, 14: 288–292, 1949.
(with S.D. Jayakar) An Enumeration of Some Human Relationships. 351
Journal of Genetics, 58: 81–107, 1962.

Linkage

(with A.D. Sprunt and N.M. Haldane) Reduplication in Mice. 381
Journal of Genetics, 5: 133–135.
The Combination of Linkage Values, and the Calculation of Distances

Between the Loci of Linked Factors. 385
Journal of Genetics, 8: 299–309, 1919.
(with C.H. Waddington) Inbreeding and Linkage. 397
Genetics, 16: 357–374, 1931.
(with D. de Winton) Linkage in the Tetraploid *Primula Sinensis*. 415
Journal of Genetics, 24: 121–144, 1931.

Biochemical Genetics and Immunogenetics

Some Recent Work on Heredity. 441
Transactions of the Oxford University Junior Scientific Club, 1 (3): 3–11, 1920.
The Genetics of Cancer. 451
Nature, 132: 265–267, 1933.
The Detection of Antigens with an Abnormal Genetic Determination. 455
Journal of Genetics, 54: 54–55, 1956.

Radiation Genetics

The Dysgenic Effect of Induced Recessive Mutations. 459
Annual of Eugenics, 14: 35–43, 1947.
The Detection of Autosomal Lethals in Mice Induced by Mutagenic Agents. 469
Journal of Genetics, 54: 327–342, 1956.
The Detection of Sublethal Recessives by the Use of Linked Marker Genes in the Mouse (appendix to T.C. Carter's paper). 485
Journal of Genetics, 55: 596–597, 1957.
The Interpretation of Carter's Results on Induction of Recessive Lethals in Mice. 487
Journal of Genetics, 57: 131–136, 1960.

Haldane's Rule

Sex-ratio and Unisexual Sterility in Hybrid Animals. 495
Journal of Genetics, 12: 101–109, 1922.

Origins of Life

The Origin of Life. 507
Rationalist Annual, pp. 1–11, 1929.

Systems of Predication

The Syādvāda System of Predication. 521
Sankhyā: The Indian Journal of Statistics, 18: 195–200, 1957.
Science Citation Index 1988 527
Bibliography of J.B.S. Haldane's Publications 529

J.B.S. Haldane is one of the towering figures in the history of twentieth-century thought. He had no peer in his foresight about the looming developments in genetics, biochemistry, and their intersection. His interests spanned the mathematical theory of populations and revolution; the genetic control and kinetics of enzymes; and the prospects of space travel and life on other worlds. His foresight was such that his writings of a half-century ago still have fresh and exciting portents. Above all, he was an unremitting optimist about the human uses of reason and science, a belief that has been confounded by ill-informed cartoon images of the evil wizard.

His papers will continue to be used and cited for many decades—a prospect assured by this readily accessible compilation.

Joshua Lederberg
Nobel Laureate
President, The Rockefeller University
New York, N.Y.

Foreword

We are all unique; but for Haldane the word seems pallid. A grizzly bear of a man, he seemed larger than life. He was a multidimensional outlier. Physically courageous to the point of foolhardiness, he did dangerous experiments on himself, and paid for it with permanent injuries. He could speak while inhaling, so he didn't have to pause for breath in a conversation. He had a near-perfect memory, and not just in English; he could recite long passages from Shakespeare, Virgil, Dante, or the Koran. He was one of the best popular science writers; somehow he could strip off unessential details without distorting the subject. He showed his contempt for things British by emigrating to India late in life. He was a prodigious writer. He contributed 345 articles to the *Daily Worker*, many of them written on the commuter train (with his memory he didn't need references). He wrote 23 books, including science fiction and children's stories, and more than 400 scientific papers. Here, alphabetized, are some of the topics: air raid protection, animal behavior, anthropology, astronomy, biochemistry, blood groups, chemical warfare, dialectics, economics, embryology, enzyme kinetics, eugenics, evolution, genetics, Hindu religion, Marxist philosophy, mathematics, mechanics, non-violent animal research, nuclear radiation, origin of life, origin of the solar system, origins of language, philosophy of science, physiology, popular science writing, probability, quantum mechanics, relativity, respiration, statistics, technology, underwater survival, zoology.

Haldane enjoyed being a "character." Stories about him abound, and improve with age. Don't let his astonishing breadth of interest, adventurous life, popular writing, politicking, and eccentricity delude you into thinking that he was superficial. But he was eclectic. In contrast to many well known, lesser scientists, Haldane's name is not associated with a single great discovery. He did too many things; he was his own dilution factor. His work on regulation of blood alkalinity is basic textbook material. He was a pioneer in the theory of enzyme kinetics, and wrote a classic book. He unified human biochemical genetics, and was the first to use the words "cis" and "trans" in a genetic context. He discovered the first case of linkage in a mammal. He derived the first gene mapping function. He instigated pioneer work on the biochemistry of flower pigments. He derived the equilibrium between mutation and selection and used it to measure for the first time the mutation rate of the gene causing hemophilia. He even showed that the mutation rate is an order of magnitude higher in males than in females, recently confirmed by others. He was the first to suggest malaria as the cause of hemoglobin polymorphisms. He pointed out that the Rhesus factor was not in stable equilibrium, and that this implied that the European population is of hybrid origin. He was the first to measure the selective advantage of a gene in a natural population, the evolution of black color in the peppered moth following industrialization. He was the first to compute the probability of fixation of a new, selectively-favored mutant gene, a finding fundamental to current discussions of molecular evolution. He found the remarkable generalization, now called "Haldane's rule," that when there is lethality or sterility in hybrids, this is in the heterogametic sex. This is far from his greatest discovery, but the only one that is routinely referred to by his name. His most famous papers, both showing the Haldane touch, are those on the mutation load ("The Effect of Variation on Fitness," 1937) and the substitution load ("The Cost of Natural Selection," 1957). In the first he showed that the fitness impact of recurrent mutation depends on the mutation rate and not on the severity of the individual mutations. In the second, he showed that the amount of reproductive excess required to carry out a gene substitution depends mainly on its initial frequency and not on the magnitude of its effect.

Haldane's best known work is in evolutionary genetics. He wrote more than one hundred papers on this subject. From 1924 to 1934 he published a series of ten papers on "The mathematical theory of natural and artificial selection," a remarkably comprehensive investigation. This work was summarized in his book, *The Causes of Evolution*, a paradigm of simple clarity (in contrast to Fisher's elegant opacity).

Haldane shares with R.A. Fisher and Sewall Wright the credit for originating the field of population genetics. There are three great mathematical theories of evolution. Fisher quantified the change of fitness in a large, panmictic population in his fundamental theorem of natural selection. Wright emphasized population structure and the effects of chance in bringing about favorable gene interactions. Kimura developed the mathematical theory of molecular evolution by mutation and random drift. The name of Haldane is not associated with any specific theory; he was too eclectic, too open-minded to push any particular view.

Haldane's popular and expository writings are remarkable for their clarity. The first article in this book, "A Defense of Beanbag Genetics," shows him at his best—spirited, sprightly, witty, and erudite. His more mathematical papers are difficult for contemporary geneticists, mainly because of his notation. Fisher and Wright used allele frequency as the basic quantity, and this has become accepted. Therefore, Haldane's use of frequency ratios seems unfamiliar and awkward. A second reason is that Haldane used an inelegant, brute-force approach; he didn't mind heavy calculations—he was a speedy calculator and I think he enjoyed them. So his mathematical papers, although not intrinsically difficult, appear daunting and require more patience than most readers will want to exercise. Nevertheless, the Haldane prose is usually clear and a lot can be learned while skipping the cumbersome mathematics.

Haldane repeatedly had new ideas. I can't think of anyone so creative in so many diverse areas. His papers abound in speculations. Naturally, many of these have turned out to be wrong. But much more remarkable are the ones that have turned out to be on target and path-breaking.

How I wish some adventurous publisher would reprint Haldane's entire output, as was done for his great contemporary R.A. Fisher! Perhaps this will happen one day. Meanwhile, this book provides a start. Herein are reprinted forty-six of Haldane's genetics papers. Dr. Dronamraju has wisely refrained from long introductions and explanations. Haldane is too well known to need an introduction, and no one can explain his writing better than himself. Those who learned genetics since Haldane's death in 1964 have a chance to encounter one of biology's most remarkable minds and one of its most remarkable characters. There is a feast ahead. Bon appétit!

James F. Crow
Genetics Department
University of Wisconsin, Madison

Acknowledgements

It is a pleasure to thank Lady Naomi Mitchison for granting permission to reproduce her brother's scientific papers. I thank Professor James F. Crow for the Foreword. I am grateful to Dr. Joshua Lederberg for his commentary and valuable advice in preparing this book.

Numerous individuals have provided ideas and suggestions over the past many years concerning the publication of Haldane's papers in genetics. These include Mrs. J.B.S. Haldane (Helen Spurway), Sewall Wright, Motoo Kimura, William J. Schull, Newton E. Morton, Elof A. Carlson, M. Nei, C. Hanis, A. G. Bearn, John Maynard Smith, J.R.S. Fincham, S.D. Jayakar, and Ajit K. Ray.

Part of the Haldane collection is catalogued and maintained at the Centre for Cellular and Molecular Biology in Hyderabad (India). I am appreciative of the cooperation received from the Director, Dr. Pushp M. Bhargava, and the assistance of Mr. G.R.N. Goudar of the CCMB/IICT library in providing some of the papers. Recent discussions of Haldane's genetical work with J.S. Murty and Yog Ahuja of Osmania University of Hyderabad have been helpful in evaluating these publications. Financial assistance was provided by the U.N.D.P. Tokten project and the Friedman Company (Steve Friedman).

My wife Lalitha has provided valuable assistance in the preparation of the manuscript. Leo Balk and Mary Ross of Garland Publishing have made valuable suggestions in preparing the book for publication. I also express my thanks to the following publishers for their cooperation in granting permission to reproduce these papers: Cambridge University Press, Indian Statistical Institute Press, University of Chicago Press, Society for the Study of Evolution (U.S.A.), Genetics of Society of America, Rationalist Press Association (London), The Illustrated Weekly of India (Bombay), MacMillan Magazines Ltd. (*Nature*), and the Royal Society of London.

Introduction

John Burdon Sanderson Haldane made important contributions to physiology, biochemistry, genetics, statistics, and biometry as well as to a number of other scientific and non-scientific disciplines. Of these, his contributions to genetics are the most significant. Although he never conducted genetic experiments to any great extent, Haldane was one of the few leaders in that field who deeply influenced the steady growth of genetics from about 1920 until 1965.[1-3]

It is desirable to understand something about his background and career before one can fully appreciate Haldane's papers in genetics in the context of his social environment and total scientific output. Haldane was born in Oxford, England, on November 5, 1892. He was the son of Dr. John Scott Haldane, eminent respiratory physiologist at Oxford, who kindled and nourished his son's scientific talent from a very young age.[4] The younger Haldane assisted in his father's physiological experiments from the age of four onwards and was rewarded with scientific training and encouragement that left a lasting impression for the rest of his life. Haldane's intellectual outlook was shaped in the pre-World War years of Oxford. His closest companions included Julian and Aldous Huxley and his own sister Naomi (later Lady Mitchison). He was educated at Eton and Oxford, graduating with honors in 1914. At Oxford, he took up mathematics at first but later switched to the study of classics. His further education was interrupted by the outbreak of World War I. After the war, he resumed his scientific career, becoming a Fellow of New College in physiology. However, he earned no degree in science. In 1923, he moved to Cambridge to accept the William Dunn Readership in Biochemistry under F. Gowland Hopkins (later President of the Royal Society) and remained there until 1933. He left Cambridge to join University College, London, at first as Professor of Genetics and later as the Weldon Professor of Biometry. In 1957, Haldane was invited by Prof. P.C. Mahalanobis, Director of the Indian Statistical Institute in Calcutta, to become a Research Professor at that institution. Promptly resigning from University College, London, Haldane accepted that position and continued his research and teaching in India. Although at first Haldane immensely enjoyed his work at the Indian Statistical Institute, soon differences with Prof. Mahalanobis forced him to resign in 1961 and seek a position elsewhere.[5] Haldane trained several young scientists in India, and wrote a number of popular articles on genetics and other sciences for the popular press. After serving a brief period with the Council of Scientific and Industrial Research, he finally found peace in Bhubaneswar, Orissa, where he founded the Genetics and Biometry Laboratory with the support of Biju Patnaik, the Chief Minister of that State. I was closely associated with Haldane both at Calcutta and Bhubaneswar. He died of cancer on December 1, 1964, at Bhubaneswar.

Haldane's Scientific Work

Haldane was noted for his versatility of scientific interests and talent. Starting in 1912, he published a number of papers in respiratory physiology. Almost simultaneously, he continued to publish a number of papers in genetics, especially on linkage and the mathematical theory of natural selection (summarized in 1932[6]), which later became one of the foundations of population genetics along with the contributions of R.A. Fisher[7] and Sewall Wright.[8] While he was Dunn Reader in Biochemistry at Cambridge, Haldane also held the part-time position of officer in charge of genetical investigations at the John Innes Horticultural Institution (now the John Innes Institute at Norwich), where he directed pioneering research on the biochemical genetics of plant pigments by Scott-Moncrieff[9] and others. After he joined University College, London, his genetical studies continued but his physiological and biochemical interests were largely replaced by statistics and biometry. He wrote twenty-four books, more than four hundred scientific papers, and numerous popular articles in his lifetime. About half his scientific papers dealt with genetics, and over one hundred dealt with population genetics. Up to the age of forty, he was professionally identified as a "biochemist." His genetical work never occupied more than fifty percent of his time at any given period during the successive phases of his life. His early scientific work was deeply influenced by his father's physiological interests. From the inception, Haldane was accustomed to view genetics from a physiological point of view. It was this outlook that led him early to discuss gene action in terms of biochemical structure as well as enzyme reactions. On the other hand, he recognized the necessity of making simplifying assumptions to conduct mathematical investigations of selection, mutation, and other aspects of genetics. In order to fully appreciate Haldane's dilemma between these two aspects, the reader must start with his combative and elegant essay, "A Defense of Beanbag Genetics," which was written during the last year of his life. Starting with this self-evaluation by Haldane, we must then work backwards to examine his early papers to form our own opinions. Some twenty-six years after his death and many more years after their publication, it should not be surprising if our outlook tends to be quite different from his. Although primarily of interest to geneticists, this collection should interest any biologist who is curious about how certain biological sciences evolved in the earlier decades of this century.

The Influence of William Bateson and R.C. Punnett

As noted in his Bateson lecture, Haldane knew Bateson well, from 1919 until Bateson's death in 1926. His early work in genetics, which was concerned with the estimation of linkage, was deeply influenced by Bateson and Punnett. When he discovered linkage as an exception in Darbishire's data on mice (at first in 1911, the first known case in vertebrates), Haldane consulted Punnett, who advised him to obtain his own experimental evidence for confirmation. This delayed the publication of his finding until 1915. When formulating his rule concerning sex-ratio in hybrid animals (Haldane's rule, expressed in "Sex-ratio and Unisexual Sterility in Hybrid Animals," 1922), Haldane consulted Bateson and later wrote that Bateson was the first person to believe in that rule, suggesting additional supportive data. In 1924, Haldane's first paper on the mathematical theory of natural selection appeared while he was under Bateson's influence. It was, in fact, stimulated by H.T.J. Norton's early calculations on the intensity of selection, which appeared in Punnett's[10] book on mimicry. In the following years, Haldane initiated biochemical genetic research on anthocyanins at the John Innes Institution, with which Bateson was closely associated.

Another instance of Bateson-Haldane connection was the *Journal of Genetics*, founded by Bateson in 1911 and continued under Punnett's editorship until 1946, when Haldane took over as its editor. During his last years in India, several of the research projects that were pursued under Haldane's direction dealt with meristic variation in nature, which was one of Bateson's major evolutionary interests.

The papers are arranged into sections, the largest of which are concerned with selection and mutation. The classification is often arbitrary. Papers on mutation and human genetics are combined into one section because of Haldane's great interest in human mutation rates and his extensive work on the estimation of the impact of mutation in human populations. Several of these papers fall under more than one category. The study of dysgenic effects of radiation (1947) could be under human genetics or mutation or radiation genetics. Finally, everyone has their own favorite Haldane papers. The criterion applied in this instance is to include papers that have had a major impact on the development of several aspects of genetics and some that have suggested lines of research still unresolved. A complete bibliography of Haldane's scientific work is also included.

Haldane's scientific approach typifies what I have called "intellectual hybridization,"[11] which appears to have played a vital role in the development of biological sciences. In numerous papers, he displayed a great talent for synthesizing concepts and methods from several different disciplines combining genetics with immunology, biochemistry, statistics, and physics. See, for instance, his discussion of meristic variation in the Bateson lecture (p. 25), where he draws analogy between the process of vertebrae formation in the tail and Turing's principle of surface tension. His early influence on the development of biochemical genetics, immunogenetics, mathematical genetics, behavior genetics, and other branches was clearly due to his ability to "cross-fertilize" on the intellectual plane. Much of the rapid expansion and evolution of biological sciences in the twentieth century has been due to his interdisciplinary synthesis. The phenomenon of so-called paradigm displacement (suggested by Kuhn[12]) does not appear to be valid in this context.

Very few scientists are outstanding writers. Haldane was an exception. He belonged to that generation of outstanding popular science writers that included Julian Huxley,[13] Bertrand Russell, J.D. Bernal, and Lancelot Hogben. Two articles included in this collection, "In Defense of Beanbag Genetics" and "An Autobiography in Brief," give us glimpses of his style. Elsewhere writing about his scientific contributions, Haldane[14] wrote: "I am a part of nature, and, like other natural objects, from a lightning flash to a mountain range, I shall last out my time and then finish. This prospect does not worry me, because some of my work will not die when I do so."

References

1. Wright, S., Haldane's contribution to population and evolutionary genetics. *Proc. XII Intern., Cong. Genet., 3*: 445–451, 1969.
2. Dronamraju, K.R., (Ed.) *Haldane and Modern Biology*, Baltimore: Johns Hopkins Uni-versity Press, 1968.

3. Dronamraju, K.R., *Haldane: The Life and Work of J.B.S. Haldane with Special Reference to India*. Aberdeen: Aberdeen University Press–Pergamon Press, 1985.
4. Haldane, L.K., *Friends and Kindred*. London: Faber and Faber Ltd., 1961. (Autobiography of his mother, Louisa Kathleen Haldane).
5. Haldane, J.B.S., An Autobiography in brief. Bombay: *Illustrated Weekly of India*, 1961; reprinted in *Persp. Biol. Med.*, *9*: 476–481, 1966.
6. Haldane, J.B.S., *The Causes of Evolution*. London: Longmans, Green, 1932.
7. Fisher, R.A., *The Genetical Theory of Natural Selection*. Oxford: Clarendon Press, 1930.
8. Wright, S., Evolution in Mendelian populations. *Genetics, 16*: 97–159, 1931.
9. Scott-Moncrieff, R., The classical period in chemical genetics: Recollections of Muriel Wheldale Onslow, Robert and Gertrude Robinson, and J.B.S. Haldane. *Notes and Records of the Royal Society of London, 36*: 125–154, 1981.
10. Punnett, R.C., *Mimicry in Butterflies*. Cambridge: Cambridge University Press.
11. Dronamraju, K.R., *The Foundations of Human Genetics*. Springfield (Ill.): Charles C. Thomas, Inc., 1989.
12. Kuhn, T.S., *The Structure of Scientific Revolutions*. Chicago: The University of Chicago Press, 1962 (second edition, 1970).
13. Dronamraju, K.R., *A Scientific Biography of Julian Huxley*. New York: Springer-Verlag (in press).
14. Haldane, J.B.S., *The Inequality of Man and Other Essays*. London: Chatto & Windus, Ltd., 1932.

Perspectives in Biology

The collection of papers included in this section have a common theme: Haldane's view of the historical perspective of a number of aspects of his life and work as well as certain aspects of evolutionary biology. In these papers he dealt with a wide-ranging series of subjects in evolutionary biology and biometry. The first one, appropriately, sums up his contributions (and those of his co-founders, Sewall Wright and R.A. Fisher) to the foundations of population genetics (see Crow[1]). This seems to provide an appropriate rationale to examine Haldane's genetic contributions. The second one is an article written for a popular newsmagazine in India, *The Illustrated Weekly of India* from Bombay, at the time of his resignation from the Indian Statistical Institute in Calcutta in 1961. He refers to his falling out with Prof. P.C. Mahalanobis, director of that Institute, in the penultimate paragraph of this article. Besides being an excellent self-evaluation of his life and work, this article is a fine example of Haldane's lucid style of popular writing for which he was well-known. In the third paper, Haldane examines the validity of Bateson's evolutionary contributions to later developments in biology. Of special interest is the role of "meristic" variation in producing such discontinuities as what were later called "quasicontinuous" variants by Gruneberg.[2] Haldane emphasized Bateson's lapidary phrase "Treasure your exceptions," which subsequently became the foundation for the development of medical genetics as well as several other sciences. Finally, in the fourth paper, he examines the status of natural selection in his presidential address delivered at the Centenary and Bicentenary Congress, which was held at the University of Malaya in Singapore in 1958.

1. Crow, J.F., The founders of population genetics. In Chakravarti, A. (Ed.): *Human Population Genetics: The Pittsburgh Symposium*, New York: Van Nostrand, 1984, pp. 177–194.
2. Gruneberg, H., Genetical studies on the skeleton of the mouse. IV. Quasi-continuous variations. *J. Genet.*, *51*: 95, 1952.

A DEFENSE OF BEANBAG GENETICS

*J. B. S. HALDANE**

My friend Professor Ernst Mayr, of Harvard University, in his recent book *Animal Species and Evolution* [1], which I find admirable, though I disagree with quite a lot of it, has the following sentences on page 263.

> The Mendelian was apt to compare the genetic contents of a population to a bag full of colored beans. Mutation was the exchange of one kind of bean for another. This conceptualization has been referred to as "beanbag genetics." Work in population and developmental genetics has shown, however, that the thinking of beanbag genetics is in many ways quite misleading. To consider genes as independent units is meaningless from the physiological as well as the evolutionary viewpoint.

Any kind of thinking whatever is misleading out of its context. Thus ethical thinking involves the concept of duty, or some equivalent, such as righteousness or *dharma*. Without such a concept one is lost in the present world, and, according to the religions, in the next also. Joule, in his classical papers on the mechanical equivalent of heat, wrote of the duty of a steam engine. We now write of its horsepower. It is of course possible that ethical conceptions will in future be applied to electronic calculators, which may be given built-in consciences!

In another place [2] Mayr made a more specific challenge. He stated that Fisher, Wright, and I "have worked out an impressive mathematical theory of genetical variation and evolutionary change. But what, precisely, has been the contribution of this mathematical school to evolutionary theory, if I may be permitted to ask such a provocative question?" "However," he continued in the next paragraph, "I should perhaps leave it to Fisher, Wright, and Haldane to point out what they consider their major contributions." While Mayr may certainly ask this question, I may not answer it at Cold Spring Harbor, as I have been officially informed that

* Address: Genetics and Biometry Laboratory, Government of Orissa, Bhubaneswar-3, Orissa, India.

I am ineligible for a visa for entering the United States.[1] Fisher is dead, but when alive preferred attack to defense. Wright is one of the gentlest men I have ever met, and if he defends himself, will not counterattack. This leaves me to hold the fort, and that by writing rather than speech.

Now, in the first place I deny that the mathematical theory of population genetics is at all impressive, at least to a mathematician. On the contrary, Wright, Fisher, and I all made simplifying assumptions which allowed us to pose problems soluble by the elementary mathematics at our disposal, and even then did not always fully solve the simple problems we set ourselves. Our mathematics may impress zoologists but do not greatly impress mathematicians. Let me give a simple example. We want to know how the frequency of a gene in a population changes under natural selection. I made the following simplifying assumptions [3]:

1) The population is infinite, so the frequency in each generation is exactly that calculated, not just somewhere near it.

2) Generations are separate. This is true for a minority only of animal and plant species. Thus even in so-called annual plants a few seeds can survive for several years.

3) Mating is at random. In fact, it was not hard to allow for inbreeding once Wright had given a quantitative measure of it.

4) The gene is completely recessive as regards fitness. Again it is not hard to allow for incomplete dominance. Only two alleles at one locus are considered.

5) Mendelian segregation is perfect. There is no mutation, non-disjunction, gametic selection, or similar complications.

6) Selection acts so that the fraction of recessives breeding per dominant is constant from one generation to another. This fraction is the same in the two sexes.

With all these assumptions, we get a fairly simple equation. If q_n is the frequency of the recessive gene, and a fraction k of recessives is killed off when the corresponding dominants survive, then

$$q_{n+1} = \frac{q_n - k q_n^2}{1 - k q_n^2}.$$

[1] In spite of this ineligibility I have, since writing this article, been granted an American visa, for which I must thank the federal government. However, I am not permitted to lecture in North Carolina, and perhaps in other states, without answering a question which I refuse to answer. Legislation to this effect does not, in my opinion, help American science.

Norton gave an equation equivalent to this in 1910, and in 1924 I gave a rough solution when selection is slow, that is to say k small. But one might hope that such a simple-looking equation would yield a simple relation between q_n and n; if not as simple as $s = \frac{1}{2} gt^2$ for fall in a uniform gravitational field, then as simple as Kepler's laws of planetary motion. Haldane and Jayakar [4] have solved this equation in terms of what are called automorphic functions of a kind which were fashionable in Paris around 1920, but have never been studied in detail, like sines, logarithms, Gamma and Polygamma functions, and so on. Until the requisite functions have been tabulated, geneticists will be faced with as much work as if a surveyor, after measuring an angle, had to calculate its cosine or whatever trigonometrical function he needed. The mathematics are not much worse when we allow for inbreeding and incomplete dominance. But they are very much stiffer when selection is of variable intensity from year to year and from place to place (as it always is) or when its intensity changes gradually with time. If we had solved such problems, our work would be impressive.

Let me add that the few professional mathematicians who have interested themselves in such matters have been singularly unhelpful. They are apt to devote themselves to what are called existence theorems, showing that problems have solutions. If they hadn't, we shouldn't be here, for evolution would not have occurred.

Now let me try to show that what little we have done is of some use, even if we have done a good deal less serious mathematics than Mayr believes. It may be well to cite the first formulation of beanbag genetics. This was by the great Roman poet Titus Lucretius Carus just over two thousand years ago (*De rerum natura*, IV, l. 1220):

> Propterea quia multa modis primordia multis
> Mixta suo celant in corpore saepe parentes
> Quae patribus patres tradunt ab stirpe profecta,
> Inde Venus varia producit sorte figuras
> Maiorumque refert vultus vocesque comasque.

A free rendering is: "Since parents often hide in their bodies many genes mixed in many ways, which fathers hand down to fathers from their ancestry; from them Venus produces patterns by varying chance, and brings back the faces, voices, and hair of ancestors." Very probably the great materialistic (but not atheistic) philosopher Epicurus had expressed the theory more exactly, if less poetically, in one of his lost books. Lucretius elsewhere described genes as "genitalia corpora" and claimed that they were immutable. What is important is that whether he called them primordia or even seeds, he always thought of them as a set of separable material bodies. When Mendel discovered most of the laws according to which Venus picks out the hidden genes from the mixture, and Bateson and Punnett further discovered linkage, we could get going; and it was Punnett [5] who first calculated the long-term effect of a very simple program of selection.

Now let me begin boasting. So competent a biologist as Professor L. T. Hogben [6] has recently written, "The mutation of chromosomes or of single genes is admittedly the pace-maker of evolution." A strong verbal argument could be made out for this statement. In racing, a "pacemaker" runs particularly fast, but I suppose Hogben means that mutation determines the rate of evolution, which would be faster if mutation were more frequent. The verbal argument might run as follows: "Evolution is the resultant of a number of processes, including adaptation of individuals during their development, migration, segregation, natural selection, and mutation. Now in this list the slowest process is mutation. The probability that a gene will mutate in one generation rarely exceeds one hundred thousandth, and may be much less than a millionth. Whereas selective advantages of one in ten are quite common, a species may spread over a continent in a few centuries, and so on. Since mutation is the slowest process, it must set the pace, or be the 'rate-determining process,' for the remainder." This is quite as good an argument as those on which most human ethical and political decisions are based. When Muller had determined a few mutation rates, Wright and I, around 1930, began to calculate the evolutionary effects of mutation. We showed that in a species with several hundred thousand members mutations could not be a pacemaker. Almost all mutations occurred several times in a generation in one member or another of a species. But this again is a verbal argument. Only algebraical argument can be decisive in such a case. No doubt Wright's original "model" or hypothesis was too simple, but it was, I believe, near enough to the truth. I put in some rather ugly algebra to show that it made no appreciable difference whether selection occurred before or after mutation in a life cycle. I do not regret this effort. It is necessary to test all sorts of possibilities in such a case. I was trying to build a mathematical theory of natural selection. In doing so I calculated the equilibria between mutation of various types of genes and selection against them. As soon as this was done it became possible to estimate human mutation rates, and I did so [7]. Later on I improved this estimate, and since then many others have done it better. The estimation of human mutation rates, which is a by-product of my mathematical work, has since assumed some political importance. Had I devoted my life to research and propaganda in this field, rather than to expanding the bounds of human knowledge, I should doubtless be a world-famous "expert." I believe that the estimation of the rate at which X-rays, gamma rays, neutrons, and so on, produce mutations in animals could be vastly improved. But what I believe to be the most accurate method [8, 9] has not been given a serious trial, probably because it involves a good deal of mathematics. However, the work of Carter [10] and of Muramutsu, Sugahara, and Okazawa [11] shows that it is practicable, but expensive.

Now, Professor Mayr might say, "We must thank Haldane for the first estimate of a human mutation rate, but his argument is very simple indeed; in his own words, 'the rates of production by mutation and elimination by natural selection [of a harmful gene] must about balance.' So if we can find out how many people die of hemophilia or sex-linked muscular dystrophy per year, we can find out how many genes for these conditions arise by mutation." Anyone can understand this argument, and it has been used to estimate many human mutation rates, even though one estimate, based on years of careful work, is out by a factor of 2 through an elementary mathematical error. But as it stands it is no better than most political arguments. Selection and mutation must balance in the long run, but how long is that? In two rather complicated mathematical papers [12, 13] I showed that while harmful dominants and sex-linked recessives reach equilibrium fairly quickly, the time needed for the frequency of an autosomal recessive to get halfway to equilibrium after a change in the mutation rate, the selective disadvantage, or the mating system, may be several thousand generations. In fact, the verbal argument is liable to be fallacious. As few people have read my papers on the spread or diminution of autosomal recessives, and still fewer understood them, the "balance" method, which I invented, is applied to situations where I claim that it leads to false conclusions.

I am in substantial agreement with David Hume when he wrote (*A trea-*

tise of human nature, Book 1, Part 3, Section 1): "There remain therefore algebra and arithmetic as the only sciences, in which we can carry on a chain of reasoning to any degree of intricacy, and yet preserve a perfect exactness and certainty." Not only is algebraic reasoning exact; it imposes an exactness on the verbal postulates made before algebra can start which is usually lacking in the first verbal formulations of scientific principles.

Let me take another example from my own work. From the records of the spread of the autosomal gene for melanism in the moth *Biston betularia* in English industrial districts, I calculated [3] that it conferred a selective advantage of about 50 per cent on its carriers. Few or no biologists accepted this conclusion. They were accustomed to think, if they thought quantitatively at all, of advantages of the order of 1 per cent or less. Kettlewell [14] has now made it probable that, in one particular wood, the melanics have at least double the fitness of the original type. As Kettlewell very properly chose a highly smoke-blackened wood where selection was likely to be intense, I do not think his result contradicts mine. The mathematics on which my conclusion was based are not difficult, but they are clearly beyond the grasp of some biologists. In a recent book [15] it was stated that this melanism must originally have been recessive, in which case even the large advantage found by Kettlewell would have taken some thousands of years to produce the changes observed in fifty years. I suspect this curious mistake is due to the fact that in an elementary exposition one may produce an argument which ignores dominance and gives a result of the right order of magnitude. But such an exposition may not stress that the argument breaks down when applied to rare recessives. I think that in this particular instance Professor Mayr may have unwittingly been a little less than fair to us beanbaggers. On his page 191 [1] he says that my "classical" calculations in a book published in 1932 were deliberately based on very small selective intensities and implies that I only reached the same conclusion for industrial melanism in 1957. In fact, it was not till 1957 that biologists took my calculation of 1924 seriously. I did not stress it in 1932 because I thought such intense selection was so unusual as to be unimportant for evolution. If biologists had had a little more respect for algebra and arithmetic, they would have accepted the existence of such intense selection thirty years before they actually did so.

When Landsteiner and Wiener discovered the genetical basis of human fetal erythroblastosis, I pointed out [16] that the death of Rh-positive babies born to Rh-negative mothers could not yield a stable equilibrium and suggested that the modern populations of Europe were the result of crossing between peoples who, like all peoples then known, possessed a majority of Rh-positive genes and peoples who had a majority of Rh-negative genes. A distinguished colleague had calculated an equilibrium but had not dipped far enough into the bag to notice that it was unstable. Since then two relict populations have been discovered, in northern Spain and in one canton of Switzerland, with a majority of Rh-negative genes. If the mortality of the babies were higher, such differences would constitute a barrier to crossing, and I do not doubt that differences of this sort play a part in preventing hybridization between mammalian species. They can, for example, kill baby mules. I therefore regard the above paper as a contribution both to anthropology and to general evolution theory.

Once one has developed a set of mathematical tools, one looks for quantitative data on which to try them out. There are perhaps three main lines of such machine tool design, which may be called the Tectonic (from Greek *τέκτων*, a Wright), the Halieutic (from Greek *ἁλιεύτης*, a Fisher), and my own. Morton and C. A. B. Smith are developing a fourth, for use in human genetics. P. A. P. Moran [17] may be starting a fifth, or he may merely have made a hard road into an impassable swamp. A worker looks for numerical data on which his own favorite tools will bite. Thus Wright has collected data on small more or less isolated populations to which his theory of genetic drift is applicable. Fisher was probably at his best with samples from somewhat larger populations, for example his brilliant demonstration [18] of natural selection in Nabours' samples of wild *Paratettix texanus*, which is still perhaps the best evidence for heterosis in wild populations. Perhaps I am at my best with still larger populations. Thus I was, I think, the first to estimate quantitatively the rate of morphological change in evolving species [19]. My estimates are of the right order of magnitude, but based on estimates of geological time less reliable than those of Simpson [20]. I therefore fully accept Simpson's emendations (his pp. 10–17) of my figures. The question was the rate at which the mean of a morphological character changes. For one tooth measurement on fossil Equidae, paracone height, the rate of increase of the mean per million years ranged from 2.4 per cent to 7.9 per cent; for another, ectoloph length, from 0.6 per cent to 3.4 per cent. The rate of increase of the ratio of these lengths, which is of greater evolutionary importance, ranged from 0.9

per cent to 5.5 per cent. The total time covered was about 50 million years. On the other hand, I suggested that human skull height had increased by over 50 per cent per million years during the Pleistocene. The fossil data could have been so analyzed earlier. If I was the first to do so it was because, as the result of my mathematical work, such numbers had come to have more meaning for me than for others.

We can now come back to the justification of mathematical genetics. I leave out the body of mathematics which has grown up around human genetics. Here we cannot experiment and must squeeze all the information out of available figures, whereas where experiment is possible, not only is experiment often easier than calculation, but its results are more certain. In the consideration of evolution, a mathematical theory may be regarded as a kind of scaffolding within which a reasonably secure theory expressible in words may be built up. I have given examples to show that without such a scaffolding verbal arguments are insecure. Let me take an example from astronomy. I do not doubt that when Newton enunciated his gravitational theory of planetary movement many people said that if the sun attracted the planets they would fall into it. This is not so naïve as might be supposed. Cotes, of whose early death Newton wrote, "If Mr. Cotes had lived, we might have known something," showed that if the system "of planets, struggling fierce towards heaven's free wilderness," as Shelley put it, were attracted by the sun with a force varying as the inverse cube of the distance, they would move in spirals, and either fall into the sun or freeze in the free wilderness. Newton felt that he had to show not only that the inverse-square law led to stable elliptic motion, but that spheres, whose density at any point was a function of distance from their center, attracted one another as if they were particles. If he had not done so, he was aware that someone might readily disprove his highly ambitious theory. This does not mean that in explaining Newtonian gravitational theory to students one need go into these or many other details.

It is, in my opinion, worth while devoting some energy to proving the obvious. Thus, suppose a population consists of two genotypes A and B, of which B is fitter than A so long as it is rare. For example, B could be a mimic only advantageous when rare compared with its model, or a self-sterile but interfertile genotype of a plant species. It is intuitively obvious that B will spread through a population till its mean fitness falls to equal that of A, and a stable equilibrium will result. But is it sure that this equilibrium will be stable? Every physicist and cybernetician knows that if regulation is too intense a system may overshoot its equilibrium and go into oscillations of increasing amplitude. Haldane and Jayakar [21] found that in several cases investigated by them there was no danger of such instability. In a microfilm on population genetics circulated in A.D. 2000 we may either find the statement, "Haldane and Jayakar showed that such equilibria are almost always stable," or, "Haldane and Jayakar believed that they had demonstrated the stability of such equilibria. They overlooked the investigations of X on termites, where, as Y later showed, the equilibrium is unstable." But even if we have given the wrong answer, we deserve a modicum of credit for asking the right question.

I could give many more examples. Thus, posterity may or may not think that my concept of the cost of natural selection—that is to say, the number of genetic deaths required to bring about an evolutionary change [22]—is important. I think it defines one of the factors, perhaps the main one, determining the speed of evolution. It has been accepted by some and criticized by others. If it is shown to be false, the demonstration of its falsity will probably reveal the truth, or at least a closer approximation to the truth. And so I could continue on a large scale. If I were on trial for wasting my life, my defense would at least be prolonged, even if unsuccessful; for I have published over 90 papers on beanbag genetics, of which over 50 contained some original statements, whether or not they were important or true, besides 200 papers on other scientific topics.

The existing theories of population genetics will no doubt be simplified and systematized. Many of them will have no more final importance than a good deal of nineteenth-century dynamical theory. This does not mean that they have been a useless exercise of algebraical ingenuity. One must try many possibilities before one reaches even partial truth. There is, however, a danger that when a mathematical investigation shows a possible cause of a phenomenon, it is assumed to be the only possible cause. Thus Fisher [23] showed that if heterozygotes for a pair of autosomal alleles are fitter than either homozygote, there will be stable polymorphism, and later work has extended this theorem to multiple alleles. Numerous cases have been discovered where such heterosis, both at single loci and for chromosomal segments, has been observed in nature. It has therefore been assumed that, except where rarity confers an obvious advantage, the Halieutic mechanism is at work. Now Haldane and Jayakar [24] have shown that, without any superiority of heterozygotes, selection of fluctuating direction will sometimes preserve polymorphism. There is no reason to think that this often happens, but it may sometimes do so. However, if I had made this calculation in 1920, as I might have done, while Fisher had published his work somewhat later, my explanation, which I do not doubt is more rarely true than Fisher's, might have been accepted as the usual explanation of stable polymorphism. It seems likely that this has happened in other cases, though naturally I do not know what these are. The best way to avoid such contingencies is to investigate mathematically the consequences following from a number of hypotheses which may seem rather farfetched and, if they would lead to observed results, looking in nature or the laboratory for evidence of their truth or falsehood.

One such possibility is the origin of "new" genes in higher animals or plants by viral transduction from species with which hybridization is impossible, conceivably even from members of a different phylum. While no doubt exaggerated claims have been made by the Michurinist school, some of its claims, such as the facilitation of hybridization by grafting, have been verified outside the Soviet Union. Transduction could account for some grafting effects which could not be regularly repeated. In terms of orthodox American genetics, such transduction would be described as a mutation leading to a neomorph. It is obvious that transduction could help to explain some cases of parallel evolution.

Let me be clear that I think the above hypothesis is improbable. But it serves to underline a fundamental point. Let us suppose that it had been proved that all evolutionary events observed in the fossil record and deduced from comparative morphology, embryology, and biochemistry could be explained on the basis of the generally accepted "synthetic theory"; this would not demonstrate that other causes were not operating. I think we have come near to showing that the synthetic theory will account for observed evolution and that a number of other superficially plausible theories, such as those of Lamarck, Osborn, and de Vries, will not do so. This does not exclude the possibility that other agencies are at work too. To take an example from astronomy, it was believed until recently that celestial mechanics were almost wholly dominated by gravitational forces. It is now believed that cosmic magnetic fields are also important.

Of course, Mayr is correct in stating that beanbag genetics do not explain the physiological interaction of genes and the interaction of genotype and environment. If they did so they would not be a branch of biology. They would be biology. The beanbag geneticist need not know how a particular gene determines resistance of wheat to a particular type of rust, or hydrocephalus in mice, or how it blocks the growth of certain pollen tubes in tobacco, still less why various genotypes are fitter, in a particular environment, than others. If he is a good geneticist he may try to find out, but in so doing he will become a physiological geneticist. If the beanbag geneticist knows that, in a given environment, genotype *P* produces 10 per cent more seeds than Q, though their capacity for germination is only 95 per cent of those of Q, he can deduce the evolutionary consequence of these facts, given further numbers as to the mating system, seed dispersal, and so on. Similarly, the paleontologist can describe evolution even if he does not know why the skulls of labyrinthodonts got progressively flatter. He is perhaps likely to describe the flattening more objectively if he has no theory as to why it happened.

The next probable development of beanbag genetics is of interest. Sakai [25] described competition between rice plants. A plant of genotype *P* planted in the neighborhood of plants of genotype Q may produce more seeds than when planted in pure stand, while its neighbors of genotype Q produce less. Roy [26] has described cases of this kind but also cases where, when *P* and Q are grown in mixture, both *P* and Q produce more seed. In such a case, if the mixed seed is harvested and sown, *P* may supplant Q, or a balanced polymorphism may result. Of course if *P* and Q interbreed, the results will be very complicated. But I have no doubt that such cases occur in nature, and are of evolutionary importance. Given quantitative data on yields of mixed crops, a beanbag geneticist can work out the consequences of such interaction, even if he does not know its causes.

Another probable development is this. It is likely [27] that as the result of duplications one locus in an ancestor can be represented by several in descendants. If so, this is one of the important evolutionary processes, and its precise "beanbag" genetics will require investigation, even though the relative fitnesses of the various types, and the reasons for them, besides the causes of duplication, are matters of physiological genetics.

I would like to make one more claim for beanbag genetics. It has been of some value to philosophy. I consider that the theory of path coefficients invented by Sewall Wright may replace our old notions of causation. A path coefficient answers the question, "To what extent is a set of events

B determined by another set A?" Path coefficients were invented to deal with problems such as the determination of piebaldness and otocephaly in guinea pigs, which are beyond the present scope of beanbag genetics. But Wright showed how to calculate them exactly in the case of inbreeding, which he treated on "beanbag" principles. Again Haldane [28] discussed how to argue back from a handful of beans to the composition of the bag. Jeffreys [29] made this paper the basis of his theory of inverse probability. Jeffreys is generally regarded as a heresiarch and takes my theory more seriously than I do myself. Nevertheless, there is presumably some measure of truth in it, and even if Birnbaum [30] has shown how to do without it, I may take some credit for stimulating him to lay a stronger foundation than my own for the theory of inverse probability.

The dichotomy between physiological and beanbag genetics is one of the clearest examples of the contrast between what my wife, Spurway [31], calls Vaiṣṇava and Śaiva[2] biology. Modern Hindus can, on the whole, be divided into Vaiṣṇavas—that is to say, worshippers of Viṣṇu, usually in one or other of his most important incarnations, Rama and Kriṣna—and Śaivas, or worshippers of Śiva. Viṣṇu has, on the whole, been concerned with preservation and Śiva with change by destruction and generation. This is a very superficial account. Spurway may be consulted for further details. Devotees of Viṣṇu do not deny the existence of Śiva, nor conversely are they necessarily exclusive in their worship, and many state that both deities are aspects of the same Being. Neither sect has actively persecuted the other. Roughly speaking, Darwin was a Śaiva when he wrote on natural selection and a Vaiṣṇava when he wrote on the adaptations of plants for cross-pollination, climbing, and so on. A biologist who is always a Śaiva, and does not worry about how living organisms achieve internal harmony and adaptation to their environment, is as narrow as a Vaiṣṇava who takes an organism as given and does not interest himself in its evolutionary past or its success in competition with other members of its species. It is very difficult to combine the two approaches in one's thought at the same moment. It may be easier a century hence. Thus, we know that human sugar metabolism depends on the antagonistic action of pancreatic insulin and one or more diabetogenic hormones from the anterior pituitary. Insulin production and anterior pituitary function are both under genetic control, but we do not know enough about this even to speculate

[2] *Ś* and *ṣ* are both near to the English *sh*.

fruitfully on the level of beanbag genetics, except to say that several different genotypes may achieve good homeostasis, while other combinations of the genes concerned are less well adapted for homeostasis, though they may have other advantages. Even this is a mere speculation. There may be only one adaptive peak in Wright's sense.

As I happen to be responsible for some of the mathematical groundwork of enzyme chemistry [32], I can say that the mathematical basis of physiological genetics is about fifty years behind that of beanbag genetics. If a metabolic process depends on four enzymes acting on the same substrate in succession, one can calculate what will happen if the amount of one of them is halved, provided that one is working with enzymes in solution in a bottle. We know far too little of the structural organization of living cells at the molecular level to predict what will happen if the amount is halved in a cell, as it is in some heterozygotes. If the enzyme molecules are arranged in organelles containing just one of each kind, the rate of the metabolic process will probably be halved. But if they are in a random or a more complicated arrangement, it may be diminished to a slight extent, or even increased; for the activities of some enzymes are inhibited by an excess of their substrate. This is a conceivable cause of heterosis, though I do not think it is likely to be common.

Now let me pass over to a counterattack. One of the central theses of Mayr's book is that speciation is rarely if ever sympatric. One species can only split into two as the result of isolation by a geographic barrier, save perhaps in very rare cases. Let me say at once that Mayr's arguments have convinced me that sympatric speciation is much rarer than some authors have believed, and a few still believe. But when, in his chapter 15, he discusses other authors' hypotheses as to how sympatric speciation might occur, his arguments are always verbal rather than algebraic. And sometimes I find his verbal arguments very hard to follow. Thus, on page 473 he makes seven assumptions, of which (1) is "Let *A* live only on plant species 1," and (4) is "Let *A* be ill adapted to plant species 2." These two assumptions seem to me to be almost contradictory. If *A* lives only on species 1, the fact that it is ill adapted to species 2 is irrelevant. If emus only live in Australia, the fact that they are ill adapted to the Antarctic has no influence on their evolution. If the assumptions had been "(1) Let *A* females only lay eggs on species 1," and "(4) Let *A* larvae (not all produced by *A* mothers) be ill adapted to species 2," I could have applied mathematical analysis to the resulting model. I propose to do so in the next few years. But I hope I have given enough examples to justify my complete mistrust of verbal arguments where algebraic arguments are possible, and my skepticism when not enough facts are known to permit of algebraic arguments.

In earlier chapters Mayr seems to show a considerable ignorance of the earlier literature of beanbag genetics. Thus, on page 215 he writes that "the classical theory of genetics took it for granted that superior mutations would be incorporated into the genotype of the species while the inferior ones would be eliminated." The earliest post-Mendelian geneticists, such as Bateson and Correns, wrote very little about this matter. Fisher [23] pointed out that if a heterozygote for two alleles was fitter than either homozygote, neither allele would be eliminated. He may well have been anticipated by Wright or some other geneticists, but at least since 1922 this has been a well established conclusion of beanbag genetics. In my first paper on the mathematical theory of natural selection [3], I ignored Fisher's result as I was dealing with complete dominance; in my second [33] I referred to it and, as I think, extended it slightly. As Mayr cites neither of these papers of mine, he can hardly mean that the first was classical and the second post-classical! I agree with him that when I first read Fisher's 1922 paper I probably did not think this conclusion as important as I now do, and that many writers on beanbag genetics ignored it for some years. But were they classical?

Mayr devotes a good deal of space to such notions as "genetic cohesion," "the coadapted harmony of the gene pool," and so on. These apparently became explicable "once the genetics of integrated gene complexes had replaced the old beanbag genetics." So far as I can see, Mayr attempts to describe this replacement in his chapter 10, on the unity of the genotype. This does not mention Fisher's fundamental paper [34] on "The correlation between relatives on the supposition of Mendelian inheritance," in which, for example, epistatic interaction between different loci concerned in determining a continuously variable character was discussed. This chapter contains a large number of enthusiastic statements about the biological advantages of large populations which, in my opinion, are unproved and not very probable. The plain fact is that small human isolates, whether derived from one "race," like the Hutterites, or two, like the Pitcairn Islanders, can be quite successful. I have no doubt that some of the statements in Mayr's chapter 10 are true. If so, they can be proved by the methods of beanbag genetics, though the needed mathematics will be exceedingly stiff. Fisher and Wright have both gone further than Mayr believes toward proving some of them. The genetic structure of a species depends largely on local selective intensities, on the one hand, and migration between different areas, on the other. If there is much dispersal, local races cannot develop; if there is less, there may be clines; if still less, local races. The "success" of a species can be judged both from its present geographical distribution and numerical frequency and from its assumed capacity for surviving environmental changes and for further evolution. I do not think that in any species we have enough knowledge to say whether it would be benefited by more or less "cohesion" or gene flow from one area to another. We certainly have not such knowledge for our own species. If inter-caste marriages in India become common, various undesirable recessive characters will become rarer; but so may some desirable ones, and the frequency of the undesirable recessive genes, though not of the homozygous genotypes, will increase. Since there is little doubt that extinction is the usual fate of every species, even if it has evolved into one or more new species, the optimism of chapter 10 does not seem justified. Sewall Wright has been the main mathematical worker in this field, and I do not think Mayr has followed his arguments. Here Wright is perhaps to blame. So far as I know, he has never given an exposition of his views which did not require some mathematical knowledge to follow. His defense could be that any such exposition would be misleading. I have given examples above to illustrate this possibility.

I am reviewing Mayr's book in the *Journal of Genetics*, and my review will, on the whole, be favorable. But if challenged, I am liable to defend myself, and have done so in this article. If I have not defended Sewall Wright, this is largely because I should like to read his defense. In my opinion, beanbag genetics, so far from being obsolete, has hardly begun its triumphant career. It has at least proved certain far from obvious facts. But it needs an arsenal of mathematical tools like the numerous functions discovered or invented to supply the needs of mathematical physics. Of course, it also needs accurate numerical data, and these do not yet exist, except in a very few cases. The reason is simple enough. Suppose we expect equal numbers of two genotypes, say, normal males and color-blind males, from a set of matings and find 51 per cent and 49 per cent; then if we are sure that this difference is meaningful, it will have evolutionary effects which are very rapid on a geological time scale. But to make sure that the difference exceeded twice its standard error (which it would do by chance once in twenty-two trials), we should have to examine 10,000 males. To achieve reasonable certainty, we should have to examine 25,000. We often base our notions of the selective advantage of a gene on mortality from some special cause. Thus babies differing from their mothers in respect of certain antigens are liable to die around the time of their birth. But this may well be balanced wholly or in part by greater fitness in some other part of their life cycle. If it were found that color-blind males had a 10 per cent higher mortality than normals from traffic accidents, this could be balanced by a very slightly greater fertility or frequency of implantation as blastocysts. One of the important functions of beanbag genetics is to show what kind of numerical data are needed. Their collection will be expensive. Insofar as Professor Mayr succeeds in convincing the politicians and business executives who control research grants that beanbag genetics are misleading, we shall not get the data. Perhaps a future historian may write, "If Fisher, Wright, Kimura, and Haldane had devoted more energy to exposition and less to algebraical acrobatics, American, British, and Japanese genetics would not have been eclipsed by those of Cambodia and Nigeria about A.D. 2000." I have tried in this essay to ward off such a verdict.

Meanwhile, I have retired to a one-storied "ivory tower" provided for me by the Government of Orissa in this earthly paradise of Bhubaneswar and hope to devote my remaining years largely to beanbag genetics.

REFERENCES

1. E. Mayr. Animal species and evolution. Cambridge, Mass.: Harvard University Press, 1963.
2. ———. Sympos. Quant. Biol., **24**:1, 1959.
3. J. B. S. Haldane. Trans. Cambridge Phil. Soc., **23**:19, 1924.
4. J. B. S. Haldane and S. D. Jayakar. J. Genet., **58**:291, 1963.
5. R. C. Punnett. J. Hered., **8**:464, 1917.
6. L. T. Hogben. *In:* M. P. Banton (ed.). Darwinism and the study of society. London: Travistock Publications, 1961; Chicago: Quadrangle Books, 1961.
7. J. B. S. Haldane. The causes of evolution. London: Longmans Green, 1932.
8. ———. J. Genet., **54**:327, 1956.
9. ———. J. Genet., **57**:131, 1960.
10. G. S. Carter. J. Genet., **56**:353, 1959.
11. S. Muramutsu, T. Sugahara, and Y. Okazawa. Int. J. Radiat. Biol., **6**:49, 1963.

12. J. B. S. HALDANE. Ann. Eugen., 9:400, 1939.
13. ———. Ann. Eugen., 10:417, 1940.
14. H. B. D. KETTLEWELL. Proc. Roy. Soc. [B.]. 297:303, 1956.
15. R. G. KING. Genetics. New York: Oxford University Press, 1962.
16. J. B. S. HALDANE. Ann. Eugen., 11:333, 1942.
17. P. A. P. MORAN. The statistical processes of evolutionary theory. Oxford: Clarendon Press, 1962.
18. R. A. FISHER. Ann. Eugen., 9:109, 1939.
19. J. B. S. HALDANE. Evolution, 3:51, 1949.
20. G. G. SIMPSON. The major features of evolution. New York: Columbia University Press, 1953.
21. J. B. S. HALDANE and S. D. JAYAKAR. J. Genet., 58:318, 1963.
22. J. B. S. HALDANE. J. Genet., 55:511, 1957.
23. R. A. FISHER. Proc. Roy. Soc. Edin., 42:321, 1922.
24. J. B. S. HALDANE and S. D. JAYAKAR. J. Genet., 58:237, 1963.
25. K. SAKAI. J. Genet., 55:227, 1957.
26. S. K. ROY. J. Genet., 57:137, 1960.
27. V. M. INGRAM. Fed. Proc., 21:1053, 1962.
28. J. B. S. HALDANE. Proc. Cambridge Phil. Soc., 38:55, 1932.
29. H. JEFFREYS. The theory of probability. London: Oxford University Press, 1948.
30. A. BIRNBAUM. J. Amer. Stat. Ass., 57:269, 1962.
31. H. SPURWAY. Zoölogische Jährbücher., 88:107, 1960.
32. J. B. S. HALDANE. Enzymes. London: Longmans Green, 1930.
33. ———. Proc. Cambridge Phil. Soc., 23:363, 1926.
34. R. A. FISHER. Trans. Roy. Soc. Edin., 52:399, 1918.

AN AUTOBIOGRAPHY IN BRIEF

*J. B. S. HALDANE**

A number of inaccurate statements have been published about me in the press—quite as many in articles favoring me as in hostile statements. So I propose to give a brief account of my scientific career. I was born in 1892. I owe my success very largely to my father, J. S. Haldane. He was perhaps best known as a physiologist, but he was so far from being a specialist that in later life he was elected president of the Institution of Mining Engineers and delivered the Gifford lectures on the "Existence and Attributes of God." I suppose my scientific career began at the age of about two, when I used to play on the floor of his laboratory and watch him playing a complicated game called "experiments"—the rules I did not understand, but he clearly enjoyed it.

At the age of eight or so I was allowed to take down numbers which I called out when reading the burette of a gas-analysis apparatus and later to calculate from these numbers the amounts of various gases in a sample. After this I was promoted to making up simple mixtures for his use and, still later, to cleaning apparatus. Before I was fourteen, he had taken me down a number of mines, and I had spent some time under water both in a submarine and in a diving dress. He had also used me as the subject in many experiments. In fact I spent a good deal of my holidays from school in learning my father's trade. Most Indian boys do this, but not the sons of scientists. After I was twelve, he discussed with me all his research before publication, and sometimes tried out a lecture course on me before delivering it to students.

At school I deserted "classics," that is to say, the study of Latin and Greek, at the age of fourteen and studied chemistry, physics, history, and biology, with my father's full backing but to the annoyance of the headmaster, who said I was becoming "a mere smatterer." The teaching of chemistry was good, and by the age of sixteen I had learned some facts discovered since my father had studied that subject, so that I could help him and C. G. Douglas; and my first scientific paper was a joint one with them, read to the Physiological Society when I was seventeen.

I went to Oxford on a mathematical scholarship in 1911 and took first-class honors in mathematical moderations (roughly the Indian B.Sc. level). But as nobody can study mathematics intensively for more than about 5 hours daily and retain sanity, I also attended the final honors course in zoölogy in my first year. One of my fellow students was the late Professor Narayan K. Bahl, who later did so much for the teaching of zoölogy in India. At a seminar for zoölogy students in 1911, I announced the discovery, from data published by others, of the first case of what is now called linkage between genes in vertebrates. My evidence was considered inadequate, and I began breeding mice with A. D. Sprunt, who was killed in 1915. In 1912 I switched over to *literate humaniores*, a course based on Latin and Greek classics, but including the study of a good deal of modern philosophy and ancient history. I took first-class honors in this subject in 1914 and had intended to go on to study physiology. But in 1914 I joined the British army and have, therefore, no scientific degree. In 1916 my mouse work with Sprunt and my sister, Mrs. Mitchison, was published.

During World War I, I was wounded twice, in France and in Iraq, after which I spent 16 months in India. I determined to come back as soon as I could associate with Indians on a footing of equality.

On returning to Oxford after the war, I was elected a Fellow of New College and began teaching physiology while myself attending Sherrington's advanced practical course in that science. Indian readers who find it incredible that I was appointed without a degree in physiology, or any other science, would do well to remember that Srinivasa Ramanujan, India's greatest mathematician since Aryabhatta, had no degree and would thus be disqualified from teaching in an Indian University were he alive today. I may not have been a good teacher, but I was a successful one. In 1922 there were about sixty candidates for honors in physiology, three from New College. These three were one-half of the six who secured first-class honors. I had 20–30 hours a week of teaching and other university duties. However, I managed to get 10 hours of private tuition done at night after 8:00 P.M. and to concentrate 9 hours on Wednesday, so I got some time for research and reading.

I worked on human chemical physiology and on genetics. Perhaps my most important discovery in physiology was that when I drank ammonium chloride solution I developed various symptoms of severe acid poisoning, including breathlessness. My main genetic discovery was the rule as to the sex of hybrid animals. In 1921 I put in a term as biochemist in the Edinburgh Royal Infirmary and learned a little medicine in the wards.

In 1922 Professor Hopkins (later president of the Royal Society, Nobel laureate, etc.) invited me to Cambridge as reader in biochemistry. I was his second-in-command for 10 years and supervised the work of about twenty graduate students—much of which was first rate. Perhaps my own most important discovery was that a substance for which carbon monoxide competes with oxygen, now called cytochrome oxidase, was found in plant seedlings, moths, and rats. The most remarkable thing about this discovery was that I was able to find out a good deal about a substance in the brains of moths without cutting them up or killing them. However, my enunciation of some of the general laws of enzyme chemistry may have been more important.

In 1924 I published what my colleagues generally think my most important paper, the first of a series on the mathematical theory of natural and artificial selection. Five of these papers have been reprinted in the United States and are available to libraries which do not possess the *Proceedings of the Cambridge Philosophical Society*. They contained calculations showing great intensity of natural selection in favor of dark color in a British moth species. This was regarded as ridiculously high, but 30 years later Kettlewell found a slightly higher figure in field studies. In 1930, in my book *The Causes of Evolution*, I published the first estimate of a human-mutation rate. Since then, this has become a matter of international politics in connection with atom-bomb tests.

Toward the end of my period at Cambridge I spent some time at the John Innes Horticultural Institution in a London suburb, directing research on plant breeding, and continued to do so after I became part-time professor of genetics in University College, London, in 1933. My most important work was with Miss de Winton on an ornamental plant, *Primula sinensis*. We were the first, for example, to study linkage in a plant with double the usual number of chromosomes. I also showed that one of the genes responsible for its color acted by changing the acidity of the petal sap.

I have always been of some use to my colleagues because I knew what was going on in several different branches of science, and it was, I think, in the autumn of 1933 that I did what posterity may regard as the best and most important action of my life. I found posts for several Jewish refugees from Germany, and I did my best to help others. One evening Dr. Boris Chain dined in my house. We talked about the work he had done in Germany, and I said, "There is a man named Florey at Oxford who is interested in that sort of thing. I advise you to visit him." Later Florey and Chain isolated penicillin, which has saved hundreds of times more lives than atomic bombs have caused deaths, a fact often forgotten by critics of science. Florey and Chain have been rewarded for this work. They shared a Nobel prize, and Florey is now president of the Royal Society. Perhaps all my discoveries will be forgotten and I shall be remembered only in the words of the ancient Greek poet Pindar: "He once nourished the contriver of painlessness, the gentle limb-guardian Asklepios (Dhanvantari), the heroic conqueror of manifold diseases." Bacteriologists, by the way, are heroic: bacteria are much more dangerous than tigers. For such activities I had the honor of figuring on the list of persons to be arrested if German armies conquered England in 1940.

In 1936 I became professor of biometry in London but never got a building for my own use. Some of my colleagues in this department did very fine work, and two became Fellows of the Royal Society, as I had in 1932. I participated in a little of their work and made some contributions to mathematical statistics, of which perhaps the most labor-saving is my calculation of the cumulants of the binomial distribution.

In 1939 the British submarine "Thetis" sank on her trials with the loss of over one hundred lives. About one-half the dead were civilians; two unions asked me to investigate the disaster. I did some experiments on myself and friends, no more drastic than I had done at Cambridge, and shed enough light on what had happened to convince the British Admiralty that their "experts" knew very little. They asked me to continue the experiments, and when war broke out I was given various assignments. E. M. Case and I, for example, were the first people to pass 48 hours shut up in a miniature submarine with apparatus which we had correctly calculated would renew the air for that time. My wife and I worked out methods for the rapid ascent of divers, and so on. During this work I made a curious discovery. Oxygen, when breathed at a pressure over about 6 atm., has quite a taste. Nevertheless, since textbooks have priority over truth, students of chemistry are well advised, when examined, to state that "oxygen is a colorless, inodorous, and tasteless gas." I advise even M.Sc. students against stating that Case and Haldane reported to the contrary in a letter to *Nature* in 1941. After breathing oxygen for five minutes or so at such pressures, one has violent convulsions; and my frequent demand for a soft chair or a cushion is due to the fact that I fractured my backbone in such convulsions.

Among the papers I wrote during the 12 years between the end of the war and my departure to India is one published in 1956 on a method for estimating the number of lethal mutations produced in mice by gamma rays and other agents causing mutation. A clear answer to this question would allow us to give a partial answer to the question, "How many human babies in future generations will die as the result of atomic-bomb tests?" I was not, of course, offered facilities for such work. G. S. Carter at Harwell began to use my method. He then resigned his post, for an undisclosed reason, and took a job with a poultry-breeding firm. However, Sugahara, Okazawa, Tutikawa, and Muramatsu have used heavy doses, like those absorbed by the survivors of Hiroshima and Nagasaki. The Japanese workers have used much smaller doses, such as might be given to workers in atomic-energy establishments or to radiologists who took precautions. They naturally got rather few mutations and cannot yet estimate the rate very accurately. According to my method, about 500 rs are needed to produce a lethal mutation, while two other methods give a somewhat lower figure of about 300, which was what I guessed in 1956. If the Japanese workers are right, the damage done to future generations by the tests so far carried out is a bit less than Pauling and Russell have stated but very much more than American official spokesmen have claimed.

In 1957 I came to India to work at the Indian Statistical Institute, and I have to thank Professor P. C. Mahalanobis for making this possible. My most important work there was, beyond doubt, starting S. K. Roy, K. R. Dronamraju, T. A. Davis, and S. D. Jayakar on their scientific careers, which are likely, in my opinion, to be illustrious. At least twenty of my pupils have become Fellows of the Royal Society, so I can probably judge fairly well. At the Indian Statistical Institute I personally published two pieces of theoretical work which may be of lasting value, besides many which are unlikely to be so. Since leaving it, and while employed by the Council of Scientific and Industrial Research, I have published jointly with Jayakar one paper on human relationships. I am grateful to Mahalanobis for giving me the opportunity of working in the Indian Statistical Institute, where I learned a great deal about what can and cannot be done in India, even though it gradually became clear that I could not carry out the kind of work I had wanted to in that institute.

I have of course done a good deal more than appears in this summary. I have taken part in politics, written a book of stories for children, and put my Latin and Greek learning to some use by commenting on biological passages in ancient writings. I may have been the first to ask the cosmological question, "Is space-time simply connected?"—though only a man of the stature of Einstein is likely to answer it. And I have made several bad mistakes. But I think this article gives some notion of my contributions to scientific knowledge.

THE THEORY OF EVOLUTION, BEFORE AND AFTER BATESON

The Bateson Lecture, delivered on July 18th, 1957, at the John Innes Horticultural Institution

By J. B. S. HALDANE
Indian Statistical Institute

(*Received July 20, 1957*)

William Bateson, as his widow emphasized, was a naturalist. He was therefore interested in the grandest of all natural processes which a biologist can contemplate, namely evolution. His work on *Balanoglossus* was an important contribution to its study. But he was then led to the study of variation, and interested himself particularly in what he called meristic variation, that is to say variation in the numbers of similar parts in like organisms. It became clear to him that much variation occurs in definite steps without intermediates, or with very rare intermediates. And he saw that this kind of variation must have been very important in evolution. In fact it was even more important than he knew. Two very similar species, all of whose taxonomic differences are, in his phrase, substantive rather than meristic, may yet differ sharply in their chromosome number, and this latter difference may account for the sterility of their hybrids.

Now many of the differences between domestic races of plant and animal species do not blend in the hybrids or in their progeny. A study of differences of this kind led inevitably to the discovery of Mendelian inheritance. But Bateson was far too honest a man not to see at a fairly early stage that his discoveries did not solve the problem of evolution. The differences between different domestic breeds are often far more striking than those between related species; but they usually only affect a limited number of organs or functions, and they do not hinder hybridization. Thus a white silkie fowl differs far more from the wild *Gallus gallus* as regards its feathers than do *Gallus sonnerati* or *Gallus varius*. But it does not differ in many other important respects, particularly in crossability. Thus Mendelism appeared to have no immediate bearing on the problem of evolution, except to show that the explanations given sixty years ago of how evolution had occurred were almost certainly false.

Bateson was almost unique among great men of science in being able to formulate his major contribution to scientific method in the lapidary phrase "Treasure your exceptions". It was this which led him to be more interested in one polydactylous cat than in ninety and nine with rather large feet. It was this which led him, though a staunch Mendelian, to investigate the exceptions to Mendel's laws which provided their explanation. The first of these exceptions was linkage, or a failure of the independent assortment of factors which Mendel had discovered. But Bateson was particularly interested in the exceptions which he classed under the heading of anisogamy. It is generally found that reciprocal crosses between two hermaphrodites give indistinguishable results. When they do not, after transient effects due to differences in the nutrition of seeds after fertilization have passed off, the female and male gametes of one or both must differ in some way as regards their genotype. In fact anisogamy can be due to at least five different causes.

1. Plastids or plasmagenes may be transmitted wholly or mainly on the female side.
2. A virus may be wholly or mainly so transmitted. No sharp line can be drawn between these first two causes. It may or may not be possible to do so in future.
3. The chromosome number may be different on the two sides, as in the *caninae* group of roses.
4. Selection may act in a different way on male and female gametes or haploid cells of different genotype. This covers such cases as pollen lethals and the Renner phenomenon in *Oenothera*. Extra chromosomes are often transmitted by nearly half the ovules and by few or no functional pollen tubes.
5. Linkage intensity between a pair of loci may differ in female and male gametogenesis.

In fact Miss Saunders hit on the genetics of double stocks (*Matthiola incana*) which involves both anisogamy due to a pollen lethal, and linkage, at a very early stage; and this was not fully elucidated during Bateson's lifetime. I want to emphasize how broad is the field opened up, once one starts systematically studying what was at first sight a single type of exception.

Besides treasuring his exceptions, Bateson was very sceptical of explanations of many facts which he accepted without question. And in particular he never accepted the word "gene" with its rather wide connotations. Mendel had used the phrase "differendierendes Merkmal", or differentiating character, for his genetical units. Here he was probably influenced by his Thomism. It is much easier for a Thomist than for adherents of most other philosophies to think of a quality being transmitted. Had Mendelism been discovered and accepted in mediaeval Europe an atomistic theory of substantial forms might have been developed. Bateson used the neutral word "factor". This word has been dropped, partly because it was used in a number of different ways. I think it could and should be revived, with a more precise definition. Later I shall try to show why it is needed for an adequate account of evolution.

Genetics is the study of a class of differences between related organisms, namely those differences which turn out to be determined genetically, that is to say not by the environments of the individuals showing them. It is however a postulate of physiological genetics that any difference which is usually determined genetically can also be determined by non-genetical causes. If that were not the case, genetics would be an inscrutable mystery. We could never know the causal path between a gene and the scorable character.

I suggest that the word factor be used for the cause of an observable difference which shows Mendelian segregation. This is often, but not always, a difference between two allelomorphic genes. Thus, a round pea differs from a wrinkled one in the following way. Both contain much the same amount of carbohydrate at corresponding stages. In their early stages both contain stachyose, a sugar composed of two glucose and two galactose residues. In a round pea this is converted into starch in the final stage, in a wrinkled pea it is not; so the pea contains a lot of soluble sugar, and collapses on drying. Very likely the wrinkled pea, like a galactosuric baby, lacks an enzyme concerned in transforming galactose into glucose. The synthesis of this enzyme in round peas is controlled by a gene at a locus in a certain chromosome, though there may be several steps between the gene and the enzyme. The wrinkled pea at the same locus contains a gene which does not make this enzyme, though it may make a similar but inactive protein. The wrinkled character is therefore recessive. It may be found, as has been found in similar cases in animals, that the homozygous round pea contains twice as much of this enzyme as the heterozygous. If so the factor would be detectable at various different levels, though it is a difference between two allelomorphic genes.

Now a gene is a material structure, and is roughly localized: but it is not exactly definable. If what seem to be the most active parts of it are transferred to a different part of a chromosome, it may alter its functions. Even if we had a precise knowledge of the chemical structure of a nucleus we could not say that changes in some parts would affect one gene and one only, and thus draw sharp boundaries between genes. The situation is quite comparable to that regarding cerebral localization. On the other hand we could define a factor exactly. We could say that because in a particular chromosome an adenine residue has been substituted for a guanine, in, say, the 25473—rd nucleotide counting from the free end of the longest chromosome, the plant makes a polyphenoloxidase with rather different properties. A factor, I suggest, can be anything from a difference of a few atoms in a single nucleotide, to an inversion or the presence of an extra chromosome; for these too are inherited in a Mendelian manner. If this is so, and a similar analysis of extranuclear factors is possible, all evolution is the accumulation or loss of factors. I think the early Mendelians perhaps went astray in taking too materialistic a view of the nature of a factor. Suppose that, as in Suskind, Yanovsky, and Bonner's (1955) work, a mutation causes the replacement of an enzyme by another protein no longer enzymatically active, but like enough to the enzyme to unite with the same antibodies. The new protein may be larger or smaller than the enzyme. The factor, which is the difference between the genes producing them, must be given a conventional sign, but is probably rarely a mere addition or substraction. It could be example be the substitution of N for C, O and H, which converts thymine into cytosine.

While, then, factors are units, though not necessarily or even usually material units, genes are not necessarily units. I do not go as far as Goldschmidt, and say that a gene can only be detected because it has mutated, and that therefore an unmutated gene is in principle unobservable, and so an hypothesis which should be eliminated from biology. On the contrary, I think that if we could isolate a normal human *X* chromosome and keep it in a suitable medium, we could observe the synthesis by it or under its influence of the globulin which is lacking in haemophilics. If we could do the same with a rabbit *X* chromosome we should be entitled to say that this chromosome, like those of men and dogs, carried a locus which, if it mutated, might be responsible for haemophilia.

The pre-Batesonian theories of evolution were, as we now see, excessively vague.

Darwin's theory was substantially correct, so far as it went. But he did not distinguish between phenotype and genotype; and we now know that within a pure line, or within what Bateson called an eversporting variety and we now call a balanced lethal system, such as double-throwing stocks, selection can continue indefinitely without evolutionary effect. What was worse, Darwin (1878, p. 10) stated that "if strange and rare deviations of structure are really inherited, less strange and commoner deviations may be freely admitted to be inheritable". The opposite is the case. If I find a *Drosophila* in an inbred line with many bristles lacking, it probably carries a mutant gene. If I find one with a rather smaller number than the average, it is probably due to an environmental effect which is not inherited. Bateson's principle of treasuring the exceptions is fully justified. Darwin also realised that heritable variations must have a cause; but he sought for this in the direct effects of use and disuse, which are rarely, if ever, so operative in the case of nuclear factors, though disuse can certainly produce extranuclear factors, such as absence of chloroplasts in algae, and adaptations due to use can be transmitted by bacteria at least for hundreds of generations.

Galton and Weismann helped to make the distinction between genotype and phenotype, but they did not achieve it, as they were unaware of the facts of dominance and epistasy. And Galton, with his emphasis on measurable characters, actually deflected genetics from its most immediately fruitful subject-matter. Karl Pearson exaggerated this emphasis, but fortunately forged mathematical tools which have been of immense value to geneticists. Bateson never used them, and it was left to Fisher and Wright to incorporate them into genetical methodology.

Let us now see how the theory of natural or artificial selection looks in its new guise. If we consider one of the simplest possible cases, the change which may take place in a single generation of sexually propagated annual higher plants or animals, we shall find that we have to consider five distinct populations. Where generations overlap matters are more complicated. I shall further assume hermaphroditism or equality in the numbers of the sexes, and that the populations studied are large. And I shall consider a closed area, into which there is no immigration. In three of these five populations we shall distinguish phenotypes and genotypes. The first of them, S, consists of all the organisms of the species in the area considered. Ideally we should like to score them at the moment of fertilization. I assume that they are actually described as early in the life cycle as is possible with the characters under consideration. They are classified by their phenotypes, and, ideally, by their genotypes. The last of our five populations, $\acute{S}$, consists of the progeny of S, counted and classified at the same stage in their life cycle as was S.

The second population, which I call the parental population P, is fictitious. It consists only of those members of S which are parents of one or more members of $\acute{S}$. But each is represented as many times as it has offspring in $\acute{S}$. So its total number is twice the number in $\acute{S}$. Thus a hermaphrodite plant which had two offspring in $\acute{S}$ as a seed parent and three as a pollen parent would be represented five times in P. Where generations overlap, Fisher's (1930) notion of reproductive value can be used.

Now P may differ from S in the frequency of phenotypes, genotypes, or both. These differences may be so small as to be explicable by random sampling, that is to say chance. If not they are attributable to selection. If a particular genotype or phenotype is significantly commoner in *P* than in *S* this can be due to three different kinds of selection. This type may have survived better than the average in the interval between the time when *S* was scored and the time when *P* produced progeny. It may have been better represented in *P* because each individual in it was, on the average, more fertile than other types. Or it may have been so because its progeny, on the whole, survived better between the moment when they were formed as zygotes and that when they were scored as members of *Ś*. If we could score *S* and *Ś* at once after fertilization we could eliminate this last kind of selection. We can sometimes, as with the characters round and wrinkled, yellow and green cotyledons, in the pea, get rather close to doing so.

The parents *P* produce a population *G* of gametes. We cannot score them except occasionally on the basis of their carbohydrates, but we can often estimate the frequencies of various genotypes among them with considerable precision. There is probably little selection among gametes in higher animals, but there is a great deal in higher plants, especially among pollen tubes, and in them we should consider a selected gametic population *H*. *G* will contain a few gametes of types not expected from the parental genotypes, due to mutation in the widest sense of that word, including such accidents as primary non-disjunction. Mutation can occur at any stage of the life cycle, but it is most convenient to consider it as concentrated in gametogenesis. The genotypic composition of *G* is so much simpler than that of *S* or *P* that it is desirable, where possible, to use it as a measure of evolutionary change. The genotypic composition of the next generation *Ś* depends not only on *H* but on the mating system. A large change in this, for example mating between two previously separate populations, or the introduction of inbreeding in a previously outbred population, can produce great changes in *S*. I assume that the mating system is not, in fact, changed.

Now if *S* and *Ś* could be classified at once after fertilization, then any differences in gene frequencies between them could only be due to selection, that is to say to differences between *S* and *P*, or *G* and *H*, apart from the very small differences due to mutation and random sampling, provided Mendelian inheritance occurs. Genotype frequencies can change through some generations towards whatever equilibria are given by the mating system. For example genes which were originally in coupling may gradually separate. Such secondary effects are rarely important. The effects of selection are hardly ever reversed except by counter-selection. Now this is not obviously true. It is a deduction from Mendelism, as I think Fisher (1930) first clearly pointed out. Karl Pearson showed that if, as he believed, Galton's law of ancestral heredity were correct, there would be a very considerable swing back after selection ceased. And in the rare cases where Mendelian segregation does not occur, for example in rye plants carrying a chromosome fragment whose descendants get into more than half the gametes, it is not true.

Unfortunately in practice there has always been some natural zygotic selection before *S* and *Ś* are scorable. However, all artificial selection is concerned in creating differences between *P* and *S*. It is also clear that only indirect methods based on genetics can reveal the nature of the selection of H from G, or that acting between fertilization and the scoring of $\acute{S}$.

It is hard enough to compare phenotype and genotype frequencies in S and P, except in animals and plants whose breeding is artificially controlled. Even if we could find how many eggs each female moth in a natural population laid, we could not estimate the relative success of different phenotypes as fathers. Only in men can we get data, still very rough, on this important question.

Darwin inevitably considered selection on the basis of phenotypes. It is, I think, important to distinguish between selection and evolution based on phenotypes and on genotypes, and my wife has suggested that, so far as possible, a different terminology should be used in the four fields. I shall therefore use Simpson's (1953) terminology for phenotype selection. Selection which alters the mean of any character between S and P he called *linear.* (I should prefer a word which expressed his meaning more clearly). If it reduces the variance of a character, weeding out extremes, he called *centripetal.* If it increases the variance he called it *centrifugal.* Centripetal selection is very common. (*cf.* Haldane, 1953). It is often to some extent also linear. Karn and Penrose (1951) found that the mean human birth weight was about 1% higher in children who survived the hazards of birth and of the first month of life than in the population originally at risk, while the variance was reduced by about 10%. Centrifugal selection is much rarer. It occurs, however, when any polymorphism is being established. If, for example, black moths are rare in a population, and owing to selection there are more blacks in P than in S, the variance of any index of colour or brightness is increased, so selection is centrifugal as well as linear.

Genotypic selection requires little special terminology. We must, however, distinguish between selection which alters gene frequencies and that which does not. I call the former *effective,* and the latter *ineffective,* even though is often strong. Selection based on heterosis, that is to say favouring heterozygotes for a pair of allelomorphic genes or chromosomal arrangements, may be effective for a while, but leads to a stable equilibrium where it is ineffective, even if, as in structurally heterozygous *Drosophila* species, it is very intense. Selection based on negative heterosis is always effective, since one allel or the other is eliminated. It is perhaps legitimate to describe selection against mutants as ineffective when it just balances mutation.

For the phenotypic evolutionary effects of selection we may use the terminology of Mather (1953) and Waddington (1953). If the mean of $\acute{S}$ differs from that of S and we think this is not due to environmental change, we may speak of *directional* evolution. If the variance of $\acute{S}$ is reduced, because there are fewer members of genotypes whose mean differs widely from the population mean, we speak of *normalizing* evolution. If it is reduced because genotypes which vary greatly in different environments are eliminated, we speak of *stabilizing* evolution. If it is increased, for whatever reason, we speak of *disruptive* evolution. I am not quite happy about this word, for the establishment of a stable polymorphism is not, in my opinion, a disruption, though it may sometimes precede one. It must also be remembered that, as Thoday (1953) has pointed out, evolution which stabilizes one character necessarily destabilizes another.

To attain uniformity in different environments organisms must react differently. If some human genotypes have a stabler temperature in a variety of environments than do others, it may be because their sweating is more increased by high temperatures and therefore more variable in a range of climates.

Finally, we have to consider genotypic evolution. And here the essential is very simple. Either gene frequencies change, or they do not. Changes in relative frequencies of genotypes without change of gene frequency are of little importance. The unit process of evolution is the substitution of a Batesonian factor.

I have used the word evolution for the difference between S and $\acute{S}$. Of course a major evolutionary change is the resultant of millions of such differences. But it is the resultant of nothing else. I think that what Waddington calls normalizing selection is better called normalizing evolution. The weeding out of phenotypically extreme genotypes, for example homozygotes at a locus, can be wholly ineffective. If so it does not normalize.

I do not wish my terminology to be adopted without full discussion. I can only hope to contribute to the terminology which will be adopted ten years hence, and perhaps be useful for another thirty years, after which it may become a menace to original thinking.

Without a knowledge of genetics we can never say that selection will be effective. Thus in all plant species the number of seeds produced is very variable, as Salisbury (1943) has shown. There must always be linear selection in favour of the plants producing most seeds. But the main cause of high seed production is a favourable environment. And evolution is probably as often directional towards the production of fewer seeds as towards the production of more. Further, selection is usually centripetal. Extremes for most characters are generally eliminated. But it may be ineffective for three reasons. Most of the variation may be due to the environment, as in a pure line or a clonal population. Or selection may favour heterozygotes or merely eliminate mutants. If so an equilibrium is reached, and evolution is neither stabilizing nor normalizing. We can, however, say with confidence that in all species selection against most mutants is occurring. If there were no selection against them the mutations would produce disruptive evolution. The selection against them is always centripetal and may be linear.

Natural selection, then, may or may not change gene frequencies. But nothing else can do so anything like as fast. Chance effects may be important in small populations, but will rarely matter to a whole species, though they may be important when one or two individuals cross a geographical barrier such as the sea between a continent and an island, and may found a new species. And they may allow for the simultaneous establishment of several factors which are harmful singly, but adaptive in combination. Mutation is at best slow, and could not usually overcome a selective disadvantage of one in ten thousand.

We are left, I think, with no alternative but to believe that natural selection has been the main evolutionary agency, and also with surprisingly little evidence for effective selection. Fortunately we have such evidence, particularly as to effective selection of insects for resistance to insecticides, and for cryptic coloration where human industrialism has changed the colour of a landscape. But in man, the best observed species, the observed selection is usually if not always at least largely ineffective, preserving an existing equilibrium either by the elimination of mutants or by favouring mediocrity, whether in intelligence, stature, or blood pressure.

If natural selection is effective, one can calculate the rate of change of gene frequencies. If an autosomal gene **A** is being favoured by selection, and the relative fitnesses and frequencies of the three genotypes are :—

	AA		**Aa**		**aa**
Fitness	$1+K$	:	1	:	$1-k$
Frequency	u^2	:	$2u$	:	1 ,

then if K and k are positive, the number of generations n, needed to change the ratio u from u_0 to u_n is

$$n = K^{-1} ln \left(\frac{k+Ku_n}{k+Ku_0} \right) - k^{-1} \; ln \left(\frac{K+ku_n^{-1}}{K+ku_0^{-1}} \right)$$

nearly, provided K and k are small.*

If u_0 is very small and u_n very large, say 10^{-4} and 10^4, which are frequencies such as would be kept in being by mutation, this becomes

$$n = K^{-1} \; ln \; u_n - k^{-1} \; ln \; u_0 + (K^{-1} - k^{-1}) \; ln(Kk^{-1})$$

nearly, which if $u_n = u_0^{-1} = 10^4$, is about 9.2 $(K^{-1} + k^{-1})$, or about 5000 generations if K and k are each .001. If, however, K or k is zero, that is say **a** or **A** is fully recessive, the time needed is very much longer, even if there is some inbreeding. 5000 generations is a short time on a geological scale.

However, another consideration limits the rate at which natural selection can act (Haldane, 1957). Consider Kettlewell's (1956) data on the spread by natural selection of the dominant gene for melanism in *Biston betularia*. On releasing equal numbers of dark and light moths in a smoke-polluted wood in the morning, and trapping on the following night, he found about two dark moths to each light one. This was due to predation of the conspicuous light form by birds. The reproductive capacity of the light moths was reduced to about a half of what it would have been in an unpolluted wood. This must have happened about 1800 A.D., in a few areas where the melanics were then very rare. So effectively the reproductive capacity of the species was halved. The species did not become extinct. But if selection of the same intensity had been going on for nine other genes it would certainly have done so, for only one moth in a thousand would have survived for a day.

If selection is by death (or relative sterility which comes to the same thing) we can calculate the total number of deaths needed to replace one gene by another, or to change the species by one Batesonian factor, or, to use his earlier phrase, one discontinuity (Haldane, 1957). This is independent of the intensity of selection when this is small, and is about equal to the population number multiplied by $ln\ p$ and by a

* *ln* means natural logarithm, or decimal logarithm multiplied by 2.3.

further factor varying from about 1 to 10 or so with the amount of dominance and inbreeding, where p is the factor by which the frequency of the originally rare gene is increased. If this is 10^4 as in the example given, the number of deaths is about 10 to 100 times the population number. I suggest 30 as a fair average. I repeat that about as many deaths are needed to establish, by Darwinian selection, a factor with very slight selective value or phenotypic effect, such as the difference between the A_1 and A_2 agglutinogens in man, as a factor with a striking effect and high selective value, such as the difference between winged and apterous forms in an insect. The deaths are spread over more generations, but their number is, in fact, slightly larger. The factor is the unit of evolution by natural selection.

If selection were such as to reduce the mean reproductive value of the population 10% below that of the fittest genotypes, this would mean that an evolving species could incorporate, on the average, about one new factor in every 300 generations. This figure is, of course, a guess at the rate of evolution. But such a rate as one factor in thirty generations would only be likely when conditions were changing very rapidly (as of course, they are at present through human interference with nature) or when an organism had recently colonised a new environment. In both these cases the original type would be in fairly serious danger of extinction.

The next step in an account of natural selection would perhaps be a guess at the number of factors by which two fairly closely related species differ. This number is probably not very different from the number by which each of them differs from their latest common ancestor, perhaps in the Pliocene. I have guessed that this number may be of the order of a thousand for two closely related mammalian species. This would accord well with the time, of the order of half a million years, which seems to be needed to form such a species. I suspect the number may be less in higher plants. Even so, Blake (1793) was nearly correct in his statement that "To create a little flower is the labour of ages", though he should perhaps have added "except by allopolyploidy".

I think that by the year 2050 or so we may be able to estimate these numbers, and I wish to suggest how it may be done. There is a strong suggestion that some proteins in living cells are very closely causally related to genes, that is to say that a change in the gene will cause a change in the protein without changes in more than a few intermediate molecules at the most, even if ribonucleic acid always acts as such an intermediate. Whether other large molecules such as antigenic polysaccharides are equally close to genes, or whether the genes control their synthesis by making special enzymes we do not yet know. The latter hypothesis seems to me a little more likely.

We know that some factors, or gene substitutions, produce quite small changes in protein molecules, even when they alter their properties a great deal. Thus, Ingram finds that normal haemoglobin and the insoluble haemoglobin of sickle cell anaemia only differ in one of the thirty peptides into which he can break both up with trypsin. The difference may be of a single amino-acid*. The work of Harris, Sanger, and Naught (1956) gives us an idea of what we may expect. Insulin is a fairly simple

* Since the lecture was delivered, Ingram (1957) has confirmed this guess.

protein consisting of 48 amino-acid residues. The homologous insulins from five mammalian species have been completely characterised. Those of the pig and whale (species not stated) are identical. The others differ from them in respect of one or more of three adjacent amino-acid residues. In one threonine is an alternative to alanine, in the second serine to glycine, in the third isoleucine to valine. At this level the factor, or difference between two residues, is a carbon atom either with two hydrogens, or with two hydrogens and an oxygen. If, as is at least possible, they are formed by different but very similar genes, the chemical differences between these genes may also consist of a few atoms.

I suggest that about the year 2000 biochemistry and genetics may have progressed so far as to make the following programme possible. Two species will be chosen sufficiently close to give fertile hybrids, but yet undoubtedly differing according to the usual criteria. All the proteins, and perhaps other large molecules, of each will be isolated and examined in detail. Some will be found to be identical while others differ. The genetics of these differences will be determined by similar examinations of the F_1, F_2, and back-crosses. We shall then know at least most of the factors by which these species differ, and at least roughly what effects they have on the chemical makeup of the species. I suggest that a hundred or so workers could carry out such a programme in thirty years. Whether such a programme will be carried out depends on the interests of future generations. I can at least imagine a society, perhaps in Africa, sufficiently interested in biology as such to carry it through. It would be as interesting to bet on the results of such an investigation as on those of the investigation of the relative speeds attained by the members of a group of perissodactyls.

Bateson would, I am sure, have endorsed Blake's (1820) statement "For Art and Science cannot exist but in minutely organized Particulars, And not in generalizing Demonstrations of the Rational Power". Some of Bateson's adversaries, such as Karl Pearson, held the opposite view, and Bateson was a little too sceptical about generalizing demonstrations for my own taste. His references to Blake in letters, by the way, are enough to show that he would not have objected to a citation of his opinions on scientific method. Bateson's (1894, p. 17) own formulation concerning the processes of evolution was as follows:—"We know much of what these processes *may* be; the deductive method has been tried, with what success we know. It is time now to try if these things cannot be seen as they are, and this is what variation may show us".

I doubt whether, even a hundred years hence, we shall be in a position to describe all the factors by which two species differ in exact biochemical terms as differences between gigantic molecules of desoxyribonucleic acid. But some of them, at least, should be so describable. And the mere discovery of how many factors there are, and how they are related to the factors which differentiate the members of a species from one another, will tell us a very great deal about the detail of evolution.

I believe, then, that a precise and complete answer to the main problem with which Bateson was concerned can be given, and I hope will be given at least in some cases. It can be precise and complete because a gamete contains a finite number of atoms, of which only a fraction are arranged in self-replicating patterns. Such an answer would not necessarily imply that an account of life had been given in chemical terms. If I can state the precise differences between two texts of the same poem I have not described the poem completely, much less elucidated its full meaning. But I may have elucidated the history of its transmission.

But supposing this problem had been solved, we should be a very long way from having solved the problem of evolution. One cannot see all the questions which posterity will ask. But already we can ask two kinds of question. What advantage, if any, did this factor confer ? And why did this factor arise; or if you prefer a different phrasing, why did this gene change in this particular way ? I shall try to show that these questions are not quite separate.

In Bateson's day Darwinism, as generally taught, showed signs of degenerating into Paleyism or Panglossism. Darwin (1878, p. 428) himself was not quite guiltless. "And as natural selection works solely by and for the good of each being, all corporeal and mental endowments will tend to progress towards perfection", he wrote in the penultimate paragraph of the Origin. Bateson was by no means convinced that all was for the best in the best of all possible worlds.

I will mention one piece of recent work which supports Bateson's scepticism as to the efficiency of natural selection. Sakai (1957) studied the competition between two varieties of rice, Red and Upland. The former is a weed, the latter an agricultural variety. A pure crop of Upland gives a much higher yield, by several different criteria, than one of Red. But Red is highly competitive. A Red plant lowers the yield of its neighbours, whether they are Upland or Red, but if surrounded by Upland, gives a higher yield than Upland in pure stand. It follows from Sakai's data that if we had a mixed crop and selected the highest yielding plants, we would usually select Red, and the end result of the selection would be a crop with a lower yield than that of the original mixed crop, or of pure Upland. The same result would occur if natural selection were based on the yields. I do not think that results of this kind are likely to be so common in competition within a species as in competition between species, but they can and do occur. The ecology of competition should be an important subject of genetical research in the future.

The second question is, I think, more fundamental. Darwin (1878, p. 125) quoted, though without reference, Walsh's (1863) "Law of equable variability". Vavilov and others have shown in more detail that comparable variations occur in related species. It was thought that, at least when their genetical determination was similar, they were usually due to mutations at homologous loci. Harland played the main part in disproving this unduly simple hypothesis, which is nevertheless, I think, fairly often true. Homologous organs may however depend on genes at different loci in closely related species. Spurway (1949) discussed this question in some detail. She pointed out that though mutations with similar phenotypic effects may, and often do, occur in related species, they may be rare or absent in one such species, and common in another. The simplest explanation of this fact is that the disturbance of a particular developmental process is more or less harmless in one species, but lethal or sublethal in another closely related one. Thus in *Drosophila subobscura* three recessives on different chromosomes give white bristles between the ommatidia, usually with some slowing down of larval development. In the very similar species *Drosophila pseudoobscura* no such mutation has been reported. Perhaps the interruption of this particular developmental process slows down development in *Drosophila pseudoobscura* so much as to be effectively lethal. If so one species but not the other has the possibility of evolving a form with bristles of this type. Again although millions of mice have been observed, no recessive yellows have been found (if we discount an ancient account by Hagedoorn) like those which are well known in guineapigs, rabbits, dogs, and so on. The dominant yellow is lethal when homozygous and gravely upsets metabolism even in heterozygotes. It seems possible that the locus which gives yellow mutants in the guineapig and *Rattus rattus* also mutates in mice but gives lethal recessives.

If an organism were completely integrated developmentally in one sense of that very vague word, any mutation would be grossly harmful or even lethal. It is not in the least obvious why, for example, two genes at different loci which block the development of yellow pigment in mouse hairs also block the reabsorption of bone by osteoclasts. If development were more integrated, such cases would be commoner. In tetrapod vertebrates polydactyly is a common variation. But only once, in the ichthyosaurs, has it been used in evolution, though one might expect to find it in other swimming groups. It is presumably harmful, perhaps because, for the reason given later, it is very hard to stabilize phenotypically. Digits and even entire limbs, can, on the other hand, be lost. Similarly the number of limbs in insect imagines is extremely constant, though *Drosophila* mutants with extra legs are known, and in my laboratory Mrs. Trent has recently found one which occasionally has only four, though such animals have not yet lived to breed.

It seems that in the course of evolution capacities for further evolution are constantly being lost. But they may be gained. For example the birds have a remarkable capacity for the evolution of combs, ceres, wattles, and such-like structures, the Orchidaceae for fantastic changes in floral morphology. I need not here repeat other examples which Spurway gave, nor her suggestions for research on this problem.

The vast majority of mammalian species have seven cervical vertebrae. Some sloth species have more or less than seven, and what is more, as Bateson (1894) pointed out, the number can vary within such a species. Here it would seem likely that the capacity for variation has been gained in evolution. It is unfortunate that the giraffe and camel, for example, did not possess this capacity.

The capacity for genetic variation of which I have spoken is very similar to what Thoday (1953) meant by genetic flexibility. I have not previously used this phrase because I am not sure that he and I are discussing quite the same fact. And a species may be very flexible as regards one group of variations, and very inflexible as regards another, so one must be careful of stating that one species is more genetically flexible than another.

Until comparative genetics have been studied from this point of view, genetics will be able to make very little contribution to the understanding of the broad outlines of evolution. The fossil record, like the human historical record, appears at first sight as a story of missed opportunities. I think this appearance is probably deceptive in both cases. We can probably see why the ancient Greeks could not develop a pan-Hellenic federal government, or the ancient Romans a democratic system for their empire, if it is less obvious why the Chinese did not develop science from their magnificent technology. We cannot yet see why the bipedal Dinosaurs failed to develop brains which would have made their hands as useful as our own or even those of a monkey, while the Synapsids did so after a hundred million years of eclipse and another hundred million of progressive evolution. We cannot guess why a number of groups in at least three different animal phyla, and a very few dioecious plants, have independently evolved morphologically differentiated sex chromosomes, while other groups have not. One can point to the advantages of this system of sex determination, and one can guess with some plausibility as to how it was evolved. But if the advantages are as great as has been suggested, and the evolutionary steps as simple, why is it absent, for example, in fish and in most Nematocera ?

My own guess is that in a few thousand years our successors may know enough genetics to be able to say that many of the major features of evolution were due to the fact that some groups kept possibilities open which others did not. This is fairly obvious at the morphological level. Tortoises and snakes have obviously fewer evolutionary possibilities than the less specialized reptilian groups, horses and whales than the less specialized mammalian groups. Sexuality seems to be an advantage because it allows for greater possibility of variation, and perhaps for no other reason. But even so I have no idea why in the vertebrates and arthropods self-sterile hermaphrodites are wholly exceptional, whereas they are the rule in the higher plants and some molluscan groups.

We have got to ask, at a higher level, the questions which Bateson asked in "Materials for the study of variation". We cannot even frame our questions correctly as yet. The suggestion which I have made here that the possibilities of genetically determined variation, and of evolution based on it, are much wider in some groups than in others, may turn out to be false. It is conceivable, say, that a single mutation perhaps with little effect by itself, could unlock the developmental processes in a lily flower, and make it as plastic under further mutations as an orchid. It is quite characteristic of genetics that the study of a single individual and its progeny may open up entirely new prospects. I think particularly of Bridges' X X Y *Drosophila* females which he used to prove the chromosome theory of heredity.

One at least, of the questions which Bateson (1894, p. 27) put in the introduction to "Materials for the study of variation" has been definitely answered. "The question" he wrote "which the Study of Variation may be expected to answer, relates to the origin of that Discontinuity of which species is the objective expression. Such Discontinuity is not in the environment; may it not, then, be in the living thing itself". Thanks to the work of Bateson and others, we can now answer this question, at least in part. There are two reasons (and perhaps more than two) for this discontinuity between species and varieties. Living things are made up of small and large molecules. Many of the small ones are common to all living things, others to most of them. But the large ones, such as proteins and polysaccharides, are characteristic of species or of genotypes within a species, though some may be found in several, or even many, different species. And their formation is controlled by large molecules or sections of large molecules, which we call genes. These are built up from the ubiquitous types of small molecule, and can only vary discontinuously. Many of the discontinuities observed by naturalists depend on discontinuities in the possible patterns of genes. We do not yet know why the number of these possible patterns is restricted, as it is: why, for example, nucleic acids do not appear to include xanthine residues. But even if they did, the atomic structure of matter forbids continuous variation at the genic level. Bateson's question has therefore been answered in principle.

There is, however, a second answer, which often applies to meristic variation. When the number of like parts, for example, teeth, vertebrae or petals, can vary, it is usual to find a whole number of such parts and unusual to find a miniature or incomplete member of the meristic series. Bateson (1894, pp. 270-272) discussed the problem of "The least size of particular teeth", but came to no very firm conclusion, though he foreshadowed the conclusion of Grüneberg. Grüneberg (1952) has studied this phenomenon in the third upper molars of a particular pure line of mice. These teeth are sometimes missing. But when they are present they are variable in size and can be decidedly smaller than the normal, though in no way rudimentary or incomplete. He concluded that the mean size of the tooth rudiment in this line was small and somewhat variable. When, at a certain critical stage, the rudiment fell below a threshold, it regressed or did not develop further. Similarly we may suppose that when a rudiment is too large at a critical stage of development it may divide into two or even more parts, giving an extra limb, for example.

The physical principle at work may in some cases be surface tension, though this theory has been heavily criticized. The mechanism may often be that propounded by Turing (1952). However that may be, the formal physical principles, and therefore the mathematical analysis, of the formation of vertebrae in a tail may be not unlike that of drops in a liquid filament, even if the forces concerned are of quite a different nature. There may be yet other physical causes of discontinuity, but they are to be looked for, I think, in the minute particulars of the chemistry and physics of living matter. This was, I think, Bateson's view. He took the comparison of a zebra's markings with ripple marks quite seriously.

From a broad philosophical point of view these two causes of discontinuity are not different. Matter consists of atoms not because electrons and atomic nuclei are the only possible forms into which it can aggregate, but because the other forms, such as mesons, are unstable and short-lived. The forces which hold an atomic nucleus together or disrupt it are like enough to those operative in a drop of water to allow argument from the latter to the former. So, I suggest, are those operative in a tooth or petal rudiment.

It is interesting that these two causes of discontinuity are independent. Genes producing meristic variation are not usually constant in penetrance and expression. This is so for example for most genes causing polydactyly and ectrodactyly. And it is to be expected. Mandeville's (1950) gene for absence of upper lateral incisors in man may reduce their size or cause their disappearance. Presumably the normal genotype produces a rudiment which hardly ever disappears or splits, and gives a tooth of a fairly uniform size. Mandeville's gene, in heterozygotes, gives a rudiment near the critical size, which may either disappear or give a small though not always obviously abnormal tooth. If, to take a possible cause, as the result of the formation of an abnormal protein, the average time between cell divisions in the rudiment is increased by five per cent, it is not to be expected that this will just be enough to bring down the size of the rudiment in question below its critical level in all cases, without any effect on the neighbouring teeth. The evolution of a human species, all of whom lacked this particular tooth and nothing else, would presumably require a particular combination of factors, Meristic variation is seldom strictly Mendelian just because these two different causes of discontinuity are operating. Bateson's (1894) generalizations about symmetry in meristic variation are a contribution to biology which is independent of his genetical work, and deserves further study and development.

To sum up, a few of Bateson's questions about evolution have been answered in some detail. The general question of the efficacy of natural selection has, I believe, been answered, though my answer involves more mathematics than Bateson would have liked, if less than Karl Pearson would have liked. But we can now begin to formulate further questions. Some of these questions can be answered on the biochemical level. For example to the question "Why are most desert beetles black, instead of being cryptically coloured ?" Kalmus (1941) after a study of *Drosophila* mutants, answered that the blackening process is a tanning of the cuticular proteins which prevents the beetles from losing water through their cuticles. It may be that our successors will be able to give equally satisfactory answers at this level to questions which still elude us, such as "Why was there a trend to reduce the formation of cartilage bones in the evolution of the Stegocephalia ?", or "Why are the morphological characters of the Solanaceae correlated with low resistance to virus infections ?"

However, as I have said, the explanation of the major features of evolution will be much more complicated, even if, as I think it will, it involves a great deal of biochemistry. It will also involve palaeogeography and palaeoclimatology. It is difficult to think that the emergence of our ancestors from the water in the Devonian was unrelated to the frequency of lagoons in that period, if in fact they were as frequent as is commonly stated. On the other hand it is not yet possible to correlate the extinction of the dinosaurs in the upper Cretaceous with any geological events. As we begin to learn about the genetics and evolution of behaviour we shall begin to ask meaningful questions on the psychological level as well as on the morphological and physiological levels. And these questions will be as important to botanists as to zoologists. The flowering plants are, on the whole, symbiotic with insects, especially Hymenoptera and Lepidoptera, and with mammals and birds. The insects mainly assist them in pollination, the mammals and birds in seed dispersal. It is, therefore, advantageous to plants to produce brightly coloured and characteristically smelling flowers and fruits, parts of which can be eaten or drunk. The origin of these structures however depended on the possibility of simultaneous morphological and biochemical evolution in plants, and psychological evolution in animals. Were the Carboniferous insects incapable of developing an instinct to visit the same kind of flower, and the Jurassic dinosaurs incapable of developing an instinct to pluck sweet fruits ? Or did the limited variability of plants limit the possibility of such evolution ? We may have to ask questions on still higher levels. But there is little chance of asking them correctly, let alone of answering them, before we have answered some of the simpler ones.

No doubt in a few thousand years, when all the questions which have yet been put have either been answered or shown to be meaningless, the theory of evolution will be as unlike Darwin's formulation of it as relativistic quantum mechanics are unlike the mechanics of Galileo and Newton. Bateson's discontinuities in evolution may be capable of description in other terms, as Newtonian particles can be described as wave packets. But I think that Bateson's fundamental notion of discontinuity in the evolutionary process, which he enunciated seven years before the rediscovery of Mendel's work, will remain, though doubtless with some modifications, a component of any theory of evolution.

I wish that time had been given me to describe Bateson as I knew him from 1919 till his death. He could be described as an angry and obstinate old man. But his anger was largely reserved for inaccuracy and loose thinking, and for certain types of injustice. His obstinacy made it difficult to convince him of the truth of theories which had previously been asserted without adequate evidence and were now being substantiated. Correns (1902) in a brilliant guess embodied in a diagram without adequate explanation, had put forward the theory of the linear arrangement of genes on chromosomes. Bateson, quite rightly, had not accepted the hypothesis. When Bridges and Sturtevant proved it, he was hard to convince, though he was finally convinced of the fact that genes were associated with chromosomes. On the other hand he instantly accepted new generalisations provided they were statements of fact not involving theoretical superstructures. Thus, he was, I think, the first person to believe my own generalisation about sex ratio and unisexual sterility in hybrid animals, though not, of course, the rather incoherent explanation of it which I gave. He then displayed a characteristic combination of anger at my ignorance with great generosity in helping me with his immense knowledge of the by-ways of entomological literature. To me, at least, he showed no signs whatever of a senile failure of original thought. On the contrary his last posthumously published paper on the genetics of bolting in root crops initiated a line of research which was later developed by Waddington in his studies on genetic assimilation.

It would be stupid to suggest that all geneticists should model themselves on Bateson. Edward Lear's autobiographical line "His mind is concrete and fastidious" applies very well to him. This made him, I think, unduly suspicious of generalizations. But it gave him an eye for detail such as perhaps only Calvin B. Bridges among his contemporary geneticists possessed. Genetics need workers of very different temperaments. But we could all benefit from imitating Bateson's good points, and above all his respect for facts, although they told, and even because they told, against the theories which he had adopted.

REFERENCES

BATESON, W. (1894). Materials for the study of variation treated with special reference to discontinuity in the origin of species. (*London: Macmillan*).

BLAKE, W. (1792). The marriage of heaven and hell. (*Privately printed*).

BLAKE, W. (1820). Jerusalem. 55. (*Privately printed*).

CORRENS, C. (1902). Modus and Zeitpunkt der Spaltung der Anlagen bei Bastarden der Erbsen-Typus. *Bot. Zeit.*, **60,** II. 65–82.

DARWIN, C. (1878). The origin of species by means of natural selection or the preservation of favoured races in the struggle for life. (Sixth edition). (*London: Murray*).

FISHER, R. A. (1930). The genetical theory of natural selection (Oxford).

GRUNEBERG, H. (1952). Genetical studies in the skeleton of the mouse. IV Quasi-continuous variation. *J. Genet.*, **51,** 95–114.

HALDANE, J. B. S. (1953). The measurement of natural selection. *Atti del IX Congresso Internazionale di Genetica.* 480–487.

HALDANE, J. B. S. (1957). The cost of natural selection. *J. Genet.*, **55,** 2.

KARN, N. & PENROSE, L. S. (1951). Birth-weight and gestation time in relation to maternal age, parity, and infant survival. *Ann. Eugen.* **16,** 147–164.

HARRIS, J. I., SANGER, F. & NAUGHT, M. A. (1956). Species differences in insulin. *Arch. Biochem. Biophys.*, **65,** 42.

INGRAM, V. M. (1957). Gene Mutations in human haemoglobin. *Nature*, **180,** 326–328.

KALMUS, H. (1941). Physiology and ecology of cuticle colour in insects. *Nature*, **148,** 428.

KETTLEWELL, H. B. D. (1956). Further selection experiments on industrial melanism in the Lepidoptera. *Heredity*, **10,** 287–303.

MANDEVILLE, L. C. (1950). Congenital absence of permanent maxillary lateral incisor teeth: a preliminary investigation. *Ann. Eugen.*, **15,** pp 1–14.

MATHER, K. (1953). The genetical structure of populations. *Symp. Soc. Exp. Biol.*, VII, 66–95.

SALISBURY, E. J. (1943). The reproductive capacity of plants. (Bell: London).

SIMPSON, G. G. (1953). The major features of evolution. (Columbia University, New York).

SPURWAY, H. (1949). Remarks on Vavilov's law of homologous variation. *Ric. Sci. Suppl.*, 18–24.

SAKAI, K. (1957). Studies on competition in plants. VII. Effect on competition of varying number of competing and non-competing individuals. *J. Genet.*, **55,** 227–234.

SUSKIND, S. R., YANOVSKY, C. & BONNER, D. M. (1955). Allelic strains of Neurospora lacking tryptophan synthetase: a preliminary immuno-chemical characterisation. *Proc. Nat. Ac. Sci. U.S.*, **41,** 577–582.

THODAY, J. M. (1953). Components of Fitness. *Symp. Soc. Exp. Biol.*, VII, 95-113.

TURING, A. M. (1952). The chemical basis of morphogenesis. *Phil. Trans. Roy. Soc.*, *B*, **237,** 37–72.

WADDINGTON, C. H. (1953). Epigenetics and Evolution. *Symp. Soc. Exp. Biol.*, VII, 186–199.

WALSH, B. S. (1863). Proc. Entomol Soc. Philadelphia, *p.* 213 (*fide* Darwin in "The variation of animals and plants under domestication.")

(Reprinted from Nature, Vol. 183, pp. 710–713, March 14, 1959)

THE THEORY OF NATURAL SELECTION TO-DAY*

By Prof. J. B. S. HALDANE, F.R.S.
Indian Statistical Institute, Calcutta

WE constantly hear that Linnæus is out-of-date, that his ideas are a danger to clear thinking, and so on. Why, then, do we not relegate them to a place in the history of science, like those of his contemporary Scheele on phlogiston ? The answer is quite clear. Whatever we may think of Linnæus's theories, we continue to use his methods. In science, methods are much more important than theories, because a theory is an attempt to describe reality in terms of symbols made by the human vocal apparatus or on paper. If we think that the properties even of an electron are inexhaustible, theories can never be adequate. But a method, that is to say, a way of dealing with reality, may be adequate for the purpose for which it was designed, even if it is based on a false theory. The transition from a fluid to a particle theory of electric conduction in metals, and the partial return to a degenerate gas theory, had no effect on the design of galvanometers.

Linnæus invented the method of describing every animal or plant in terms of two, and only two, words. A group sharing the same two names is called a species. A group sharing the first only is called a genus. Genera are grouped together in higher categories, such as families, orders, classes and, more recently, phyla.

It is worth comparing this with some other methods of classification. To identify a particular star we give its right ascension and declination. In order to group stars which are judged to be similar, we use another two-dimensional classification. One co-ordinate is the surface temperature or a character highly correlated with it, such as the spectral type or colour. The other is the absolute luminosity. We then find that stars which agree in both these respects usually agree in others, for example, their period if they pulsate, their probable age, and so on. Linnæus tried such a two-dimensional classification of flowering plants, and it was one of his least-valuable contributions to biology.

The Linnæan system of classification is much more valuable in the tropics than in temperate or arctic

* Substance of the presidential address delivered at the Centenary and Bicentenary Congress, University of Malaya, Singapore, on December 2, 1958. (See also p. 723.)

climes, for the simple reason that there are many more different species of animals and plants. Linnæus's flora of Lapland was probably fairly complete. I am sure that nobody supposes that we have yet a complete list even of the flowering plants, let alone the ferns, mosses and liverworts, of Malaya. So it is no reproach to tropical biologists that they are still at the Linnæan stage when those of temperate climates have gone beyond Linnæus. One might as well reproach students of proteins because they cannot yet describe the structure of proteins with the accuracy possible for sodium chloride. It is therefore entirely fitting that we should be commemorating Linnæus on the equator.

If Linnæus's method of assigning every living organism to a species is so useful, why do we attack his species concept ? The species concept, like the concept of a molecule, is not always true ; but even where not true, both can be useful. Sodium chloride does not exist as molecules either in crystals or in solution. But it is convenient to use the same terminology to describe sodium chloride and carbon tetrachloride, though the latter is a true molecule. Similarly, we can describe a silicate the anion of which is a lattice of indefinite extent in terms appropriate to a small molecule. By the end of this century I expect that our chemical vocabulary will be brought up to date. I do not think the Linnæan terminology will be abandoned for several centuries.

The Linnæan species concept often breaks down when we extend our studies over a large enough space. Classical cases are the circum-Tibetan distribution of *Parus* and the circumpolar distribution of *Larus*. Here differences, which are at best subspecific, add up to a specific difference. The principal postulate of evolutionary theory is that all, or almost all, specific differences disappear if we trace the ancestry of two species far enough back. Thus, the horse and ass are believed to be descended from one ancestral species in the Pliocene, the horse and any bird from a common ancestral species in the Carboniferous. Finally, recent work on the transfer of substances (perhaps always deoxyribonucleic acid) responsible for hereditary differences, between bacteria not only of the same but also of different species, suggests that the species concept is only roughly applicable to bacteria.

But most biologists, and particularly experimental biologists, are dealing with organisms living in the present and obtained in a particular locality. The determination of their Linnæan species is a prerequisite to description of other observations. It may be said that the Linnæan system is merely a convenience of human communication. This is perhaps true, but it raises the question whether any scientific theory, or for that matter any philosophical theory, is anything more than such a convenience.

It is not a trivial fact that Linnæus worked on the periphery of the area where science was studied in his time. This meant that rather few of the plants and animals of his native country had been described either by the scientists of the ancient Mediterranean culture such as Aristotle and Theophrastus, or by such men as Aldrovandus and Gessner. Two centuries earlier, when Britain was similarly peripheral, Turner had realized that the plants and animals of his country required special study and special names.

It is not trivial that Darwin and Wallace were stimulated to formulate the theory of evolution as they did by observing the plants and animals of countries very distant from their own. A four-year voyage around the world gave Darwin enough facts inexplicable without a theory of evolution to last him a life-time, but in his case the theory germinated slowly. Wallace had spent much longer in the tropics, and produced a theory equivalent to Darwin's in a shorter time. It is not impossible that some resident in a scientifically peripheral area such as Singapore or Calcutta may to-day be making observations which will form the basis of an advance in biology comparable to those made by Linnæus two centuries ago, and by Darwin and Wallace a hundred years since. I shall later suggest reason to hope that Calcutta may be the locus of such a discovery.

Darwin and Wallace not only championed the notion of evolution, but also produced a coherent theory as to how it had occurred. To-day almost all biologists believe in evolution, that is to say, they believe that the plants and animals alive to-day, including men, are descended from ancestors very unlike themselves, and that many very different living forms are descended from one ancestral species. However, by no means all living biologists believe that the main agency of evolution has been natural selection. Indeed, Wallace in his old age concluded that a decisive step in the evolution of man could not be so explained.

Darwin thought that evolution occurred by imperceptibly small steps. To-day we know that some of the steps have been fairly abrupt ; and this is the main modification to which the account of evolution given a century ago must be subjected. These steps are of three main kinds. Mendel showed that on crossing races of peas certain characters showed no blending. Even when a character disappeared in the first generation it might reappear in a fraction of the next. We know that some evolutionary steps are due to the selection of characters inherited according to Mendel's law. About seventy species of British Lepidoptera have evolved black varieties since the industrial revolution, and some have almost completely replaced the original light form in the smokiest areas. In the best-studied case, *Biston betularia*, the dark form differs from the light by a single dominant gene. I shall later describe why the population evolved as it did. At present I merely wish to point out that the evolutionary process was not gradual, in the sense that the population did not pass through a phase of intermediate colour.

Secondly, the chromosomes, on which the genes responsible for Mendelian inheritance are carried, change abruptly. The number in a species is usually constant, and must be an integer, usually an even one. Not only does the number change, but also when a new species evolves, parts of two different chromosomes can be exchanged, so that in the hybrid the normal process of gamete production by meiosis is disturbed. This is not the only cause of hybrid sterility, perhaps not the main one, but it is one cause of this important biological fact.

Thirdly, and most important, we now know that a new species can arise in one step by the formation of a sterile or nearly sterile hybrid followed by a doubling of the chromosomes which renders it fertile but still vigorous. Such hybrids, which are called allopolyploids, breed very nearly true. While Winge and others must take much credit for this discovery, the most decisive steps were probably taken by the Japanese botanist Kihara, who recently crowned his life's work by discovering growing as a weed in wheat fields in Afghanistan the grass which, by crossing with a wheat like the macaroni wheats of to-day, gave rise to the bread wheats in or near Afghanistan about 6,000 years ago. It is probable that Kihara has made the most important amendment to Darwin and Wallace's account of evolution as a historical fact.

Finally, Garstang, Bolk, de Beer, and others have pointed out an evolutionary process at which Darwin and his immediate successors had not guessed. Many animals pass through a larval stage, and this may be highly specialized for its own kind of life. You have only to think of such familiar larvæ as a caterpillar and a tadpole. If the timing of development is shifted so that reproduction occurs when some or most of the non-reproductive organs are still in the larval stage, this may lead to the evolution of a wholly new adult type. Such are, for example, the Larvacea, or swimming tunicates, which resemble the larvæ of the sessile forms, but never attach themselves to rocks. It is probable that the Copepod Crustacea, a very successful order, are essentially larvæ of prawns or crabs which never grow up. A similar process has played a great part in human evolution. The development of our nearest relatives is very slow. A chimpanzee is not mature until about eight years. A human being is not mature until about sixteen, and never develops many of the characters of adult apes, let alone adults of other mammalian groups. In particular, we have kept the embryonic character of cranial flexure, so that our eyes are directed forwards and not upwards or even backwards. A change in the timing of sexual maturity may occur quite suddenly, as it does in the axolotl, and have very great evolutionary effects.

Nevertheless, palæontological research has, on the whole, fully confirmed Darwin and Wallace. Among the more spectacular 'missing links' which must have lived if their account of evolution is substantially correct, and are no longer missing, though they were so in Darwin's time, are amphibians with four legs but a fish-like tail with bone-supported fins, birds with long tails, teeth, and many other primitive features, and later short-tailed but still toothed birds. Our picture of vertebrate evolution is now so complete that one can make a list of dozens of discoveries, any one of which would go far to disprove the theory of evolution. For example, if the skeleton of a man or a horse were discovered in the Cretaceous, or that of a reptile or a bird in the Devonian, I, for one, would regard most of my life's work as having been as futile as that of an astrologer. Every year in which such discoveries are not made strengthens the evidence for the theory of evolution, and makes it less possible for biologists to accept any other theory.

Although both Darwin and Wallace made major contributions to the study of variation (and Darwin did some very important genetical work), we now know so much more than they did on these matters that their account of how evolution occurs must be restated. In my opinion, most of what they wrote is true : but the fact that they reached the truth on the meagre evidence before them is a proof of their genius.

Let me try to state the theory of natural selection as I hold it in language which they would have understood. "All species vary. But not all variation is inherited. Natural selection discourages most variations from the structures and functions normal in a species. It encourages a few variations ; and if these are inherited, evolution will take place."

The main objection to this formulation is to the word 'inherit', which is applied to property and to characters. For example, I have inherited my father's watch, his baldness, and a growth of bristles on the nose. We could not both possess the watch

5

simultaneously, but we were simultaneously bald. It may be incorrect to speak of possessing baldness, but we certainly possessed the nasal bristles simultaneously. A character is not an object like a watch, and it is misleading to use the same word about it. The physical basis of heredity is now fairly well understood. Certain patterns in cells are copied with great fidelity when a cell divides. The most important are the molecular patterns which we call genes, and which determine what kinds of proteins will be built in the new cells, and thus may have a great effect on the structure and function of descendant cells and organisms. However, a character, such as tallness, hairiness, or capacity for distinguishing between green and grey, can only be said to be inherited if it depends in a fairly simple way, either on genes in the nucleus, or on the rarer copiable molecular patterns outside the nucleus. A change in one of these copied patterns, whether it is due to copying error or alteration between copyings, is called mutation.

Heredity can be defined statistically as a positive correlation between characters in a group of ancestors and their descendants, which is not due to a positive correlation between the environments of ancestors and descendants. My skin colour is hereditary in the biological sense, my linguistic habits are not. My mother taught me to speak English ; but if I had been handed over to a Malay foster-mother as an infant, I could just as easily have learned to speak Malay.

An example of a biological and genetically determined character which is not inherited is the complete sterility of some so-called double-flowered plants such as the double *Matthiola incana*. Other characters, such as size within a pure line, are not inherited, because they are not genetically determined any more than are human languages.

Natural selection may be defined as a statistical difference between the parents of the next generation and the population from which they are drawn, each parent being counted once for each of its progeny. Darwin and Wallace thought mainly in terms of selection by survival, but fully recognized selection by fertility, parental care, and other means. We now see that selection, whether natural or artificial, is not always effective. For example, roan cattle (which, by the way, are common in England and very rare in India, though they exist, but may be unknown in Singapore) do not breed true, and selection in favour of roan may increase the frequency of roan to about 50 per cent, but cannot raise it above this level.

But as soon as biologists began to study natural

selection they found something much more surprising. Natural selection is generally centripetal, that is to say, it favours individuals near the norm of the population in question, at the expense of those which deviate from it. In other words, the parents of the next generation are usually less variable than the generation of which they form a part. This is difficult to prove formally, because one cannot often determine parenthood in animals or plants under natural conditions, but it has been abundantly proved for many episodes of selection by killing. Perhaps the first case was Bumpus's observation in the late nineteenth century that of a number of sparrows picked up immobile with cold after a blizzard, those which did not recover were more variable in several measurable characters, such as wing-span, than those which did.

In the human species, centripetal selection occurs at all stages. For example, babies which are lighter or heavier than the average have a higher death-rate than the average. So have adults with very high or low weight or systolic pressure. When it comes to intelligence, the very stupid, who are classed as mental defectives, have a much higher death-rate than the average, and the survivors are less fertile than others, as they are largely confined in special institutions or in prisons. The very intelligent are probably longer-lived than the average, but are less fertile.

Centripetal selection acts partly by eliminating mutant genes, and partly by eliminating homozygotes, that is to say, organisms which have a like pair of genes, instead of an unlike pair, in a particular region of a chromosome. Thus, the first observations certainly confirmed Darwin and Wallace that natural selection occurs, but showed, contrary to their belief, that its main effect was to prevent species from changing. Only much later was natural selection with an evolutionary effect discovered.

The reason for this is clear enough. Evolution is a very slow process, how slow only Darwin guessed. He estimated the age of the Wealden, or upper Jurassic, at about 300 million years. His contemporaries, if they believed the theologians, put it at 6,000 years; if they believed the physicists, at about a million. The correct figure is about 130 million. In a fairly steadily evolving line such as the ancestors of horses, the average rate of change of a character, such as length of tooth, is about 4 per cent per million years. In 1924 I calculated the intensity of selection needed to make such changes. An advantage of one-thousandth for one type over another would be much more than enough; and this could only be detected on a sample of several millions, whereas a 10 per cent advantage could be detected on a sample of a few hundred.

In fact, natural selection with evolutionary consequences has only been observed where men have created drastically new conditions which impose a heavy selection pressure. The most striking is the use of insecticides such as DDT. This causes intense selection in favour of resistance to it, and relatively resistant races of mosquitoes arise in a few years. The best-studied case is that of the moth *Biston betularia*. In the smoke-polluted parts of Britain the original light form is conspicuous when resting on tree trunks, as these moths do during the day. In the unpolluted areas the dark form is equally conspicuous. Kettlewell found that birds ate the form which is conspicuous to human eyes at such a rate that if equal numbers of the two forms are released at dawn, the ratio of inconspicuous to conspicuous moths caught in flight the next night is 2 : 1. Thirty years earlier I had calculated, from the rate at which the numbers of the black form had increased, that the fitness of the light form in smoke-polluted areas was about 70 per cent of that of the black. This may well be true on an average, for Kettlewell chose a highly blackened wood near Birmingham for his experiment.

I have no doubt that natural selection of much less intensity, but yet with an intensity far greater than that which has been usual in the past, is going on in many species. But it would be difficult for a single worker to collect the data.

Can natural selection explain evolution ? If Darwin thought that it could, this was perhaps because he thought that members of a species varied in all possible directions, and natural selection could favour any kind of variation. This is probably not so. Only certain kinds of heritable variations seem to be possible in any particular species. The course of evolution is not (except perhaps in very rare cases) determined by the frequency with which a particular type of mutation occurs ; and the vast majority of mutations are rejected as useless, the process of rejection being called centripetal selection. No important event has only one cause. Houses would not be burned down if they were all made of ferroconcrete, or if the air only contained 17 per cent of oxygen. If there were no mutation, natural selection would be ineffective ; if there were no natural selection, every species would become a collection of freaks. Only in this rather restricted sense can it be claimed that natural selection explains evolution.

However, it does not follow that the claim is true. In contradistinction to Wallace, I think it probably is true. Let us take such an organ as the eye of a man or a bird. It has been argued that it could not have evolved by natural selection, because it would

8

seem that any improvement, in the later stages at least, would require simultaneous changes in several of its measurable magnitudes. I think a careful study of the eyes of living molluscs greatly weakens this argument, as we can find among them a dozen or so stages from a mere light-sensitive spot to an eye with a lens and retina much like our own. Wright has shown how, in small animal or plant communities, several changes, each slightly harmful, but beneficial in combination, may occur together.

Wallace regarded the origin of certain characters which he considered to be specifically human as inexplicable by natural selection. Many such characters, including a disposition to monogamy and a respect for property, both of which human moralists might envy, have since been found in animals. I have also shown, or at least suggested, how a mode of behaviour originated by the initiative of a single individual, and then converted, by imitation, into a tradition, may become instinctive as the result of natural selection. Until it has been shown that my arguments are worthless, it may be rash to say that natural selection cannot account for such changes. It is equally rash to assert dogmatically that it can.

If this celebration were merely concerned with eulogies of three great men, it would be worse than useless. If it helps us to imitate them, it is of the greatest value. Linnæus, Darwin and Wallace had this in common, that they did not use complicated apparatus. Any student to-day would turn up his nose at Darwin's microscope. Now we in India find it difficult to get apparatus. This discourages us from some lines of biological research. We cannot get electron microscopes, highly purified amino-acids, and so forth. But we can get land and labour to grow plants or keep animals, we can collect them on a large scale, and we can at least travel all over India. I want to tell you what I am trying to do in these circumstances.

I have already acted as a catalyst in getting one of the world's leading palæontologists (Dr. Pamela L. Robinson, University College, London) over here: and, with Indian colleagues, she has, in about ten weeks work, obtained reptilian and fish fossils, some of which are new to science, while others date some mesozoic formations with considerable precision (*Nature*, 182, 1722: 1958). Similarly, I hope shortly to catalyse the visit of one of the world's leading systematists to attack a group of animals the Indian representatives of which are practically unknown. My own junior colleagues are at last continuing the study of variation where Karl Pearson and Bateson left it fifty years ago.

Perhaps I may begin with a discovery made by a

colleague, Mr. K. Dronamraju. Darwin directed attention to heterostylism in *Primula* and other genera. In many species there are two types of plant, in one of which the flowers have long styles, in the other short. The position of the anthers also differs. The phenomenon is called heterostylism. Darwin found that crosses between flowers of the different types gave far more seed than the so-called illegitimate unions between plants of the same morphological type. As no work of this kind has been done in the tropics, I asked Mr. Dronamraju to look for a suitable plant near the Indian Statistical Institute; for the assessments of fertility and of the viabilities of seeds in such cases raise some interesting statistical problems. Mr. Dronamraju discovered something much more important. He found both long-styled and short-styled flowers growing together on each of five trees of *Bauhinia acuminata*. So far, his results are merely statistical. In a year or two I hope that he will have physiological results also. This observation would most certainly have excited Darwin, who did not attempt to hide his emotions, so that his books are full of such adjectives as 'wonderful' and 'beautiful'. It is at least possible that heterostylism started as a variation between flowers on the same plant, and that, later, genes which controlled it were evolved.

Another colleague, Mr. S. K. Roy, is also almost slavishly imitating Darwin's interests. He has measured the amount of earth brought up by earthworms in Bengal and Bihar, and his measurements are the first to be made in Asia. A proper understanding of Asian soils demands that they be repeated in a thousand different places. I hope that some will be in Singapore or Malaya. He is now working, among other things, on variation in the like parts of the same plant. In a number of individuals of three different species he has reached the startling conclusions that while the mean number of petals per flower does not alter much during a season, the variance usually increases, and may be doubled. If the size of pots made by a potter became more variable at the end of a day, we should say that he was getting tired. I do not know what we are to say about a plant. To reach this conclusion, Mr. Roy has examined about 200,000 flowers. It is an interesting coincidence that Dr. A. K. Sharma, with his wife and other colleagues in the University of Calcutta, are working on differences in chromosome number in different organs of the same plant.

The point which I want to make is this. Apart from genetics, which can scarcely be understood without some special knowledge, no work is going on under my supervision which Darwin or Wallace would not have readily understood, and which is not, in fact, a continuation of a line of work started by one of them. Nevertheless, most of it is original in the sense that it is not an attempt to extend to tropical animals and plants principles which have already been established as holding in Europe, North America or Japan. It was Wallace, above all, who saw that certain biological problems are forced on one by a study of tropical life, which are by no means so obvious in temperate climates. The converse is, of course, true. Many ecological questions are fairly simple in the arctic regions, where a biotic community may consist of only twenty or thirty species; more difficult in the temperate zone, where a hundred or more species must be considered; and extremely complicated in a tropical rain forest, where it might be necessary to consider thousands of species, many as yet undescribed.

Printed in Great Britain by Fisher, Knight & Co., Ltd., St. Albans.

Selection

Haldane's early papers in population genetics typified what has been called "beanbag" genetics. In his first paper on the mathematical theory of natural selection, Haldane (1924) derived formulae for measuring the intensity of selection operating in a population under various biological situations. Prior to Haldane's work, H.T.J. Norton[1] conducted some simpler studies of this nature but Haldane, through a series of systematic studies of the intensity of selection, established an elaborate selection theory. From 1924 to 1934, he published a series of papers on different aspects of this subject. Four of these papers, which were published in 1924 (part I), 1927a (part IV), 1927b (part V), and 1931 (part VIII) are included in this section. In part IV, he analysed the effects of selection when generations overlap, stating that Norton had independently arrived at similar results. This paper's importance lies in the fact that Haldane was the first to integrate mode of selection into demographic structures. He considered the problem of selection in the context of population growth, showing that the oscillations of the population number around an exponential function of the time. The significance of this paper has been recognized by those working in demographic genetics.[2]

In part V he showed that the probability that a single mutation with selective advantage k will not be lost by accidents of sampling but will ultimately become established is only about 2k, if more or less dominant, and only of the order k/N if completely recessive, where N is the population size. In part VIII Haldane (1931) investigated situations where mutant genes are disadvantageous singly but become advantageous in combinations. This paper, dealing with "metastable" populations, anticipated Wright's shifting balance theory.[3]

Among a number of diverse evolutionary studies, Haldane dealt with both the statics and the dynamics of natural selection. In one interesting paper (1932), he considered the evolutionary implications of the time of action of genes, citing several examples where the time of action of a gene may be distributed over more than one life-cycle. He made the interesting suggestion that selection tends to make life-cycles more and more variegated, thus increasing the possibility of fixing the time of action of genes, as in the case of parasites that live in widely different hosts. Throughout his life, Haldane continued to make suggestions for quantitative studies of evolution, and suggested the unit *darwin* (1949) for measuring evolutionary rates. Papers written during the last two decades of his life include an update of his early calculation in the light of Kettlewell's work on melanism and the conflict between inbreeding and selection. The most noteworthy paper of that period was that dealing with the cost of natural selection, in which he showed that, in horotelic evolution, the mean time taken for each gene substitution is about 300 generations, the number of deaths needed to secure the substitution being about 30 times the number of organisms in a generation. Haldane's cost estimate provided a rationale for Kimura's neutral theory of evolution.[4]

1. Norton, H.T.J., in Punnett, R.C.: *Mimicry in Butterflies*, Cambridge: Cambridge University Press, 1915.

2. Sutter, J., Haldane and demographic genetics. In: Dronamraju, K.R. (Ed.), *Haldane and Modern Biology*, Baltimore: Johns Hopkins University Press, 1968.
3. Wright, S., Evolution in Mendelian populations. *Genetics, 16*: 97–159, 1931.
4. Kimura, M., Evolutionary rate at the molecular level. *Nature, 217*: 624–626, 1968.

II. *A Mathematical Theory of Natural and Artificial Selection.*

PART I.

By J. B. S. HALDANE, M.A.
Trinity College, Cambridge.

A SATISFACTORY theory of natural selection must be quantitative. In order to establish the view that natural selection is capable of accounting for the known facts of evolution we must show not only that it can cause a species to change, but that it can cause it to change at a rate which will account for present and past transmutations. In any given case we must specify:

(1) The mode of inheritance of the character considered,
(2) The system of breeding in the group of organisms studied,
(3) The intensity of selection,
(4) Its incidence (e.g. on both sexes or only one), and
(5) The rate at which the proportion of organisms showing the character increases or diminishes.

It should then be possible to obtain an equation connecting (3) and (5).

The principal work on the subject so far is that of Pearson (1), Warren (2), and Norton. Pearson's work was based on a pre-Mendelian theory of variation and heredity, which is certainly inapplicable to many, and perhaps to all characters. Warren has only considered selection of an extremely stringent character, whilst Norton's work is as yet only available in the table quoted by Punnett (3).

In this paper we shall only deal with the simplest possible cases. The character dealt with will be the effect of a single completely dominant Mendelian factor or its absence. The system of breeding considered will be random mating on the one hand or self-fertilization, budding, etc. on the other. Moreover we shall confine ourselves to organisms such as annual plants, and many insects and fish in which different generations do not interbreed. Even so it will be found that in most cases we can only obtain rigorous solutions when selection is very rapid or very slow. At intermediate rates we should require to use functions of a hitherto unexplored type. Indeed the mathematical problems raised in the more complicated cases to be dealt with in subsequent papers seem to be as formidable as any in mathematical physics. The approximate solutions given in this paper are however of as great an order of accuracy as that of the data hitherto available.

It is not of course intended to suggest that all heredity is Mendelian, or all evolution by natural selection. On the other hand we know that besides non-Mendelian differences between species (e.g. in chromosome number) there are often Mendelian factor-differences. The former are important because they often lead to total or partial sterility in crosses, but their somatic expression is commonly less striking than that of a single factor-difference. Their behaviour in crosses is far from clear, but where crossing does not occur evolution takes place according to equations (1·0)—(1·2).

SPECIFICATION OF THE INTENSITY OF SELECTION.

If a generation of zygotes immediately after fertilization consists of two phenotypes A and B in the ratio $pA : 1B$, and the proportion which form fertile unions is $pA : (1-k)B$, we shall describe k as the coefficient of selection. Thus if $k = \cdot 01$, a population of equal numbers of A and B would survive to form fertile unions in the proportion $100A : 99B$, the A's thus having a slight advantage. k may be positive or negative. When it is small selection is slow. When $k = 1$ no B's reproduce, when $k = -\infty$ no A's reproduce. It will be convenient to refer to these two cases as "complete selection." They occur in artificial selection if the character is well marked.

If the character concerned affects fertility, or kills off during the breeding period, we can use just the same notation. In this case each B on the average leaves as many offspring as $(1-k)$ A's, e.g. if $k = \cdot 01$ then 100 B's leave as many as 99 A's. The effect is clearly just the same as if one of the B's had died before breeding. It will be observed that no assumption is made as to the total number of the population. If this is limited by the environment, natural selection may cause it to increase or diminish. It will for example tend to increase if selection renders the organism smaller or fitter to cope with its environment in general. If on the other hand selection increases its size, or merely arms it in the struggle with other members of its species for food or mates, the population will tend to diminish or even to disappear.

Warren (2) considered the case where the total population is fixed. He supposes that the parents produce l times their number of offspring, and that type A is p times as numerous as type B, but $\frac{1}{m}$ as likely to die. In this case it can be shown that

$$k = \frac{(l-1)(m-1)(p+1)}{lm - l + p + 1}.$$

Hence the advantage of one type over the other as measured by k is not independent of the composition of the population unless $m-1$ is very small, when $k = (l-1)(m-1)$ approximately. Hence when selection is slow—the most interesting case—the two schemes of selection lead to similar results. On the other hand the mathematical treatment of selection on our scheme is decidedly simpler.

FAMILIAL SELECTION.

The above notation may easily be applied to the cases, such as Darwinian sexual selection, where one sex only is selected. There is however another type of selection which so far as I know has not been considered in any detail by former authors, but which must have been of considerable importance in evolution. So far we have assumed that the field of struggle for existence is the species as a whole, or at least those members of it living within a given area. But we have also to consider those cases where the struggle occurs between members of the same family. Such cases occur in many mammals, seed-plants, and nematodes, to mention no other groups. Here the size of the family is strictly limited by the food or space available for it, and more embryos are produced than can survive to enter into the struggle with members of other families. Thus in the mouse Ibsen and Steigleder (4) have shown that some embryos of any litter perish in utero. Their deaths are certainly sometimes selective. In litters from the mating yellow × yellow one-quarter of the embryos die in the blastula stage, yet as Durham (5) has shown, such litters are no smaller than the normal, because the death of the YY embryos allows others to survive which would normally have perished.

The above is a case of complete selection. Where the less viable type of embryo, instead of perishing inevitably, is merely at a slight disadvantage, it is clear that selection will only be effective, or at any rate will be much more effective, in the mixed litters. Thus let us consider 3 litters of 20 embryos each, the first consisting wholly of the stronger type, the second containing 10 strong and 10 weak, the third wholly of the weaker type. Suppose that in each case there is only enough food or space for 10 embryos, and that the strong type has an advantage over the weak such that, out of equal numbers, 50 °/₀ more of the strong will survive, i.e. $k = \frac{1}{3}$. Then the survivors will be 10 strong from the first litter, 6 strong and 4 weak from the second, and 10 weak from the third, or 16 strong and 14 weak. If the competition had been free, as with pelagic larvae, the numbers would have been 18 strong and 12 weak. Clearly with familial selection the same advantage acts more slowly than with normal selection, since it is only effective in mixed families.

The "family" within which selection acts may have both parents in common, as in most mammals, or many different male parents, as in those plants whose pollen, but not seeds, is spread by the wind. In this case the seeds from any one plant will fall into the same area, and unless the plants are very closely packed, will compete with one another in the main. In rare cases familial sexual selection may occur. Thus in *Dinophilus* the rudimentary males fertilize their sisters before leaving the cocoon. Clearly so long as every female gets fertilized before hatching selection can only occur in the male sex between brothers, and must tend to make the males copulate at as early a date as possible.

The survival of many of the embryonic characters of viviparous animals and seed-plants must have been due to familial selection.

Selection in the absence of amphimixis.

The simplest form of selection is uncomplicated either by amphimixis or dominance. It occurs in the following cases:

(1) Organisms which do not reproduce sexually, or are self-fertilizing.

(2) Species which do not cross, but compete for the same means of support.

(3) Organisms in which mating is always between brother and sister.

(4) Organisms like *Bryophyta* which are haploid during part of the life cycle, provided that selection of the character considered only occurs during the haploid phase.

(5) Heterogamous organisms in which the factor determining the character selected occurs in the gametes of one sex only. For example Renner (6) has shown that *Oenothera muricata* transmits certain characters by the pollen only, others by the ovules only. Schmidt (7) has found a character in *Lebistes* transmitted by males to males only, and Goldschmidt (8) has postulated sex-factors in *Lymantria* transmitted only by females to females. As far as the characters in question are concerned there is no amphimixis, and these organisms behave as if they were asexual. Other species of *Oenothera* which are permanently heterozygous for other reasons would probably be selected in much the same way.

Let the nth generation consist of types A and B in the ratio $u_n A : 1B$, and let the coefficient of selection be k, i.e. $(1-k)$ B's survive for every A. Then the survivors of the nth generation, and hence the first numbers of the $(n+1)$th, will be $u_n A : (1-k) B$.

$$\therefore \quad u_{n+1} = \frac{u_n}{1-k}, \qquad \text{.......................................(1·0)}$$

and if u_0 be the original ratio $u_n = (1-k)^{-n} u_0$.

3—2

Now if we write y_n for the proportion of B's in the total population of the nth generation,

$$y_n = \frac{1}{1 + u_n} = \frac{1}{1 + (1-k)^{-n} u_0} = \frac{y_0}{y_0 + (1-k)^{-n}(1-y_0)},$$

or if we start with equal numbers of A and B, $y_0 = \frac{1}{2}$, and

$$y_n = \frac{1}{1 + (1-k)^{-n}}. \qquad \text{.................................. (1·1)}$$

If k is very small, i.e. selection slow, then approximately

$$\left.\begin{aligned} y_n &= \frac{1}{1 + e^{kn}} \\ \text{or} \qquad kn &= \log_e \left(\frac{1-y_n}{y_n}\right) \end{aligned}\right\}. \qquad \text{.................................. (1·2)}$$

Hence the proportion of B's falls slowly at first, then rapidly for a short time, then slowly again, the rate being greatest when $y = \frac{1}{2}$. Before $y = \frac{1}{2}$, n is of course taken as negative. So long as k is small the time taken for any given change in the proportions varies inversely as k. The curve representing graphically the change of the population is symmetrical about its middle point, and is shown in Fig. 1 for the case where $k = \cdot 001$, i.e. 999 B's survive for every 1000 A's. 9,184 generations are needed for the proportion of A's to increase from 1 °/o to 99 °/o. Equation (1·2) gives an error of only 4 in this number.

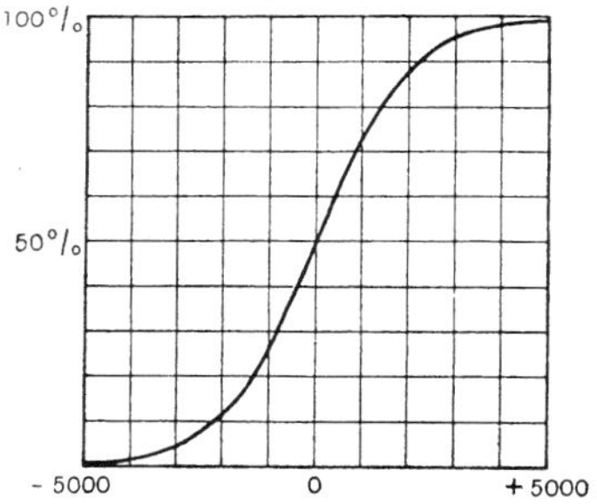

Fig. 1. Effect of selection on a non-amphimictic character. $k = \cdot 001$.
Abscissa = generations.
Ordinate = percentage of population with the favoured character.

As will be shown below, selection proceeds more slowly with all other systems of inheritance. In this case the speed must compensate to some extent for the failure to combine advantageous factors by amphimixis. Where occasional amphimixis occurs, as for example in wheat, conditions are very favourable for the evolution of advantageous combinations of variations.

SELECTION OF A SIMPLE MENDELIAN CHARACTER.

Consider the case of a population which consists of zygotes containing two, one, or no "doses" of a completely dominant Mendelian factor A, mating is at random, and selection acts to an equal degree in both sexes upon the character produced by the factor. Pearson (9) and Hardy (10) have shown that in a population mating at random the square of the number of heterozygotes is equal to four times the product of the numbers of the two homozygous classes. Let $u_n A : 1a$ be the proportion of the two types of gametes produced by the $(n-1)$th generation. Then in the nth generation the initial proportions of the three classes of zygotes are:

$$u_n^2 AA : 2u_n Aa : 1aa.$$

The proportion of recessives to the whole population is:

$$y_n = (1+u_n)^{-2}. \quad \text{.......................................(2·0)}$$

Now only $(1-k)$ of the recessives survive to breed, so that the survivors are in the proportions:

$$u_n^2 AA : 2u_n Aa : (1-k)\, aa.$$

The numbers of the next generation can be most easily calculated from the new gametic ratio u_{n+1}. This is immediately obvious in the case of aquatic organisms which shed their gametes into the water. If each zygote produces N gametes which conjugate, the numbers are clearly:

$$(Nu_n^2 + Nu_n)\, A, \text{ and } (Nu_n + N\overline{1-k})\, a.$$

So the ratio

$$u_{n+1} = \frac{u_n(1+u_n)}{1+u_n-k}. \quad \text{.......................................(2·1)}$$

It can easily be shown that this result follows from random mating, for matings will occur in the following proportions:

$AA \times AA$		$u_n^2 \times u_n^2$	or u_n^4,
$AA \times Aa$	and reciprocally,	$2 \times u_n^2 \times 2u_n$	,, $4u_n^3$,
$AA \times aa$	,, ,,	$2 \times u_n^2 \times (1-k)$	,, $2(1-k)\,u_n^2$,
$Aa \times Aa$		$2u_n \times 2u_n$	,, $4u_n^2$,
$Aa \times aa$	and reciprocally,	$2 \times 2u_n \times (1-k)$	,, $4(1-k)\,u_n$,
$aa \times aa$		$(1-k) \times (1-k)$	,, $(1-k)^2$.

Hence zygotes are formed in the following proportions:

AA	$u_n^4 + 2u_n^3 + u_n^2$	or $u_n^2(1+u_n)^2$,
Aa	$2u_n^3 + 2(1-k)\,u_n^2 + 2u_n^2 + 2(1-k)\,u_n$	,, $2u_n(1+u_n)(1+u_n-k)$,
aa	$u_n^2 + 2(1-k)\,u_n + (1-k)^2$	,, $(1+u_n-k)^2$.

These ratios may be written:

$$\left[\frac{u_n(1+u_n)}{1+u_n-k}\right]^2 AA : \frac{2u_n(1+u_n)}{1+u_n-k} Aa : 1aa,$$

or

$$u^2_{n+1} AA : 2u_{n+1} Aa : 1aa,$$

where

$$u_{n+1} = \frac{u_n(1+u_n)}{1+u_n-k}, \quad \text{.......................................(2·1)}$$

as above. It is however simpler to obtain u_{n+1} directly from the ratio of A to a among the gametes of the population as a whole, and this will be done in our future calculations.

Now if we know the original proportion of recessives y_0, we start with a population:

$$u_0^2 AA : 2u_0 Aa : 1aa,$$

where

$$u_0 = y_0^{-\frac{1}{2}} - 1,$$

and we can at once calculate

$$u_1 = \frac{u_0(1+u_0)}{1+u_0-k},$$

and thence u_2 and so on, obtaining y_1, y_2, etc. from equation (2·0). Thus if we start with 25 °/₀ of recessives, and $k = ·5$, i.e. the recessives are only half as viable as the dominants, then $u_0 = 1$, and

$$u_1 = \frac{1(1+1)}{1+1-\frac{1}{2}} = \tfrac{4}{3},$$

$$y_1 = (1+\tfrac{4}{3})^{-2} = \tfrac{9}{49} = ·184, \text{ or } 18·4\ °/_{\circ}.$$

Similarly $y_2 = 13{\cdot}75\ \%$, $y_3 = 10{\cdot}9\ \%$, and so on. Starting from the same population, but with $k = -1$, so that the recessives are twice as viable as the dominants, we have $y_1 = 36\ \%$, $y_2 = 49{\cdot}8\ \%$, $y_3 = 64{\cdot}6\ \%$, $y_4 = 77{\cdot}5\ \%$, $y_5 = 87{\cdot}0\ \%$, and so on. If k is small this method becomes very tedious, but we can find a fairly accurate formula connecting y_n with n.

The case of complete selection is simple. If all the dominants are killed off or prevented from breeding we shall see the last of them in one generation, and $y_n = 1$. Punnett (11) and Hardy have solved the case where the recessives all die. Here $k = 1$, and

$$u_{n+1} = \frac{u_n(1+u_n)}{1+u_n-1} = 1 + u_n.$$

$$\therefore\ u_n = n + u_0;$$

$$\therefore\ y_n = (n+1+u_0)^{-2}$$

$$= (n + y_0^{-\frac{1}{2}})^{-2}$$

$$= y_0(1 + ny_0^{\frac{1}{2}})^{-2}. \qquad \text{.......(2·2)}$$

Thus if we start with a population containing $\frac{1}{4}$ recessives the second generation will contain $\frac{1}{9}$, the third $\frac{1}{16}$, the nth $\frac{1}{(n+1)^2}$. Thus 999 generations will be needed to reduce the proportion to one in a million, and we need not wonder that recessive sports still occur in most of our domestic breeds of animals.

When selection is not very intense, we can proceed as follows:

$$u_{n+1} = \frac{u_n(1+u_n)}{1+u_n-k}; \qquad \text{.......(2·1)}$$

$$\therefore\ \Delta u_n \equiv u_{n+1} - u_n = \frac{ku_n}{1+u_n-k}.$$

When k is small we can neglect it in comparison with unity, and suppose that u_n increases continuously and not by steps, i.e. take $\Delta u_n = \frac{du_n}{dn}$.

$$\therefore\ \frac{du_n}{dn} = \frac{ku_n}{1+u_n}\ \text{approximately};$$

$$\therefore\ kn = \int_{u_0}^{u_n} \frac{1+u}{u}\,du$$

$$= u_n - u_0 + \log_e\left(\frac{u_n}{u_0}\right). \qquad \text{.......(2·3)}$$

If we start from or work towards a standard population containing 25 % of recessives, and hence $u_0 = 1$, we have

$$kn = u_n + \log_e u_n - 1. \qquad \text{.......(2·4)}$$

This equation is accurate enough for any practical problem when $|k|$ is small, and as long as k lies between $\pm 0{\cdot}1$, i.e. neither phenotype has an advantage of more than 10 %, it may be safely used. When $|k|$ is large the equation

$$kn = u_n + (1-k)\log_e u_n - 1 \qquad \text{.......(2·5)}$$

is fairly accurate for positive values of n. Thus when $k = \frac{1}{2}$, the error is always under 4 %. For large values of $|k|$ and negative values of n the equation

$$kn = u_n + \left(1 - \frac{k}{2}\right)\log_e u_n - 1 \qquad \text{.......(2·6)}$$

gives results with a very small error. But for every case so far observed equation (2·4) gives results within the limits of observational error.

In the above equations we have only to make k negative to calculate the effects of a selection which favours recessives at the expense of dominants. For the same small intensity of selection the same time is clearly needed to produce a given change in the percentage of recessives whether dominants or recessives are favoured. Fig. 2 shows graphically the rate of increase of dominants and recessives respectively when $k = \pm \cdot 001$, i.e. the favoured type has an advantage of one in a thousand, as in Fig. 1. In each case 16,582 generations are required to increase the proportion of the favoured type from 1 °/₀ to 99 °/₀, but dominants increase more rapidly than recessives when they are few, more slowly when they are numerous. The change occurs most rapidly when y_n, the proportion of recessives, is 56·25 °/₀. When selection is ten times as intense, the population will clearly change ten times as fast, and so on.

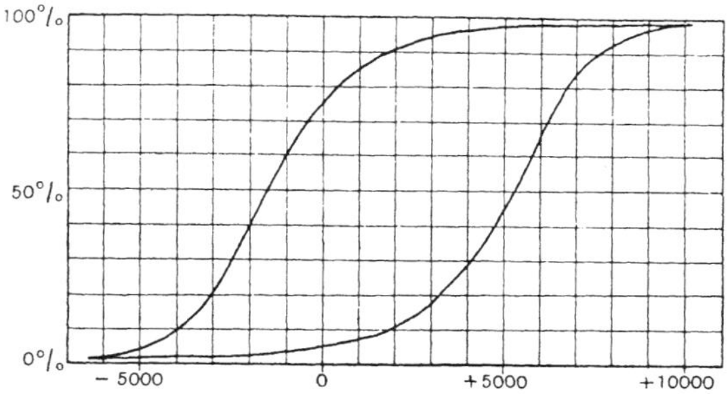

Fig. 2. Effect of selection on an autosomal Mendelian character. $k = \cdot 001$.
Upper curve, dominants favoured; lower curve, recessives favoured.
Abscissa = generations. Ordinate = percentage of population with the favoured character.

TABLE I.

Effect of slow selection on an autosomal Mendelian character.

kn (number of generations × *k*)	− 1000	− 100	− 50	− 20	− 15	− 10						
°/₀ of recessives when dominants are favoured	...	...	...	...	99·9998	99·975						
,, ,, ,, recessives ,, ,,	·0001	·0105	·0427	·2773	·4215	1·036						
kn	− 9	− 8	− 7	− 6	− 5	− 4·5	− 4	− 3·5	− 3	− 2·5	− 2	− 1·5
dominants favoured	99·933	99·82	99·50	98·68	96·50	94·38	91·14	86·36	79·71	71·24	61·53	50·68
recessives favoured	1·254	1·545	1·940	2·497	3·308	...	4·537	...	6·528	...	9·718	12·11
kn	− 1	− 0·5	0	0·5	1	1·5	2	2·5	3	3·5	4	4·5
dominants favoured	40·98	32·05	25·0	19·53	15·30	12·11	9·718	...	6·528	...	4·537	...
recessives favoured	15·30	19·53	25·0	32·05	40·98	50·68	61·53	71·24	79·71	86·36	91·14	94·38
kn	5	6	7	8	9	10	15	20	50	100	1000	
dominants favoured	3·308	2·497	1·940	1·545	1·254	1·036	·4215	·2773	·0427	·0105	·0001	
recessives favoured	96·50	98·68	99·50	99·82	99·933	99·975	99·9998	...	...	...	...	

In Table I the values of y_n calculated from equations (2·4) and (2·0) are given in terms of kn. In Table II kn is given in terms of y_n. The number of generations (forwards or backwards) is reckoned from a standard population containing 75 °/₀ of dominants and 25 °/₀ of recessives. A few examples will make the use of these tables clear.

1. Detlefsen (12) has shown that in a mixed population of mice about 95·9 without the factor *G*, causing light bellies and yellow-tipped hair, survive for every 100 with it. Hence $k = ·041$. It is required to find how many recessives will be left after 100 generations, starting from a population with 90 °/₀ of recessives, and assuming that different generations do not interbreed.

From Table II, when $y = ·9$, $kn = -3·863$, $\therefore n = -94·2$. So 94·2 generations of selection will bring the recessives down to 25 °/₀. The remaining 5·8 generations give $kn = ·238$, and from Table I by interpolation we find $y = ·224$, i.e. only 22·4 °/₀ of recessives remain.

2. In the same case how many generations are needed to reduce the number of recessives to 1 °/₀? $y_n = ·01$, hence, from Table II, $kn = 10·197$, $\therefore n = 248·7$. So 248·7 generations after 25 °/₀ is reached, or 343 in all, will be required.

3. The dominant melanic form *doubledayaria* of the peppered moth *Amphidasys betularia* first appeared at Manchester in 1848. Some time before 1901 when Barrett (13) described the case, it had completely ousted the recessive variety in Manchester. It is required to find the least intensity of natural selection which will account for this fact.

TABLE II.

Effect of slow selection on an autosomal Mendelian character.

°/₀ of favoured type	·0001	·001	·01	·05	·1	·2	·5
kn when dominants are favoured	− 15·51	− 13·21	− 10·90	− 9·294	− 8·600	− 7·905	− 6·996
kn ,, recessives ,, ,,	− 1005	− 320·0	− 102·60	− 45·50	− 33·04	− 23·42	− 14·72

°/₀ of favoured type	1	2	3	5	10	15	20	25	30	35	40
kn when dominants are favoured	− 6·286	− 5·580	− 5·161	− 4·624	− 3·863	− 3·290	− 2·979	− 2·712	− 2·439	− 2·180	− 1·964
kn when recessives are favoured	− 10·197	− 6·875	− 4·976	− 3·717	− 1·933	− 1·041	− ·448	0	+ ·366	+ ·681	+ ·962

°/₀ of favoured type	45	50	55	60	65	70	75	80	85	90	95
kn when dominants are favoured	− 1·708	− 1·467	− 1·220	− ·962	− ·681	− ·366	0	+ ·448	+ 1·041	+ 1·933	+ 3·717
kn when recessives are favoured	+ 1·220	+ 1·467	+ 1·708	+ 1·964	+ 2·180	+ 2·439	+ 2·712	+ 2·979	+ 3·290	+ 3·863	+ 4·620

°/₀ of favoured type	97	98	99	99·5	99·8	99·9	99·95	99·99	99·999	99·9999
kn when dominants are favoured	+ 4·976	+ 6·875	+ 10·197	+ 14·72	+ 23·42	+ 33·04	+ 45·50	+ 102·60	+ 320·0	+ 1005
kn when recessives are favoured	+ 5·161	+ 5·580	+ 6·286	+ 6·996	+ 7·905	+ 8·600	+ 9·294	+ 10·90	+ 13·21	+ 15·51

Assuming that there were not more than 1 °/₀ of dominants in Manchester in 1848, nor less than 99 °/₀ in 1898, we have, from Table II, $kn = 16·58$ as a minimum. But $n = 50$, since this moth usually has one brood per year. $\therefore k = ·332$ at least, i.e. at least 3 dominants must survive for every 2 recessives, and probably more; or the fertility of the dominants must be 50 °/₀ greater than that of the recessives. Direct calculation step by step from equation (2·1) shows that 48 generations are needed for the change if $k = ·\dot{3}$. Hence the table is sufficiently accurate. After only 13 generations the dominants would be in a majority. It is perhaps instructive, in view of the fact that attempts have been made to explain such cases by epidemics of mutation due either to the environment or to unknown causes, to note that in such a case one recessive in every five would have to mutate to a dominant. Hence it would be impossible to obtain true breeding recessives as was done by Bate (14). Another possible explanation would be a large excess of dominants begotten in mixed families, as occurs in human night-blindness according to Bateson (15). But this again does not agree with the facts, and the only probable explanation is the not very intense degree of natural selection postulated above.

FAMILIAL SELECTION OF A SIMPLE MENDELIAN CHARACTER.

Consider the case of a factor A whose presence gives any embryo possessing it an advantage measured by k over those members of the same family which do not possess it. In this case the Pearson-Hardy law does not hold in the population. Each family may have both parents in common, as in mammals, or only the mother, as in cross-pollinated seed-plants. In the first case let the population consist of

$$p_n AA : 2q_n Aa : r_n aa, \text{ where } p_n + 2q_n + r_n = 1.$$

Then in a mixed family where equality was to be expected the ratio of dominants to recessives will be $1 : 1 - k$. But since the total is unaltered, the actual number of dominants will be to the expected as $2 : 2 - k$, of recessives as $2 - 2k : 2 - k$, and similarly for a family where a $3 : 1$ ratio was to be expected. The nth generation mating at random will therefore produce surviving offspring in the following proportions:

	AA	Aa	aa
From mating $AA \times AA$ ...	p_n^2	0	0
,, ,, $AA \times Aa$ ...	$2p_n q_n$	$2p_n q_n$	0
,, ,, $AA \times aa$ ...	0	$2p_n r_n$	0
,, ,, $Aa \times Aa$ ...	$\frac{4q_n^2}{4-k}$	$\frac{8q_n^2}{4-k}$	$\frac{(4-4k)\,q_n^2}{4-k}$
,, ,, $Aa \times aa$ ...	0	$\frac{2q_n r_n}{2-k}$	$\frac{(2-2k)\,q_n r_n}{2-k}$
,, ,, $aa \times aa$ ...	0	0	r_n^2

$$\left.\begin{aligned} \therefore\ [AA] = p_{n+1} &= (p_n + q_n)^2 + \frac{kq_n^2}{4-k} \\ \tfrac{1}{2}[Aa] = q_{n+1} &= (p_n + q_n)(q_n + r_n) + kq_n\left(\frac{q_n}{4-k} + \frac{r_n}{2-k}\right) \\ [aa] = r_{n+1} &= (q_n + r_n)^2 - kq_n\left(\frac{3q_n}{4-k} + \frac{2r_n}{2-k}\right) \end{aligned}\right\} \quad \text{............(3·0)}$$

With complete selection, when $k = 1$, we have $r_{n+1} = r_n^2$, so the proportion of recessives, starting from $\frac{1}{4}$, will be $\frac{1}{16}$, $\frac{1}{64}$, etc., in successive generations, provided of course that all-recessive families survive, as in *Oenothera*. So recessives are eliminated far more quickly than in the ordinary type of selection. Clearly however dominants are not eliminated at once when $k = -\infty$ (provided that they survive in all-dominant families), for

$$p_{n+1} = p_n(1 - r_n) = p_n p_{n-1}(2 - p_{n-1}).$$

Starting from the standard population, successive proportions of recessives are 25 %, 56·25 %, 66·02 %, 84·25 %, etc.

In the more interesting case when k is small we can solve approximately, as follows. From equation (3·0) we see that $q^2_{n+1} - p_{n+1}r_{n+1}$ and hence $q_n^2 - p_n r_n$ is a small quantity of the order kq_n^2, i.e. is less than k. Hence if we write $u_n = \frac{p_n + q_n}{q_n + r_n}$, then q_n only differs from $\frac{u_n}{(1+u_n)^2}$ by a small quantity of the order of k.

Now

$$u_{n+1} = \frac{p_{n+1} + q_{n+1}}{q_{n+1} + r_{n+1}}$$

$$= \frac{p_n + q_n + kq_n\left(\dfrac{2q_n}{4-k} + \dfrac{r_n}{2-k}\right)}{q_n + r_n - kq_n\left(\dfrac{2q_n}{4-k} + \dfrac{r_n}{2-k}\right)}$$

$$= \frac{p_n + q_n + \frac{1}{2}kq_n(q_n + r_n)}{q_n + r_n - \frac{1}{2}kq_n(q_n + r_n)} \text{ approximately}$$

$$= \frac{u_n + \frac{1}{2}kq_n}{1 - \frac{1}{2}kq_n}$$

$$= u_n + \tfrac{1}{2}kq_n(1 + u_n) \text{ approximately}$$

$$= u_n + \frac{ku_n}{2(1 + u_n)}. \qquad (3{\cdot}1)$$

Solving as for equation (2·1) we find

$$\tfrac{1}{2}kn = u_n + \log_e u_n - 1. \qquad (3{\cdot}2)$$

And since as above r_n (the proportion of recessives) $= (1 + u_n)^{-2}$, it follows that the species changes its composition at half the rate at which it would change if selection worked on the species as a whole, and not within families only.

If each family has its mother only in common, but the fathers are a random sample of the population, we assume the nth generation to consist of

$$p_n AA : 2q_n Aa : r_n aa, \text{ where } p_n + 2q_n + r_n = 1.$$

Let $u_n = \dfrac{p_n + q_n}{q_n + r_n}$, hence $p_n + q_n = \dfrac{u_n}{1 + u_n}$, $q_n + r_n = \dfrac{1}{1 + u_n}$.

Then families will be begotten as follows:

	AA	Aa	aa
From AA females ...	$\dfrac{p_n u_n}{1 + u_n}$	$\dfrac{p_n}{1 + u_n}$	0
,, Aa ,, ...	$\dfrac{q_n u_n}{1 + u_n}$	q_n	$\dfrac{q_n}{1 + u_n}$
,, aa ,, ...	0	$\dfrac{r_n u_n}{1 + u_n}$	$\dfrac{r_n}{1 + u_n}$

After selection and replacement the proportions will be:

	AA	Aa	aa
From AA females ...	$\dfrac{p_n u_n}{1 + u_n}$	$\dfrac{p_n}{1 + u_n}$	0
,, Aa ,, ...	$\dfrac{q_n u_n}{1 + u_n - \frac{1}{2}k}$	$\dfrac{q_n(1 + u_n)}{1 + u_n - \frac{1}{2}k}$	$\dfrac{q_n(1-k)}{1 + u_n - \frac{1}{2}k}$
,, aa ,, ...	0	$\dfrac{r_n u_n}{1 + u_n - k}$	$\dfrac{r_n(1-k)}{1 + u_n - k}$

With complete selection, where $k = 1$, recessives are eliminated at once, provided families are large enough. Where $k = -\infty$, dominants are not eliminated at once if pure dominant families survive, since $p_{n+1} = \frac{p_n(1-p_n)}{1+p_n}$. Starting from the standard population, successive values of r_n are 25 %, 75 %, 87·5 %, 99·7 %, etc. Where k is small we obtain approximate equations analogous to (3·0) whose solution is

$$\tfrac{3}{4}kn = u_n + \log_e u_n - 1. \qquad \text{(3·3)}$$

Thus selection proceeds at $\frac{3}{4}$ of the rate given by equation (2·4).

Sex-limited characters and unisexual selection.

We have next to deal with characters which only appear in one sex, for example milk yield or other secondary sexual characters; or on which selection at least is unisexual, as for example in Darwinian sexual selection. Let the $(n-1)$th generation form spermatozoa in the ratio $u_n A : 1a$, eggs in the ratio $v_n A : 1a$. Then the nth generation consists of zygotes in the ratios

$$u_n v_n AA : (u_n + v_n)\,Aa : 1aa,$$

$$\therefore\ y_n = (1+u_n)^{-1}(1+v_n)^{-1}. \qquad \text{(4·0)}$$

If only $1-k$ recessive ♀ survives for every dominant ♀, whilst ♂'s are not affected by selection, we have

$$\left.\begin{aligned} u_{n+1} &= \frac{2u_n v_n + u_n + v_n}{u_n + v_n + 2} \\ v_{n+1} &= \frac{2u_n v_n + u_n + v_n}{u_n + v_n + 2 - 2k} \end{aligned}\right\}. \qquad \text{(4·1)}$$

With complete selection, when $k = -\infty$, and all dominants of one sex are weeded out, we have $v_n = 0$, and $u_{n+1} = \frac{u_n}{2+u_n}$.

$$\therefore\ u_n = \left[2^{n-1}\left(1+\frac{1}{u_0}\right) - 1\right]^{-1},$$

and

$$y_n = 1 + 2^{1-n}(y_0^{\frac{1}{2}} - 1). \qquad \text{(4·2)}$$

Hence the proportion of dominants is halved in every successive generation. When $k = 1$, and all the recessives of one sex die childless, the proportions of recessives in successive generations, starting from the standard population, are 25 %, 16·7 %, 12·5 %, 9·56 %, 7·94 %, and so on.

When k is small, since

$$v_{n+1} - u_{n+1} = \frac{2k(2u_n v_n + u_n + v_n)}{(u_n + v_n + 2)(u_n + v_n + 2 - 2k)}$$

and

$$\Delta u_n = \frac{(1+u_n)(v_n - u_n)}{u_n + v_n + 2},$$

and hence the differences between u_n, u_{n+1}, v_n, v_{n+1} may be neglected in comparison with themselves;

$$\therefore\ v_n - u_n = \frac{ku_n}{1+u_n} \text{ approximately,}$$

and

$$\Delta u_n = \frac{ku_n}{2(1+u_n)} \text{ approximately.}$$

$$\therefore\ \tfrac{1}{2}kn = u_n + \log_e u_n - 1, \qquad \text{(4·3)}$$

and selection proceeds at half the rate given by equation (2·4), a result stated by Punnett (3).

4—2

SELECTION OF AN ALTERNATIVELY DOMINANT CHARACTER.

A few factors, such as that determining the presence or absence of horns in Dorset and Suffolk sheep, according to Wood (16) are dominant in one sex, recessive in the other. Consider a factor dominant in the male sex, recessive in the female. Let the nth generation be produced by

$$\text{spermatozoa } u_n A : 1a, \quad \text{eggs } v_n A : 1a.$$

It consists of

$$\text{zygotes} : u_n v_n AA : (u_n + v_n) Aa : 1aa,$$

and the survivors after selection are in the ratios

$$♂ \quad u_n v_n AA : (u_n + v_n) Aa : (1-k)\, aa,$$

$$♀ \quad \frac{u_n v_n}{1-k} AA : (u_n + v_n) Aa : 1aa.$$

$$\left.\begin{aligned} \therefore\ u_{n+1} &= \frac{2u_n v_n + u_n + v_n}{u_n + v_n + 2 - 2k} \\ v_{n+1} &= \frac{\frac{2}{1-k} u_n v_n + u_n + v_n}{u_n + v_n + 2} \end{aligned}\right\} \quad \text{.............................(5·0)}$$

Whilst $\quad y_n \text{ (for males)} = (1+u_n)^{-1}(1+v_n)^{-1}$. ....(5·1)

With complete selection, when all members of the type dominant in the female sex are weeded out, $k = 1$.

$$\therefore\ v_{n+1} = \infty, \text{ and } u_{n+1} = 1 + 2u_n, \text{ after the first generation.}$$

$$\therefore\ 1 + u_n = 2^{n-1}(1 + u_1),$$

and if z_n be the proportion of the weeded out type occurring in the female sex,

$$\left.\begin{aligned} \therefore\ y_n &= 0 \\ z_n &= 2^{1-n} z_1 \end{aligned}\right\}. \quad \text{......................................(5·2)}$$

So this type disappears in the male sex, and is halved in successive female generations. If $k = \infty$ the type recessive in the female sex disappears in that sex and is halved in successive male generations.

When k is small,

$$\therefore\ v_{n+1} - u_{n+1} = \frac{k u_n (u_n - 1)}{1 + u_n} \text{ approximately,}$$

and $\Delta u_n = \frac{1}{2} k u_n$.

$$\therefore\ kn = 2 \log_e u_n \quad \text{......................................(5·3)}$$

if $u_0 = 1$, so selection occurs on the whole more rapidly than by equation (2·4). (See Table V.) y_n is given by equation (2·0).

SEX-LINKED CHARACTERS UNDER NO SELECTION.

The events in an unselected population whose members differ with regard to a sex-linked factor have been considered by Jennings (17) but can be treated more simply. We suppose the male to be heterozygous for sex, but the argument is the same where the female is heterozygous. Consider a fully dominant factor A, such that the female may be AA, Aa, or aa, the male Aa or aa (or in Morgan's notation, which will be adopted, A or a). As Jennings showed, a population with

$$♀\text{'s } u^2 AA : 2uAa : 1aa; \quad ♂\text{'s } uA : 1a$$

is stable during random mating, and other populations approach it asymptotically. In any population let the eggs of the $(n-1)$th generation be $u_n A : 1a$, the ♀-producing spermatozoa $v_n A : 1a$. Then the nth generation will be: ♀'s $u_n v_n AA : (u_n + v_n) Aa : 1aa$; ♂'s $u_n A : 1a$.

$$\left.\begin{aligned} \therefore\ u_{n+1} &= \frac{2u_n v_n + u_n + v_n}{2 + u_n + v_n} \\ v_{n+1} &= u_n \end{aligned}\right\}, \qquad (6\cdot 0)$$

and if y_n be the proportion of recessive ♀'s, z_n of recessive ♂'s,

$$\left.\begin{aligned} y_n &= (1 + u_n)^{-1}(1 + v_n)^{-1} \\ z_n &= (1 + u_n)^{-1} \end{aligned}\right\}, \qquad (6\cdot 1)$$

$$\therefore\ z^{-1}_{n+1} = 1 + u_{n+1} = \frac{2(1 + u_n)(1 + u_{n-1})}{2 + u_n + u_{n-1}} = \frac{2}{z_n + z_{n-1}}.$$

$$\therefore\ 2z_n = z_{n-1} + z_{n-2}.$$

Solving as usual for recurring series, we have

$$\left.\begin{aligned} 3z_n &= z_0 + 2z_1 + (-\tfrac{1}{2})^n (2z_0 - 2z_1) \\ y_n &= z_n z_{n-1} \end{aligned}\right\}, \qquad (6\cdot 2)$$

$$\left.\begin{aligned} \therefore\ z_\infty &= \tfrac{1}{3}(z_0 + 2z_1) = \tfrac{1}{3}(z_n + 2z_{n+1}) \\ y_\infty &= z_\infty^2 \end{aligned}\right\}. \qquad (6\cdot 3)$$

Hence from the proportion of males in two successive generations, or both sexes in one, we can calculate the final values. Successive values of y_n and z_n oscillate alternately above and below their final values, but converge rapidly towards them.

Bisexual selection of a sex-linked character.

If the conditions are as above, except that in each generation one dominant survives for every $(1 - k)$ recessives in each sex, then

$$\left.\begin{aligned} u_{n+1} &= \frac{2u_n v_n + u_n + v_n}{u_n + v_n + 2 - 2k} \\ v_{n+1} &= \frac{u_n}{1 - k} \end{aligned}\right\}, \qquad (7\cdot 0)$$

and

$$\left.\begin{aligned} y_n &= (1 + u_n)^{-1}(1 + v_n)^{-1} \\ z_n &= (1 + u_n)^{-1} \end{aligned}\right\}. \qquad (6\cdot 1)$$

With complete selection if $k = -\infty$, and no dominants survive to breed, selection is complete in one generation. If $k = 1$, and no recessives survive to breed,

$$u_{n+1} = 1 + 2u_n, \text{ and } v_n = \infty.$$

$$\therefore\ 1 + u_n = 2^n(1 + u_0),$$

and

$$\left.\begin{aligned} z_n &= 2^{-n} z_0 \\ y_n &= 0 \end{aligned}\right\}. \qquad (7\cdot 1)$$

So no recessive females are produced and the number of recessive males is halved in each generation. Selection is therefore vastly more effective than on an autosomal character. If colour-blind or haemophilic persons were prevented from breeding, these conditions could be almost abolished in a few generations, which is not the case with feeble-mindedness. If selection is slow we solve as for equations (4·1), and find approximately

$$v_n - u_n = \frac{2ku_n^2}{3 + 3u_n},$$

$$\Delta u_n = \frac{ku_n(3 + u_n)}{3 + 3u_n}.$$

So, reckoning generations to or from a standard population where $u_0 = 1$, and 50 °/₀ of the males and 25 °/₀ of the females are recessives,

$$kn = \log_e u_n + 2 \log_e\left(\frac{3 + u_n}{4}\right), \qquad \text{(7·2)}$$

$$\left.\begin{aligned} y_n &= (1 + u_n)^{-2} \\ z_n &= (1 + u_n)^{-1} \end{aligned}\right\}. \qquad \text{(7·3)}$$

Table III and Fig. 3 are calculated from these equations. Within the limits covered by the figure selection acts more rapidly on a sex-linked character in the homozygous sex than on an

TABLE III.

Effect of slow selection in both sexes on a sex-linked character, dominants being favoured.

°/₀ of recessives of homozygous sex	99·998	99·98	99·80	99·60	99·00	98·01
,, ,, ,, heterozygous sex	99·999	99·99	99·9	99·8	99·5	99
kn (number of generations × k) ...	− 12·09	− 9·786	− 7·481	− 6·787	− 5·866	− 5·164

96·04	90·25	81	64	49	36	25	16	10	6·25	4
9·8	95	90	80	70	60	50	40	31·62	25	20
− 4·454	− 3·485	− 2·700	− 1·802	− 1·156	− ·580	0	·619	1·282	1·910	2·506

2	1	·5	·25	·1	·01	·001	·0001	$\cdot 0_5 1$	$\cdot 0_7 1$
14·14	10	7·071	5	3·162	1	·3162	·1	·01	·001
3·441	4·394	5·366	6·353	7·679	11·07	14·50	17·95	24·86	31·76

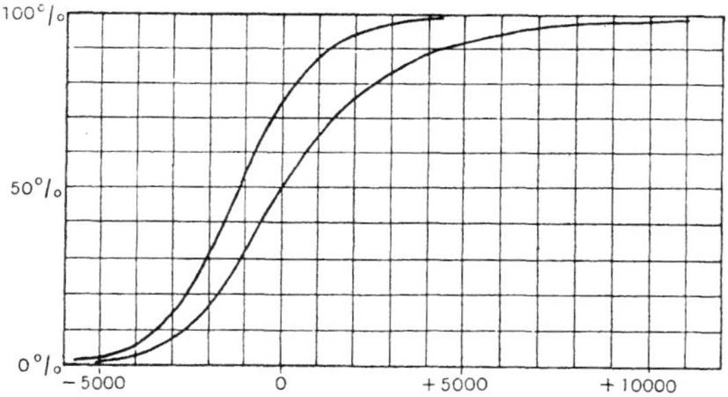

Fig. 3. Effect of selection on a sex-linked character. $k = \cdot 001$. Dominants favoured. Upper curve, homozygous sex; lower curve, heterozygous sex. Abscissa = generations. Ordinate = percentage of sex with the favoured character.

autosomal character. In the heterozygous sex selection occurs at about the same rate in the two cases. However, as appears from Table V, sex-linked recessive characters increase far more rapidly in the early stages, and sex-linked dominants in the late stages of selection, the autosomal characters.

Table III is not quite accurate unless selection is very slow, the error being of the order of k. Thus when $k = 0·2$ the error in n is nearly 10 °/₀. Still even for these large values it furnishes a useful first approximation.

BISEXUAL FAMILIAL SELECTION OF A SEX-LINKED CHARACTER.

Here we need only consider the case where the family within which selection occurs has both parents in common. Sex-linkage of the animal type is rare in plants, and families with many fathers per mother are rare in animals. Let the nth generation be

$$♀\ p_n AA : 2q_n Aa : r_n aa ; \quad ♂\ s_n A : t_n a,$$

where $p_n + 2q_n + r_n = s_n + t_n = 1$. Let the dominants have an advantage of $1 : 1 - k$ over the recessives in the mixed families. Then the $(n + 1)$th generation occurs in the following proportions, after selection has operated :

From mating	AA ♀	Aa ♀	aa ♀	A ♂	a ♂
$AA \times A$ ...	$p_n s_n$	0	0	$p_n s_n$	0
$Aa \times A$ ...	$q_n s_n$	$q_n s_n$	0	$\frac{2q_n s_n}{2-k}$	$\frac{2(1-k)q_n s_n}{2-k}$
$aa \times A$ ...	0	$r_n s_n$	0	0	$r_n s_n$
$AA \times a$ ...	0	$p_n t_n$	0	$p_n t_n$	0
$Aa \times a$ ...	0	$\frac{2q_n t_n}{2-k}$	$\frac{2(1-k)q_n t_n}{2-k}$	$\frac{2q_n t_n}{2-k}$	$\frac{2(1-k)q_n t_n}{2-k}$
$aa \times a$ ...	0	0	$r_n t_n$	0	$r_n t_n$

Hence, writing $k' = \frac{k}{2-k}$,

$$\left.\begin{aligned} p_{n+1} &= (p_n + q_n) s_n \\ 2q_{n+1} &= (p_n + q_n) t_n + (q_n + r_n) s_n + k' q_n t_n \\ r_{n+1} &= (q_n + r_n) t_n - k' q_n t_n \\ s_{n+1} &= p_n + q_n + k' q_n \\ t_{n+1} &= q_n + r_n - k' q_n \end{aligned}\right\} \quad \text{......................(8·0)}$$

With complete selection, when the recessives are eliminated, $k' = k = 1$, and

$$r_{n+1} = r_n t_n,$$
$$t_{n+1} = r_n,$$
$$\therefore\ r_n = r_0^{\phi(n+1)} t_0^{\phi(n)},$$

where
$$\phi(n) = \frac{2^{-n}}{\sqrt{5}} [(1 + \sqrt{5})^n - (1 - \sqrt{5})^n], \quad \text{..........................(8·1)}$$

i.e. $\phi(n)$ is the nth term of Fibonnacci's series 1, 2, 3, 5, 8, 13, 21, etc. So the recessives disappear very fast. When dominants are eliminated $k' = -1$, $k = -\infty$, and the equations are less tractable. The percentages of recessives in succeeding generations, starting from a standard population, are :

♀	25	37·5	56·25	66·80	82·97	etc.
♂	50	75	75	89·06	93·16	etc.

When k is small we solve as in equations (3·0), and find

$$\Delta u_n = \frac{k'u(2 + u)}{3 + 3u} \text{ approximately.}$$

$$\left.\begin{aligned} \therefore\ kn &= 3\log_e\left[\frac{u_n(2+u_n)}{3}\right] \\ r_n &= (1+u_n)^{-2} \\ t_n &= (1+u_n)^{-1} \end{aligned}\right\}, \qquad (8{\cdot}2)$$

starting from the standard population, and p_n, q_n have very nearly the values for a population in equilibrium. Selection therefore proceeds much as in racial selection but at from a half to a third of the rate. Some figures are given in Table V.

SELECTION OF A SEX-LINKED CHARACTER IN THE HOMOZYGOUS SEX ONLY.

Several sex-linked factors are known which have a much more marked effect on the homozygous than the heterozygous sex. Thus in *Drosophila melanogaster* "fused" females are sterile, males fertile; whilst the character "dot" occurs in 8 °/₀ of the genetically recessive females, but only 0·8 °/₀ of the males. [Morgan and Bridges (18).] But the chief evolutionary importance of this type of selection must have been in the Hymenoptera and other groups where the males are haploid and all amphimictic inheritance sex-linked. The characters of the diploid females and neuters are generally more important (especially in the social species) than those of the males. On the other hand it must be remembered that for a few drone characters selection must be very intense, and largely familial. Using the usual notation

$$\left.\begin{aligned} u_{n+1} &= \frac{2u_n v_n + u_n + v_n}{u_n + v_n + 2 - 2k} \\ v_{n+1} &= u_n \end{aligned}\right\}. \qquad (9{\cdot}0)$$

With complete selection, if all dominants are eliminated and $k = -\infty$, all dominants disappear in two generations. If all recessives are eliminated $k = 1$, and starting with a standard population the percentages of recessives in successive generations are:

♂ (heterozygous sex)	50	33·3	30	23·2	21·4	18·6
♀ (homozygous sex)	25	16·7	10	6·96	5·14	3·95

So elimination is vastly slower than when selection occurs in both sexes (equation (7·1)). When k is small we solve as in (7·0), and find

$$3\Delta u_n = \frac{2ku_n}{1+u_n} \text{ approximately.}$$

$$\therefore\ \tfrac{2}{3}kn = u_n + \log_e u_n - 1, \qquad (9{\cdot}1)$$

$$\left.\begin{aligned} y_n &= (1+u_n)^{-2} \\ z_n &= (1+u_n)^{-1} \end{aligned}\right\}. \qquad (7{\cdot}3)$$

So selection of the homozygotes proceeds as in Fig. 2 and Tables I and II, but 1·5 times as many generations are needed for a given change. The heterozygous sex changes rather more slowly.

SELECTION OF A SEX-LINKED CHARACTER IN THE HETEROZYGOUS SEX ONLY.

In certain cases sex-linked factors appear only or mainly in the heterozygous sex. Thus in *Drosophila melanogaster* "eosin" eye-colour is far more marked in the male than the female, and the sex-linked fertility factor L_2 postulated by Pearl (19) in poultry can only show in the female sex. If selection is limited to the heterozygous sex,

$$\left.\begin{aligned} u_{n+1} &= \frac{2u_n v_n + u_n + v_n}{u_n + v_n + 2} \\ v_{n+1} &= \frac{u_n}{1-k} \end{aligned}\right\}. \qquad (10{\cdot}0)$$

With complete selection, if all dominants are eliminated, $k = -\infty$, and

$$u_{n+1} = \frac{u_n}{2 + u_n} \text{ (after the second generation)},$$

$$v_n = 0.$$

$$\therefore u_n = \left[2^{n-1}\left(1 + \frac{1}{u_1}\right) - 1\right]^{-1}, \text{ but } u_1 = u_0;$$

$$\therefore y_n = z_n = 1 - 2^{1-n} z_0. \quad \text{.......} (10 \cdot 1)$$

So the number of dominants is halved in each generation after the second. If recessives are eliminated, $k = 1$, and

$$u_{n+1} = 1 + 2u_n \text{ (after the second generation)},$$

$$v_{n+1} = \infty.$$

$$\therefore u_n = 2^{n-1}(1 + u_1) - 1;$$

$$\left.\begin{array}{l} \therefore y_n = 0 \\ \quad z_n = 2^{1-n} z_0 \end{array}\right\}, \quad \text{.......} (10 \cdot 2)$$

the proportion of recessives being halved in each generation. If selection is slow

$$\Delta u_n = \tfrac{1}{3} k u_n \text{ approximately};$$

$$\therefore kn = 3 \log u_n \quad \text{.......} (10 \cdot 3)$$

if $u_0 = 1$; and y_n, z_n are given by equations (7·3). Hence selection in the heterozygous sex proceeds as in Fig. 1, but at one-third of the pace, whilst selection in the homozygous sex is slightly faster.

Certation, or gametic selection of an autosomal character.

The work of Renner (6) and Heribert-Nilsson (20) shows that gametes or gametophytes may be selected according to what factors they carry. The field of such selection may be wide, as in wind pollination, but is more often restricted, and mainly familial, i.e. among the gametes of the same individual. Except in homosporous plants the intensity must be different in gametes of different genders, and we shall here only consider the case where one is affected. Let the nth generation be formed from gametes carrying $u_n A : 1a$, this proportion being reduced by selection in one gender to $u_n A : (1 - k) a$, the selection being general and not familial. Then the nth generation will be $u_n^2 AA : (2 - k) u_n Aa : (1 - k) aa$.

$$\therefore u_{n+1} = \frac{u_n (2u_n + 2 - k)}{(2 - k) u_n + 2 - 2k}. \quad \text{.......} (11 \cdot 0)$$

With complete selection, if all dominant-carrying gametes are eliminated, $k = -\infty$, and

$$u_{n+1} = \frac{u_n}{2 + u_n};$$

$$\therefore y_n = \frac{1}{1 + u_n} = 1 - 2^{1-n}(1 - y_1). \quad \text{.......} (11 \cdot 1)$$

So the proportion of dominants is halved in each generation. If recessive-carriers are eliminated, no recessive zygotes appear, and the proportion of heterozygotes is halved in each generation. If selection is slow,

$$\Delta u_n = \tfrac{1}{2} k u_n \text{ approximately};$$

$$\therefore kn = 2 \log_e u_n, \quad \text{.......} (11 \cdot 2)$$

$$y_n = (1 + u_n)^{-2}. \quad \text{.......} (2 \cdot 0)$$

If the gametes are replaced in heterozygous organisms, as must happen in a large batch of pollen-grains or spermatozoa from the same source, let the nth zygotic generation be formed from unselected gametes (say megagametes) $u_n A : 1a$, and selected gametes (say microgametes) $v_n A : 1a$, so its proportions are $u_n v_n AA : (u_n + v_n) Aa : 1aa$.

$$\left.\begin{aligned} \therefore\ u_{n+1} &= \frac{2u_n v_n + u_n + v_n}{u_n + v_n + 2} \\ v_{n+1} &= \frac{2u_n v_n + u_n + v_n + k'(u_n + v_n)}{u_n + v_n + 2 - k'(u_n + v_n)} \end{aligned}\right\}, \quad \text{.........(11·3)}$$

where $k' = \frac{k}{2-k}$, as in equation (8·0). With complete selection (when for example there is a very great disparity between growth-rates of pollen-tubes, though both types are viable), if dominant gametes are eliminated, $k' = -1$, and the percentages of recessive zygotes in successive generations, starting from a standard population, are:

25, 37·5, 54·69, 71·48, 84·16, 91·83, etc.

If recessive gametes are eliminated, $k' = 1$, and the percentages of recessive zygotes in successive generations are:

25, 12·5, 4·56, 1·14, 0·17, ·014, etc.

When selection is slow, $\Delta = \frac{1}{4} k u_n$ approximately.

$$\therefore\ kn = 4 \log_e u_n \quad \text{.........(11·4)}$$

if $u_0 = 1$, so selection proceeds at half the rate given by equation (11·2), y_n being given by (2·0).

Gametic selection of a sex-linked character.

This is not known to occur, and at all complete gametic selection is very unlikely in animals, so we need only consider slow selection. Let selection occur among the gametes of the homozygous sex, with no replacement within heterozygous organisms. Let the nth generation be formed from eggs in the ratio $u_n A : 1a$ before, or $u_n A : (1-k) a$ after selection, and ♀-producing spermatozoa in the ratio $v_n A : 1a$. Then the nth generation is

♀ $u_n v_n AA : (u_n + v_n - kv_n) Aa : (1-k) aa$; ♂ $u_n A : (1-k) a$.

$$\left.\begin{aligned} \therefore\ u_{n+1} &= \frac{2u_n v_n + u_n + v_n - kv_n}{u_n + v_n + 2 - kv_n - 2k} \\ v_{n+1} &= \frac{u_n}{1-k} \end{aligned}\right\}; \quad \text{.........(12·0)}$$

$$\therefore\ \Delta u_n = \tfrac{2}{3} k u_n \text{ approximately.}$$

$$\therefore\ \tfrac{2}{3} kn = \log_e u_n, \quad \text{.........(12·1)}$$

whilst y_n and z_n are given by equation (7·3), so selection proceeds twice as fast as in equation (10·3). In the more important case of familial selection (replacement in heterozygous individuals), if $k' = \frac{k}{2-k}$, then

$$\left.\begin{aligned} u_{n+1} &= \frac{2u_n v_n + u_n + v_n + k'(u_n + v_n)}{u_n + v_n + 2 - k'(u_n + v_n)} \\ v_{n+1} &= u_n \end{aligned}\right\}, \quad \text{.........(12·2)}$$

u_n being here the gametic ratio after selection.

$$\therefore\ \Delta u_n = \tfrac{2}{3} k' u_n = \tfrac{1}{3} k' v_n;$$

$$\therefore\ \tfrac{1}{3} kn = \log_e u_n, \quad \text{.........(12·3)}$$

so selection proceeds as in equation (10·3).

If selection occurs among the gametes of the heterozygous sex there is clearly no effect if they are replaced, whilst otherwise the effects are the same as those of zygotic selection, and are given by equation (10·3).

Comparative results of complete (artificial) selection.

The results of complete selection in the more important cases are summarized in Table IV. In every case the field of selection considered is the whole population. Complete familial selection occasionally occurs through natural causes, but never through human agency. Column 3 gives the sex to which the numbers in columns 4 and 5 refer. Selection is supposed to begin on

TABLE IV.

Effects of complete selection.

Character eliminated	Type of selection	Sex	% after 5 generations from 50 %	% after 10 generations from 50 %	Equation
Non-amphimictic ...	Any	Both	0	0	—
Autosomal dominant	Bisexual	,, ...	0	0	—
,, recessive	,, ...	,, ...	2·44	0·768	2·2
,, dominant	Unisexual... ...	,, ...	1·83	0·0572	4·2
,, recessive	,, ...	,, ...	8·88	3·27	—
Sex-linked dominant	Bisexual	Homozygous	0	0	—
		Heterozygous	0	0	—
,, recessive	,, ...	Homozygous	0	0	7·1
		Heterozygous	1·56	0·0484	7·1
,, dominant	In homozygous sex	Homozygous	0	0	—
		Heterozygous	0	0	—
,, recessive	,, ,, ,,	Homozygous	5·34	1·74	—
		Heterozygous	18·5	13·28	—
,, dominant	In heterozygous sex	Homozygous	1·83	0·0572	10·1
		Heterozygous	3·125	0·0977	10·1
,, recessive	,, ,, ,,	Homozygous	0	0	—
		Heterozygous	3·125	0·0977	10·2
Autosomal dominant	Gametic unisexual	Both	1·83	0·0572	11·1
,, recessive	,, ,, ,,	,, ...	0	0	—

a population in equilibrium containing equal numbers of dominants and recessives of the sex considered. It is worth noting that in the case of sex-linked characters, and autosomal recessives when selection is gametic, individuals of types which have wholly disappeared reappear if selection ceases. With many types of heredity dominants are eliminated in one or two generations, and where this is not the case they generally decrease more rapidly than recessives.

Applications to slow selection.

With the exception of (1·1) the equations found for the rate of slow selection are not rigorously accurate. n is in general a higher transcendental function of u, but of what nature is not clear. It will be shown later that the finite difference equations found in this paper are special cases of integral equations which may possibly prove more tractable. The values for kn found in terms of u all have inexactitudes of the order k^2n. Thus if one type has an advantage of 1 %, the number of generations required for a given change can also be found within about 1 %.

5—2

Table V shows the effect of slow selection in the various cases considered. The third column gives the sex to which the subsequent figures apply. Selection is throughout supposed to give the favoured type an advantage of $\frac{1}{1000}$, i.e. 1000 of this type survive for 999 of the other. If the advantage is $\frac{1}{100}$, one-tenth of the number of generations is required for a given change, and so on, but when selection is very rapid the numbers are somewhat inaccurate.

It will at once be seen that selection is most rapid when amphimixis is avoided by any of the means cited above. Moreover selection is ineffective on recessive characters when these are rare, except in the case of sex-linked factors, when selection is effective in the heterozygous sex, and in gametic selection. It seems therefore very doubtful whether natural selection in random-mating

TABLE V.

Generations required for a given change with various types of slow selection. $k = \cdot 001$.

Dominant factor favoured	Type of selection	Sex	·001—1 %	1—50 %	50—99 %	99—99·999 %	Equations
Non-amphimictic	Bisexual racial	Both ...	6,921	4,592	4,592	6,921	1·1
Autosomal ...	,, ,,	,, ...	6,920	4,819	11,664	309,780	2·0, 2·4
,, ...	Unisexual racial / Bisexual familial	,, ...	13,841	9,638	23,328	619,560	2·0, 3·2, 4·3
,, ...	,, familial*	,, ...	9,227	6,425	15,522	413,040	2·0, 3·3
,, † ...	,, racial	♂	13,831	8,819	6,157	7,112	2·0, 5·3
Sex-linked ...	,, ,,	Homozygous	6,916	4,668	5,593	10,106	7·2, 7·3
		Heterozygous	6,928	5,164	11,070	20,693	
,, ...	,, familial	Homozygous	20,753	13,785	13,785	20,753	8·2
		Heterozygous	20,768	14,987	24,332	41,450	
,, ...	Racial of homozygous sex	Homozygous	10,380	7,228	17,496	464,670	7·3, 9·1
		Heterozygous	10,392	8,378	153,893	149,860,377	
,, ...	Racial of heterozygous sex	Homozygous	20,746	13,228	9,236	10,668	7·3, 10·3
		Heterozygous	20,753	13,785	13,785	20,753	
Autosomal ...	Unisexual gametic	Both ...	13,831	8,819	6,157	7,112	2·0, 11·2
,, ...	,, ,, ‡	,, ...	27,661	17,638	12,314	14,224	2·0, 11·4
Sex-linked ...	Gametic of homozygous sex	Homozygous	10,373	6,619	4,618	5,334	7·3, 12·1
		Heterozygous	10,377	6,892	6,892	10,377	
,, ...	Gametic of homozygous sex‡	Homozygous	20,746	13,228	9,236	10,668	7·3, 12·3
		Heterozygous	20,753	13,785	13,785	20,753	

* The families have only one parent in common.

† Dominant in ♂, recessive in ♀.

‡ In heterozygous individuals gametes are replaced (as zygotes in familial selection).

The effect of selection on recessive characters may be found by inverting the order of the four numerical columns. Thus 309,780 generations are needed for an autosomal recessive to increase from ·001 % to 1 %, 11,664 generations to increase from 1 % to 50 %, and so on.

organisms can cause the spread of autosomal recessive characters unless they are extraordinarily valuable to their possessors. Such characters appear far more frequently than dominant mutations, but in their early stages are selected infinitely more slowly. It is thus intelligible that none of the melanic varieties of Lepidoptera which are known to have spread should be recessive.

There are at least four ways out of this impasse:

A. In a species which adopts self-fertilization or very close inbreeding advantageous autosomal recessive characters can spread rapidly. Thus supposing that in each of two otherwise similar species, one of which is mainly self-fertilizing, an advantageous recessive mutation occurs, it will spread far more quickly in the self-fertilizing species, and this species will tend to replace the other. This fact may well account for the widespread presence of self-fertilization and close inbreeding, in spite of the fact that they seem often to be physiologically harmful, and must certainly check the combination of useful variations which have arisen independently.

B. Recessives may be helped to spread by assortative fertilization. This may take place in the following ways:

1. Psychological isolation. Thus Pearson and Lee (21) have shown that a tall man is more likely to marry a tall woman than a short woman if presented with equal numbers of each. Of course the recessives must not be so repulsive to the dominants as to escape mating altogether at first. In plants psychological isolation may be due to the psychology of the insect or other pollinating organism. Thus a mutant plant with a new colour, scent, or shape may be isolated because it attracts a different insect from the type plant.

2. Anatomical isolation. Pearl (22) and Crozier and Snyder (23) have shown that in *Paramoecium* and *Gammarus* there is a strong tendency for organisms of like size to mate. This will be effective provided mutations are not so great as to leave the first mutants unmated.

3. Temporal isolation. If the recessive factor causes (or is very closely coupled with a factor causing) a change in the breeding or flowering time, this will serve as an effective barrier against crossing.

4. Spatial isolation. If the recessive has a different habitat, e.g. a different range of soil or temperature conditions to which it is adapted, some of its individuals will be spatially isolated from the dominants.

5. Selective fertilization. If the results of Jones (24) are due to this cause, as seems almost certain, we have here a *vera causa*, though it must be remembered that he did not work with single factor-differences. He found that when either of two races of maize is fertilized with a mixture of pollen the proportion of hybrids was less than was to be expected from random fertilization. This does not seem to have been due to inviability of the hybrids, which were more vigorous and fertile than the parent races. Clearly if the hybrid zygotes are inviable or sterile the rarer form of the species will be weeded out whether it is dominant or recessive, weak or vigorous. But if there is selective fertilization due for example to increased activity of pollen-tubes in tissue of the type which produced them, the increase of the rare form, especially if it is recessive, will be facilitated.

All these types of isolation, then, will favour the replacement of a type species by a recessive mutant. May it not be that in many cases mutual infertility is the cause and not the effect of specific differences? A new mutant form arises within a species. If it crosses freely with the type we call it a variety, and a moderately advantageous recessive variety will only spread very slowly indeed. But if it does not cross freely we call it a new species, and it is much more likely to establish itself. Possibly then interspecific sterility is partly to be explained by its having a selective value.

C. The increase of recessives is greatly facilitated, as will be shown later, by incomplete dominance. Thus if there is only one recessive in a million, and the recessives have an advantage of ·001, their rate of increase will be speeded up elevenfold if the heterozygotes have an advantage of ·00001 over the pure dominants.

D. If heterozygotes have any advantage *as such* this will tend to favour any new factors so long as they are rare. But no "stimulus of heterozygosis" has yet been demonstrated in cases of single factor-differences.

Whether the isolation of small communities, or what comes to much the same thing, great immobility of individuals at all stages of their lives, will help or hinder the spread of a new recessive type in the species as a whole is a nice question. It will certainly slow the spread of a dominant.

At first sight the selection of dominant factors would not seem to be a probable cause of the origin of species rather than new varieties. But it must be remembered that dominant mutations are very often lethal in the homozygous condition. Under certain circumstances, to be discussed later, their selection may lead to the establishment of a system of balanced lethals, and a probable change in the chronosome number.

The theory so far developed gives a quantitative account of the spread of a new advantageous type within a population under certain simple conditions, and demonstrates that inbreeding, homogamy, and inter-varietal sterility may sometimes be of selective value, and therefore preserved by natural selection. It is proposed in later papers to discuss the selection of semi-dominant, multiple, linked, and lethal factors, partial inbreeding and homogamy, overlapping generations, and other complications.

SUMMARY.

Mathematical expressions are found for the effect of selection on simple Mendelian populations mating at random. Selection of a given intensity is most effective when amphimixis does not affect the character selected, e.g. in complete inbreeding or homogamy. Selection is very ineffective on autosomal recessive characters so long as they are rare.

REFERENCES.

1. PEARSON. *Proc. Roy. Soc.* 54—72.
2. WARREN. *Genetics*, 2, p. 305, 1917.
3. PUNNETT. *Mimicry in Butterflies*, p. 154.
4. IBSEN and STEIGLEDER. *Am. Nat.* 51, p. 740, 1917.
5. DURHAM. *Journ. Genetics*, 1, p. 107, 1911.
6. RENNER. *Zeit. Ind. Abst. u. Ver.* 18, p. 121, 1917.
7. SCHMIDT. *Comptes rendus trav. Lab. Carlsberg*, 14, 1920.
8. GOLDSCHMIDT. *Zeit. Ind. Abst. u. Ver.* 23, p. 1, 1920.
9. PEARSON. *Phil. Trans. Roy. Soc.* A, 203, p. 53, 1904.
10. HARDY. *Science*, 28, p. 49, 1908.
11. PUNNETT. *Journ. Hered.* 8, p. 464, 1917.
12. DETLEFSEN. *Genetics*, 3, p. 573, 1918.
13. BARRETT. *Lepidoptera of the British Islands*, 7, p. 130.
14. BATE. *Ent. Rec.* 1895, p. 27.
15. BATESON. *Mendel's Principles of Heredity*, p. 221.
16. WOOD. *Journ. Agric. Science*, 1, p. 364.
17. JENNINGS. *Genetics*, 1, p. 53, 1915.
18. MORGAN and BRIDGES. *Carn. Inst. Wash. Pub.* 237, 1916.
19. PEARL. *Am. Nat.* 46, p. 130.
20. HERIBERT-NILSSON. *Hereditas*, 1, p. 41, 1920.
21. PEARSON and LEE. *Biometrika*, 2, p. 371, 1903.
22. PEARL. *Biometrika*, 5, p. 213, 1907.
23. CROZIER and SNYDER. *Proc. Soc. Exp. Biol. & Med.* 19, p. 327, 1922.
24. JONES. *Biol. Bull.* 38, p. 251, 1920.

A mathematical theory of Natural and Artificial Selection. Part IV. By Mr J. B. S. HALDANE, Trinity College.

[*Received* 11 November, *read* 22 November 1926.]

In such organisms as annual plants, in which successive generations do not overlap, the composition of the $n+1$th generation can be calculated from that of the nth, and the resulting finite difference equation investigated. Where generations overlap we may obtain a similar relation between the compositions of the population at times t and t', but the finite difference equation is now represented by an integral equation. This fact was first pointed out in 1910 by Mr H. T. J. Norton of Trinity College. At a much later date I arrived at the same conclusion, and Mr Norton showed me his results in 1922, stating that he would publish them shortly. He has been prevented from doing so by illness, and, although I believe that all the results here given were reached by me independently, there can be no question that Mr Norton had obtained many of them previously, and had treated the problem rigorously, which I have not done.

The only case considered here is the very simple one in which the intensity of selection is independent of the size of the population. A preliminary lemma will first be discussed.

The growth of a population.

If the death-rate and birth-rate of a population are not functions of its density, its number at any time may be calculated as follows:

Let $N(t)$ be the number at time t. Only the female sex need be considered if the sexes are separate.

$S(x)$ be the probability of an individual surviving to the age x.

$U(t)\,\delta t$ be the number of individuals produced between times t and $t+\delta t$.

$K(x)\,\delta x$ be the probability of an individual between the ages x and $x+\delta x$ producing one (female) offspring. All individuals of this age, both alive and dead, are considered, so that if $P(x)$ be the corresponding function for living individuals only, $K(x)=S(x)\,P(x)$. Then

$$\left.\begin{aligned} N(t) &= \int_0^t U(t-x)\,S(x)\,dx \\ U(t) &= \int_0^x U(t-x)\,K(x)\,dx \end{aligned}\right\} \qquad (1\cdot 0).$$

Instead of infinity any upper limit exceeding the maximum life of the organism may be taken. Equation (1·0) has been considered by Herglotz*. Let $U(t) = ce^{zt}$. Then

$$\int_0^\infty e^{-zx} K(x)\,dx = 1, \text{ or } \int_0^a e^{-zx} K(x) = 1 \quad \ldots\ldots\ldots (1 \cdot 1),$$

where a is sufficiently large. Since $K(x)$ is always real and zero or positive, the above integral is a monotone function of z when z is real, and can have any real positive value. Hence it has one and only one real root for z, say α_0. The complex roots clearly occur in pairs $\alpha_r \pm i\beta_r$. Then

$$\int_0^\infty e^{-\alpha_r x} K(x)\,dx > \int_0^\infty e^{-(\alpha_r + i\beta_r)x} K(x)\,dx$$
$$= 1.$$

Therefore $$\alpha_r < \alpha_0.$$

If any two functions of t are solutions of (1·0) so is their sum. Therefore

$$\left.\begin{aligned} U(t) &= a_0 e^{\alpha_0 t} + \sum_{r=1}^{\infty} a_r e^{\alpha_r t} \cos \beta_r (t - b_r) \\ N(t) &= c_0 e^{\alpha_0 t} + \sum_{r=1}^{\infty} c_r e^{\alpha_r t} \cos \beta_r (t - d_r) \end{aligned}\right\} \quad \ldots\ldots (1 \cdot 2).$$

In general there will be an infinite number of terms. The values of a_r and b_r, and hence of c_r and d_r, depend on the initial conditions. Where multiple roots occur there will be periodic terms including powers of t as factors. Since $\alpha_r < \alpha_0$, all the periodic terms become negligible compared with the first after the lapse of a sufficient time. That is to say, oscillations of the population about an exponential function of the time are either damped or at least increase less rapidly than the population itself. In particular, if $\int_0^\infty K(x)\,dx = 1$, so that the population is in equilibrium, oscillations are damped and the equilibrium is stable. We are therefore justified in neglecting periodic terms in the solution of equations which only differ by small terms from (1·0), and which occur in the subsequent analysis. It is proposed to discuss the stability of the equilibrium when $S(x)$ and $K(x)$ depend on the number of the population in a subsequent paper.

Incidentally, if $C(x)\,\delta x$ be the probability of any member of the population being between the ages x and $x + \delta x$, then

$$C(x) = \frac{U(t-x)\,S(x)}{N(t)}.$$

* Herglotz, *Math. Ann.* 65, p. 87.

Hence, when oscillations have died down

$$C(x) = \frac{e^{-\alpha_0 x} S(x)}{\int_0^x \epsilon^{-\alpha_0 x} S(x)\, dx}$$

This constitutes a new proof of Lotka's* theorem on the stability of the normal age distribution.

Selection of an autosomal factor.

Consider a population consisting, at time t, of $D(t)$ female zygotes possessing a dominant factor A, $R(t)$ female recessives. The sex-ratio at birth is taken as fixed.

Let $F(t)\,\delta t$ be the number of fertile A ova produced between times t and $t+\delta t$.

$f(t)\,\delta t$ be the number of fertile a ova produced between times t and $t+\delta t$.

$M(t)\,\delta t$ be the number of A spermatozoa produced between times t and $t+\delta t$.

$m(t)\,\delta t$ be the number of a spermatozoa produced between times t and $t+\delta t$.

$S(x)$ be the probability of a female dominant reaching the age x.

$s(x)$ be the probability of a female recessive reaching the age x.

$K(x)\,\delta x$ be the probability of a female dominant (alive or dead, as above) producing a female offspring between the ages x and $x+\delta x$.

$[K(x)-k(x)]\,\delta x$ be the same probability for a female recessive.

$L(x)\,\delta x$ be the same probability for a male dominant.

$[L(x)-l(x)]\,\delta x$ be the same probability for a male recessive.

$$S = \int_0^x S(x)\,dx, \quad s = \int_0^x s(x)\,dx$$

$$K = \int_0^x K(x)\,dx, \quad K' = \int_0^x xK(x)\,dx, \quad k = \int_0^x k(x)\,dx.$$

$$L = \int_0^x L(x)\,dx, \quad L' = \int_0^x xL(x)\,dx, \quad l = \int_0^x l(x)\,dx.$$

In general the functions $S(x)$, $s(x)$, $K(x)$, etc., will not be functions of age alone, but of $D(t)$, $R(t)$, etc. We make the assumption however that selection and population growth are proceeding so slowly that $k(x)$ and $l(x)$, and $K-1$ are small, and $S(x)$, etc., do not vary appreciably in the course of a generation.

* Lotka, *Proc. Nat. Ac. Sci.* 8, p. 339, 1922.

If mating be at random, the rates of production of the three female phenotypes at time t are

$$AA,\ \frac{F(t)\,M(t)}{M(t)+m(t)};\quad Aa,\ \frac{F(t)\,m(t)+f(t)\,M(t)}{M(t)+m(t)};\quad aa,\ \frac{f(t)\,m(t)}{M(t)+m(t)}.$$

The group aged x at time t was hatched or born at time $t-x$. Therefore

$$\left.\begin{aligned}
F(t) &= \tfrac{1}{2}\int_0^t \frac{2F(t-x)\,M(t-x)+F(t-x)\,m(t-x)+f(t-x)\,M(t-x)}{M(t-x)+m(t-x)}\,K(x)\,dx\\
f(t) &= \tfrac{1}{2}\int_0^t \frac{F(t-x)\,m(t-x)+f(t-x)\,M(t-x)+2f(t-x)\,m(t-x)}{M(t-x)+m(t-x)}\,K(x)\,dx\\
&\qquad -\int_0^t \frac{f(t-x)\,m(t-x)\,k(x)\,dx}{M(t-x)+m(t-x)}\\
M(t) &= \tfrac{1}{2}\int_0^t \frac{2F(t-x)\,M(t-x)+F(t-x)\,m(t-x)+f(t-x)\,M(t-x)}{M(t-x)+m(t-x)}\,L(x)\,dx\\
m(t) &= \tfrac{1}{2}\int_0^t \frac{F(t-x)\,m(t-x)+f(t-x)\,M(t-x)+2f(t-x)\,m(t-x)}{M(t-x)+m(t-x)}\,L(x)\,dx\\
&\qquad -\int_0^t \frac{f(t-x)\,m(t-x)\,l(x)\,dx}{M(t-x)+m(t-x)}
\end{aligned}\right\}\quad\ldots(2\cdot0).$$

Since selection and population growth are slow, we may put $F(t-x)=F(t)-xF'(t)$, etc., $M(t)=\lambda F(t)$, $m(t)=\lambda f(t)$, all to the first order of small quantities. Hence, to this degree of approximation,

$$\begin{aligned}
F(t) &= \tfrac{1}{2}KF(t)+\frac{\tfrac{1}{2}K[F(t)+f(t)]\,M(t)}{M(t)+m(t)}-\tfrac{1}{2}K'F'(t)-\frac{\tfrac{1}{2}K'[F'(t)+f'(t)]\,M(t)}{M(t)+m(t)}\\
&\qquad -\frac{\tfrac{1}{2}K'[F(t)+f(t)]\,[M'(t)\,m(t)-M(t)\,m'(t)]}{[M(t)+m(t)]^2}\\
&= \tfrac{1}{2}KF(t)+\frac{\tfrac{1}{2}K[F(t)+f(t)]\,M(t)}{M(t)+m(t)}-K'F'(t).
\end{aligned}$$

Similarly

$$f(t)=\tfrac{1}{2}Kf(t)+\frac{\tfrac{1}{2}K[F(t)+f(t)]\,m(t)}{M(t)+m(t)}-K'f'(t)-\frac{k[f(t)]^2}{F(t)+f(t)}$$

$$M(t)=\tfrac{1}{2}LF(t)+\frac{\tfrac{1}{2}L[F(t)+f(t)]\,M(t)}{M(t)+m(t)}-L'F'(t)$$

$$m(t)=\tfrac{1}{2}Lf(t)+\frac{\tfrac{1}{2}L[F(t)+f(t)]\,m(t)}{M(t)+m(t)}-L'f'(t)-\frac{l[f(t)]^2}{F(t)+f(t)}$$

all approximately. Therefore

$$\begin{aligned}
\frac{M(t)}{m(t)} &= \frac{\left[2LF(t)-Lf(t)-2L'F'(t)\right]\dfrac{M(t)}{m(t)}-LF(t)-2L'F'(t)}{\left[LF(t)-2L'f'(t)-\dfrac{2l[f(t)]^2}{F(t)+f(t)}\right]\dfrac{M(t)}{m(t)}+LF(t)-2Lf(t)-2L'f'(t)-\dfrac{2l[f(t)]^2}{F(t)+f(t)}}\\
&= \frac{L[2F(t)-f(t)]\dfrac{M(t)}{m(t)}-LF(t)-\dfrac{2L'F'(t)[F(t)-f(t)]}{f(t)}}{Lf(t)\dfrac{M(t)}{m(t)}-LF(t)-2Lf(t)-\dfrac{2L'f'(t)[F(t)+f(t)]}{f(t)}-2lf(t)}
\end{aligned}$$

approximately.

$$\frac{F(t)}{f(t)} = \frac{2L'[F(t)f'(t) - F'(t)f(t)]}{L[F(t)+f(t)]} + \frac{lF(t)[f(t)]^2}{L[F(t)+f(t)]^2}$$

approximately, by solving the quadratic. Therefore

$$(K-1)F(t) - K'F'(t) - \frac{L'[F(t)f'(t) - F'(t)f(t)]}{L[F(t)+f(t)]} + \frac{lF(t)[f(t)]^2}{L[F(t)+f(t)]^2} = 0$$

$$(K-1)f(t) - K'f'(t) + \frac{L'[F(t)f'(t) - F'(t)f(t)]}{L[F(t)+f(t)]} - \frac{lF(t)[f(t)]^2}{L[F(t)+f(t)]^2} - \frac{k[f(t)]^2}{F(t)+f(t)} = 0 \quad \text{......(2·1).}$$

If $$u(t) = F(t)/f(t),$$

$$\frac{d}{dt}u(t) = \frac{(l+kL)\,u(t)}{(L'+K'L)[1+u(t)]} \quad \text{............(2·2).}$$

This is equivalent to equation (2·1) of Part I*, $\frac{l+kL}{L'+K'L}$ being the coefficient of selection. In general this quantity is not independent of t, hence the equation cannot be integrated, but if its upper and lower limits are known, the march of the composition of the population can be roughly calculated from equation (2·3) of Part I. If, however, the population is very nearly in equilibrium, and either dominants or recessives are very rare, more accurate results are possible.

When recessives are rare, $F(x)$ is large and equal to a constant F, $D(x)$ being also large and equal to a constant N. $K = 1$, and $F'(t)$ is negligible, while $f(t)$ is small. Therefore

$$K'f''(t) + \frac{L'}{L}f'(t) + \left(\frac{l+kL}{L}\right)\frac{[f(t)]^2}{F} = 0,$$

and $$f(t) = \frac{(L'+K'L)F}{(l+kL)(t-t_0)},$$

where t_0 is an integration constant. But

$$N = D(t) = \int_0^\infty F(t-x)\,S(x)\,dx = FS.$$

$$R(t) = \int_0^\infty \frac{[f(t-x)]^2\,s(x)\,dx}{F(t-x)+f(t-x)} = \frac{(L'+K'L)^2 Fs}{(l+kL)^2(t-t_0)^2}.$$

$$R(t) = \frac{(L'+K'L)^2 sN}{(l+kL)^2 S(t-t_0)^2} \quad \text{..............(2·3).}$$

Hence selection proceeds at the same rate as when generations are separate with a selection coefficient equal to

$$\left(\frac{l+kL}{L'+K'L}\right)\left(\frac{S}{s}\right)^{\frac{1}{2}}.$$

* Haldane, *Trans. Camb. Phil. Soc.* 23, p. 19, 1924

When dominants are rare, $f(x)$ is large and equal to a constant l, $K = 1 + k$, and $F(x)$ is small. Therefore

$$\left(k + \frac{l}{L}\right) F(t) + \left(K' + \frac{L'}{L}\right) F'(t) = 0,$$

$$F(t) = e^{\frac{(l + kL)(c - t)}{L' + K'L}},$$

where c is a constant of integration. Therefore

$$D(t) = \int_0^\infty 2F(t - x)\, S(x)\, dx = 2SF(t)$$

$$= e^{\frac{(l + kL)(t_0 - t)}{L' + K'L}} \qquad \ldots\ldots\ldots\ldots\ldots\ldots\ldots\ldots\ldots\ldots (2\cdot4),$$

where t_0 is an arbitrary constant. Selection therefore proceeds as when generations are separate, but with a selection coefficient

$$\frac{l + kL}{L' + K'L}.$$

When the death rates and fertility rates are the same in the two sexes, or in a hermaphrodite species, we have in general,

$$\frac{d}{dt} u(t) = \frac{k u(t)}{K' [1 + u(t)]} \qquad \ldots\ldots\ldots\ldots\ldots\ldots (2\cdot5),$$

when recessives are rare,

$$R(t) = \frac{K'^2 s N}{k^2 S (t - t_0)^2} \qquad \ldots\ldots\ldots\ldots\ldots\ldots (2\cdot6),$$

when dominants are rare,

$$D(t) = e^{\frac{k(t_0 - t)}{K'}} \qquad \ldots\ldots\ldots\ldots\ldots\ldots (2\cdot7).$$

Now k has approximately the same meaning as when generations are separate, provided $K' = 1$. Hence the two cases become comparable if we choose our unit of time, or "generation," so as to make K' or $\int_0^\infty xK(x)\, dx = 1$, as in the calculations of Dublin and Lotka* on the rate of increase of a population. In each case, if functions analogous to $S(x)$, $s(x)$ are known for the males, their numbers can be calculated.

* Dublin and Lotka, *Journ. Amer. Stat. Assoc.* 1925, p. 306.

Selection of a sex-linked factor.

Here, using the same notation as above, we find

$$\left.\begin{aligned} (K-1)F(t) - K'F'(t) + \frac{L'[F(t)f'(t) - F'(t)f(t)] + lF(t)f(t)}{2L[F(t) - f(t)]} &= 0 \\ (K-1)f(t) - K'f'(t) - \frac{L'[F(t)f'(t) - F'(t)f(t)] + lF(t)f(t)}{2L[F(t) + f(t)]} - \frac{k[f(t)]^2}{F(t) - f(t)} &= 0 \end{aligned}\right\} \quad \ldots(3\cdot1).$$

In general, if $u = F(t)/f(t)$,

$$(L' + 2K'L)\frac{d}{dt}u(t) = lu(t) + \frac{2kLu(t)}{1 + u(t)} \quad \ldots\ldots(3\cdot2),$$

an equation analogous to (2·0) of Part III *.

When recessives are rare,

$$(L' + 2K'L)f'(t) + lf(t) + \frac{2kL[f(t)]^2}{F} = 0,$$

where F is the birth-rate of dominants. Three cases occur:

(*a*) If kL is negligible compared with lN, which will be the case if selection is of the same order of intensity in the two sexes, or more intense among males, then

$$f(t) = e^{\frac{l(t_0 - t)}{L' + 2K'L}} \quad \ldots\ldots\ldots\ldots\ldots\ldots\ldots(3\cdot31).$$

The number of recessive males is proportional to $f(t)$, of recessive females to its square.

(*b*) If kL is of the same order of magnitude as lF, then

$$\frac{2kLf(t)}{2kLf(t) + lF} = e^{\frac{l(t_0 - t)}{L' + 2K'L}} \quad \ldots\ldots\ldots\ldots\ldots(3\cdot32).$$

Hence if V, v are quantities corresponding to S, s for the male sex, the proportion of recessive males is

$$\frac{lv}{2kLV\left(e^{\frac{l(t - t_0)}{L' + 2K'L}} - 1\right)},$$

of recessive females

$$\frac{l^2 s}{4k^2L^2S\left(e^{\frac{l(t - t_0)}{L' + 2K'L}} - 1\right)^2}.$$

* Haldane, *Proc. Camb. Phil. Soc.* 23. p. 363. 1926.

(*c*) If kL is much larger than lF, i.e. selection is confined to females, then

$$f(t) = \frac{(2K'L + L')F}{2kL(t - t_0)} \qquad \text{..............(3·33).}$$

Hence the proportion of recessive males is

$$\frac{(L' + 2K'L)r}{2kLV(t - t_0)},$$

of recessive females

$$\frac{(L' + 2K'L)^2 s}{4k^2L^2S(t - t_0)^2}.$$

When dominants are rare,

$$F(t) = e^{\frac{(l + 2kL)(t - t_0)}{L' + 2K'L}} \qquad \text{..................(3·4).}$$

The number of male dominants is proportional to $F(t)$, that of females being double that of males.

When the intensity of selection is equal in both sexes, these equations simplify to

$$\frac{d}{dt}u(t) = \frac{ku(t)[3 + u(t)]}{3K'[1 + u(t)]} \qquad \text{...............(3·5).}$$

$$f(t) = e^{\frac{k(t_0 - t)}{3K'}} \qquad \text{..........................(3·6).}$$

$$F(t) = e^{\frac{k(t_0 - t)}{K'}} \qquad \text{..........................(3·7).}$$

analogous to equation (7·2) of Part I.

Discussion.

The most satisfactory table of $K(x)$ known to me is that given by Dublin and Lotka* for certain American women. Here the population is growing, and $K = 1·17$, while $\frac{K'}{K}$, the length of a "generation," is 28·45 years. No satisfactory values of k are known in the present state of genetics, though the data on mice discussed in Part I suggest that here $k = ·04$ approximately. In man mating is highly assortative for age, and the above formulae cannot be applied. Moreover, a change in the coefficient of correlation between the ages of spouses would undoubtedly affect the values of $K(x)$, etc., if other conditions remained equal. Thus old men would beget more children if they were more likely to have young

* Dublin and Lotka, *loc. cit.*

wives. It is thus impossible to calculate the effect of this correlation on selection. But a consideration of the extreme case when the age of the wife fixes that of the husband makes it clear that selection must follow equations of the type here arrived at, with changes in the parameters only.

Summary.

Expressions are found for the progress of slow selection in a Mendelian population where generations overlap. The changes are very similar to those which occur when generations are separate.

A Mathematical Theory of Natural and Artificial Selection, Part V: Selection and Mutation. By Mr J. B. S. HALDANE, Trinity College.

[*Received* 21 May, *read* 25 July, 1927.]

New factors arise in a species by the process of mutation. The frequency of mutation is generally small, but it seems probable that it can sometimes be increased by changes in the environment (1, 2). On the whole mutants recessive to the normal type occur more commonly than dominants. The frequency of a given type of mutation varies, but for some factors in Drosophila it must be less than 10^{-6}, and is much less in some human cases. We shall first consider initial conditions, when only a few of the new type exist as the result of a single mutation: and then the course of events in a population where the new factor is present in such numbers as to be in no danger of extinction by mere bad luck. In the first section the treatment of Fisher (3) is followed.

In a large population let p_r be the chance that a factor present in a zygote at a given stage in the life-cycle will appear in r of its children in the next generation. If the individual considered is homozygous, this is the chance of leaving r children, if mutation is neglected. Let $\sum_{r=0}^{\infty} p_r x^r = f(x)$. Therefore $f(1) = 1$, $f(0) = p_0$, the probability of the factor disappearing, while $f'(1) = \sum_{r=0}^{\infty} rp_r$, *i.e.*, the probable number of individuals possessing the factor in the next generation. The probability of m individuals bearing one each of the factors considered leaving r descendants is clearly the coefficient of x^r in $[f(x)]^m$, if we neglect the possibility of a mating between two such individuals, which we may legitimately do if m is small compared with the total number of the population. If then the probability of the factor being present in r zygotes of the nth generation be the coefficient of x^r in $F(x)$, the corresponding probability in the $(n+1)$th generation is the same coefficient in $F[f(x)]$. Hence if a single factor appears in one zygote, the probability of its presence in r zygotes after n generations is the coefficient of x^r in $S_f^n(x)$, *i.e.* $f(f(f\ldots f(x)\ldots))$, the operation being repeated n times. The probability of its disappearance is therefore $\operatorname{Lt}_{n\to\infty} S_f^n(0)$. By Koenigs' theorem (4) this is the root of $x = f(x)$ in the neighbourhood of zero.

Now in the case of a dominant factor appearing in a population in equilibrium, and conferring an advantage measured by k, as in Part I (5), $f'(1) = 1 + k$. Since $f'(x)$ and $f''(x)$ are positive when x is positive, and $f(0)$ is positive, $x = f(x)$ has two and only two real positive roots, one equal to unity, the other lying between 0 and 1, but near the latter value if k be small. Hence any advantageous dominant factor which has once appeared has a finite chance of survival, however large the total population may be.

If a large number of offspring is possible, as in most organisms, the series p_n approximates to a Poisson series, provided that adult organisms are counted, and since $f'(1) = 1 + k$, $f(x) = e^{(1+k)(x-1)}$. Hence the probability of extinction $1 - y$ is given by

$$1 - y = e^{-(1+k)y}.$$

Hence $$(1 + k)y = -\log(1 - y) \quad \text{.............} (1 \cdot 0),$$

and $$k = \frac{y}{2} + \frac{y^2}{3} + \frac{y^3}{4} + \ldots,$$

and if k be small, $y = 2k$ approximately. Hence an advantageous dominant gene has a probability $2k$ of survival after only a single appearance in an adult zygote, and if in the whole history of a species it appears more than $\frac{\log_e 2}{2k}$ times it will probably spread through the species. But, however large k may be, the factor may be extinguished after a single appearance. Thus if $k = 1$, so that the new type probably leaves twice as many offspring as the normal, the probability of its extinction is still ·203. If in any generation there are m dominant individuals the probability of extinction is reduced to y^m, where y is the smaller positive root of $x = f(x)$. When k is small this reduces to $(1 - 2k)^m$. Hence if in any generation more than $\frac{\log_e 2}{2k}$ adult dominants exist, the factor will probably spread through the whole population.

On the other hand a recessive factor whose phenotype is advantageous has a quite negligible advantage in a random mating population provided that the number of its bearers is small compared with the square root of the total population. This is best seen by considering the case of a hermaphrodite: in a dioecious organism the argument, though similar, is more complicated. Let N be the fixed number of the population, and z_n the number of heterozygotes plus double the number of recessives for the factor A in the nth generation. It therefore produces gametes in the ratio $(2N - z_n) A : z_n a$. If now the recessives have a small advantage measured by k, the probabilities of production of each genotype in the next generation are

$$(2N - z_n)^2 AA : 2z_n(2N - z_n) Aa : (1 + k) z_n^2 aa.$$

Hence if, as above, $f(x)$ be the function defining the probable number of offspring of a dominant, so that $f'(1) = 1$, the probability of r heterozygotes in the $(n + 1)$th generation is the coefficient of r in

$$[f(x)]^{\frac{2Nz_n(2N - z_n)}{4N^2 + kz_n^2}},$$

that of r recessives the same coefficient in

$$[f(x)]^{\frac{N(1 + k)z_n^2}{4N^2 + kz_n^2}}.$$

Hence the probability of z_{n+1} in the next generation is the coefficient of $x^{z_{n+1}}$ in

$$[f(x)]^{\frac{2Nz_n(2N + kz_n)}{4N^2 + kz_n^2}},$$

or, approximately, if z_n be small compared with N, in

$$[f(x)]^{z_n\left(1 + \frac{kz_n}{2N}\right)}.$$

The corresponding expression for a dominant factor is

$$[f(x)]^{z_n(1 + k)}.$$

Hence provided that z_n is small the probability of escaping extinction is much smaller than k. I have been unable to evaluate it exactly, but it seems from a comparison with the case of a dominant factor, that the value of z_n such that the factor is as likely to survive as to be extinguished, is of the order of $\left(\frac{N}{k}\right)^{\frac{1}{2}}$, *i.e.* generally $>N^{\frac{1}{2}}$. So if N is sufficiently large the probability of a single mutation leading to the establishment of a recessive factor is negligible.

When the population is wholly self-fertilized or inbred by brother-sister mating, on the other hand, a recessive factor has almost as good a chance of survival as a dominant. With partial self-fertilization or inbreeding it can be shown by methods similar to those of Part II (6) that an advantageous recessive factor has a finite chance of establishment after one appearance, however large be the population.

If mutation occurs with a finite frequency any advantageous or not too disadvantageous factor will certainly be established. Consider a random mating population in which, in each generation, a proportion p of the A genes mutate to a, a proportion q of the a genes to A, and the coefficient of selection is k. Let u_n be the gametic ratio of the nth generation. But for mutation we should have

$$u_{n+1} = \frac{u_n(u_n + 1)}{u_n + 1 - k};$$

allowing for mutation

$$u_{n-1} = \frac{(1-p)(u_n^2+u_n)+q(u_n+1-k)}{(1-q)(u_n+1-k)+p(u_n^2+u_n)}.$$

Hence
$$\Delta u_n = \frac{ku_n^2 - pu_n(u_n+1)^2 + q(u_n+1)(u_n+1-k)}{u_n+1-k+pu_n(u_n+1)-q(u_n+1-k)} \quad \ldots(2{\cdot}0)$$

$$= \frac{ku_n}{u_n+1} - pu_n(u_n+1) + q(u_n+1) \quad \ldots\ldots\ldots\ldots\ldots(2{\cdot}1)$$

approximately, if p, q, and k are small, as is generally the case. It is clear that u_n must lie between $\frac{1-p}{p}$ and $\frac{q}{1-q}$, *i.e.* between $\frac{1}{p}$ and q approximately, and that when near these values it alters rapidly. But as p and q may be less than 10^{-6} these limits are very wide. The population is in equilibrium when

$$pu^3 + (2p-q)u^2 + (p-2q-k+kq)u - q + kq = 0.$$

There is always one real positive root since p and q are positive and less than unity. If k be positive there is only one such root, defining a stable condition towards which the population tends when dominants have the advantage. If k or q be large compared with p this root approximates to $\left(\frac{k}{p}\right)^{\frac{1}{2}}$ or $\frac{q}{p}$ as the case may be, *i.e.* recessives nearly disappear. If p be of the same order of magnitude as the larger of k and q, u has a moderate value and the population is dimorphic. If p be much larger than k or q, u is small and approximates to $\frac{q}{p}$, *i.e.* dominants are rare.

If k be negative all the roots are positive if they are real, provided $q > 2p$ and $-k(1-q) > 2q-p$. They are real if $\frac{\Delta}{3k}$, *i.e.*

$$4(p+q)^3 + [-27p^2+18p(p+q)(1-q)+(p+q)^2(1-q)^2]k + 4p(1-q)^3k^2$$

is positive, that is to say, when q is small, if

$$4pk^2 + (-8p^2+20pq+q^2)k + 4(p+q)^2$$

is positive. All these three conditions can rarely be fulfilled, but such cases may presumably occur. Thus if $p = {\cdot}000{,}001$, $q = {\cdot}0004$, $k = -{\cdot}008$; $u^3 - 398u^2 + 7197{\cdot}8u - 403{\cdot}2 = 0$. Therefore $u = {\cdot}057$, $18{\cdot}93$, or $379{\cdot}0$, giving $89{\cdot}5$ %, $0{\cdot}252$ %, or ${\cdot}000{,}693$ % of recessives. In such a case the middle root defines an unstable equilibrium, the other two equilibria being stable. Thus the above considered population would be stable with only about seven recessives per million, the small tendency of dominant genes to mutate to recessive being balanced by reverse mutation. But if a group containing more than one recessive gene in twenty were isolated from it, selection would be effective, and it would pass into a condition where only 10·5 °/$_\circ$ were dominants, this number being kept up by mutation.

Usually when k is negative there is only one real root. If p or $-k$ be large compared with q, it is small and approximates to $\frac{q}{p}$ or $\frac{-q}{k}$ as the case may be, so that dominants are rare. If q be of the same order of magnitude as the larger of p and $-k$, the root has a moderate value and the population is dimorphic. If q be larger than p or $-k$, u is large and approximates to $\frac{q}{p}$, so that recessives are few.

The rate of approach to equilibrium is given by

$$\frac{du_n}{dn} = \frac{ku_n}{u_n+1} - pu_n(u_n+1) + q(u_n+1) \quad \text{......(2·2)},$$

provided that the constants are small. The exact expression for n in terms of u_n depends on the nature of the roots and the side from which an equilibrium is being approached, but it always contains logarithmic terms. Hence the numbers of the rarer type of the population in succeeding generations always lie between two geometric series until equilibrium is nearly reached. That is to say, the march of events is comparatively rapid.

In a self-fertilizing population we can similarly show that

$$\Delta u_n = ku_n - pu_n(u_n+1) + q(u_n+1) \quad \text{.........(2·3)}.$$

Only one equilibrium is possible, and the course of events can readily be calculated in any given case. Similarly for a sex-linked factor

$$\Delta u_n = \frac{ku_n(u_n+3)}{3(u_n+1)} - pu_n(u_n+1) + q(u_n+1) \quad \text{......(2·4)}.$$

In this case if k be negative, three equilibria are sometimes found, and selection is more effective than in the autosomal case when recessives are rare.

To sum up, if selection acts against mutation, it is ineffective provided that the rate of mutation is greater than the coefficient of selection. Moreover, mutation is quite effective where selection is not, namely in causing an increase of recessives where these are rare. It is also more effective than selection in weeding out rare recessives provided that it is not balanced by back mutation of dominants. Mutation therefore determines the course of evolution as regards factors of negligible advantage or disadvantage to the species. It can only lead to results of importance when its frequency becomes large.

Addendum. Equilibrium and selection in Sciara and similar animals.

In Part I of this series all the then known types of single-factor Mendelian inheritance were discussed. Since then Metz (7) has discovered a new type in Sciara which is here treated on the lines of Part I. Gametogenesis is normal in the female, but spermatozoa are formed from maternal chromatin only. Hence there are two types of heterozygous male, which may be symbolized by $A(a)$ and $(A)a$ according as the A is received from the mother or father. They yield A and a spermatozoa respectively, the other genotypes behaving normally.

In the absence of selection let eggs and spermatozoa be produced by the mth generation in the proportions $u_m A : 1a$ and $v_m A : 1a$, respectively. The next generation is therefore:

$$♀\ u_m v_m AA : (u_m + v_m)Aa : 1aa.$$

$$♂\ u_m v_m AA : u_m A(a) : v_m (A)a : 1aa.$$

Hence

$$\left.\begin{aligned} u_{m+1} &= \frac{2u_m v_m + u_m + v_m}{u_m + v_m + 2} \\ v_{m+1} &= u_m \end{aligned}\right\} \qquad \text{.............. (3·0)},$$

which is the same as equation (6·0) of Part I (5). Hence, as in the above equation, we find, if y_m be the proportion of recessives in the mth generation.

$$y_m = y_\infty - \left(\frac{-1}{2}\right)^m c^{\frac{1}{2}} y_\infty^{\frac{1}{2}} + \left(\frac{-1}{2}\right)^{2m-1} c \quad \text{...... (3·1)},$$

where c is a constant depending on the initial conditions. Hence equilibrium is rapidly approached, the values in successive generations being alternately greater and less than the final value.

If selection occurs with a coefficient k in ♀s, l in ♂s, then

$$\left.\begin{aligned} u_{n+1} &= \frac{2u_n v_n + u_n + v_n}{u_n + v_n + 2 - 2k} \\ v_{n+1} &= \frac{u_n(v_n + 1)}{v_n + 1 - l} \end{aligned}\right\} \qquad \text{............ (3·2)}.$$

If the population is nearly in equilibrium apart from selection and k and l are small, so that u_n and v_n are nearly equal,

$$\Delta u_n = \frac{v_n - u_n}{2} + \frac{ku_n}{u_n + 1},$$

$$\Delta v_n = u_n - v_n + \frac{lu_n}{u_n + 1}, \text{ both approximately.}$$

Hence
$$\Delta u_n = \frac{2k+l}{3} \frac{u_n}{u_n+1},$$

and
$$\frac{2k+l}{3} n = u_n - u_0 + \log_e \left(\frac{u_n}{u_0}\right) \quad \text{.........(3·3)},$$

approximately. Selection therefore occurs much as with a normally inherited autosomal factor.

REFERENCES.

1. HARRISON and GARRETT. *Proc. Roy. Soc.* B, 99, p. 241, 1926.
2. GAGER and BLAKESLEE. *Proc. Nat. Ac. Sci.* 13, p. 75, 1927.
3. FISHER. *Proc. Roy. Soc. Edin.* 42, p. 321, 1922.
4. KOENIGS. *Darb. Bull.* (2) 7, p. 340, 1883.
5. HALDANE. *Trans. Camb. Phil. Soc.* 23, p. 19, 1924.
6. HALDANE. *Biol. Proc. Camb. Phil. Soc.* 1, p. 158, 1924.
7. METZ. *Proc. Nat. Ac. Sci.* 12, p. 690, 1926.

Reprinted from THE AMERICAN NATURALIST, Vol. LXIV,
January–February, 1930.
"PRINTED IN U. S. A."

A NOTE ON FISHER'S THEORY OF THE ORIGIN OF DOMINANCE, AND ON A CORRELATION BETWEEN DOMINANCE AND LINKAGE

R. A. FISHER (28 a, b) has suggested that, on its first appearance, a mutant gene usually produces a marked effect in the heterozygous condition, and becomes recessive to the wild type only as the result of natural selection acting over very long periods. He regards this process as due to the selection of specific modifying genes which render the appearance and viability of the heterozygote approximately the same as those of the wild type. S. Wright (29) has criticized this process on the ground of its slowness. The present note raises the question of whether it is possible in the manner suggested by Fisher.

Consider, with Wright, a population mostly of composition AAmm, and that Aamm have a viability $1-k$, compared with the proportion of Aa in the population is $\frac{2u}{k}$ (Haldane, 27a). Next consider a modifier M, which increases the viability of Aa to normal (the most favorable case for Fisher's theory). It is clear that AAMm can not have a viability greater than normal, or M would spread through the population apart from its modifying effect. Hence its presence in the species would have nothing to do with the mutability of A. Suppose the viability of AAMm to be $1-k'$, then it carries a disadvantage $-k'$ in most cases, an advantage $+k$ in a fraction $\frac{2u}{k}$ of all cases; *i.e.*, when combined with Aa. If it is to spread, $\frac{2u}{k} \cdot k > k'$, *i.e.*, $k' < 2u$. If we take u as 10^{-6}, the viability of AAMm must lie between .999998 and 1.0. Now suppose a number of M genes exist which raise the viability of Aa nearly to normal. I suspect that the viabilities of the AAMm zygotes will be fairly evenly distributed over values between 1.0 and .99, even if lower viabilities are rarer. If so, the chances are over 5,000 to 1 against any given one of them being selected as a result of the Fisher effect.

If an infinite number of possible modifiers were available, this would not matter, but the number of loci at which mutation can occur is finite. Hence I conclude that it is only in rare cases that suitable modifiers will be found. If, however, they do exist, then owing to the very nearly normal viability of AAMm they will be fairly common in the population as the result of mutation, and will spread somewhat more rapidly than would otherwise be the case. The fact that modifiers rapidly appear in an inbred mutant race does not dispose of this argument, unless it can be shown that these modifiers have no adverse effect on the viability of the wild type.

I suspect that the Fisher effect has operated in a different manner. Adopting Goldschmidt's (27) view that genes are catalysts acting at a definite rate, there is, as pointed out elsewhere (Haldane, 27b) no obvious way of distinguishing those which act at more than a certain rate. *E.g.*, if an enzyme can oxidize a certain substance as quickly as it is formed, no visible result arises from doubling the amount of that enzyme. Hence, while a minus mutation (diminution of activity) of a normal gene may yield a recessive type, a plus mutation is often unobservable. Now on this hypothesis we have to explain why a wild-type gene generally has a factor of safety of at least 2, as is shown by the fact that one wild-type gene has nearly the same effect as two. If we imagine a race whose genes were only just doing the work required of them, then any inactivation of one of a pair of genes would lead to a loss of total activity. Thus if A_1A_1 can just oxidize all of a certain substrate as fast as it is formed, its inactivation will produce a zygote A_1a which can only oxidize about half. If now A_1 mutates to A_2, which can oxidize at twice or thrice the rate of A_1, if necessary, no effect will be produced, *i.e.*, A_1A_2 and A_2A_2 zygotes will be indistinguishable from A_1A_1. But A_2a will be normal. Hence A_2a zygotes will have a better chance of survival than A_1a, and A_2 will be selected.

In other words the modifiers postulated by Fisher are probably the normal allelomorphs of mutant genes, and the Fisher effect is rather to accentuate the activity of genes already present than to call up new modifiers. This hypothesis would not, of course, explain the behavior of the "crinkled dwarf" type of Sea Island cotton, which behaves as a recessive within the species, but gives intermediates in F_1 and F_2 with other New World cottons. Now the haploid number in these cottons is 26, as opposed to 13 in Old World cottons. They are therefore tetraploids, and failures of Mendelian inheritance are to be expected on crossing them. Several equally plausible hypotheses as to their genetical nature would explain the results cited by Fisher.

No theory of dominance can be complete which does not take cognizance of the fact that there are certain organisms in which mutant types are generally dominant, and not recessive to the normal type. For example, Nabours (17, 25) found eleven "genes" dominant to the most frequently occurring type of *Apotettix eurycephalus*, and none recessive; fourteen dominant and no recessive in *Paratettix texanus*. Similarly Winge (27) found eighteen "genes" dominant to the normal and none recessive in *Lebistes reticulatus*. A few other cases, less completely studied, fall into the same class. Now these organisms all share another peculiarity, namely, that the number of linkage groups is much smaller than the number of chromosomes. *Apotettix* has one autosomal linkage group, with seven pairs of chromosomes, *Paratettix* three linkage groups with six or seven pairs of chromosomes. *Lebistes* has twenty-three pairs of chromosomes, with one autosomal "gene" and the other seventeen sex-linked.

Haldane (20) and Demereč (28) have suggested that these results are due to linkage between chromosomes. A study of Nabours' (25) linkage map for *Apotettix* suggests the possibility that his eleven "genes" lie in four or five chromosomes, and that crossing over within a chromosome is extremely rare. How are we to explain the correlation between dominance of mutant types and excessive linkage? My friends Mr. C. D. Darlington and Mr. C. L. Huskins have suggested that these dominant mutant types differ from the normal, not by single genes, but by duplication or translocation of whole sections of chromosome. Translocation will account for linkage between chromosomes, on the lines of the theory developed by Darlington (29) for *Oenothera*. Thus both features can be explained if the chromosomes have an unusual tendency to break up and reunite in novel ways.

The cytological facts known in other Orthoptera and notably the work of Carothers (17, 21) support this view. Differences which are probably translocations or duplications have been seen, and behave in a Mendelian manner. There is no obvious ring formation, but it must be remembered that in *Oenothera*, where this occurs, interchromosomal linkage is nearly, if not quite, absolute. The rarity of crossing over within a chromosome is readily explained by the postulated differences between nearly homologous chromosomes.

Now on Fisher's theory there is no obvious reason why modifiers should not be able to suppress the effect of a duplication as easily as that of a gene. On the theory here adopted we need only suppose that some of the genes in the duplication have a greater effect when three or four are present than when two only are found, as in the normal type.

To sum up, it is suggested that dominance may be due to either of three causes: the Fisher effect in rare cases, the overactivity of normal genes due to a modified Fisher effect in most cases and duplication of a section of chromosome in still a third small group.

J. B. S. HALDANE

JOHN INNES HORTICULTURAL INSTITUTION,
MERTON, ENGLAND

LITERATURE CITED

Carothers, E. E.

1917. "The Segregation and Recombination of Homologous Chromosomes as Found in Two Genera of *Acrididae*," *Journ. Morph.*, 28: 445–521.

1921. "Genetical Behavior of Heteromorphic Homologous Chromosomes of *Circotettix* (Orthoptera)," *Journ. Morph.*, 35: 457–483.

Darlington, C. D.

1929. "Ring-formation in *Oenothera* and other Genera," *Journ Gen.*, 20: 345–365.

Demereč, M.

1928. "A Possible Explanation for Winge's Findings in *Lebistes reticulatus*," AMER. NAT., 62: 90–94.

Fisher, R. A.

1928a. "The Possible Modifications of the Responses of the Wild Type to Recurrent Mutations," AMER. NAT., 62: 115–126.

1928b. "Two Further Notes on the Origin of Dominance," AMER. NAT., 62: 571–574.

Goldschmidt, R.

1927. "Physiologische Theorie der Vererbung."

Haldane, J. B. S.

1920. "Note on a Case of Linkage in *Paratettix*," *Journ. Gen.*, 10: 47–52.

1927a. "A Mathematical Theory of Natural and Artificial Selection, Pt. V," *Proc. Cam. Phil. Soc.*, 23: 838.

1927b. "The Comparative Genetics of Color in Rodents and Carnivores," *Biol. Rev.*, 2: 199.

Nabours, R. K.

1917. "Studies of Inheritance and Evolution in Orthoptera, II," *Journ. Gen.*, 7: 1–47.

1925. "Studies of Inheritance and Evolution in Orthoptera, V," Kansas Agr. Exp. Station, *Technical Bulletin* 17.

Winge, O.

1927. "The Location of Eighteen Genes in *Lebistes reticulatus*," *Journ. Gen.*, 18: 1–43.

Wright, Sewall

1929. "Fisher's Theory of Dominance," AMER. NAT., 63: 274–279.

A Mathematical Theory of Natural Selection. Part VIII. Metastable Populations. By Mr J. B. S. HALDANE, Trinity College.

[*Received* 20 November, *read* 8 December 1930.]

Almost every species is, to a first approximation, in genetic equilibrium; that is to say no very drastic changes are occurring rapidly in its composition. It is a necessary condition for equilibrium that all new genes which arise at all frequently by mutation should be disadvantageous, otherwise they will spread through the population. Now each of two or more genes may be disadvantageous, but all together may be advantageous. An example of such balance has been given by Gonsalez(1). He found that, in purple-eyed *Drosophila melanogaster*, arc wing or axillary speck (each due to a recessive gene) shortened life, but the two together lengthened it.

Consider the case of two dominant genes A, B, where the relative chances of producing offspring by the four phenotypes are as follows: AB 1, aaB $1-k_1$, Abb $1-k_2$, $aabb$ $1+K$. k_1 and k_2 are small and positive. K is small, and if negative its absolute value is less than k_1 or k_2.

Consider a random mating population where in the nth generation the genic ratios are $u_n A : 1a$; $v_n B : 1b$.

Then

$$u_{n-1} = \frac{(u_n^2 + u_n)\{1 - k_2(1+v_n)^{-2}\}}{u_n\{1 - k_2(1+v_n)^{-2}\} + 1 + \{K - k_1(v_n^2 + 2v_n)\}(1+v_n)^{-2}},$$

whence

$$\Delta u_n = \frac{u_n\{k_1(1+v_n)^2 - K - k_1 - k_2\}}{(1+u_n)(1+v_n)^2}, \text{ approximately.}$$

So, taking a generation as the unit of time,

$$\frac{du}{dt} = \frac{u\{k_1(1+v)^2 - K - k_1 - k_2\}}{(1+u)(1+v)^2}, \text{ approximately.}$$

Let $x = 1/(1+u)$ (the proportion of recessive genes) and $y = 1/(1+v)$, so that $1 > x > 0$, $1 > y > 0$.

Then
$$\frac{dx}{dt} = x^2(1-x)[(K + k_1 + k_2)y^2 - k_1].$$

Similarly
$$\frac{dy}{dt} = y^2(1-y)[(K + k_1 + k_2)x^2 - k_2].$$

Clearly $x = 0$, $y = 0$; and $x = 1$, $y = 1$ are the only stable equilibria, though Fisher(2) appears to regard a mixed population as stable in such a case. Putting

$$\frac{k_1}{K + k_1 + k_2} = a^2, \quad \frac{k_2}{K + k_1 + k_2} = b^2,$$

we have

$$\frac{dy}{dx} = \frac{y^2(1-y)(x^2-a^2)}{x^2(1-x)(y^2-b^2)}.$$

So

$$\int_{y_0}^{y} \frac{(s^2-b^2)\,ds}{s^2(1-s)} = \int_{x_0}^{x} \frac{(s^2-a^2)\,ds}{s^2(1-s)},$$

whence $\quad f(y, b) - f(x, a) = c = f(y_0, b) - f(x_0, a),$

where x_0, y_0 represent the initial conditions, and

$$f(x, a) = a^2/x - a^2 \log x + (a^2 - 1)\log(1 - x).$$

Each value of $f(y_0, b) - f(x_0, a)$ determines a trajectory passing to (0, 0) or (1, 1), which represent populations composed entirely of double dominants or double recessives respectively. The minimum value of $f(x, a)$ occurs when $x = a$ and is

$$a - a^2 \log a + (a^2 - 1)\log(1 - a),$$

and $f(x, a)$ is always real and positive, becoming infinite when $x = 0$ or 1. If $c > f(b, b) - f(a, a)$, there are two values of x corresponding to each value of y, but some values of x are excluded. Hence the trajectories fall into four families divided by the two branches of the curve whose equation is

$$f(y, b) - f(x, a) = f(b, b) - f(a, a).$$

This consists of two trajectories running from (0, 1) and (1, 0) to (a, b) and two from (a, b) to (0, 0) and (1, 1). These are represented by the dotted lines in Fig. 1, where $a = \frac{1}{2}$, $b = \frac{1}{4}$. The former divides the whole area into two portions. Populations in the one tend to the values $x = y = 0$, in the other to the values $x = y = 1$. Some examples of trajectories are given. It is clear that a population consisting mainly of *AABB* or *aabb* tends, as the result of selection, to return to those compositions. If the signs of K, k_1, and k_2 be changed, the same trajectories will be described in the reverse direction.

If the original population is *AABB*, the factors *A* and *B* will generally have a small tendency to mutate to *a* and *b* respectively. Let p_1 and p_2 be the probabilities that *A* will mutate to *a* and *B* to *b* in the course of a generation. These appear to be generally small numbers of the order of 10^{-6} or less. The population is in equilibrium when $x = p_1/k_1$, $y = p_2/k_2$ (Haldane(3)). In general x will be much smaller than a, and y than b, but from time to time chance fluctuations may isolate a population where this is no longer the case. Its representative point will lie in the area whose stable type is *aabb*, and the whole population will be transformed into this type, apart from rare exceptions due to back mutation. In such a population modifying factors will be selected in such a way as to increase the viability of the *aabb* type, i.e. the value of K. But even so it may be expected to be swamped by hybridisation on coming into contact with the original *AABB* population, unless one of two things has happened.

aabb may possess or develop characters which render mating with *AABB* rare. For example, it may have a different flowering time if a plant, or a different psychology if an animal. In this case the species will divide into two. Or chromosome changes may occur to cause close linkage of A and B when the populations are crossed. Thus if the loci of A and B are in the same chromosome an inversion of the portion containing them will lead to their behaving as a single factor on crossing. In this case if K is positive the whole species will be transformed into the type *aabb*. A species which is liable to transformations of this kind may be called metastable. Possibly metastability is quite a general phenomenon, but it is only rarely that the circumstances arise which favour a change of the type considered.

In a population which is mainly self-fertilised, conditions are probably more favourable. Were self-fertilisation universal, the proportion of *aaBB* zygotes, when mutation and selection were in equilibrium, would be $\frac{1}{2}p_1/k_1$. So that of *aabb* would be $p_1p_2/(4k_1k_2)$ or less. This is presumably a small number, probably of the order 10^{-9}, and when such individuals occur, they will generally be wiped out by chance. But their probability of spreading through the population, though small, will be finite, and roughly equal to $2K$ (Haldane (3)). Hence, within a geologically short period we may expect evolution to occur in such cases.

The theory may be extended in two different ways. We may consider m genes. In this case any population can be represented by a point in m-dimensional space, all populations being represented by the points of a regular orthotope, or hypercube. Each of the 2^m apices of this figure represents a homozygous population. Clearly the condition for stability of any such population is that no change in a *single* factor should yield a more viable type. In other words, no adjacent apices can both represent stable populations. The maximum number of stable populations is thus 2^{m-1}, represented by the vertices of the polytope arising from the omission of alternate vertices of the regular orthotope. This is not regular but only semi-regular if $m > 3$. In general the numbers of stable genotypes will be much smaller than this, and may not exceed 1.

If there is more than one stable population the orthotope is divided into two or more regions analogous to the two areas of Fig. 1. A population in any given region tends to the same point of stable equilibrium. The regions are separated by a variety (surface or hyper-surface) of $m-1$ dimensions. If we take as our variables x_1, x_2, x_3, etc. not the proportions of recessive genes, but their squares, i.e. the proportion of recessive zygotes, we have

$$\frac{dx_1}{dt} = x_1^{\frac{3}{2}}(1 - x_1^{\frac{1}{2}})\, f_1(x_2, x_3, x_4, \ldots),$$

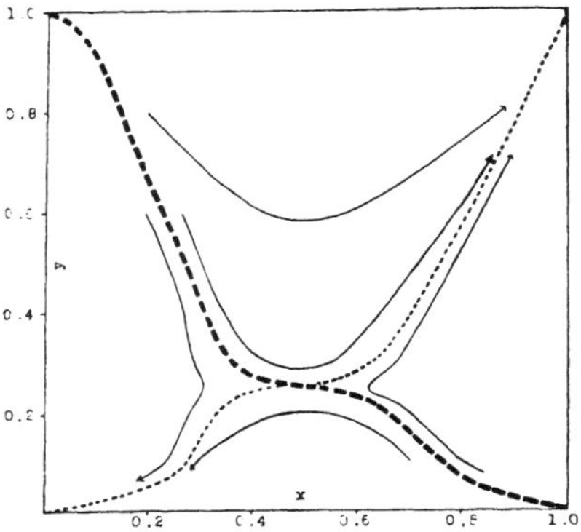

Fig. 1. Abscissa and ordinate. Proportions of genes *a* and *b* in a population. Trajectories of points representing populations are represented by continuous lines, and boundaries between families of trajectories by dotted lines.

where $f_1(x_2, x_3, x_4, \ldots)$ is linear in each of x_2, x_3, etc. and has 2^{m-1} constant coefficients; and $m-1$ similar equations. The $(m-1)$-dimensional space defined by x_2, x_3, etc. is thus divided into two regions, in one of which x_1 increases with time, whilst it diminishes in the other. These are not necessarily connected, as is obvious in the case where there are only three variables, and $f_1(x_2, x_3)$ may define a hyperbola which divides the unit square into three regions, in two of which dx_1/dt has the same sign. Hence in the course of a trajectory dx_1/dt may change sign several times. I have been unable to obtain the general equation for the trajectories or for the boundaries of the regions in which they lie.

So far we have only considered cases of complete dominance. If the heterozygotes are exactly intermediate in viability between the corresponding homozygous types, we have, in the terminology of the case first considered,

$$\frac{dx}{dt} = \tfrac{1}{2}x(1-x)\{(K+k_1+k_2)y-(K+k_1)\},$$

$$\frac{dy}{dt} = \tfrac{1}{2}y(1-y)\{(K+k_1+k_2)y-(K+k_2)\}.$$

Thus

$$\frac{dy}{dx} = \frac{y(1-y)(x-a)}{x(1-x)(y-b)}, \text{ where } a = \frac{K+k_2}{K+k_1+k_2}, \quad b = \frac{K+k_1}{K+k_1+k_2}.$$

Hence
$$\frac{x^a(1-x)^{1-a}}{x_0{}^a(1-x_0)^{1-a}} = \frac{y^b(1-y)^{1-b}}{y_0{}^b(1-y_0)^{1-b}}.$$

By an argument similar to that used above we can show that the trajectories fall into two families, separated by one branch of the curve whose equation is

$$\left(\frac{x}{a}\right)^a\left(\frac{1-x}{1-a}\right)^{1-a} = \left(\frac{y}{b}\right)^b\left(\frac{1-y}{1-b}\right)^{1-b}.$$

The general case where heterozygotes are of any arbitrary viability is rather complicated. But where a heterozygote has a greater viability than any genotype differing from it in respect of a single gene only, there will be a stable population including some of these heterozygotes. Thus if *aabb* has a viability $1+K$, *AABb* of $1+K_2$, all other genotypes having unit viability,

$$\frac{dx}{dt} = xy(1-x)\{K_1xy-K_2(1-x)(1-y)\},$$

$$\frac{dy}{dt} = y\{K_1x^2y-K_2(1-x)^2(2y-1)\}.$$

The stable equilibria are at $x=1$, $y=1$ and $x=0$, $y=\frac{1}{2}$. But I have not been able to integrate these equations, since the variables are not readily separable. Nevertheless it is clear that the trajectories fall into two groups bounded by a curve passing through $(0, 1)$ and $\left(\frac{K_2}{K_1+2K_2}, \frac{1}{2}\right)$.

In the case of m genes, if heterozygotes have an advantage as such there may be points of stable equilibrium anywhere in the m-dimensional space, but it seems fairly clear that their number cannot exceed 2^{m-1}.

It is suggested that in many cases related species represent stable types such as I have described, and that the process of species formation may be a rupture of the metastable equilibrium. Clearly such a rupture will be specially likely where small communities are isolated. I have to thank Mr C. H. Waddington for calculating and drawing the figure.

REFERENCES.

(1) B. M. GONSALEZ, *Am. Nat.*, 57, p. 289 (1923).

(2) R. A. FISHER, *The Genetical Theory of Natural Selection*, p. 102 (1930).

(3) J. B. S. HALDANE, *Proc. Camb. Phil. Soc.*, 23, p. 838 (1927).

Reprinted from THE AMERICAN NATURALIST, Vol. LXVI,
January–February, 1932.
PRINTED IN U. S. A.

THE TIME OF ACTION OF GENES, AND ITS BEARING ON SOME EVOLUTIONARY PROBLEMS

PROFESSOR J. B. S. HALDANE
JOHN INNES HORTICULTURAL INSTITUTION, MERTON, LONDON

ANY classification of variations must at present be provisional, largely because of the extremely limited sources of information which we possess. To take two simple examples, the white flowers on dark-stemmed races of *Primula sinensis* contain flavone. This gives a bright or faint yellow color with ammonia, according as the plant does or does not carry a gene B which modifies anthocyanin color when anthocyanin is present. If our vision extended far enough into the ultra-violet to reach the flavone absorption bands, it would be possible to distinguish these whites without using ammonia. In the same plant a gene R, apparently by causing an acidity of the cell sap greater than that found in rr plants, converts blue flowers into red, the anthocyanin acting as an indicator, but produces no visible effect in the absence of anthocyanin. A genetically minded caterpillar, which regarded the taste of the petals as more interesting than their color, would (one may suppose) readily detect the gene R in white-petalled plants, just as we classify cherries into sweet and sour by their taste. It is highly probable that many morphological differences between varieties are caused by chemical differences appearing earlier in the life-cycle, which could be detected by suitable methods, so that the stage in the life-cycle at which a character appears is necessarily a function of our means of observation. Indeed with a sufficiently fine technique it would be theoretically possible to observe the genes in the nucleus of any cell from any organ, except where some of the chromatin is eliminated in somatic cells. Nevertheless, we are justified in classifying genes by their effects observable with our present technique.

Any chemical or morphological classification would be very complex were it possible. But a classification in time simplifies matters, because variations can be arranged in a nearly (though not quite) linear order by the time of their appearance in the life-cycle, and in another order by the time of their disappearance. A given gene (and throughout this paper what is said of genes may be applied, *mutatis mutandis,* to other nuclear, and sometimes cytoplasmic, structures concerned in inheritance) may affect any six distinct organisms:

(1) The gamete carrying it.
(2) The zygote carrying it.
(3) The endosperm carrying it.
(4) The mother (not necessarily carrying it) of the zygote carrying it.
(5) A gamete (not necessarily carrying it) formed by a zygote carrying it.
(6) A zygote (not necessarily carrying it) produced by a mother carrying it.

This list is not of course exhaustive. Thus in metazoa with alternation of generations, such as the Anthozoa or Aphididae it may be expected that the action of certain genes will be confined to one of these generations. We could also distinguish genes according as they affect one or both sexes of zygote, or genders of gamete.

There are still further possibilities. A variation in the composition of milk might be detected by its effects on foster-children, a variation in the blood-corpuscles by the effect of injecting it into another individual, and so on. However, in principle it would seem that all such variations could be detected by other methods. But genes (or sets of genes) are known which can only be detected by their action on one or another of the six organisms listed. It is further convenient to subdivide genes acting on the zygote by the time at which their effects are evident. We can then classify the genes of higher plants and animals according to Table I.

TABLE I

Designation	Action in plant	Action in animal
G	Gametophyte and gametic	Gametic
E	Endospermal	
MZ	Affecting maternal zygote	Affecting maternal zygote
Z1	Embryonic	Embryonic
Z2	Affecting seedling	Larval or late embryonic
Z3	Affecting immature plant, or non-productive organs of mature plant	Affecting immature animal, or characters of mature animal not connected with reproduction
Z4	Affecting reproductive organs (diploid tissue only) flowering time, etc.	Affecting reproductive organs or behavior, or secondary sexual characters
Z5	Affecting maternal seed and fruit structures	Affecting egg-shell, egg-white or other maternal egg or uterine structures
DG	Delayed gametophytic (affecting gametes, not necessarily carrying them, borne by zygotes carrying them)	Delayed gametic
DZ	Delayed zygotic (affecting zygotes, not necessarily carrying them, produced by mothers carrying them)	Delayed zygotic

The different stages in the zygote are of course arbitrary, and sharp distinctions can not be drawn. A different classification would be desirable in the Bryophyta, and perhaps even in the Pteridophyta. Thus Wettstein ('24) was able to observe the effects of one of four genes in *Funaria hygrometrica* in the protonema stage, of others not till later. So if we were dealing with Bryophyta we should want to break up group G into several subgroups. The same applies to the genes of the Protista and Thallophyta. Examples will now be given of the different types of gene.

G. Besides the above-mentioned genes in mosses, certain genes of the higher plants affect only gametes which carry them. Such are the genes which determine the type of polysaccharide in the endosperm of *Oryza* (Parnell, '21) and *Zea* (Brink and Abegg, '26). In each case the dominant form has ordinary starch, the recessive ("glutinous" and "waxy") contains a polysaccharide of different physical properties and giving a red color with iodine. The pollen grains contain the same polysaccharide as the endosperm in pure lines. But in heterozygous plants half the pollen grains contain each type of polysaccharide, and there can be little doubt that the type is determined by the gene carried by the pollen grain concerned. Parnell found that the immature pollen grains immediately after meiosis contain no starch. This develops gradually, under the influence of the particular gene carried by the grain. Similarly, in some but not all species, a pollen grain borne by a zygote with irregular meiosis attains to a size roughly proportional to the numbers of its chromosomes.

The genes determining membership of an intrasterile group in such plants as *Nicotiana* (East and Mangelsdorf, '26) fall into this class, and also into class Z4. Genes falling into class G only are indeed rather rare, but include the gene Ga for pollen tube growth-rate in *Zea Mays* (Mangelsdorf and Jones, '27). I do not know of any single gene in class G which affects megaspore characters. It is not yet clear whether the effects of Renner's "complexes" in *Oenothera,* which influence both microspores and megaspores, are due to single genes or gene groups. It is a noteworthy fact that no genes of this class are known in animals. Muller and Settles ('27) showed that the viability of the spermatozoa of *Drosophila* did not depend on genes either in the X-chromosome or in a section of the second chromosome which is essential for the life of the zygote. It is, moreover, known that apyrene spermatozoa may be fully motile, and it seems unlikely that the chromatin of a spermatozoon has any relation other than a purely mechanical one to its other constituents. Doubtless this difference between higher animals and plants is due to the fact that in the latter the gamete represents a suppressed generation, which still preserves its own specific physiology. The difference is important from the evolutionary point of view because it implies that certation between gametes, which is an important type of natural selection in plants, is relatively unimportant in animals. It is also probably one reason why no animal is known whose genetics correspond to those of *Oenothera*.

E. Numerous genes are known affecting the endosperm in *Zea Mays*. Some, *e.g.*, "waxy," also fall into class G. Others, such as the gene for carotene (provitamin A) formation, are not known to act except in the endosperm. These genes have, of course, no analogies in animals, though possibly genes may be found controlling the structure and function of the tissue formed from the polar bodies in such forms as *Litomastix*.

MZ. This is the least studied group of genes with which we have to deal. Metaxenia, *i.e.*, difference between the influence exerted by different kinds of pollen on diploid maternal tissue, is quite a well-known phenomenon. Thus Crane and Lawrence ('29) showed that in *Prunus* and *Rubus* drupes or drupels generally require the formation of an embryo, and abort if it perishes early enough. But the differences in embryonic development thus influencing the maternal tissue were due, not to single genes, but to abnormalities involving whole chromosomes. Nixon ('28) and Swingle ('28) showed that in *Phoenix dactylifera* the pollen had a considerable influence on the fruit, fruit size and seed size being correlated. Here the effect is more probably to be ascribed to genes, though no analysis has been made. Metaxenia is of course only part of the action of genes of group MZ. If the mother is heterozygous for genes of this group, we shall find variation in fruit size due to this fact even if pollen of a homozygote is used. Tschermak ('31) gives a bibliography of MZ and Z1 action in plants.

There can be little doubt that (although no MZ genes are known in animals) genes of the MZ type have been of extreme importance in mammalian evolution. The foetus has a great influence on the mother, which must have been evolved by successive steps, and until such genes have been observed in mammals a large chapter in their evolution will remain obscure. Thus the placenta is known to contain hormones capable of acting on the mother, but nothing is known as to their variation. Nor do we know whether genetic factors in the foetus may not transform it into a chorion-epithelioma which kills the mother.

Z1. This group includes a number of well-known plant genes, such as Mendel's gene-pairs for round and wrinkled, yellow and green, cotyledons in *Pisum*. Some characters show at this stage, and are confined to it (*e.g.*, round and wrinkled). Others persist through life (*e.g.*, the sap color gene in *Matthiola,* Frost, '28). In animals the situation is not so good. Some lethal genes are known which act at this stage, but they may be regarded as acting throughout the rest of the life-cycle, as adults bearing them are conspicuous by their non-existence. An example of a gene acting at this stage is Toyama's ('13) recessive gene for crimson serosa color and reddish larval head color in *Bombyx mori.* The importance of purely embryonic variation in evolution is clear when we consider the extreme divergence of the early embryonic forms of species in which the adults are fairly similar, such as *Lepus* and *Cavia.* We do not know if this is due to Z1 or DZ genes, or possibly to extranuclear plasmons. The study of genes whose action is confined to the Z1 stage in higher animals is an important but difficult field for future research. A beginning has been made by Gregory and Castle ('31). They showed that in the eggs of a race of large rabbits, the number of blastomeres at 40 hours after mating was $9.94 \pm .24$, in a small race $8.29 \pm .19$. In hybrids derived from the eggs of a large female and spermatozoa of a small male the number was $8.44 \pm .40$. In this case it is clear that Z1 genes carried by the spermatozoon had an important influence on cleavage rate, which was not mainly determined by DZ genes.

Z2. Apart from lethals, and genes for leaf shape and chlorophyll which show at this stage and persist through life, genes of this class are not very common in the higher plants, where seedlings are on the whole more uniform than adults. There is a little evidence for heritable variation in cotyledon shape not due to genes whose action is apparent in the adult, in *Primula sinensis.*

In animals such as holometabolous insects with a well-marked larval stage, differences confined to this stage are not uncommon, *e.g.,* several genes for larval color in *Lymantria monacha* (Goldschmidt, '27).

Z3. This class includes the majority of genes studied in animals, and all those in plants which affect the leaf and stem. These latter may or may not influence the flower.

Z4. This group includes the genes for flower character in plants; and a good many animal characters, *e.g.,* intersexuality, milk yield and egg yield fall into it. Perhaps the genes governing feather characters in birds which depend for their expression on the sex hormones (*e.g.,* henny feathers in poultry) should properly be included here.

Z5. This is perhaps merely a sub-group of Z4, but assumes a special importance in plant genetics, owing to the importance of fruits. Genes of class Z5 interact with E, Z1, MZ, and possibly DZ genes. Thus the shape of peas is conditioned by Z5 genes such as "indent," which acts on the maternal seed coat, and to a greater extent by Z1 genes, such as "wrinkled," which act on the cotyledon; and the pod character is mainly determined by Z5 genes. On the other hand, in the cherry and date Z1 genes are relatively unimportant except in so far as they also fall into group MZ.

In animals Z5 genes are not so important, but for the sake of symmetry such characters as those of the egg-shell and albumen, which depend on secretions of the oviduct, may be included here. In the evolution of the mammal a critical part was doubtless played by Z5 genes which interact with MZ genes in the foetus to determine a suitable response of the uterus to its contents. We have not, of course, the faintest idea which group played the principal part in the evolutionary process.

DG. Delayed gametic characters are not uncommon in plants. Sometimes a gene is only known to act on gametes, *e.g.*, the gene for round as opposed to oblong pollen in *Lathyrus odoratus*. Sometimes it acts at other periods in the life-cycle. *E.g.*, the gene S in *Primula sinensis* produces a short style and long anthers, and also large pollen grains. Usually these genes seem to act wholly or mainly on the pollen, but the "polymitotic" gene in maize (Beadle, '30) causes extra nuclear divisions in gametes of both genders.

It must be emphasized that these genes act on all the gametes of zygotes carrying them, whether or not they are present in the gametes concerned. In some cases, *e.g.*, where size or shape of the grains is affected, their action does not continue in grains which do not contain them. But the normal allelomorph of the polymitotic gene suppresses supernumerary divisions of gametes borne by heterozygotic plants, even when those gametes carry the polymitotic gene. It clearly has a lasting influence on the surrounding cytoplasm.

Lesley and Frost ('27) describe a gene L in *Matthiola incana* which is on the borderline between Z4 and DG. LL and Ll plants have normal meiosis, with short chromosomes during meiosis. ll plants have long chromosomes during this period. Philp and Huskins ('31) regard the extra length as due to a delay in the onset of prophase contraction. This gene also has a DG effect, in that ll plants produce an unusually large proportion of gametes with chromosomal irregularities. Chromosomes may be lost or fragmented, or extra chromosomes may enter gametes, giving rise to trisomics.

If, therefore, the cytology of ll plants were not known, l might be regarded as a recessive DG gene for "bad pollen."

No cases are known with certainty of DG genes in animals, though it should be possible to detect the action of some DZ genes in the unfertilized egg. Thus it would almost certainly be possible to ascertain the color of silk-worm egg-yolks in the ovary before fertilization. Since, as we saw above, it appears that genes do not function in spermatozoa, it is probable that the main differences between spermatozoa of different species are determined by genes of this class.

DZ. Genes of this group do not appear to be known with certainty in plants, though Miss Pellew informs me that the size of adult *Pisum* plants depends to a considerable extent on seed size determined by the mother and not the father. However, in this species inheritable variation in seed size occurs among peas in the same pod, *i.e.*, some of the genes determining size fall into group Z1. We have then not only to reckon with the fact that, besides environmental effects, genes of both these classes determine seed size, but with the possibility that the same gene may fall into both groups Z1 and DZ. If this is so the genetics of seed size will prove exceedingly complicated.

In animals DZ genes are well known. The classical case in *Bombyx mori* was described by Toyama ('13) as "maternal inheritance." This phrase might be taken to cover extra-nuclear inheritance, in which all inheritance takes place through females only. The tendency of modern genetics is to describe genetical facts in terms of gene action rather than heredity. So possibly "delayed gene action" is a more lucid phrase than "maternal inheritance." Some of Toyama's characters, such as spindle-shape and roughness of egg-shell, are Z5 characters due to a purely maternal structure. Others, such as yellowness of yolk, associated with yellow blood in the mother, are presumably DG. Others, however, such as blueness, are due to pigment formed in the serosa, a zygotic structure, but do not seem to be at all influenced by the father. Along with these occur Z1 genes such as that for crimson eggs.

Since then Boycott, Diver, Garstang and Turner ('31), have shown that dextrality and sinistrality in *Limnaea peregra* are DZ characters, presumably depending on the structure of the unfertilized egg. Redfield ('26) discovered a lethal DZ gene in the second chromosome of *Drosophila melanogaster* affecting female embryos much more than males.

Experiments on interspecific hybridization in fish and echinoderms show that the rate and type of cleavage is mainly conditioned by the cytoplasm. If so it is controlled either by plasmons (characters inherited outside the nucleus) or by DZ genes. The evidence from species crosses yielding fertile hybrids shows that on the whole plasmons are far less important than genes in determining early development, not only in species where the cytoplasm of the egg is obviously differentiated, as in molluscs, but also where this is not the case, as in echinoderms. In mammals and other viviparous animals some maternal genes doubtless have a DZ action on the embryo through the uterus, and it would be hard to distinguish them from DZ genes of the normal type.

The range in time covered by a single gene is a matter of some interest, though data are scanty, because only very striking differences in the gamete and embryo are noticed at all. Thus C in *Pisum* is necessary for anthocyanin formation in the axils, color in the petals, the pods, and also in the seed-coat, *i.e.*, ranges from Z3 to Z5. But its detection depends on the presence of other genes. It does not for example affect the axil unless a special gene is present, or the seed-coat unless one of several genes is present. Perhaps a suitable chemical technique might detect its presence at earlier or later stages.

Frost ('28) gives an example of a gene acting over more than a life-cycle, so that a Z1 gene of one generation interacts with a DZ gene of its predecessor. BB and Bb *Matthiola incana* (provided the color genes C and R and a plastid gene W are present) have purple flowers, bb being red. BB plants have black seeds, and bb brown. On the whole a Bb plant selfed gives 3 black (BB and Bb) to 1 brown (bb) seeded. But among the black seeds a few give red-flowered (bb) plants. Clearly the main action of B is to blacken embryos carrying it. But it may have a slighter effect in blackening bb embryos borne by zygotes carrying it. Fortunately, B can be scored unambiguously on flower color, but if it only affected seed color the genetic analysis would be very difficult. We must be prepared to find characters presenting this difficulty. Hogben ('31) thinks that in man blue sclerotics are due to a dominant gene of this type.

From the point of view of this paper certain evolutionary problems appear in a rather new light. As a general rule the embryos of related organisms are more alike than the adults. This merely means that the genes which determine interspecific differences mostly come into action rather late in the life cycle. The gill-clefts of embryo fish persist throughout life. Those of *Amniota* are transformed or disappear. The genes responsible for this difference must be present throughout the life-cycle, but only come into action during the stage Z2. The opposite is occasionally the case. The adult forms of many animals resemble one another more than the larval forms. Examples are the larva of *Unio* as compared with that of related salt-water mussels, the larvae of *Culex, Chironomus* and *Corethra,* and so on. These presumably differ by genes whose action is mainly confined to stage Z2.

There has been a common tendency in evolution for development to accelerate, *i.e.,* for certain characters to appear progressively earlier in the life cycle. Thus in the *Ammonoidea* complicated types of suture line first appear in the adult, and then progressively earlier in development. This presumably means that the time of first action of certain genes has tended to be pushed back from stage Z4 or Z3 to Z2 and Z1. Although the genes may have been somewhat modified in the course of ages, this seems a simpler hypothesis than that quite new genes arose which produced an effect similar to that of the ancestral genes, but at an earlier stage.

Another common tendency has been a retardation of certain characters relative to the life-cycle, so that originally embryonic characters persist in the adult. This is known as neoteny or sometimes paedogenesis. In a neotenic animal such as man many adult ancestral characters, *e.g.*, the straightening out of the cranial flexure, do not occur. Presumably the genes causing cranial flexure, which in most mammals are confined in their action to stages Z1 and Z2, act for longer in man. Or alternatively various genes which act in stage Z3 of most mammals have either been lost or never come into action in man.

These are of course well-known examples. But so far the existence of G, DG and DZ genes has been forgotten in their discussion. In acceleration Z3 genes come to act in stage Z2, in neoteny the opposite process occurs. The result is then the sudden appearance in an adult form of new characters, which have evolved in ancestral embryos. De Beer ('30) to whose book I am indebted throughout this paper, describes this process as clandestine evolution. I think that the same processes may have an even wider scope. G genes may come to act in stage Z1 and conversely. Z3 and Z4 genes may come to act in stages DG and DZ and conversely.

It is possible that some of the more mysterious of evolutionary phenomena may be explained in this way. Very early *Ammonoidea* such as the Devonian *Bactrites* were straight, and the inner whorls of its contemporary *Mimoceras* did not meet. These primitive forms were replaced by organisms with normally coiled shells. But in later periods of degeneration the shells of a number of genera were coiled during the early part of the life cycle, but later uncoiled. Such were the Triassic *Choristoceras* and *Rhabdoceras*, the Cretaceous *Lytoceras* and *Bactrites*. The general tendency in Ammonoid evolution had been to push back the action of genes from Z3 to Z2, and so on. I suggest that the gerontic straightness of degenerate forms was due to the pushing back of DZ genes governing embryonic development into the Z4 and Z3 stages. The adult *Bactrites* formed an uncoiled shell for the same reason that its ancestors formed a straight protoconch. The same argument could be applied to other cases where, after a long evolutionary history of acceleration, embryonic characters appear in the later stage of life-history.

The opposite process of caenogenesis may also perhaps occur in three ways, of which only the first has apparently been recognized. New Z1 or Z2 genes may appear. New DZ genes may appear. And finally Z3, Z4 or DG genes may come to act in stage DZ. We should expect the last to happen in connection with a general process of retardation. To take an example, Garstang ('28) has suggested that gastropod asymmetry began as a larval adaptation. We know that it is largely conditioned by DZ genes. These may have first appeared as such. But they may also have at first been Z3 or Z4 genes responsible for relatively trivial asymmetry in the adult or its cells, whose action was retarded in relation to the life-cycle, and thus came to produce larval asymmetry.

Whereas the change in time of action of a gene from Z2 to Z3, or conversely, presumably has effects which can at least be roughly predicted, this is not in general true for the changes from Z3 to DG or DZ, and conversely. Such changes are likely to lead to violent evolutionary novelties. A G or DG gene responsible for a lipase or protease in the spermatozoon might render uterine implantation possible for extending its action to cover stage Z1 or DZ. A DZ gene for rapid growth might cause malignancy if it came to act in stage Z4, and so on. The possibilities of clandestine evolution have probably been underestimated.

It may be objected that the above point of view is somewhat superficial. A DZ gene for shell straightness in an Ammonite, if its action were accelerated, would come into action of some kind, it might be urged, in the oocytes of the ovary, but not in the somatic cells responsible for shell form. I doubt if this objection can stand. Presumably during the life-cycle the protoplasm of the cells in the germ-track passes through a cycle of chemically definable stages, each being associated with a particular pattern of metabolism, and each being to a large extent the cause of the next. It is, however, possible, within certain limits, to alter the timing of one event relative to others, just as the time of ignition in an internal combustion engine may be altered relatively to the piston stroke. The cells lying off the germ-track seem to remain fixed for a long time in one stage of the cycle. If, however, other processes were accelerated in relation to meiosis, this might mean that not only oocytes, but somatic cells, passed into a chemical condition which had hitherto only been found in the embryo.

Acceleration or retardation can occur in two different ways. Thus in the case of acceleration the appearance or disappearance of one or many characters may occur at an earlier stage in the life-cycle in a descendant than in an ancestor. If only one or a few characters are concerned it is reasonable to suppose that the essential event was the acceleration of the action of the genes determining them (*e.g.*, the heart in birds or the horns in *Titanotheria*). But where the acceleration was general, as in certain lines of *Ammonoidea*, it is simpler to regard the process at work as a retardation of maturity in relation to other events. Such a retardation would of course allow DG and DZ genes to come into action before instead of after meiosis.

The reduction to vestiges of organs present in the adult ancestor and retained in the embryo (*e.g.*, notochord or pronephros) may often be due to acceleration. In some fish the notochord only ceases growing with the body as a whole. In other fish, and all *Amniota*, it ceases to grow (apart from cases of chordoma) in an embryonic stage. This may be due to the presence of inhibitory genes, or merely to a pushing backwards of the time of activity of some gene or genes involved in notochord growth. In view of the large number of other vestigial organs which have shared the notochord's fate, the latter hypothesis is perhaps simpler.

So with the retardation of the appearance or disappearance of characters. This is most usually part of the general phenomenon of neoteny, which can be regarded as due to accelerated maturity in some cases (paedogenesis) and general retardation of structural development in relation to maturity in others (*e.g.*, man). It probably occurs also for individual characters in the absence of any general neoteny, but I do not know of any clear examples of this.

In the evolutionary speculations of the last century hypermorphosis played an important part. The descendant was supposed to go through all the stages of its ancestor, and a final stage in addition. As de Beer ('30) and others have pointed out, many of the alleged examples of this process can be equally well explained by deviation. From the genetic point of view such a process involves one of two events. Either a large number of new genes must come into being which act in stage Z3 or Z4, and simultaneously maturity must be delayed; or, by a general acceleration, DG and DZ genes must come to act in stages Z3 or Z4. The former process is a complex one needing many simultaneous adjustments. It is difficult to believe that it has occurred very often. The latter would be simpler, but might lead to racial "second childhood."

Underlying all the above speculations is the tacit assumption that the same process may accelerate or retard the appearance or disappearance of the activity of a large number of genes at once. I believe that this is justifiable. In many cases genes seem to act, not directly, but by producing enzymes. Whether these latter can be effective depends on circumstances. For example, catalase is essential for the well-being of bacteria in presence of oxygen, but in its absence forms with and without catalase may do equally well. Koller ('30) found that rabbits with the gene E^D produced more (or a more resistant)

dioxyphenylalanine oxidase than EE rabbits. But the question whether or not this gene will have any visible effect depends on the presence or otherwise of the inhibitor G, which produces little effect on rabbits with E^D. Now enzymes depend particularly on the pH and salt content of their medium. The latter at any rate often varies greatly during development. The growing tadpole absorbs proportionately much more water than salts from its environment. This process will affect a whole group of enzymes (*e.g.*, amylase, fumarase and catalase) and have very little effect on others. Thus a change in permeability due to a single gene would affect the time of action of many others. The same substance may be required for several quite separate processes, *e.g.*, glutathione for oxidation (Hopkins and Elliott, '31) proteolysis (Waldschmidt-Leitz, Purr, and Balls, '30), and starch hydrolysis (Pringsheim, Borchardt, and Hupfer, '31). So the biochemical effects of one gene may accelerate or retard the action of a whole group of others.

Equally important is the fact that at least in vertebrates the development of many characters is conditioned by hormones, *e.g.*, thyroxin and various gonadic secretions. So several processes exist by which the time of action of a number of genes could be accelerated or retarded simultaneously.

The gradual acceleration or retardation of a number of genes will lead to orthogenetic evolution. In many cases, as Goldschmidt ('27) has pointed out, the sooner a gene starts work, the more it can do. So that selection for a character will not merely cause the spread through a population of genes directly causing that character, but of genes accelerating their action. These latter will probably accelerate the action of other genes as well, leading to apparently useless evolution.

Two types of selection can be mentioned which probably cause general acceleration and retardation, respectively. When a number of embryos or larvae are competing in a limited area, *e.g.*, embryos in a mouse uterus, or seedlings from seeds dropped by the same tree, rapid growth will commonly be of great selective value, and the slower growing individuals will be weeded out. There will be a tendency to cut short the period of intense competition, and to push back the first appearance of characters as early as possible. So Z2 genes will begin to act in stage Z1, Z3 in Z2 and so on. This will react on the adult form both by giving certain genes longer to act, and possibly by accelerating the action of DG or DZ genes.

On the other hand, where a larva or embryo is well adapted to its surroundings, and can go on growing in relatively slight danger, there will be a tendency to prolong the embryonic phase. Examples may be found in the human embryo, which rarely suffers from twin competition, and in a savage country may well be safer than a new-born baby, or the aquatic larvae of many insects, which are well adapted to their surroundings, and do not generally compete directly with one another. In such cases the appearance of adult characters may be delayed. Z2 genes will not begin to act till stage Z3, and so on. There will be a tendency to neoteny, and possibly a retardation of Z3 and Z4 genes to act in stages DG or DZ. This can of course be counterbalanced by intercalating, as in the holometabolous insect, a period of catastrophic metamorphosis, during which genes act with very great speed. This again may lead to unpredictable results. Genes particularly adapted to the chemical environment of the chrysalis will assume particular importance. Others will cease to have selective value. As the metamorphosis becomes more and more pronounced there will probably be a tendency to select, on the one hand, genes acting only at this time, on the other, genes whose action abruptly ceases then. The more the time of action of genes can be limited, the more the possibility of combining adaptation in the larva and adult.

In general the more limited is the period of action of a gene, the more unalloyed will be its benefits if it is useful at a certain period. There is no reason to suppose that the same type of polysaccharide is desirable in pollen and endosperm in maize, but so long as one gene controls both, the adaptation of the endosperm will be subordinated to that of the pollen grain, or conversely. The greater the difference in cell chemistry at different stages of the life-cycle the greater should be the possibility of limiting gene action. It would therefore seem that within limits natural selection will tend to make life-cycles more and more variegated, as every increase in complexity will increase the possibility of fixing the time of action of genes. Clearly there are limits to the process, but it may be a partial explanation of some of the apparently useless complexities of biology, such as the tendency of parasites to live in widely different hosts. We must consider the possibility that a liver-fluke is well adapted to its very different environments just because on changing from a diet of *Limnaea* to a diet of *Ovis* at a higher temperature, the chemical conditions in it are so changed as to allow a new set of genes to come into action, and it can thus possess two sets of genes, one acting in each host, and each capable of evolving in almost complete independence of the other.

Another way of fixing the time of action of genes is by elimination of part of the chromatin in somatic cells, as in *Ascaris* and *Miastor*. This method has, however, rarely been adopted. It must involve the localization together of all genes whose action is limited to an early stage of development, and are not essential later on. In view of the lack of correlation between the location of genes and their function, it is surprising that such elimination ever occurs, and intelligible that it is rare, although it is the mechanism which one would obviously adopt in designing a "synthetic animal."

We see, then, that the time of action of genes not only merits further study by the geneticist, but is essential for a detailed discussion of evolution.

Summary

(1) Genes can be classified according to their time of action. Not only can they act in diploid zygotes, endosperms or gametes carrying them, but their action can be manifested in the following organisms which do not carry them: mothers of zygotes carrying them, and gametes or embryos borne by zygotes carrying them. Their time of action is therefore distributed over more than one life-cycle.

(2) It is contended that change in the time of action of genes has been an important factor in evolution, and that some cases of orthogenesis, including degeneration, can be explained by it.

(3) In an organism undergoing metamorphosis the adaptive efficiency of a gene depends on the limitation in time of its action.

LITERATURE CITED

Beadle, G. W.
1930. "A Gene in Maize for Supernumerary Cell Divisions Following Meiosis." *Cornell Univ. Agr. Exp. Station Mem.* 135.

Boycott, A. E., C. Diver, S. L. Garstang and F. M. Turner
1931. "The Inheritance of Sinistrality in *Limnaea peregra*." *Phil. Trans. Roy. Soc. B*, 219: 51–131.

Brink, R. A. and F. A. Abegg
1926. "Dynamics of the Waxy Gene in Maize. I. The Carbohydrate Reserves of Endosperm and Pollen." *Genetics*, 11: 163–199.

Crane, M. B. and W. J. C. Lawrence
1929. "Genetical and Cytological Aspects of Incompatibility and Sterility in Cultivated Fruits." *J. Pomol. and Hort. Sci.*, 7: 276–301.

de Beer, G. R.
1930. "Embryology and Evolution." Oxford University Press.

East, E. M. and A. J. Mangelsdorf
1926. "Studies on Self-Sterility. VII. Heredity and Selective Pollen-tube Growth." *Genetics*, 11: 466–481.

Frost, H. B.
1928. "Chromosome-mutant Types in Stocks. II. Putting a Tramp Chromosome to Work." *J. Hered.*, 19: 105–111.

Garstang, W.
1928. "The Origin and Evolution of Larval Forms." *Rep. Brit. Ass. Adv. Sci. D.*

Goldschmidt, R.
1927. "Physiologische Theorie der Vererbung." Berlin, Springer.

Gregory, P. W. and W. E. Castle
1931. "Further Studies on the Embryological Basis of Size Inheritance in the Rabbit." *J. Exper. Zool.*, 59: 199–211.

Hopkins, F. G. and K. A. C. Elliott
1931. "The relation of Glutathione to Cell Respiration with Special Reference to Hepatic Tissue." *Proc. Roy. Soc. B*, 109: 58–87.

Hogben, L.
1931. "Genetic Principles in Medicine and Social Science." London (Williams and Norgate), pp. 62–65.

Koller, P.
1930. "On Pigment Formation in the D-black Rabbit." *J. Genet.*, 22: 103–109.

Lesley, M. M. and H. B. Frost
1927. "Mendelian Inheritance of Chromosome Shape in Matthiola." *Genetics*, 12: 449–460.

Mangelsdorf, P. C. and D. F. Jones
1926. "The Expression of Mendelian Factors in the Gametophytes of Maize." *Genetics*, 11: 423–455.

Muller, H. J. and F. Settles
1927. "The Non-functioning of the Genes in Spermatozoa." *Zeits. Abst. u. Vererb.*, 43: 285–312.

Nixon, R. W.
1928. "Immediate Influence of Pollen in Determining the Size and Time of Ripening of the Fruit of the Date-palm." *J. Hered.*, 19: 241–255.

Parnell, F. R.
1921. "Note on the Detection of Segregation by Examination of the Pollen of Rice." *J. Genet.*, 11: 209–212.

Pringsheim, H., H. Borchardt and H. Hupfer
1931. "Über Glutathion als Aptivator der fermentative Stärkeverzuckerung." *Biochem. Zeit.*, 238: 476–477.

Redfield, H.
1926. "The Maternal Inheritance of a Sex-limited Lethal Effect in *Drosophila melanogaster*." *Genetics* 11: 482–502.

Swingle, W. T.
1928. "Metaxenia in the Date Palm. Possibly a Hormone Action by the Embryo or Endosperm." *J. Hered.*, 18: 257–268.

Toyama, K.
1913. "Maternal Inheritance and Mendelism." *J. Genet.*, 2: 351–405.

Tschermak, E.
1931. "Über Xenien beim Leguminosen." *Zeit. f. Züchtung. A*, 16: 73–81.

Waldschmidt-Leitz, E., A. Purr and A. R. Bulls
1930. "Über der natürlichen Aktivator der Katheptischen Enzyme." *Naturwiss.*, 28: 644.

Wettstein, F. v.
1924. "Morphologie und Physiologie des Formwechsels der Moose auf genetische Grundlage. I." *Zeits. Abst. u. Vererb.*, 33: 1–236.

Reprinted from EVOLUTION, Vol. III, No. 1, March, 1949
Printed in U. S. A.

SUGGESTIONS AS TO QUANTITATIVE MEASUREMENT OF RATES OF EVOLUTION

J. B. S. HALDANE
Dept. of Biometry, University College, London

Received November 5, 1948

The best known recent work on rates of evolution is probably that of Simpson (1944), though Small's (1945, 1946) work on diatoms is more extensive. Small is concerned with the origin of species, which in this group seems to be a sudden or almost sudden process. Simpson compares evolutionary rates in different groups mainly by means of data on the origin and extinction of genera. Now among living animals and plants the distinction between genera is much less objective than that between species. On the other hand the paleontologist often finds it hard to be sure of differences less than generic. Moreover the criteria of generic distinction are certainly different in different groups. For example good systematists from Linnaeus onward have assigned the polecat (*Mustela putorius*) and the ferret (*Martes furo*) to different genera, while in fact they give quite fertile hybrids and are probably to be regarded as at most subspecifically different. On the other hand I know of no viable, let alone fertile, hybrids between animals assigned to different genera of Diptera or Amphibia. This sugests that animals are rather more readily placed in different genera among mammals than in some other classes. And in view of the incomplete character of the best fossil remains, the systematics of extinct animals are certainly less uniform than that of living ones.

On the other hand the dimensions of a solid organ, such as a tooth, a shell, or a bone, are often measureable with great precision; and when we have a series of fossil populations believed to form a lineage, we can calculate the rate of change of the mean value of any measure. In specifying a rate we must have scales for the time and for the character. From data on radioactivity we have a fairly precise measure of the duration of the whole tertiary period, and less accurate dates within it; and estimates of ten million years during this period are not likely to be out by much more than 25%. The precisely dated strata from earlier rocks are not so common. The error is likely to be a good deal greater in paleozoic or mesozoic marine deposits where we have continuous records over some millions of years, as in the English chalk or Lias. Here estimates of time may very well be out by a factor of 2, but are hardly likely to be so by a factor of 10.

As biologists we should like to be able to measure time in generations. In a fair number of insects the generation is exactly a year, in others there are two generations per year, and so on. Where generations overlap, as in most vertebrates, we can theoretically define a mean generation length exactly by definite integrals if we have life and fertility tables. In fact we can never do so for fossil forms. But we can be fairly sure that for a small rodent the mean generation length was less than a year, for most ungulates more so. For mammals not larger than a cow we may be fairly sure that it was under ten years. The longest mean interval between sexual generations is probably to be found in clonally propagated invertebrates such as corals, where it may possibly extend over centuries.

If evolutionary rates depend on mutation rates (which is doubtful), the year is as natural a unit as the generation. For it seems possible that the intensity of natural radiation produces a minimum mutation rate per unit of time which is often exceeded (as in *Drosophila*) but below which mutation cannot fall (Haldane, 1948). If however evolution depends more on selection, the generation seems the more suitable unit of time, though it is of course less accurate.

In the case of a metrical character the simplest and most accurate measurements are linear. Even if we have as few as ten specimens of an adult mammalian tooth we can often state their mean value with a standard error of as little as 2%. For an index, that is to say a ratio of lengths, the precision is often somewhat greater. If we wish to compare the rates of change of different organs, or of the same organ in different genera, it is clearly best to do so by comparing changes on a basis of percentage rather than absolute length. That is to say we shall do better to say that one bone length has increased by 10% and another by 20% in a million years than that one has increased by 1 cm and another by 30 cm.

Now suppose that in the time t the mean length of a structure has increased from x_1 cm to x_2 cm, the mean value of the proportional rate of change

$$\frac{1}{x}\frac{dx}{dt} \quad \text{or} \quad \frac{d}{dt}(\log_e x)$$

is

$$\frac{\log_e x_2 - \log_e x_1}{t}.$$

Thus if a tooth length doubles in ten million years, the natural logarithm increases by .693, and its mean length increases by a factor of $1 + .693 \times 10^{-7}$ per year, or with a 5-year generation, by $1 + 3.5 \times 10^{-7}$ per generation. The figure 7×10^{-8} can be regarded as a measure of its rate of evolution.

If our measures are made on mammalian adult teeth, the inner whorls of ammonites, or other structures not subject to growth or reabsorption, we can work with linear measures or more rarely areas or weights. If however we are concerned with vertebrate bones it will be better, where possible, to choose a measure of shape which does not change much with the age of the animal concerned. Where this is a ratio of lengths, such as a cranial index, matters are simple. Where it is an angle or an index of allometric growth, we shall meet with complications. Thus although our measure of evolutionary change would be the same if we measured our angle in degrees or radians, it would be altered if we measured the change in tan θ instead of θ. And in the case of the allometric equation $y = \beta x^\alpha$ it would be better to measure α rather than $\log_e \alpha$, since α is effectively a logarithm.

We may also take as our unit of change the increase or decrease of a mean value through one standard deviation of the character in question as determined from a population found at a single horizon. Such standard deviations are not so accurately known as the means. But since coefficients of variation of dimensions of homologous structures are generally nearly equal in related species, we can use this fact with some confidence when populations are too small for their variance to be determined accurately.

The use of the standard deviation as a yardstick has a certain interest because, on any version of the Darwinian theory, the variation within a population at any time constitutes, so to say, the raw material available for evolution. It must however be added that since the fossil record consists mainly of the hard parts of adults which have already undergone some natural selection, this selection will already have reduced their variance appreciably. It may be noted that if two fossils differ by more than about four times the standard deviation of the populations from which either is drawn they would be regarded as almost certainly derived from different species, on the basis of the metrical character under consideration alone.

Evolutionary Rates in Horses and Dinosaurs

Any measures of evolutionary rate made in this way will refer to particular metrical characters, and paleontologists are natu-

TABLE 1. *Mean annual rates of increase of two lengths and their ratio*

	Paracone	Ectoloph	Ratio
Hyracotherium-Mesohippus	3.6×10^{-8}	2.3×10^{-8}	1.3×10^{-8}
Mesohippus-Merychippus	10.0×10^{-8}	3.7×10^{-8}	6.3×10^{-8}
Mesohippus-Hypohippus	5.8×10^{-8}	4.4×10^{-8}	1.4×10^{-8}
Merychippus-Neohipparion	8.6×10^{-8}	0.8×10^{-8}	7.8×10^{-8}

rally most interested in those which are evolving most rapidly. Others however remain stationary over very long periods. For example the constants α and β in the allometric equation $y = \beta x^{\alpha}$, where x is a "horse's" skull length and y its preorbital length, did not change appreciably from *Hyracotherium* to *Equus*, while the ratio of lateral digit length to cannon bone length was also constant over the same range, except for one very abrupt change (Robb 1935, 1936).

Let us now evaluate some rates on these lines. I use the data of Simpson's (1944) table I concerning the paracone height and ectoloph length of unworn M^3 of five "horse" species, *Hyracotherium borealis, Mesohippus Bairdi, Merychippus paniensis, Hypohippus osborni*, and *Neohipparion occidentale*. I take the time intervals from *Hyracotherium* to *Mesohippus* to be 16 million years, from *Mesohippus* to *Merychippus* and *Hypohippus* 14 million years, from *Merychippus* to *Neohipparion* 5 million years. The first two figures, at least, are probably not more than 25% out.

The mean rates per year are given in table 1.

The calculation is as follows. In 16 million years the mean paracone height increased from 4.67 to 8.36 mm. The natural logarithms are 1.5412 and 2.1235. The rate is therefore $0.5823/16 \times 10^6$ or 3.6×10^{-8}. As Simpson points out, the ratio, which is a measure of hypsodonty, is the most interesting of the quantities considered, since it is likely to be little affected by a mere increase in the animals' size. All the evolutionary rates are positive in this case, but that of ectoloph length from *Merychippus* to *Neohipparion* is not significantly so on the samples quoted by Simpson. The figure 3.6×10^{-8} means that the paracone height increased on an average by 3.6% per million years, and so on. The median is about 4×10^{-8}.

The average length of a generation is unknown, but it can hardly have been less than 2 years in *Hyracotherium* nor more than 8 years in *Neohipparion*. To obtain the evolutionary rate per generation we must therefore multiply these figures by factors of 2 to 8, giving a median rate per generation of about 2×10^{-7}. The coefficient of variation of the tooth measurements was about 5% (4.6% to 6.2%) except in *Hypohippus* of which there were only 4 specimens with the high value of 14%. The coefficients of variation of the ratios varied between 2% and 4.5%, with a median value of 3.4%. If $100\,V$ is the coefficient of variation, the time taken to move the mean through one standard deviation is approximately[1]

$$\frac{Vt}{\log_e x_2 - \log_e x_1}.$$

[1] When the mean, x, moves through one standard deviation we may consider that x moves from $x = m$ to $x = m + \sigma x$ but $V = \frac{\sigma x}{m}$ by definition, hence $\sigma x = mV$, $m + \sigma x = m + mV = m(1 + V)$, hence x moves from m to $m(1 + V)$ and $\log_e x$ from $\log_e m$ to $\log_e m + \log_e (1 + V)$. Expanding $\log_e(1 + V)$ by Maclaurin's theorem we have:

$$\log_e(1 + V) = V - \tfrac{1}{2} V^2 + \tfrac{1}{3} V^3 - \tfrac{1}{4} V^4 + \cdots$$

Now as V is much less than one, V^2, V^3, V^4, etc. are very small numbers and we may safely write the approximation $\log_e (1 + V) = V$. The log of the mean thus moves through a distance V and as the time taken to move a given distance may be expressed as distance divided by rate, the above formula is obtained.

In the case of the evolution of the paracone of *Mesohippus* from *Hyracotherium*, the mean value of V is .055, so the time needed was 1.5×10^6 years or about half a million generations. Similar calculations could be made in the other cases, but this value is representative. About five times as long would be needed before a specific distinction could be made with confidence on the basis of a few metrical characters evolving at this rate, though of course if there were numerous diagnostic characters the time would be considerably less. Since the indices are less variable than the linear measurements, their rates of evolution, measured in standard deviations, are about as high as those of the linear measurements.

Data are given by Colbert (1948) on the increase in length of six suborders of Dinosaurs during the mesozoic era. The figures are taken from his graphs of figs. 4 and 5, and are probably rather less accurate than Simpson's data.

Suborder	Annual rate	Time in million years
Sauropoda	3.0×10^{-8}	35
Stegosauria	2.1×10^{-8}	30
Theropoda	2.0×10^{-8}	97
Ornithopoda	2.2×10^{-8}	60
Ankylosauria	0.26×10^{-8}	40
Ceratopsia	6.1×10^{-8}	22

Further among the Ceratopsia the mean rate of evolutionary length increase from *Protoceratops* to *Monoclonius* was 15×10^{-8} over 7 million years, from *Monoclonius* to *Triceratops* 1.7×10^{-8} over 18 million (the dates of *Triceratops* given in the two graphs are slightly different). These figures are slightly less than the figures for Equidae, with one exception. However a generation was probably considerably longer in the large dinosaurs at least than in the Equidae. Since Colbert's graphs are given on a basis of actual length, the increase of the Ceratopsians from 1.7 to 6.5 meters in 22 million years appears less impressive than that of the Sauropoda from 6 to 17 meters in 35 million years. On my reckoning he is fully justified in stressing the rapidity of their evolution.

Evolutionary Rates in Hominids

Another example may be taken from the evolution of our own species. Some workers regard *Sinanthropus* as a possible ancestor of *Homo*. Others think that more advanced forms typified by *Eoanthropus* were contemporaneous with *Sinanthropus* and nearer our ancestral line. If so the evolutionary rates were less, perhaps by a factor of 2, but hardly by a factor of 5, than those which may be calculated on the hypothesis that *Sinanthropus* was actually ancestral. Weidenreich (1943) gave a number of exact figures for linear measurements of skulls of *Sinanthropus pekinensis* and *Homo soloensis*, with more conjectural ones for cranial capacity.

The majority of measures of length do not differ significantly from those of *Homo sapiens*. Thus the mean maximum length (glabella to opisthocranion) is 193.6 mm in *Sinanthropus* and 185.6 in *H. sapiens*. The mean "maximum" breadths are given as 141.0 and 133.6 On the other hand the heights are very different. Unfortunately basibregmatic height in *Sinanthropus* can only be estimated from a reconstruction. But 4 heights (2 doubtful) of the opisthion above the Frankfurt horizontal averaged 104.6 as compared with 136.1 in *H. sapiens*, while 5 auricular heights above the same plane averaged 98.4 as compared with 113.5 in *H. sapiens*. The greater cranial capacity of *H. sapiens* is partly due to increased height and partly to reduction of the bone which leaves more room for the brain.

Since the sex of the *Sinanthropus* skulls is not known with certainty, it is not certain what figures for *H. sapiens* should be taken as comparable. It is better therefore to compare height-length indices, which are almost independent of sex and cranial capacity in modern man (Pearson and Davin, 1924). We find that the ratio of length to opisthion height has risen from .541 ± .013 to .736. There is another reason for choosing this index. Weidenreich gives it for *Pithecanthropus* (one skull), *Homo soloensis* (six skulls) and *H. neanderthalensis* (six skulls). The values are .521, .518, and .596. That is to say *Sinanthropus* was nearer to modern man in this respect than was *Homo soloensis,* although the latter is attributed to the upper Pleistocene. The difference of the natural logarithms of .541 and .736 is .3078. If with Zeuner (1946) we take the date of *Sinanthropus* as − 500,000, we obtain a mean annual evolutionary rate of -6.2×10^{-7} for the length/height index. Even if we supposed that the common ancestor of *Sinanthropus* and *Homo sapiens* lived in the upper pliocene a million years ago, and that since his separation from our ancestral stock the skull height of *Sinanthropus* had not increased at all, we should be left with the high annual rate of 3×10^{-7}.

If we use the standard deviation yardstick, we find that length/height indices have coefficients of variation of about 4% in modern populations, so the number of years needed to move through a standard deviation is about 70,000. But the most striking evidence of the rapidity of human evolution in this respect is obtained if we try to reckon time in generations. The age of human or sub-human puberty may have increased considerably in the last million years. But it is hard to suppose that the mean length of a generation, even of *Sinanthropus,* was much under 20 years. If we allow this very short period, the number of generations needed for the mean to change through a standard deviation is 3500, and only 7000 if we put back the equivalent stage in human evolution to a million years. This is to be compared with a minimum value of about 200,000 generations in the Equidae.

Standards of Evolutionary Change

I do not suggest that any particular weight should be given to this comparison. This would only be justified when quite a number of different structures had been compared, and particularly homologous structures in different lineages. However I believe that our knowledge both of absolute geological time and of some paleontological lineages is sufficient to allow many further calculations of this type to be made. It is equally clear that they can only be made satisfactorily by paleontologists. And it is likely that better indices of evolutionary rate can be made than any which I have suggested. It will be particularly important to characterize slow rates of evolution. Thus if a length or an index in a brachiopod line has not doubled or halved since the middle Cambrian, its annual evolutionary rate is less than 1.5×10^{-9}. It may be found desirable to coin some word, for example a *darwin,* for a unit of evolutionary rate, such as an increase or decrease of size by a factor of *e* per million years, or, what is practically equivalent, an increase or decrease of 1/1000 per 1000 years. If so the horse rates would range round 40 millidarwins, and rates much under a millidarwin would be hard to measure. Rates of one darwin would be exceptional in nature. But domesticated animals and plants have changed at rates measured in kilodarwins, though not megadarwins.

If the mean rate of change in linear measurements per generation is fairly often of the order of 10^{-7}, but rarely very much greater, we can draw some tentative conclusions. Genes are known in mammals which alter skeletal measurements by several per cent, without any obvious pathological effect. For example the gene b (brown) in mice increases body length by about 1.5% when homozygous (Castle, 1941). If genes with such a large effect played a part in the evolution of the Equidae, the substitution of such a gene for its allelomorph cannot have occurred more often than once per 300,000 years in the history of this family. It is more probable that most of the genes concerned had smaller effects.

Again the median figure of 4×10^{-8}

(40 millidarwins) for the Equidae implies that the means were increased by a standard deviation in about half a million generations. That is to say if selection was acting at much the same rates on most of the genes responsible for variation, a majority of them were replaced by allelomorphs in a few million generations. Such calculations are extremely rough, but they suggest the remarkably small order of magnitude of the selective "forces" which are at work if natural selection is largely responsible for evolution, and the extreme difficulty of demonstrating them in action. It is in no way surprising that progressive changes in gene frequencies in nature have only been observed in a few species. The fact that they have been observed at all is indeed probably only due to man's alteration of natural conditions.

The slowness of the rate of change also makes it clear that agencies other than natural selection cannot be neglected because they are extremely slow by laboratory standards or even undetectable during a human lifetime. The observed rates of mutation are quite large enough to account for evolutionary changes. Thus a mutation rate of 1 in a million at the brown locus in mice would, if unopposed, give a rate of change in the length of mice reaching a maximum of 7×10^{-9} per year, a quite substantial rate. The reason why most biologists do not believe in mutation as a driving force is because such a gene would be expected to confer a selective advantage or disadvantage of much more than one millionth; and therefore natural selection, rather than mutation, would decide the direction of evolution. We are not yet in a position to deny the possibility that under some environmental circumstances particular genes may mutate in nature with frequencies of 10^{-3} per generation, as a few genes do in cultivated plants, or that cytoplasmic changes of equal or greater rapidity may occur. Such rates cannot be frequent, or evolution would be quicker than it is. But they might determine the course of evolution in particular cases. It is premature to suggest that they do so, but not perhaps to suspect that they may.

I have to thank Mr. K. A. Kermack for valuable advice and criticism.

Summary

Suggestions are made for the measurement of evolutionary rates of metrical characters. The unit of time may be the year or the generation. The unit for the character may be a unit increase in the natural logarithm of a variate, or alternatively one standard deviation of the character in a population at a given horizon. Examples are given from mammalian paleontology of the calculation of such rates.

Literature Cited

Castle, W. F. 1941. Influence of certain color mutations on body size in mice, rats, and rabbits. Genetics, 26: 177–191.

Haldane, J. B. S. 1948. The formal genetics of man. Proc. Roy. Soc. B., 135: 147–170.

Pearson, K., and A. G. Davin. 1924. On the biometric constants of the human skull. Biometrika, 16: 328–363.

Robb, R. C. 1935, 1936. A study of mutations in evolution, Pts. 1–4. Journ. Genet., 31: 39–46, 47–52; 33: 267–273; 34: 477–486.

Simpson, G. G. 1944. Tempo and mode in evolution. Columbia University Press.

Small, J. 1945. Quantitative evolution. VII. The diatoms. Proc. Roy. Soc. Edin. B., 62: 128–131.

Small, J. 1946. Quantitative evolution. VIII. Numerical analysis of tables to illustrate the geological history of species number in diatoms; an introductory summary. Proc. Roy. Soc. Irish Acad., 51: B., 53–80.

Weidenreich, F. 1943. The skull of *Sinanthropus pekinensis*. Palaeontologica Sinica N.S. D. 10.

Zeuner, F. E. 1946. Dating the past. London, Methuen.

THE MEASUREMENT OF NATURAL SELECTION

by

J. B. S. HALDANE

Although nearly a century has elapsed since DARWIN and WALLACE formulated the theory of evolution by natural selection, it is remarkable that no agreement exists as to how it should be measured. Ideally we should wish to follow a sufficient number of members of every genotype (including gametes) of a species through a life cycle, and discover what advantages or disadvantages each possesses at every stage. This is clearly impossible. But it would also be insufficient. For natural or artificial selection acts on phenotypes. It is ineffective unless it favours one genotype at the expense of another. But it may occur without doing so. If we only breed from the heaviest 1% of members of a pure line, this intense artificial selection has no effect on the distribution of weights in the next generation. Nor would natural selection of comparable intensity have any effect. This is indeed the usual criterion for a pure line, though it may break down if there are strong maternal influences.

We must not judge the intensity of natural selection by its effect on the next generation, but by a comparison of the actual parents of the next generation with the population of which they are a sample, biassed by the very fact of selection. In this communication I shall only consider selection by differential mortality over a certain part of the life cycle, and I shall mainly be concerned with continuously variable metrical characters such as weight. How shall we measure the intensity of selection?

If, over the period considered, 10% of the population die, it is reasonable to assume that the intensity of natural selection cannot exceed 10%, or, if a logarithmic scale is used, $-\log_e(.9)$ or .1054. If all phenotypes and genotypes have the same mortality, we say that the deaths are entirely accidental, and there is no natural selection. If one phenotype has no mortality at all, but all the deaths occur in others, we say that the intensity of selection is .1054. If we can distinguish several phenotypes, there is an optimal phenotype, or set of phenotypes, of which a fraction s_o survives, while of the total population a smaller fraction S survives. If all the population had belonged to the optimal phenotype, then a fraction s_o of it would have survived. The extra mortality due to natural selection is $s_o - S$. I define the intensity of natural selection as $I = \log_e s_o - \log_e S$. For example if $S = .9$ and $s_o = .95$, that is to say 10% of the whole population dies, but only 5% of the optimal phenotype, then $s_o - S = .05$, and $I = .0541$. The two measures are nearly the same when death rates are small.

In practice we generally consider only one measurable character x, say weight at birth, at a time. We can then roughly determine the value of x for which the mortality is a minimum. This is not usually, if ever, an extreme value, and is often close to the mean. Within this optimal phenotype we could doubtless pick out a still more «favoured» phenotype, to use DARWIN'S word, by other criteria. For example ducks' eggs have an optimal weight, but within the group of optimal weight there is presumably a group with optimal water content, if this could be determined without killing the eggs, and so on. Similarly there is an optimal genotype.

This measure of the intensity of selection for a metrical character is quite different from that of LUSH (1953). If the mean value of x is the same in the survivors as in the original population, LUSH puts the intensity of selection as zero. This may be justifiable when artificial selection is being measured. It is not so in the case of natural selection, which may have no effect on the mean, while considerably reducing the variance.

In some cases full data are available which enable us to measure S and s_0. Thus KARN and PENROSE (1951) recorded the birth weights of 13,730 babies, and the fractions in various weight groups which survived the hazards of birth and of the first 28 days of life. I shall only consider their data on the 6693 females. The mortality rates for males were slightly higher. The overall survival S was $.959 \pm .002$. The survival for weights between 7.5 and 8.5 pounds was $.985 \pm .003$. It fell to $.414 \pm .037$ for babies weighing under 4.5 pounds, and to $.905 \pm .064$ for weights over 10 pounds. Although the latter figure does not differ significantly from the optimal survival, there is no doubt of the lower viability of heavy babies. Although the distribution of birth-weights is decidedly negatively skew, and that of the weights of the dead babies is even bimodal, the ratio of survivors to dead, when plotted against weight at birth, has a very nearly normal (Gaussian) distribution. For KARN and PENROSE's Fig. 3 shows that its logarithm, when plotted against birth weight, is well fitted by a parabola. That is to say if s_x is the fraction of babies of birth weight x which survives, $\frac{s_x}{1-s_x}$ gives a parabolic graph: and in the neighbourhood of the maximum value s_o, s_x gives a parabolic graph. The optimal survival s_o can be calculated with considerable accuracy, though the optimal birth-weight x_o is less precisely known. We find s_o = .9828, or very close to the survival frequency of the optimal group. That is to say only 1.7% of the babies would have died if all had been of the optimal weight, while, in fact 4.1% did so. Thus 58% of all the deaths were selective, on the sole criterion of weight, and the intensity of natural selection for weight was:

$$I = .0240 \pm .004.$$

These data do not, of course, show that any of the differences in weight were genetically determined. PENROSE (1953) has produced evidence that they depend to a considerable extent on the mother's genotype.

The effect of this natural selection on the population was to increase the mean birth weight from 7.06 to 7.13 pounds, that is to say by 1%, but to decrease the standard deviation of birth weights from 1.22 to 1.10, that is to say by 10%. Its effect in reducing the variance was therefore far greater than its effect in increasing the mean.

This appears to be true in every case where natural selection for a metrical character has been observed. A little of this selection against extremes may be due to the elimination of mutants. Thus the majority of human achondroplasic dwarfs result from recent mutation, and a large fraction of these die at birth or in the first month of life. But the intensity of natural selection on such a gene throughout the whole life cycle is less than the frequency in the population, and about equal to the mutation rate. Natural selection against achondroplasics contributes about 2×10^{-5} to KARN and PENROSE's value of .024, that is to say about one thousandth. I believe that a large fraction of the selection is of homozygotes for pairs of genes at loci where the heterozygous genotype is fitter than either homozygote. That is to say selection is not mainly counterbalancing the effects of mutation, but those of segregation.

It is possible to calculate the intensity I of natural selection even when the fraction S of survivors is unknown, provided that the distributions of x among the population originally at risk, and among the survivors, is known. For if the distribution fuction for the original popul-ation is $dF = f_1(x)dx$.

and that for the survivors is

$$dF = f_2(x)dx,$$

then the fraction surviving for any given value of x is

$$s_x = \frac{Sf_2(x)}{f_1(x)}.$$

Hence if x_0 is the optimal value of x, for which s_x is greatest,

$$I = \log_e f_2(x_0) - \log_e f_1(x_0).$$

In particular if x has a normal distribution among the original population and among the survivors, and their means are m_1, m_2, their standard deviations σ_1 and σ_2, then

$$I = \log_e\left(\frac{\sigma_1}{\sigma_2}\right) + \frac{(m_1 - m_2)^2}{2(\sigma_1^2 - \sigma_2^2)}.$$

If m_1 and m_2 do not differ significantly, the last term may be neglected. And where it is not negligible it may often be made so by a change in the scale of x, for example by taking logarithms.

RENDEL (1943) weighed 960 ducks' eggs of the N.P.I. breed. Of these 619 hatched, so S = .6448. The mean weight of the original population was 73.92 ± 0.23 gms., that of those which hatched was 73.78 ± 0.27 gms. The difference is insignificant. On the other hand the variance of weights was reduced from 52.72 ± 2.18 to 43.87 ± 3.02, which was highly significant. This gives I = .094. However, the distributions were both rather positively skew and leptokurtic. The distributions of the logarithms of the weights were much more nearly normal, and give I = .100 ± .032. In this case about 30% of the total deaths during the period considered were selective for weight. Many of the rest may have been selective for other measurable characters.

However RENDEL made similar observations at the same time on 930 eggs of the Allport breed. Here S was .6269, but s_0 was only .6445, and I only .0276, which is not significantly positive, though probably so. The variance was in fact reduced from 44.62 to 41.32, but the reduction was not significant at the 5% level.

WELDON (1901, 1904) and his pupil DI CESNOLA (1907) worked on snails as follows. The earliest formed whorls of a snail's shell are preserved in the adult. So if we make measurements on the shells of young snails, and on the early formed whorls of those adult snails, we can see whether natural selection has been occurring. WELDON proved that this had occurred, but could not measure its intensity. In *Clausilia laminata* he measured the distance from the apex to the external groove between two whorls at various angular distances measured backwards towards the apex from the point where the columellar distance from the apex was 5 millimetres. This gave him a shape parameter for the shell, measuring the increase in size with each successive coil.

He found that the mean values differed by less than 1% in 100 young snails and in the juvenile parts of 100 old ones. But the standard deviations were always less in the adults, on the average less by 11.4%. It follows that the intensity of natural selection for this character was about .12. DI CESNOLA's somewhat less consistent data for *Helix arbustorum* give a value of about .10 for I.

WELDON's sample of *Clausilia laminata* came from a fairly ancient German forest. When he repeated the work on a population of *Clausilia itala* from the citadel of Brescia, he found no evidence of natural selection. We now see that this could be explained if this population were very homogeneous genetically, being derived from one or a few individuals which had colonized the citadel. It would clearly be of great interest if an Italian biologist repeated this work, comparing the Brescia population with one less isolated.

A number of results of other workers are concordant with those here cited. We can, of course, apply the same methods to populations studied over the whole life cycle. Thus DOBZHANSKY (1953) described a population of *Drosophila pseudoobscura* which had reached equilibrium under laboratory conditions, and which was polymorphic for two chromosomal configurations, ST and CH. The relative fitnesses, or adaptive values, of $\frac{ST}{ST}$, $\frac{ST}{CH}$ and $\frac{CH}{CH}$ were as 0.90 : 1.00 : 0.41. If these fitnesses are as $1-h : 1 : 1-k$, it can easily be shown that under random mating the frequencies of the three genotypes at fertilization are:

$$\frac{k^2}{(h+k)^2},\quad \frac{2hk}{(h+k)^2},\ \text{and}\ \frac{h^2}{(h+k)^2}.$$

If selection were entirely by mortality before maturity, the extra deaths of homozygotes would be $\frac{hk^2}{(h+k)^2} + \frac{kh^2}{(h+k)^2}$ or $\frac{hk}{h+k}$. Since $h = 0.1$, $k = 0.59$, $\frac{hk}{h+k} = .0855$, and $I = .089$, a value close to those found above.

In fact much of the selection was for fertility rather than for viability. This makes no difference to the value of I arrived at. The fact that the value found is close to those found above by quite different methods suggests that DOBZHANSKY's results do not refer to a special case, but to a phenomenon which is occurring in many or most outbred populations.

It is entirely possible to apply WELDON's method, with suitable modifications, to populations of shells of fossil molluscs, such as ammonites, and thus perhaps to discover that natural selection was occurring in Palaeozoic times.

The interpretation of such data must vary in different cases. If, for example, as withy some of SALISBURY's (1943) data on plants, the larger individuals contribute up to 800 times more seeds than the smaller, this may well be (as he showed to be the case for *Dianthus prolifer*) because the differences in growth were mainly determined by soil differences. There is no reason to assume selection for genotypes making for large sized plants. On the other hand when the mean of parents, or of survivors, differs little from that of the original population, this kind of explanation is much less probable. It is difficult to suppose that the heavy babies or eggs, which had a higher death rate than those of the mean weight, were due to unfavourable environmental conditions, and it is reasonable to suppose that they were due to unfavourable genotypes, in these two cases maternal rather than individual. It is further reasonable to suppose that a good deal of the selection was not for weight as such, but for heterozygosity for genes at a number of loci which, among other things, control weight.

In all the cases considered selection reduced the variance, that is to say it was of the type described as stabilizing or normalizing. Probably almost all natural selection for a quantitative character is of this type. Even when the mean of x is appreciably higher in the parents of the next generation it is probable that selection occurs against very high values of x. This seems to be so in a good many cases of artificial selection. The individuals showing the selected character with the highest intensity are often weak or sterile. If this is so, natural selection, even when it is altering the genetic composition of a population, is probably usually weeding out homozygotes at a number of loci.

If a population is in equilibrium under selection for heterozygosis for genes at a number of loci, the mean value of a metrical character determinable in early life will not, in general, be quite the same in the parents of the next generation as in the population of which they are a sample biassed by natural selection, though it may not be very different. But this selective differential will not alter the genetical composition of the next generation.

The examples which I have discussed, apart from DOBZHANSKY's data, all refer to natural selection by differential survival over a fraction of the life cycle. It is theoretically possible that this selection could be reversed over another part of the life cycle. But this is improbable, as it would usually involve a bimodal distribution of fitness, such as could occur if, for example, a structural heterozygote were viable but infertile. But even among these few examples there were very great differences in the intensities of selection. In RENDEL'S case the difference was certainly due to genetical differences between the two populations. In WELDON'S it may have been.

Similar work could and should be done on a number of different human, animal, and plant populations, for example by following up the survival and fertility of some thousands of men measured at school or in the army, by measurements on fossil populations, by following the birds which hatched from eggs of different weights through a life cycle, and so on. Only when this has been done shall we have a satisfactory knowledge concerning phenotypic natural selection. Genotypic natural selection will, of course, be still harder to follow. At present we merely know that both of them occur. We know very little about their intensity.

SUMMARY

When any phenotypic character is measured or otherwise determined, there is usually an optimal phenotype, whose fitness, either over the whole life cycle or a portion of it, exceeds that of other phenotypes. The intensity of natural selection for the character in question is defined as the logarithm of the ratio of the fitness of the optimal phenotype to that of the whole population. This can sometimes be determined from frequency distributions, even when the actual fitnesses are unknown. The values found for the intensity of natural selection range from near zero to about 12%. In all cases natural selection reduces variance by weeding out extreme forms.

BIBLIOGRAPHY

DI CESNOLA A. P., 1907. — *A first study of natural selection in « Helix arbustorum »* (Helicogena). Biometrika, *5:* 387-399.

DOBZHANSKY T., 1953. — *Evolution as a creative process.* Proc. IXth Int. Gen. Congress (in press).

KARN M. N. & PENROSE L. S., 1951. — *Birth weight and gestation time in relation to maternal age, parity, and infant survival.* Ann. Eugen. *16:* 147-164.

LUSH J. L., 1953. — *Rates of genetic change in populations of farm animals.* Proc. IXth Int. Cong. Genetics (in press).

PENROSE L. S. 1953. — *Some recent trends in human genetics.* Proc. IXth Int. Cong. Genetics (in press).

RENDEL J. M., 1943. — *Variations in the weights of hatched and unhatched ducks' eggs.* Biometrika, *33:* 48-58.

SALISBURY E. J., 1943. — *The reproductive capacity of plants.* [Bell, London].

WELDON W. F. R., 1901. — *A first study of natural selection in* Clausilia laminata (*Montagu*). Biometrika. *1:* 109-124.

—, 1904. — *Note on a Race of* Clausilia itala (*von Martens*). Biometrika, *3:* 299-307.

Reprinted without change of pagination from the
Proceedings of the Royal Society, B, *volume* 145, pp. 303–308, 1956

The theory of selection for melanism in Lepidoptera

By J. B. S. Haldane, F.R.S.
Department of Biometry, University College, London

Dr Kettlewell's proof that the dark form *carbonaria* of *Biston betularia* has replaced the type, at least in part as the result of selection by bird predators, gives me the right to bring my calculation (Haldane 1924) on this matter up to date.

Assuming random mating, if the relative fitnesses of the genotypes CC, Cc and cc are as $1 : 1-k : 1-K$, and the gene frequencies are $pC+qc$, then the annual change in the value of p is

$$\Delta p = \frac{pq(kp-kq+Kq)}{1-2kpq-Kq^2}.$$

But K and k are not constants, even in a constant environment. They change with the frequency of other genes (or possibly plasmons). At present in industrial areas, K is positive and k nearly zero, since C is apparently fully dominant. However, on the genetic background of unpolluted areas, Cc is intermediate and k may be about $\frac{1}{2}K$ (Ford 1955).

Before industrial pollution began, C was a rare mutant, rendering the moth conspicuous to birds, and K and k were negative. If μ was the mutation rate of c to C, p was about $\frac{2\mu(1-K)}{k-K}$, or perhaps 3 or 4 times the value of μ, say 10^{-5}. If k is zero the final state in an industrial area would be given by $q^2 = \nu K^{-1}$, where ν is the rate of mutation of C to c. Thus q would be of the order of 10^{-2} to 10^{-3}, with one recessive per 10000 or per million. This, however, would not be achieved until after over $K^{-1}q^{-1}$ years, that is to say, several centuries or millennia, of selection. Dr Kettlewell tells me that at present about 1% to 10% of recessives are commonly found in industrial areas, so that $q = 0{\cdot}2$ approximately.

If $1-K = (1-k)^2$, that is to say, the fitness of the heterozygotes is the geometric mean of that of the homozygotes, the time needed for p to increase from 10^{-5} to 0·8 is $-\frac{11{\cdot}20}{\log_{10}(1-K)}$ years, or 37 years if $K = \frac{1}{2}$, as Kettlewell's Table 3 suggests. If $k = 0$ it is

$$\frac{4-(1-K)\ln 5}{K} - \frac{\ln(8\times 10^4)}{\ln(1-K)} \quad \text{(Haldane 1932)},$$

or 27 years if $K = \frac{1}{2}$. The effect of dominance is to double the rate of selection at first, but to slow it down greatly when recessives become rare.

I conclude, either that selection is usually much less intense than Kettlewell found, that immigration from unpolluted areas is important (which is unlikely) or that selection has slowed down for a reason which I consider.

It appears that during the last century genes have been selected which have no effect of *CC*, but make *Cc* nearly as dark as *CC*. Now such genes will only confer an advantage if they are present in *Cc* animals, and, as shown in the Appendix, the total number of *Cc* moths, on the hypotheses so far considered, will be of the order of 4 to 6 times the annual population at most, so the frequency of a modifying gene is unlikely to increase even twentyfold. On this hypothesis the selection of modifiers of heterozygotes cannot be explained.

A possible hypothesis is that heterozygotes are or were physiologically fitter than either homozygote. Ford (1940) showed that when partially starved, *Cc* survived better than *cc*. There is no evidence as to whether *Cc* is fitter than *CC*. If it is so, or was so for a number of years, then we can suggest that the primary selective process in the more polluted industrial areas was complete by about 1890, leading to a balanced polymorphism with $p = 0{\cdot}86$ or some neighbouring value, giving about 74 % *CC*, 24 % *Cc*, 2 % *cc* at hatching. If the fitness of *cc* was $\frac{1}{2}$ that of *Cc*, as Kettlewell's results suggest, that of *CC* would have been about 92 % that of *Cc*. In this case selection has had a reasonable opportunity of favouring genes which increase the dominance of *C*. It should be possible to test this hypothesis, at least on genetic backgrounds where *C* is not fully dominant.

I wish then to emphasize that the problem is not yet fully solved, and that numerical calculations of the type here given are of a certain value if only as suggesting further experiments.

References (Haldane)

Ford, E. B. 1940 *Ann. Eugen., Lond.*, **10**, 227–252.
Ford, E. B. 1955 *Moths*. London: Collins.
Haldane, J. B. S. 1924 *Trans. Camb. Phil. Soc.* **23**, 10–41.
Haldane, J. B. S. 1932 *Proc. Camb. Phil. Soc.* **28**, 244–248.

Appendix (Haldane)

The selection of modifiers of heterozygotes

Consider any case of transient polymorphism, where a population passes from being almost all *cc* to being almost all *CC* under the influence of selection. In each generation there is a fraction h of heterozygotes. We ask what is the total value H of all these fractions? For only if H is fairly large will natural selection have much opportunity to increase the frequency of genes which are only of value in so far as they act on heterozygotes, by increasing the dominance of *C* or otherwise. For example, if $H = 10$, such genes will only have increased as much as they would have done had selection acted on a population consisting entirely of *Cc* during 10 years. I neglect the small numbers of heterozygotes kept in being by mutation before and after the change.

Let the relative fitnesses of CC, Cc and cc be as $1:1-k:1-K$, where $K>k>0$, and let q be the frequency of c in a random mating population. Then if K is small $dq/dt = -q(1-q)(k+Kq-2kq)$ approximately, taking the generation as the unit of time. If K is not small the rate is somewhat greater, so H will be less than the number here calculated. The total fraction of heterozygotes is approximately

$$\begin{aligned} H &= \int_0^\infty 2q(1-q)\,dt \\ &= \int_0^1 \frac{2dq}{k+Kq-2kq} \\ &= \frac{2}{K-2k}\ln\left(\frac{K-k}{k}\right) \quad \text{if } K>2k \\ &= \frac{2}{2k-K}\ln\left(\frac{k}{K-k}\right) \quad \text{if } K<2k \\ &= \frac{4}{K} \quad \text{if} \quad K=2k. \end{aligned}$$

Putting $k=\lambda K$, where $1>\lambda>0$

$$\begin{aligned} H &= \frac{2\ln\left(\frac{1-\lambda}{\lambda}\right)}{(1-2\lambda)K} \quad \text{if} \quad \lambda<\tfrac{1}{2} \\ &= \frac{2\ln\left(\frac{\lambda}{1-\lambda}\right)}{(2\lambda-1)K} \quad \text{if} \quad \lambda>\tfrac{1}{2} \\ &= 4K^{-1} \quad \text{if} \quad \lambda=\tfrac{1}{2}. \end{aligned}$$

H has a minimum when $\lambda=\frac{1}{2}$, and becomes infinite when $\lambda=1$ or 0. However, even if λ is near to 1 or 0, H is not very large. Thus if $\lambda = 0{\cdot}1$ or $0{\cdot}9$,

$$H = 5\ln 3K^{-1} = 5{\cdot}5K^{-1}.$$

Let us investigate the infinite values of H which arise when $k=0$, or $k=K$, that is to say, dominance is complete. Suppose C to be completely dominant, so that $k=0$, but the final value of q is Q, where Q is small but not zero. Then

$$\begin{aligned} H &= -\int_Q^1 \frac{2dq}{Kq} \\ &= -2K^{-1}\ln Q. \end{aligned}$$

Thus if $Q=0{\cdot}1$, giving 1 % of recessives, $H=4{\cdot}6K^{-1}$. However, this case does not concern us, for if k is zero there is no selective pressure tending to select modifiers of heterozygotes.

Now if a modifier M present in a small fraction x of the gametes increases the fitness of Cc from $1-k$ to unity, then $\Delta x = 2kq(1-q)x(1-x)$ approximately. That is to say, x is increased by a factor of approximately $1-2kq(1-q)$ or $1+kh$. If x is not small the increase is less. So during the whole selective process, x will be increased by about e^{kH}. This is e^2 when $\lambda = \frac{1}{2}$, and in general $\left(\frac{1-\lambda}{\lambda}\right)^{2\lambda/(1-2\lambda)}$ or $\left(\frac{\lambda}{1-\lambda}\right)^{2\lambda/(2\lambda-1)}$. The value rises from 1·73 when $\lambda = 0{\cdot}1$ to 7·39 when $\lambda = 0{\cdot}5$, 27 when $\lambda = 0{\cdot}75$, and 140·3 when $\lambda = 0{\cdot}9$. However, if λ were initially 0·5 except in the presence of a rare modifying gene, a twenty-fold increase in the frequency of the modifier might raise it to 0·6, if the frequency of the modifier rose from 1 to 20 %. But this would not greatly accelerate the selection of the modifier. I conclude that it is improbable that the frequency of a modifier would increase as much as 20 times, though it might increase 10 times.

The above calculations are only based on the selection of a rare gene with full dominance as a modifier. The process would be slower if the modifier were not rare or not dominant.

The relation between density regulation and natural selection

By J. B. S. Haldane, F.R.S.

Department of Biometry, University College, London

Darwin (1859) introduced the notion of natural selection by showing that if the density of a species is to remain steady, most of the individuals in each generation must die prematurely. Nicholson (1954) has analyzed the factors determining the density of a species in great detail. Haldane (1953) did so more summarily. It is simplest to consider annual plants or animals. Their increase or decrease from one year to another is a function, among other things, of their density. A factor which leads to increase as the density increases is called density-disturbing (Nicholson), or positive density-dependent (Haldane). Such factors include all forms of mutual aid, from the mutual protection of trees from storms and the greater ease of finding mates if the population is not too sparse, to various forms of social behaviour. Density-regulating (Nicholson) or negative density-dependent (Haldane) factors include all forms of competition, including competition for food and space, and disease facilitated by overcrowding. Other factors, which Nicholson calls density-legislative and density-inactive, are independent of density. Examples are the effects of heat and cold, in so far as they are not modified by competition or co-operation.

Clearly at high densities some negative density-dependent factor must come into action, or density would increase indefinitely. Positive density-dependent factors may be important at low densities. If so there may be an unstable equilibrium, and populations which fall below it decrease further and die out, for example, sessile bisexual or self-sterile organisms with juvenile dispersal. They always make for instability of equilibrium. Negative density-dependent factors may do so if their effect increases very sharply with density, or if it is delayed (Nicholson & Bailey 1935).

All these factors are, or may be, agents of natural selection. Parasitism is the main negative density-dependent factor regulating the density of many insect species. If so, as Nicholson & Bailey showed, other adverse factors may actually cause the population density to increase. For example, increased predation of larvae by birds, provided the same fraction of parasitized and unparasitized larvae are killed, will cause an increase of density if the parasite is fairly specific, so that predation diminishes its numbers nearly as much as those of the host. A gene causing cryptic coloration of larvae and thus protecting them from predators will spread through a population as the result of natural selection. It will, however, lower the population density in areas or in years where, owing to high density, parasites are the main controlling factor. But it will raise the population density in areas where, owing to density-independent factors, the population is sparse.

The range of a species includes many types of habitat. But it can roughly be divided into favourable areas where the density is high, and from which, on the whole, there is emigration, and unfavourable areas of low density into which there is, on balance, immigration. The latter will usually include the marginal geographical areas such as the hottest and coldest in which the species is found. In these marginal areas selection is mainly against density-independent factors such as frost, and in favour of positive density-dependent factors such as sexual recognition at a distance or self-fertility. In the central areas selection is against density-dependent factors such as disease and the effects of various kinds of competition, and of course against the local density-independent factors.

But just because there is a net migration from central to peripheral areas, adaptation in the latter must be incomplete. If there are adequate geographical barriers, or if a species is sufficiently immobile, it may break up into subspecies, some of which are potentially new species. Let me take a concrete example. Several moth species such as *Peridroma saucia* and *Agrotis ypsilon* winter over in southern England. But large numbers occasionally migrate from the south. This must make it hard or impossible for a race adapted to our climate to establish itself. If the English Channel were as broad as the Straits of Mozambique, rare migrants might have given rise to a local race or subspecies.

Matthew (1926) observed that contemporaneous species of *Hipparion* could be advanced in their dentition or their leg skeleton, but not in both. A species which had made both advances would presumably have eliminated all its competitors. Kermack (1954) similarly found that in a fossil echinoid population, characters which were found together in populations some million years later were negatively correlated. It was presumably impossible or at least difficult to achieve both in the same organism with the available genes.

Applying the Matthew–Kermack principle to an existing species, it appears that selection in the central areas for protection against density-dependent factors must make it difficult to achieve the resistance to density-independent factors which is needed in the peripheral areas. The converse tendency may operate to some extent, as there is often some migration back into the central areas.

If a species is insufficiently mobile it will be unable to exist in areas where the birth-rate does not suffice to balance the death-rate. If it is too mobile there will be no chance for specialization to develop in such areas. This is just one of the conflicts between opposing tendencies which must be, and have been, overcome in the course of evolution, but which have slowed down evolution.

But, owing to the net direction of population flow, a species must, I think, usually tend to be overadapted to conditions in the area where its density is greatest, including negative density-dependent factors, and underadapted to conditions where it can barely hold its own, but which it could conquer with the aid of new adaptations.

References (Haldane)

Darwin, C. 1859 *The origin of species.* London: Murray.

Haldane, J. B. S. 1953 *New Biol.* **15**, 9–24.

Kermack, K. A. 1954 *Phil. Trans.* B, **237**, 375–428.

Matthew, W. D. 1926 *Quart. Rev. Biol.* **1**, 139–185.

Nicholson, A. J. 1954 *Aust. J. Zool.* **2**, 9–65.

Nicholson, A. J. & Bailey, V. A. 1935 *Proc. Zool. Soc. Lond.* (3), pp. 551–598.

PRINTED IN GREAT BRITAIN AT THE UNIVERSITY PRESS, CAMBRIDGE
(BROOKE CRUTCHLEY, UNIVERSITY PRINTER)

[From JOURNAL OF GENETICS, Vol. 54, No. 1,
pp. 56–63, January 1956.]

THE CONFLICT BETWEEN INBREEDING AND SELECTION
I. SELF-FERTILIZATION

By J. B. S. HALDANE
Department of Biometry, University College, London

(With One Text-figure)

On the whole, inbred populations become more homozygous in successive generations. But occasionally heterozygosis is preserved, either at a locus or for a pair of chromosomal orders, permanently or for longer than would be expected unless heterozygotes were at a great advantage. Hollingsworth & Maynard Smith (1955) give an example.

Hayman & Mather (1953) have discussed this question. However, their principal results appear to me to be incorrect, and they have only considered a very few of the ways in which selection may act. It is therefore desirable to deal with the matter afresh.

In any system of complete inbreeding, as opposed to inbreeding varied by an occasional outcross, the population is divided into a number of lines. In each generation a line is represented by one or more individuals, one in the case of self-fertilization, two in that of sib-mating, and so on. It is convenient to consider a population consisting of a fairly large and constant number of lines. In fact this number is often far from constant in practice. Thus Hollingsworth & Maynard Smith inform me that in their O line the number of pairs set up per generation between F_2 and F_{17} varied irregularly from 13 to 55, with mean 24·6.

It is theoretically possible to keep the number of lines constant, breeding from only one individual, pair, trio, etc., of each line in each generation, provided the depression due to inbreeding is not too severe. In this case there is no selection between lines. More usually some lines die out owing to inbreeding depression, or are discarded either because they show signs of weakness or sterility, or because they do not conform to some desired standard (Fig. 1). In this case there is voluntary or involuntary selection between lines.

In this series of papers I shall mainly consider selection acting on a single pair of alleles at one locus, or on a pair of alternative chromosome orders. Either may be denoted by A and a. It is not assumed that a is recessive. Selection is supposed to favour Aa at the expense of one or both homozygotes, but this selection is assumed not to be complete, as it can be when heterozygotes can be picked out with certainty, or in the case of balanced lethals. I shall also neglect mutation, which I have considered earlier (Haldane, 1936).

It follows that in every line there is in each generation a finite chance that the next generation will consist entirely of like homozygotes. This is not necessarily so if numerous alleles or chromosome orders are present in a population. For example, the mating $a^1a^2 \times a^3a^4$ cannot give rise to homozygotes. But a line consisting of like homozygotes will always give rise to like homozygotes. Hence no amount of selection within lines can prevent the population from ultimately consisting of homozygotes in the case of self-fertilization, and of sets of like homozygotes in the more complicated cases. It may of course slow this process down considerably.

If, however, there is selection between lines, there are two possibilities. The homozygous, or like homozygous, lines may die out or be discarded so rapidly, and the heterozygous, or partly heterozygous, lines expanded so rapidly, that heterozygosis never disappears. Or the heterozygotes may ultimately disappear, as with selection within lines. There will be a critical value of selection for which heterozygotes just disappear, as Hayman & Mather pointed out.

However, this critical value is a little deceptive. Supposing that we were keeping twenty-five lines in each generation, some being discarded, and others split into two or more, and that calculation showed that in a large number, N, of lines $0{\cdot}08N$ would be expected to remain wholly or partly heterozygous. We should expect two out of twenty-five to remain so. But if so the probability of finding no heterozygous or partly hetero-

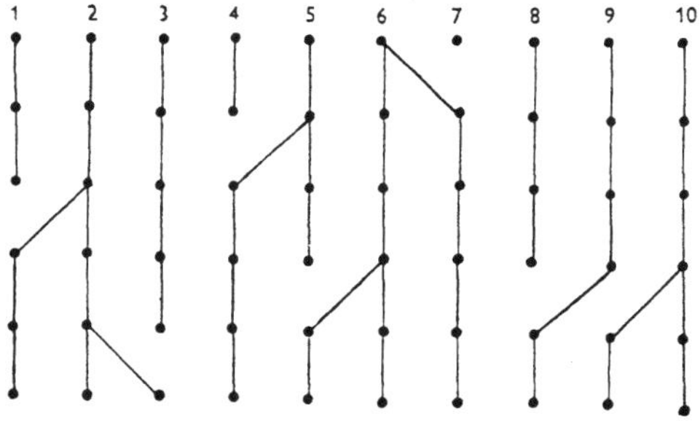

Fig. 1. Hypothetical diagram of selection between lines. Ten selfed individuals or mated sib pairs are grown in each generation, represented by the points. But lines 1, 3, 4, 7 and 8 are extinguished, while line 10 is finally represented by two lines, and lines 2 and 6 by three lines each.

zygous lines would be $(0{\cdot}92)^{25}$, or $0{\cdot}12$. Thus in the course of time heterozygotes would be bound to disappear. In fact, therefore, homozygosis is ultimately achieved with intensities of selection well below the critical values calculated. I shall neglect this complication in what follows. In consequence the results are only valid in the case of selection between lines if the number of lines is pretty large.

The present paper deals entirely with self-fertilization. I suppose that, in the nth generation, the breeding population consists of: $Nx_n\,AA$, $Ny_n\,Aa$, $Nz_n\,aa$, with $x_n+y_n+z_n=1$, where N is large, but not necessarily constant. As measures of selection I use k and l, which correspond with Hayman & Mather's parameters $1-x$ and $1-y$.

SELECTION WITHIN LINES ONLY

Suppose that in a progeny from Aa selfed, AA and aa are at disadvantages given by k and l. Then the probabilities that AA, Aa and aa will be the genotype of the next parent in a heterozygous line are not $\frac{1}{4}$, $\frac{1}{2}$ and $\frac{1}{4}$, but

$$\frac{1-k}{4-k-l},\quad \frac{2}{4-k-l}\quad \text{and}\quad \frac{1-l}{4-k-l}.$$

On the other hand, *AA* and *aa* lines are at no disadvantage. k and l are assumed to be positive, but cannot exceed unity. Then

$$\left.\begin{aligned} x_{n+1}&=x_n+\frac{(1-k)\,y_n}{4-k-l},\\ y_{n+1}&=\frac{2y_n}{4-k-l},\\ z_{n+1}&=z_n+\frac{(1-l)\,y_n}{4-k-l}.\end{aligned}\right\} \qquad (1)$$

Clearly $y_n=\left(\frac{2}{4-k-l}\right)^n y_0$. So since it is assumed that both k and l are not unity, that is to say, that homozygotes of at least one sort have a chance, heterozygotes ultimately disappear. Also

$$\begin{aligned} x_n&=x_0+\frac{1-k}{4-k-l}(y_0+y_1+y_2+\dots+y_{n-1})\\ &=x_0+\frac{1-k}{2-k-l}\left[1-\left(\frac{2}{4-k-l}\right)^n\right]y_0.\end{aligned}$$

The population therefore tends to an equilibrium given by

$$\left.\begin{aligned} X&=x_0+\frac{(1-k)\,y_0}{2-k-l},\\ Y&=0,\\ Z&=z_0+\frac{(1-l)\,y_0}{2-k-l}.\end{aligned}\right\} \qquad (2)$$

And in the nth generation

$$\left.\begin{aligned} x_n&=X-\frac{1-k}{2-k-l}\left(\frac{2}{4-k-l}\right)^n y_0,\\ y_n&=\left(\frac{2}{4-k-l}\right)^n y_0,\\ z_n&=Z-\frac{1-l}{2-k-l}\left(\frac{2}{4-k-l}\right)^n y_0.\end{aligned}\right\} \qquad (3)$$

SELECTION BETWEEN LINES ONLY

I next suppose that there is no selection within each progeny of a self-fertilized heterozygote, but that there is selection between lines. This could occur, for example, if *A* and *a* had no effect on viability, but the *Aa* plants were, on an average, somewhat superior to *AA* and *aa* as regards an economically important character. I suppose that an *AA* line has only $1-k$ times the chance of a segregating line of being perpetuated, and an *aa* line $1-l$ times the chance. Some homozygous lines are discarded in each generation, and some heterozygous lines split. This is what happens in the early stages of wheat breeding, though there is usually selection within lines also. In fact k and l probably tend to increase with time, since as other loci become homozygous, it is easier to pick out Aa lines. I neglect this complication. We find

$$\left.\begin{aligned} x_{n+1} &= \frac{(1-k)\,x_n + \frac{1}{4}y_n}{1 - kx_n - lz_n}, \\ y_{n+1} &= \frac{\frac{1}{2}y_n}{1 - kx_n - lz_n}, \\ z_{n+1} &= \frac{(1-l)\,z_n + \frac{1}{4}y_n}{1 - kx_n - lz_n}. \end{aligned}\right\} \tag{4}$$

Now suppose that at equilibrium the frequencies are X, Y and Z. Then if $Y \neq 0$, $1 - kX - lZ = \frac{1}{2}$, from the second of equations (4), or $kX + lZ = \frac{1}{2}$. Hence the first of equations (4) becomes $X = 2(1-k)X + \frac{1}{2}Y$, or $X = \dfrac{Y}{2(2k-1)}$. Similarly $Z = \dfrac{Y}{2(2l-1)}$. This implies that $k > \frac{1}{2}$, $l > \frac{1}{2}$. Hence

$$\begin{aligned} 1 &= X + Y + Z \\ &= \left[\frac{1}{2(2k-1)} + 1 + \frac{1}{2(2l-1)}\right] Y. \end{aligned}$$

The equilibrium frequencies are thus

$$\left.\begin{aligned} X &= \frac{2l-1}{2(4kl-k-l)}, \\ Y &= \frac{(2k-1)(2l-1)}{4kl-k-l}, \\ Z &= \frac{2k-1}{2(4kl-k-l)}. \end{aligned}\right\} \tag{5}$$

Next suppose that $l > \frac{1}{2}$, but $k < \frac{1}{2}$, that is to say, that there is strong selection against aa, but not very strong against AA. The only possible equilibrium is $X = 1$, $Y = 0$, $Z = 0$, that is to say, the whole population comes to consist of AA. If $k < \frac{1}{2}$ and $l < \frac{1}{2}$, heterozygotes first disappear, and then the less fit homozygote.

The progress towards homozygosis can readily be calculated in the artificially simple case where $l = k$. If so

$$1 - kx_n - kz_n = 1 - k + ky_n.$$

Hence from (4)

$$y_{n-1} = \frac{y_n}{2(1-k) + 2ky_n}. \tag{6}$$

This is a non-linear equation, and we cannot hope, save in exceptional cases, to obtain linear equations describing selection. It is, however, readily soluble. For

$$\frac{1}{y_{n-1}} = \frac{2(1-k)}{y_n} + 2k.$$

So

$$\frac{1}{y_{n-1}} + \frac{2k}{1-2k} = 2(1-k)\left(\frac{1}{y_n} + \frac{2k}{1-2k}\right).$$

and

$$\frac{1}{y_n} + \frac{2k}{1-2k} = (2-2k)^n\left(\frac{1}{y_0} + \frac{2k}{1-2k}\right).$$

Hence
$$
\left.\begin{aligned}
y_n &= \frac{(1-2k)\,y_0}{(2-2k)^n(1-2k+2ky_0)-2ky_0} \quad \text{if} \quad k<\tfrac{1}{2},\\
&= \frac{(2k-1)\,y_0}{2ky_0+(2-2k)^n(2k-1-2ky_0)} \quad \text{if} \quad k>\tfrac{1}{2},\\
&= Y - \frac{(2k-1)(2-2k)^n(2k-1-2ky_0)}{2k[2ky_0+(2-2k)^n(2k-1-2ky_0)]} \quad \text{if} \quad k>\tfrac{1}{2}.
\end{aligned}\right\} \tag{7}
$$

Another simple case occurs if $l=1$, that is to say, no *aa* plants are bred from. In practice the progeny of plants segregating for *aa*, that is to say, of *Aa* plants, would probably be discarded also. However, the case is perhaps worth working out. Equations (4) become $z_n=0$, $x_n+y_n=1$, and $y_{n+1}=\dfrac{y_n}{2(1-k)+2ky_n}$. Hence equation (7) holds in this case also.

The general case is only a little more difficult. I write equations (4) as

$$
\left.\begin{aligned}
4u_nx_{n+1} &= 4(1-k)x_n+y_n,\\
2u_ny_{n+1} &= y_n,\\
4u_nz_{n+1} &= 4(1-l)z_n+y_n.\\
u_n &= 1-kx_n-lz_n.
\end{aligned}\right\}
$$

From the last of these equations

$$
\begin{aligned}
u_n &= 1-kx_n-l(1-x_n-y_n)\\
&= 1-l-(k-l)x_n+ly_n,
\end{aligned}
$$

or

$$
\begin{aligned}
(k-l)x_n &= ly_n+1-l-u_n\\
&= ly_n+1-l-\frac{y_n}{2y_{n+1}}.
\end{aligned} \tag{8}
$$

Substituting in the first equation

$$
(k-l)y_n+4(1-k)\left(ly_n+1-l-\frac{y_n}{2y_{n+1}}\right)-\frac{2y_n}{y_{n+1}}\left(ly_{n+1}+1-l-\frac{y_{n+1}}{2y_{n+1}}\right)=0,
$$

or $$(k+l-4kl)y_{n+2}y_{n+1}y_n+4(1-k)(1-l)y_{n+2}y_{n+1}-2(2-k-l)y_{n+2}y_n+y_{n+1}y_n=0.$$

Hence
$$
\frac{1}{y_{n+2}}-\frac{2(2-k-l)}{y_{n+1}}+\frac{4(1-k)(1-l)}{y_n}+k+l-4kl=0 \tag{9}
$$

If
$$
\frac{1}{y_n}=t_n+\frac{4kl-k-l}{(2k-1)(2l-1)},
$$

then
$$
t_{n+2}-2(2-k-l)t_{n+1}+4(1-k)(1-l)t_n=0.
$$

Hence
$$
t_n=A(2-2k)^n+B(2-2l)^n.
$$

Substituting the values of t_0 and t_1 we find

$$
\begin{aligned}
A &= \frac{x_0}{y_0}+\frac{1}{2(1-2k)},\\
B &= \frac{z_0}{y_0}+\frac{1}{2(1-2l)}.\\
y_n &= 2(2k-1)(2l-1)y_0[2(4kl-k-l)y_0-(2-2k)^n(2l-1)\{y_0-2(2k-1)x_0\}\\
&\qquad -(2-2l)^n\{y_0-2(2l-1)z_0\}]^{-1}.
\end{aligned} \tag{10}
$$

The expressions for x_n and z_n are readily found from (8). The difference from the equilibrium value soon approximates to a geometric series whose common ratio, if $l > k$, is $(2-2k)$ if $k > \frac{1}{2}$, and $(2-2k)^{-1}$ if $k < \frac{1}{2}$. I have given this calculation in what is perhaps needless detail, as others have clearly found it difficult.

SEED SELECTION

Let us next suppose that seeds are sown at random, and the relative fitnesses of AA, Aa and aa are $1-k:1:1-l$. This appears to correspond to Hayman & Mather's hypothesis, and is also an approximation to what might happen in nature, though rarely under artificial conditions. We find

$$\left.\begin{aligned} u_n x_{n+1} &= (1-k)(x_n + \tfrac{1}{4}y_n), \\ u_n y_{n+1} &= \tfrac{1}{2}y_n, \\ u_n z_{n+1} &= (1-l)(z_n + \tfrac{1}{4}y_n), \\ u_n &= 1 - k(x_n + \tfrac{1}{4}y_n) - l(z_n + \tfrac{1}{4}y_n). \end{aligned}\right\} \quad (11)$$

At equilibrium, provided Y is not zero, $U = \frac{1}{2}$. So

$$2(2k-1)X = (1-k)Y \quad \text{or} \quad X = \frac{(1-k)Y}{2(2k-1)},$$

and similarly

$$Z = \frac{(1-l)Y}{2(2l-1)}.$$

This implies that $k > \frac{1}{2}$, $l > \frac{1}{2}$. Hence

$$\tfrac{1}{2} = 1 - \frac{kY}{4(2k-1)} - \frac{lY}{4(2l-1)},$$

from the last of equations (11); and at equilibrium, if $k > \frac{1}{2}$, $l > \frac{1}{2}$,

$$\left.\begin{aligned} X &= \frac{(1-k)(2l-1)}{4kl-k-l}, \\ Y &= \frac{2(2k-1)(2l-1)}{4kl-k-l}, \\ Z &= \frac{(1-l)(2k-1)}{4kl-k-l}. \end{aligned}\right\} \quad (12)$$

If k or $l < \frac{1}{2}$, only the fitter homozygote survives. If $k = l = \frac{1}{2}$ there is an unstable equilibrium, and in the long run one homozygote or the other will prevail.

Again the solution of (11) is simple if $k = l$, or $l = 1$. If $l = k$,

$$y_{n+1} = \frac{y_n}{2(1-k) + ky_n},$$

and solving as before

$$\left.\begin{aligned} y_n &= \frac{(1-2k)y_0}{(2-2k)^n(2-2k+ky_0) - ky_0} \quad \text{if} \quad k < \tfrac{1}{2}, \\ y_n &= \frac{(2k-1)y_0}{ky_0 + (2-2k)^n(2k-1-ky_0)} \quad \text{if} \quad k > \tfrac{1}{2}. \end{aligned}\right\} \quad (13)$$

If $l=1$, so that aa is eliminated at once,

$$y_{n+1}=\frac{y_n}{2(1-k)+\frac{1}{2}(3k-1)y_n}.$$

So

$$\left.\begin{aligned} y_n&=\frac{2(1-2k)\,y_0}{(2-2k)^n[2-4k+(3k-1)y_0]-(3k-1)y_0} \quad \text{if} \quad k<\tfrac{1}{2},\\ y_n&=\frac{2(2k-1)y_0}{(3k-1)y_0+(2-2k)^n[4k-2-(3k-1)y_0]} \quad \text{if} \quad k>\tfrac{1}{2}.\end{aligned}\right\} \tag{14}$$

In the general case we find, by the same method as before,

$$\frac{1}{y_{n+2}}-\frac{2(2-k-l)}{y_{n+1}}+\frac{4(1-k)(1-l)}{y_n}=\tfrac{1}{2}(4kl-k-l).$$

Hence

$$y_n=\frac{2(2k-1)(2l-1)\,y_0}{(4kl-k-l)\,y_0+(2-2k)^n\,(2l-1)[2(2k-1)\,x_0-(1-k)\,y_0]+(2-2l)^n(2k-1)[2(2l-1)\,z_0-(1-l)y_0]} \tag{15}$$

The corresponding values of x_n and z_n can easily be calculated. Again the difference from the equilibrium value falls off in an approximately geometrical series.

If we think of this situation in terms of lines, we see that there is selection both between lines and within lines.

A consideration of Hayman and Mather's analysis

Hayman & Mather (1953, pp. 167–70) have dealt with the case when a generation consisting of a fraction p of homozygotes and q of heterozygotes, is selfed. Denoting the corresponding values in the next generation by p' and q', the upper matrix on their p. 168 is equivalent to

$$p'=p+\tfrac{1}{2}q,$$
$$q'=\quad \tfrac{1}{2}q,$$

which is correct. They then suppose that 'all the heterozygotes have the same viability, and... only x of any of the homozygotes survive for each one of the heterozygotes'. They give a second matrix which is equivalent to

$$p'=xp+\tfrac{1}{2}xq,$$
$$q'=\quad \tfrac{1}{2}q.$$

This is incorrect. For

$$p'+q'=xp+\tfrac{1}{2}(1+x)q=1-(1-x)(p+\tfrac{1}{2}q).$$

They state in a footnote that this 'need cause no trouble'. However the correct equations are

$$p'=\frac{x(p+\frac{1}{2}q)}{xp+\frac{1}{2}(1+x)\,q},$$

$$q'=\frac{\frac{1}{2}q}{xp+\frac{1}{2}(1+x)\,q}.$$

These equations, which are equivalent to my (11) with $k=l=1-x$, are non-linear, and cannot be solved by matrix methods, though they are readily solved by the methods given in this paper. All Hayman & Mather's subsequent calculations both as regards self-fertilization and other forms of inbreeding seem to be based on similar errors. However, they give the correct critical values of $\frac{1}{2}$ for k and l, or x. This is because when y_n is approaching zero in equations (11) the value of u_n becomes almost constant.

On the other hand, Hayman's (1953) calculations as to the equilibrium reached under a mixed system of self-fertilization and random mating, which are not based on matrix algebra, appear to be correct.

DISCUSSION

I hope that I have proved two points. First, if there is any such complication as that referred to in the footnote of Hayman & Mather's p. 168 it is always desirable to write out the equations to be solved in full, rather than as a matrix. In my experience it is quite unusual to obtain a set of linear recurrence equations such as my equations (1) in connexion with a problem of selection. Secondly, it is desirable to specify the conditions of selection as carefully as possible. If so, it will often turn out that, as in this paper, such an expression as 'a disadvantage of homozygotes equal to $1-k$' may have a number of different meanings.

Thus I agree with Hayman & Mather that the critical fitness of homozygotes is half that of heterozygotes if there is selection between lines. But if x (in their terminology) is the relative fitness of homozygotes, they find that the frequency of heterozygotes at equilibrium is $\frac{1-2x}{1-x}$, whereas I find that in different circumstances it may be zero (equations (2)), $\frac{1-2x}{2(1-x)}$ (equations (5)), or $\frac{1-2x}{1-x}$ (equations (12)).

I have not considered the situation where selection of unequal intensity against homozygotes occurs within lines and between lines. It can be discussed by the methods developed here, but I doubt if enough biological data exist to warrant its discussion. I also postpone a general discussion of inbreeding as it occurs in practice until the publication of calculations of the same type as those here set out, on sib mating.

I must thank Dr B. I. Hayman and Dr E. Reeve for correcting an error in my algebra.

SUMMARY

Reason is given for doubting the validity of Hayman & Mather's results on this question. Selection in favour of heterozygotes within lines slows down the onset of homozygosis, but cannot prevent it, if any homozygotes are allowed to breed. Similar selection between lines leads to different equilibria in different circumstances.

REFERENCES

HALDANE, J. B. S. (1936). The amount of heterozygosis to be expected in an approximately pure line *J. Genet.* **32**. 375–91.

HAYMAN, B. I. (1953). Mixed selfing and random mating when homozygotes are at a disadvantage. *Heredity*. 7. 185–92.

HAYMAN, B. I. & MATHER, K. (1953). The progress of inbreeding when homozygotes are at a disadvantage. *Heredity*, 7, 165–83.

HOLLINGSWORTH, M. J. & MAYNARD SMITH, J. (1955). The effects of inbreeding on rate of development and on fertility in *Drosophila subobscura*. *J. Genet.* **53**, 295.

THE COST OF NATURAL SELECTION

By J. B. S. HALDANE

University College, London, and Indian Statistical Institute, Calcutta

(*Received* 10 *January*, 1957)

Introduction

It is well known that breeders find difficulty in selecting simultaneously for all the qualities desired in a stock of animals or plants. This is partly due to the fact that it may be impossible to secure the desired phenotype with the genes available. But, in addition, especially in slowly breeding animals such as cattle, one cannot cull even half the females, even though only one in a hundred of them combines the various qualities desired.

The situation with respect to natural selection is comparable. Kermack (1954) showed that characters which are positively correlated in time may be negatively correlated at any particular horizon. The genes available do not allow the production of organisms which are advanced in respect of both characters. In this paper I shall try to make quantitative the fairly obvious statement that natural selection cannot occur with great intensity for a number of characters at once unless they happen to be controlled by the same genes.

Consider a well-investigated example of natural selection, the spread of the dominant *carbonaria* gene through the population of *Biston betularia* in a large area of England (Kettlewell, 1956*a*, *b*). Until about 1800 the original light type, which is inconspicuous against a background of pale lichens, was fitter than the mutant *carbonaria* due to a gene **C**. Then, as a result of smoke pollution, lichens were killed in industrial regions, and the tree trunks on which the moths rest during the day were more or less completely blackened. The **cc** moths became more conspicuous than **Cc** or **CC** and the frequency of the gene **C** increased, so that **cc** moths are now rare in polluted areas. During the process of selection a great many **cc** moths were eaten by birds. Kettlewell (1956*b*) showed that the frequency of the more conspicuous phenotype may be halved in a single day.

Now if the change of environment had been so radical that ten other independently inherited characters had been subject to selection of the same intensity as that for colour, only $(\frac{1}{2})^{10}$, or one in 1024, of the original genotype would have survived. The species would presumably have become extinct. On the other hand, it could well have survived ten selective episodes of comparable intensity occurring in different centuries. We see, then, that natural selection must not be too intense. In what follows I shall try to estimate the effect of natural selection in depressing the fitness of a species.

The principal unit process in evolution is the substitution of one gene for another at the same locus. The substitution of a new gene order, a duplication, a deficiency, and so on, is a formally similar process. For the new order behaves as a unit like a gene in inheritance. The substitution of a maternally inherited self-reproducing cytoplasmic factor by a different such factor is formally similar to the substitution of a gene by another gene in a haploid or of a gene pair by another gene pair in a self-fertilized diploid. I shall show that the number of deaths needed to carry out this unit process by selective survival is independent of the intensity of selection over a wide range.

Natural selection may be defined as follows in a population where generations are separate. The animals in a population are classified as early as possible in their life cycle for phenotypic characters or for genotypes. Some of them become parents of the next generation. A fictitious population of parents is then constituted, in which a parent of n progeny (counted at the same age as the previous generation) is counted n times. If the sex ratio is not unity a suitable correction must be made. If generations overlap Fisher's (1930) reproductive value can be used instead of a count of offspring. Natural selection is a statement of the fact that the fictitious parental population differs significantly from the population from which it was drawn. For example, with respect to any particular metrical character it may differ as regards the mean, variance, and other moments. A difference in means is called a selective differential (Lush, 1954).

Selection may be genotypic or phenotypic. Phenotypic selection may or may not result in genotypic selection. By definition it does not do so in a pure line. Nor need it do so in a genetically heterogeneous population. If underfed individuals are smaller than the mean, and also on an average yield less progeny as a result of premature death or infertility, there is phenotypic selection against small size. But this could be associated with genotypic selection for small size, if organisms whose genotypes disposed them to small size were less damaged by hunger.

In what follows I shall consider genotypic selection; that is to say, selection in which some genotypes are more frequent in the parental population than in the population from which it was drawn.

We can measure the intensity of natural selection as follows. First let us consider selection by juvenile survival. For any range of phenotypes there is a phenotype with optimal survival, s_0, compared with S in the whole population, and similarly for a range of genotypes which includes the whole population. The intensity of selection is defined (Haldane, 1954) as $I = \ln (s_0/S)$. Thus Karn & Penrose (1951) found that about 95·5% of all babies born in a London district and 98·5% of those weighing 7·5–8·5 lb. survived birth and the first month of life: $s_0 = 0{\cdot}985$, $S = 0{\cdot}955$, $I = 0{\cdot}03$. The notion is even simpler for genotypes where they can in fact be distinguished. If all genotypes had survived as well as the optimal genotype, s_0 individuals would have survived for every S which did so. That is to say, of the $1-S$ deaths, $s_0 - S$ were selective. When s_0 and S are nearly equal, $I = s_0 - S$ approximately.

If selection is measured by comparing the parental population with the one from which it is derived, suppose that a number of genotypes are distinguished. Let f_r be the frequency of the rth genotype in the original population, F_r its frequency in the parental population:

$$\Sigma f_r = \Sigma F_r = 1.$$

Let $F_r f_r^{-1}$ be maximal when $r = 0$. The 0th genotype is called the optimal. If all genotypes had been as well represented in the parental population it would have contained $F_0 f_0^{-1}$ individuals for every one which it contained in fact. Thus the intensity of selection is $I = \ln (F_0/f_0)$.

It is convenient to think of natural selection provisionally in terms of juvenile deaths. If it acts in this way, by killing off the less fit genotypes, we shall calculate how many must be killed while a new gene is spreading through a population. This supplements my earlier calculation (Haldane, 1937) as to the effect of variation on fitness. I pointed out that, in a stable population, genetic variation was mainly due to mutation and to the lesser fitness of homozygotes at certain loci. I calculated that each of these agencies might lower the mean fitness of a species by about 5–10 %. In fact the effect of sublethal homozygotes is much greater than this in such organisms as *Drosophila subobscura* and *D. pseudo-obscura*. I did not deal with the dynamic effect of Darwinian natural selection in lowering fitness.

Loss of fitness in genotypes whose frequency is being lowered by natural selection will have different effects on the population according to the stage of the life cycle at which it occurs, and the ecology of the species concerned. In some species the failure of a few eggs or seeds to develop will have little effect on the capacity of the species for increase. This is perhaps most obvious in such polytokous animals as mice, where a considerable prenatal elimination occurs even when no lethal or sublethal genes are segregating. But we can judge of the effect of elimination of a fraction of seeds from Salisbury's (1942, p. 231) conclusion that 'for ecologically comparable species, the magnitude of the reproductive capacity is associated with the frequency and abundance of which it is probably one of the determining factors'. Failure to germinate lowers the reproductive capacity. But death or sterility at a later stage is probably more serious in species whose members compete with one another for food, space, light and so on, or where overcrowding favours the prevalence of disease.

Natural selection, or any other agency which lowers viability or fertility, lowers the reproductive capacity of a species. This is sometimes called its 'natural rate of increase', but this expression is unfortunate, since in nature a population very rarely increases at this rate. Haldane (1956*a*) pointed out that in those parts of its habitat where climate, food, and so on are optimal, the density of a species is usually controlled by negative density-dependent factors, such as disease promoted by overcrowding, competition for food, and space, and so on. In such areas a moderate fall in reproductive capacity has little effect on the density. In exceptional cases, such as control by a parasite affecting no other species, it can even increase the density (Nicholson & Bailey, 1935). But in the parts of the habitat where the population is mainly regulated by density-independent factors such as temperature and salinity, the species can only maintain its numbers by utilizing its reproductive capacity to the full. A fall in reproductive capacity will lead to the disappearance of a species in these marginal areas, except in so far as it is kept up by migration from crowded areas. Birch (1954) showed very clearly that in some cases species with a similar ecology compete on the basis of their reproductive capacities.

It must, however, be emphasized that natural selection against density-independent factors is quite efficient in populations controlled by density-dependent factors. If in some parts of its range *Biston betularia* is so common as to be controlled mainly by parasites favoured by overcrowding, selective predation is not abolished. If 90 % of the larvae die of disease, the 10 % of imagines which emerge are still liable to be eaten by birds. Negative density-dependent factors must, however, slightly lower the overall efficiency of natural selection in a heterogeneous environment. If as the result of larval disease due to overcrowding the density is not appreciably higher in a wood containing mainly *carbonaria* than in a wood containing the original type, the spread of the gene C by migration is somewhat diminished.

A serious complication arises in bisexual organisms if the selective killing or sterilization is of different intensity in the two sexes. In any particular species and environment there is presumably an optimal sex ratio which would give the most rapid possible rate of increase. This would be near equality for monogamous animals, whereas an excess of females might be optimal where a male can mate with many females. But if males are smaller than females or have to search for them intensively an excess of males might be optimal. There is little reason to think that the sex ratio found in nature is closely adjusted to the optimum.

In a species with considerable embryonic or larval competition, and an excess of males above the optimum, the early death of some males might be advantageous. But even in this case an increased death-rate of males soon before maturity or during maturity would be of no advantage. Before dying they would have eaten the food which might have nourished other members of the species, and would have infected them, and so on. There seems no good reason why natural selection should fall more heavily on males than on females except in so far as males are haploid or hemizygous. But even if it fell wholly on males, it would not in general be harmless to the species.

I shall investigate the following case mathematically. A population is in equilibrium under selection and mutation. One or more genes are rare because their appearance by mutation is balanced by natural selection. A sudden change occurs in the environment, for example, pollution by smoke, a change of climate, the introduction of a new food source, predator, or pathogen, and above all migration to a new habitat. It will be shown later that the general conclusions are not affected if the change is slow. The species is less adapted to the new environment, and its reproductive capacity is lowered. It is gradually improved as the result of natural selection. But meanwhile a number of deaths, or their equivalents in lowered fertility, have occurred. If selection at the ith selected locus is responsible for d_i of these deaths in any generation the reproductive capacity of the species will be $\Pi(1-d_i)$ of that of the optimal genotype, or $\exp(-\Sigma d_i)$ nearly, if every d_i is small. Thus the intensity of selection approximates to Σd_i.

Let D_i be the sum of the values of d_i over all generations of selection, neglecting the very small values when the eliminated gene is only kept in being by mutation. I shall show that D_i depends mainly on p_0, the small frequency, at the time when selection begins, of the gene subsequently favoured by natural selection. I shall assume that the frequency of the phenotype first kept rare, and later favoured, by natural selection is about 10^{-4}, a value typical for disadvantageous but not lethal human phenotypes. If so p_0 would be about 5×10^{-5} for a partially or wholly dominant gene, and about 0·01 for a fully recessive one. The former are probably the more important in evolution. All the known genes responsible for industrial melanism are at least partially dominant, and most gene pairs which are responsible for variation of metrical characters in natural populations (as opposed to laboratory or 'fancy' mutants) seem to give heterozygotes intermediate between the homozygotes.

Selection in haploid, clonal, or self-fertilizing organisms, or for maternally inherited cytoplasmic characters

Let the nth generation, before selection, occur in the frequencies

$$p_n\mathbf{A},\ q_n\mathbf{a},\quad \text{where}\quad p_n+q_n=1.$$

Here **A** and **a** are allelomorphic genes in a haploid, genotypes in clonal or self-fertilizing organisms, or different types of cytoplasm. If $1-k$ of **a** survive for every one of **A**, then the fraction of selective deaths in the nth generation is

$$d_n = kq_n. \tag{1}$$

Also

$$q_{n+1} = \frac{(1-k)q_n}{1-kq_n}.$$

So

$$\Delta q_n = \frac{-kp_n q_n}{1-kq_n}. \tag{2}$$

Hence $q_n = [1+(1-k)^{-n}(q_0^{-1}-1)]^{-1}$, which tends to zero with $(1-k)^n$. So the total of the fractions of selective deaths is

$$D = k\sum_{n=0}^{\infty} q_n,$$

which is finite. When k is small, taking a generation as a unit of time,

$$\frac{dq}{dt} = -kq(1-q),$$

approximately. This is also true if generations overlap. So, approximately,

$$\begin{aligned} D &= k\int_0^{\infty} q\,dt \\ &= \int_0^{q_0} -q\frac{dt}{dq}\,dq \\ &= \int_0^{q_0} \frac{dq}{1-q} \\ &= -\ln p_0 + O(k). \end{aligned} \tag{3}$$

If greater accuracy is required, we note that

$$\begin{aligned} \int_{q_{n+1}}^{q_n} \frac{dq}{1-q} &= \ln\left(\frac{1-q_{n+1}}{1-q_n}\right) \\ &= -\ln(1-kq_n) \\ &= kq_n + \tfrac{1}{2}k^2q_n^2 + \tfrac{1}{3}k^3q_n^3 + \ldots. \end{aligned}$$

We require the sum of the first term of this series, namely,

$$D = \sum_{n=0}^{\infty} kq_n.$$

We must subtract suitable terms from the integrand.

$$\begin{aligned} \int_{q_{n+1}}^{q_n} q^r\,dq &= (r+1)^{-1}(q_n^{r+1} - q_{n+1}^{r+1}) \\ &= (r+1)^{-1} q_n^{r+1}(1-kq_n)^{-r-1}[(1-kq_n)^{r+1} - (1-k)^{r+1}] \\ &= kq_n^{r+1}(1-q_n)(1-kq_n)^{-r-1}[1 - \tfrac{1}{2}kr(1+q_n) + \tfrac{1}{6}k^2r(r-1)(1+q_n+q_n^2) + \ldots]. \end{aligned}$$

Hence we find

$$\int_{q_{n+1}}^{q_n} [(1-\tfrac{1}{2}k-\tfrac{1}{12}k^2)(1-q)^{-1} + \tfrac{1}{2}k + \tfrac{1}{12}k^2 - \tfrac{1}{6}k^2q]\,dq = kq_n + O(k^4).$$

So
$$D=\int_0^{q_0}[(1-\tfrac{1}{2}k-\tfrac{1}{12}k^2)(1-q)^{-1}+\tfrac{1}{2}k+\tfrac{1}{12}k^2-\tfrac{1}{6}k^2q]\,dq$$
$$=-(1-\tfrac{1}{2}k-\tfrac{1}{12}k^2)\ln(1-q_0)+(\tfrac{1}{2}k+\tfrac{1}{12}k^2)\,q_0-\tfrac{1}{12}k^2q_0^2+O(k^3)$$
$$=(1-\tfrac{1}{2}k-\tfrac{1}{12}k^2)\ln(p_0^{-1})+\tfrac{1}{2}k-(\tfrac{1}{2}k-\tfrac{1}{12}k^2)\,p_0+O(k^3)+O(k^2p_0^2). \quad (4)$$

To obtain the coefficient of k^3 we have only to use the method of undetermined coefficients, adding $k^3[\alpha(1-q)^{-1}+\beta+\gamma q+\delta q^2]$ to the integrand, and equating the coefficient of k^4 to zero.

Clearly if k is small, D is almost independent of k, while if k is large, D is less than $-\ln p_0$. When $k=1$, that is to say, the fitness of **a** is zero, $D=q_0$, for selection is complete after one generation; that is to say, $D=1$, very nearly. If $p_0=10^{-4}$, as suggested, $D=9{\cdot}2$, provided selection is slow. If p_0 were as high as 0·01, or 1 %, D would still be 4·6, while if it were as low as 10^{-6}, D would only be 13·8.

The correction to be made for the fact that q_n does not become zero, but reaches a small value set by the rate of back mutation, is negligible. If the final small value is Q, (3) becomes

$$D=-\ln p_0+\ln(1-Q)$$
$$=-\ln p_0-Q,$$

very nearly. If Q is about 10^{-4} the error is of this order, though, of course, a slight loss of fitness equal to the back mutation rate will go on indefinitely. The same is true for other expressions such as (7).

We may, therefore, take it that when selection is fairly slow, the total number of selective deaths over all generations is usually 5–15 times the total number in the population in each generation, 10 times this number being a representative value. When k exceeds $\tfrac{1}{3}$, this number is appreciably reduced.

During the course of selection the value of k may vary. If the environment is changing progressively it will, on the whole, increase. But provided it is small this makes no difference to the result. The cost of changing q from q_1 to q_2 is

$$\int_{q_2}^{q_1}\frac{dq}{1-q}+O(k)=\ln\left(\frac{1-q_2}{1-q_1}\right)+O(k),$$

which is nearly independent of the value of k.

Selection at an autosomal locus in a diploid

Consider an autosomal pair of allels **A** and **a** in a large random mating population, with frequencies p_n and q_n in the nth generation. Let their relative fitnesses be as below:

Genotype	AA	Aa	aa
Frequency	p_n^2	$2p_nq_n$	q_n^2
Fitness	1	$1-k$	$1-K$

where $K \geqslant k \geqslant 0$. Let $k=\lambda K$. If $\lambda=1$, **a** is dominant as regards fitness. If $\lambda=0$, $k=0$, and **a** is recessive as regards fitness. λ is usually between 1 and 0. I assume $\lambda \leqslant 1$, for if $k<0$, the gene **A** will not displace **a** completely, but an equilibrium will be reached, while if $k>K$ selection will not occur. For the reasons given above I assume $p_0=5\times10^{-5}$ unless λ is very small or zero, in which case p_0 may be about 0·01.

The fraction of selective deaths in the nth generation is

$$d_n = 2kp_n q_n + Kq_n^2$$
$$= Kq_n[2\lambda + (1-2\lambda)\, q_n]. \tag{5}$$

So the total deaths are the population number multiplied by

$$D = K \sum_{n=0}^{\infty} [2\lambda q_n + (1-2\lambda)\, q_n^2].$$

Also

$$\Delta q_n = \frac{-p_n q_n[k(p_n - q_n) + Kq_n]}{1 - 2kp_n q_n - Kq_n^2}$$
$$= -Kp_n q_n\, [\lambda + (1-2\lambda)\, q_n], \tag{6}$$

approximately. Using the same approximation as before,

$$D = \int_0^{q_0} \frac{[2\lambda + (1-2\lambda)\, q]\, dq}{(1-q)\,[\lambda + (1-2\lambda)\, q]}$$
$$= \frac{1}{1-\lambda} \int_0^{q_0} \left[\frac{1}{1-q} + \frac{\lambda(1-2\lambda)}{\lambda + (1-2\lambda)\, q}\right] dq$$

(provided $\lambda < 1$)

$$= \frac{1}{1-\lambda}\left[-\ln p_0 + \lambda \ln\left(\frac{1-\lambda-p_0}{\lambda}\right)\right]$$
$$= \frac{1}{1-\lambda}\left[-\ln p_0 + \lambda \ln\left(\frac{1-\lambda}{\lambda}\right)\right], \tag{7}$$

nearly. If, however, $\lambda = 1$,

$$D = \int_0^{q_0} \frac{(2-q)\, dq}{(1-q)^2}$$
$$= \int_0^{q_0} \left[\frac{1}{1-q} + \frac{1}{(1-q)^2}\right] dq$$
$$= p_0^{-1} - \ln p_0 + O(k). \tag{8}$$

If $\lambda = 0$ (**A** dominant), then from (7), $D = -\ln p_0$, if $\lambda = \frac{1}{2}$, $D = -2 \ln p_0$, if $\lambda = \frac{3}{4}$, $D = -4 \ln p_0 - 3{\cdot}3$, and if $\lambda = 0{\cdot}9$, $D = -10 \ln p_0 - 19{\cdot}8$. Thus if $p_0 = 5 \times 10^{-5}$, $\ln p_0 = 9{\cdot}9$, and D ranges from 9·9 to about 79. However, when **A** is nearly recessive, p_0 is probably somewhat larger than 5×10^{-5}, and when it is fully recessive p_0 is more probably about 0·01, giving $D = 105$ approximately, from (8). Thus D usually lies between 10 and 100, with 30 as a representative value.

We can find corrections to be made when K is not small. They are analogous to (4). In the limiting cases when $K = 1$, $k = 0$, $D = 1$ approximately. While if $K = k = 1$,

$$D = 1 + \frac{1}{2^2} + \frac{1}{3^2} + \frac{1}{4^2} + \dots$$
$$= \tfrac{1}{6}\pi^2$$
$$= 1{\cdot}645.$$

Once again the value of D is not affected by the intensity of selection provided this is small, and is not very sensitive to the value of p_0.

SELECTION AT AN AUTOSOMAL LOCUS WITH INBREEDING

If inbreeding is almost complete, as in self-fertilized crop plants, the deaths of heterozygotes can be neglected, and equation (3) holds with sufficient accuracy. If there is partial inbreeding, suppose that gene frequencies and genotypic fitnesses are as in the last section, but the mean coefficient of inbreeding in the population is f instead of zero. Then the survivors of selection occur in the ratios

$$(p_n^2+fp_nq_n)\,\mathbf{AA}:2(1-k)(1-f)\,p_nq_n\,\mathbf{Aa}:(1-K)(fp_nq_n+q_n^2)\,\mathbf{aa}.$$

Hence
$$d_n=q_n[2k(1-f)\,p_n+K(fp_n+q_n)],$$

$$\Delta q_n=\frac{-p_nq_n[k(1-f)(p_n-q_n)+K(fp_n+q_n)]}{1-2k(1-f)\,p_nq_n-K(fp_nq_n+q_n^2)}.$$

Hence
$$D=\int_0^{q_0}\frac{2(1-f)\,k+fK+(1-f)(K-2k)\,q}{(1-q)\,[(1-f)\,k+fK+(1-f)(K-2k)\,q]}\,dq,\quad\text{nearly}$$

$$=[K-(1-f)\,k]^{-1}\int_0^{q_0}\left[\frac{K}{1-q}+\frac{(1-f)^2\,k(K-2k)}{(1-f)\,k+fK+(1-f)(K-2k)\,q}\right]dq$$

$$=[K-(1-f)\,k]^{-1}\left[-K\ln p_0+(1-f)\,k\ln\left(\frac{K-k+fk}{K+fK-fk}\right)\right]\qquad(9)$$

nearly. If $(1-f)\,k=\mu K$,

$$D=(1-\mu)^{-1}\left[-\ln p_0+\mu\ln\left(\frac{1-\mu}{\mu}\right)-\ln\left(1+\frac{f}{\mu}\right)\right].$$

That is to say, the effect of partial inbreeding is very nearly to replace λ by $(1-f)\,\lambda$ in equation (7). The value of D is slightly reduced, as if the heterozygotes were a little fitter. But D is never as small as the value given by equation (3). If $k=\frac{1}{2}K$, D is divided by $(1+f)$. Partial inbreeding thus saves a few deaths, but has little effect on the value of D unless **A** is recessive, when it reduces it drastically.

SELECTION AT A SEX-LINKED LOCUS IN A DIPLOID

I assume males to be heterogametic. The results are the same, *mutatis mutandis*, if females are so. I assume that selection is so slow that the gene frequencies are very nearly the same in both sexes. Let the frequencies and relative fitnesses be

Genotype	AA		Aa		aa		A		a
Frequency	p_n^2		$2p_nq_n$		q_n^2		p_n		q_n
Fitness	1	:	$1-k$	:	$1-K$	:	1	:	$1-l$

In fact the frequencies of **a** differ in the two sexes by a quantity of the order of the largest of k, K and l, but this can provisionally be neglected. The selective death-rates in females and males are respectively:

$$\left.\begin{aligned}d_{f,n}&=2kp_nq_n+Kq_n^2,\\ d_{m,n}&=lq_n.\end{aligned}\right\}\qquad(10)$$

And
$$\Delta q_n=-\tfrac{1}{3}p_nq_n[2k(p_n-q_n)+Kq_n+l],\qquad(11)$$

since there are twice as many loci in female as in male gametes forming the next generation. Thus, the total of female selective death-rates approximates to

$$D_f = 3\int_0^{q_0} \frac{[2k+(K-2k)q]\,dq}{(1-q)[2k+l+2(K-2k)q]}.$$

Provided $2K+l>2k$,

$$D_f = \frac{3}{2K-2k+l}\int_0^{q_0}\left[\frac{K}{1-q}+\frac{(K-2k)(2k-l)}{2k+l+2(K-2k)q}\right]dq$$
$$= \frac{3}{2K-2k+l}\left[-K\ln p_0+\tfrac{1}{2}(2k-l)\ln\left(\frac{2k+l}{2K-2k+l}\right)\right],$$

and similarly the total for males is

$$D_m = \frac{3l}{2K-2k+l}\left[-\ln p_0+\ln\left(\frac{2k+l}{2K-2k+l}\right)\right]. \tag{12}$$

If, however, $2K+l=2k$, which implies that $k>K$, unless $l=0$, in which case **A** is fully recessive as regards fitness in females,

$$\left.\begin{aligned} D_f &= \frac{3}{2}\left(\frac{K}{K+l}p_0-\ln p_0\right),\\ D_m &= \frac{3lp_0}{2(K+l)}.\end{aligned}\right\} \tag{13}$$

It is possible that almost all the selective mortality should be concentrated on the males. This will be so if K is small, provided $2K+l>2k$. This is unlikely but not impossible. For the reasons discussed earlier this would probably not ease the burden on the species very greatly.

The value of p_0 would be about 10^{-4} provided that in the preliminary period **A** males were at an appreciable disadvantage. The mean of D_f and D_m is

$$D = \frac{3}{2(2K-2k+l)}\left[-(K+l)\ln p_0+(k+\tfrac{1}{2}l)\ln\left(\frac{2k+l}{2K-2k+l}\right)\right], \tag{14}$$

unless $2K+l=2k$, when $\quad D=\tfrac{3}{2}(p_0-\ln p_0).$ (15)

If $2k>2K+l$ an equilibrium is reached.

We see that the cost of selection at a sex-linked locus depends, as at an autosomal locus, on $-\ln p_0$, and on the ratios of selective intensities, provided these are small. The factor multiplying $-\ln p_0$ will seldom be large. It is, for example, 3 if $K=k=l$, and 1 if $K=l$, $k=0$. Thus a representative value of D is 20, and it will probably be between 10 and 40 in most cases. It will not be greatly increased if the gene selected is completely recessive in females, provided that it is of selective advantage in males.

SELECTION OF HETEROZYGOTES

The total death-rates of heterozygotes at an autosomal locus are given by

$$D_h = \Sigma\, 2kp_nq_n$$
$$= 2\lambda K\Sigma q_n(1-q_n).$$

This approximates to

$$2\lambda K\int_0^\infty q(1-q)\,dt = 2\lambda K\int_{q_0}^{q_n} q(1-q)\frac{dt}{dq}\,dq$$

$$= 2\lambda\int_{q_n}^{q_0}\frac{dq}{\lambda+(1-2\lambda)q}$$

$$= \frac{2\lambda}{1-2\lambda}\Big[\ln\{\lambda+(1-2\lambda)q\}\Big]_{q_n}^{q_0}.$$

If $1>\lambda>0$, $$D_h = \frac{2\lambda}{1-2\lambda}\ln\left(\frac{1-\lambda}{\lambda}\right),$$

except when $\lambda=\frac{1}{2}$, when $$D_h = 2.$$

If $\lambda=1$, $$D_h = -2\ln p_0. \qquad (16)$$

Over the range considered D_h is a monotone increasing function of λ, being 0·549 when $\lambda=0{\cdot}1$, and 4·944 when $\lambda=0{\cdot}9$. That is to say unless λ is very nearly unity, or **A** almost recessive as regards adaptive value, D_h is small. And it is always a small fraction of D. During most of the course of a gene substitution heterozygotes are rare.

It can easily be shown that in the case of a sex-linked locus the total deaths of heterozygous females are

$$D_h = \frac{3k}{K-2k}\ln\left(\frac{2K-2k+l}{2k+l}\right),$$

unless $K=2k$, when $D_h=3K/(K+l)$. These are also relatively small numbers.

In a recent discussion on natural selection (Haldane, 1956*b*) I gave the total numbers of heterozygotes produced in the course of a gene substitution, or $k^{-1}D_h$. The results are equivalent. Since so few heterozygotes are killed, there can, in the course of a gene replacement, be little selection in favour of genes raising the fitness of heterozygotes by altering dominance or otherwise, unless they affect homozygotes also.

Discussion

The unit process of evolution, the substitution of one allel by another, if carried out by natural selection based on juvenile deaths, usually involves a number of deaths equal to about 10 or 20 times the number in a generation, always exceeding this number, and perhaps rarely being 100 times this number. To allow for occasional high values I take 30 as a mean. If natural selection acts by diminished fertility the effect is equivalent.

Suppose then that selection is taking place slowly at a number of loci, the average rate being one gene substitution in each n generations, the fitness of the species concerned will fall below the optimum by a factor of about $30n^{-1}$ so long as this is small. If the depression is larger we reason as follows. If a number of loci are concerned, the ith depressing fitness by a small quantity δ_i, the mean number of loci transformed per generation is $D^{-1}\Sigma\delta_i$ or about $\frac{1}{30}\Sigma\delta_i$. The fitness is reduced to $\Pi(1-\delta_i)$ or about $\exp(-\Sigma\delta_i)$. But $n=30/\Sigma\delta_i$, roughly. Thus, the fitness is about $e^{-30n^{-1}}$, or the intensity of selection $I=30n^{-1}$.

To be concrete, if a species had immigrated into an environment where its reproductive capacity was half that obtainable after selection had run its course, so that $I=\ln 2=0{\cdot}69$,

n would be 43. This represents, in my opinion, fairly intense selection, of the order of that found in *Biston betularia*, where it has had a rapid effect because it was concentrated on a phenotypic change due mainly to a single gene. I doubt if such high intensities of selection have been common in the course of evolution. I think $n = 300$, which would give $I = 0{\cdot}1$, is a more probable figure. Whereas, for example, $n = 7{\cdot}5$ would reduce the fitness to e^{-4}, or 0·02, which would hardly be compatible with survival.

We do not know at how many loci two 'good' but fairly closely related species differ. Their taxonomic characters may depend mainly on as few as twenty gene substitutions. But there is every reason to think that substitutions have occurred at a great many other loci. Punnett (1932) showed that among eighteen fully recessive mutants in *Lathyrus odoratus* which he studied the viability increased with the time which had elapsed since the mutation occurred. In Table 1 I have presented the data of his Table VI in a different form. The second column is the estimated viability. If d dominants and r

Table 1. *Punnett's data on sweet peas*

	Mutant	Viability	S.E.
g_1	White	1·037	0·024
a_1	Red	1·021	0·017
b_1	Light axil	1·011	0·017
f_1	White	0·996	0·038
d_5	Picotee	0·996	0·022
a_2	Round pollen	0·990	0·024
b_2	Sterile	0·988	0·017
a_3	Hooded	0·977	0·021
e	Cupid	0·976	0·032
f_2	Bush	0·936	0·030
d_2	Blue	0·931	0·024
g_3	Mauve	0·917	0·031
d_1	Acacia	0·964	0·020
d_4	Smooth	0·940	0·020
d_3	Copper	0·909	0·040
h	Spencer	0·897	0·030
b_3	Cretin	0·886	0·048
f_3	Marbled	0·821	0·023

recessives are found out of n, this is $3r/(d+1)$ (Haldane, 1956*c*) and its standard error is $3\sqrt{(rn/d^3)}$. The standard errors are given in the third column. The first group of mutants occurred in wild populations, in the eighteenth, or possibly in the early nineteenth, century. The second group originated between 1880 and 1899. The third group originated between 1901 and 1912. In each group the order is that of viabilities. None of the viabilities in the first group differs significantly from unity, nor does their mean. I know of no equally satisfactory series of data in any other organism. It seems that a mutant on appearance is generally somewhat inviable. But intense selection exercised by breeders accumulates 'modifiers' which, in the course of fifty years or so, raise its viability in F_2 to normal.

Presumably the same kind of process occurs in evolution. The number of loci in a vertebrate species has been estimated at about 40,000. 'Good' species, even when closely related, may differ at several thousand loci, even if the differences at most of them are very slight. But it takes as many deaths, or their equivalents, to replace a gene by one producing a barely distinguishable phenotype as by one producing a very different one. If two species differ at 1000 loci, and the mean rate of gene substitution, as has been suggested, is one per 300 generations, it will take at least 300,000 generations to generate an interspecific difference. It may take a good deal more, for if an allel a^1 is ultimately replaced by a^{10} the population may pass through stages where the commonest genotype at the locus is a^1a^1, a^2a^2, a^3a^3, and so on, successively, the various allels in turn giving maximal fitness in the existing environment and the residual genotype. Simpson (1953) finds the mean life of a genus of Carnivora to be about 8 million years. That of a species in horotelic vertebrate evolution may average about a million.

Zeuner (1945), after a very full discussion of the Pleistocene fossil record, concluded that in mammals about 500,000 years were required for the evolution of a new species, though in the vole genera *Mimomys* and *Arvicola* the rate was somewhat greater. Some insects seem to have evolved at about the same rate, while other insects, and all molluscs, evolved more slowly. He estimated the total duration of the Pleistocene at 600,000 years, but some later authors would about halve this figure. On the other hand environmental changes during the Pleistocene were unusually rapid, and evolution, therefore, probably also unusually rapid. The agreement with the theory here developed is satisfactory.

Some writers, such as Fisher (1930, 1931), appear to assume that the number of loci at which 'modifiers', for example, genes affecting the dominance of other genes, may be selected, is indefinitely large. The number of loci is, however, finite. But even if enough modifiers were available, the selection of, say, ten modifiers which between them caused a previously dominant mutant to become recessive, would involve the death of a number of individuals equal to about 300 generations of the species concerned. Even the geological time scale is too short for such processes to go on in respect of thousands of loci. Renwick (1956) has made it very probable that dominance modifiers occur at the mutant locus, and if so recessivity may often be assured by strengthening the 'wild-type' allel (Wright, 1934; Haldane, 1939).

Can this slowness be avoided by selecting several genes at a time? I doubt it, for the following reason. Consider clonally reproducing bacteria, in which a number of disadvantageous genes are present, kept in being by mutation, each with frequencies of the order of 10^{-4}. They become slightly advantageous through a change of environment or residual genotype. Among 10^{12} bacteria there might be one which possessed three such mutants. But since the cost of selection is proportional to the negative logarithm of the initial frequency the mean cost of selecting its descendants would be the same as that of selection for the three mutants in series, though the process might be quicker. The same argument applies to mutants linked by an inversion. Once several favourable mutants are so linked the inversion may be quickly selected. But the rarity of inversions containing several rare and favourable mutants will leave the cost unaltered.

There can, of course, be other reasons for the slowness of evolution. In some cases several genes must be substituted simultaneously before fitness is increased. This process can perhaps occur in two ways. On the one hand in a species broken up into small endogamous groups such a combination of genes may be established by a random process of 'drift' (Wright, 1934 and earlier) or a single founder crossing a geographical barrier may possess them (Spurway, 1953). Or they may be linked by an inversion. But such events are not perhaps very frequent even on an evolutionary time scale. On the other hand, each gene may change by a number of small successive steps. Fisher's (1930, pp. 38–40) argument is applicable here, though he may have envisaged changes at a large number of loci, rather than successive changes at a few. In either case the cost is high and the process must, therefore, be slow. The slowness of evolution of such an organ as the vertebrate eye is thus intelligible.

Evolution by natural selection can be very rapid if a species, like the first land vertebrates, or the first colonists of an island, finds itself in an environment to which it is very ill-adapted, but in which it has no competition, and perhaps no predators and few parasites. If so selection might be so intense as to reduce the capacity for increase to one-tenth of that of its adapted descendants, and it could yet hold its own. Such episodes have doubtless been important, and account for tachytelic (Simpson, 1953) evolution. But they are probably exceptional.

On the whole it seems that the rate of evolution is set by the number of loci in a genome, and the number of stages through which they can mutate. If pre-Cambrian organisms had much fewer loci than their descendants, they may have evolved much quicker, though the possibilities open to them were more limited.

The calculations regarding heterozygotes enable us to answer certain questions. Kettlewell (1956*b*) has evidence that **C** in *Biston betularia* is now more dominant than it was in the nineteenth century. **CC** is now usually indistinguishable from **Cc** by human beings, and probably by birds. This is thought to be due to selection of one or more genes which modify dominance. The value of λ in equations (5) to (8) has decreased from about $\frac{1}{2}$ to nearly zero. If λ was originally $\frac{1}{2}$, the total number of **Cc** moths killed selectively was about twice the number in a generation, and since λ diminished, it can hardly be as many as this.

Now supposing a modifier **M** which made **Cc** as dark as **CC** had been selected by deaths of heterozygotes which did not carry it, the natural logarithm of its frequency would have increased by about 4, from equation (7). That is to say its frequency would have increased about e^4, or 55 times. This is certainly an overestimate, since fewer heterozygotes would have been killed as soon as the modifier became at all common. Probably a twenty-fold increase is the most that could be expected. This is not enough to make **C** almost always dominant when it was previously semi-dominant.

However, two other possibilities are open. It is quite possible that at the present time **Cc** has a higher adaptive value than **CC**, and this accounts for the persistence of **cc** in all populations studied. If so the proportion of **Cc** moths may be much higher that it would be if **CC** had a higher adaptive value than **Cc**. In fact λ may sometimes at least be negative in equation (5), leading to balanced polymorphism. Another possibility is that **M** improves the physiological adjustment of **CC**. Suppose, for example, that **C** is responsible for a tyrosinase or a similar enzyme absent in **cc**, and that **CC** moths produce twice as much of this enzyme as **Cc**. Then if the substrate concentration is low, it may not be possible for **Cc** moths to make enough melanin to become fully black. However, **CC** moths may use up most of the available phenolic substrate, and the resulting shortage may lead to ill-health. There will then be selection for a gene **M** which leads to the synthesis of more substrate, and incidentally permits **Cc** moths to make enough melanin to appear as black as **CC**. This is, of course, only one of many hypotheses. But it is important to realize that a dominance modifier may be selected for its effect on homozygotes.

To conclude, I am quite aware that my conclusions will probably need drastic revision. But I am convinced that quantitative arguments of the kind here put forward should play a part in all future discussions of evolution.

SUMMARY

Unless selection is very intense, the number of deaths needed to secure the substitution, by natural selection, of one gene for another at a locus, is independent of the intensity of selection. It is often about 30 times the number of organisms in a generation. It is suggested that, in horotelic evolution, the mean time taken for each gene substitution is about 300 generations. This accords with the observed slowness of evolution.

REFERENCES

BIRCH, L. C. (1954). Experiments on the relative abundance of two sibling species. *Aust. J. Zool.* **2**, 66–74.

FISHER, R. A. (1930). *The Genetical Theory of Natural Selection.* Oxford: Clarendon Press.

FISHER, R. A. (1931). The evolution of dominance. *Biol. Rev.* **6**, 345–68.

HALDANE, J. B. S. (1937). The effect of variation on fitness. *Amer. Nat.* **71**, 337–49.

HALDANE, J. B. S. (1939). The theory of the evolution of dominance. *J. Genet.* **37**, 365–74.

HALDANE, J. B. S. (1954). The measurement of natural selection. *Proc. 9th Int. Congr. Genet.* pp. 480–7.

HALDANE, J. B. S. (1956*a*). The relation between density regulation and natural selection. *Proc. Roy. Soc.* B, **145**, 306–8.

HALDANE, J. B. S. (1956*b*). The theory of selection for melanism in Lepidoptera. *Proc. Roy. Soc.* B, **145**, 303–6.

HALDANE, J. B. S. (1956*c*). The estimation of viabilities. *J. Genet.* **54**, 294–6.

KARN, N. & PENROSE, L. S. (1951). Birthweight and gestation time in relation to maternal age, parity and infant survival. *Ann. Eugen.* **16**, 147–64.

KERMACK, K. A. (1954). A biometrical study of *Micraster coranguinum* and *M.* (*Isomicraster*) *senonensis*. *Phil. Trans.* B, **237**, 375–428.

KETTLEWELL, H. B. D. (1956*a*). A resumé of investigations on the evolution of melanism in the Lepidoptera. *Proc. Roy. Soc.* B, **145**, 297–303.

KETTLEWELL, H. B. D. (1956*b*). Further selection experiments on industrial melanism in the Lepidoptera. *Heredity*, **10**, 287–303.

LUSH, J. L. (1954). Rates of genetic change in populations of farm animals. *Proc. 9th Int. Congr. Genet.* pp. 589–99.

NICHOLSON, A. J. & BAILEY, V. A. (1935). The balance of animal populations, Part I. *Proc. Zool. Soc. Lond.*, pp. 551–98.

PUNNETT, R. C. (1932). Further studies of Linkage in the Sweet pea. *J. Genet.* **26**, 97–113.

RENWICK, J. H. (1956). Nail-patella syndrome: evidence for modification by alleles at the main locus. *Ann. Hum. Genet.* **21**, 159–69.

SALISBURY, E. (1942). *The Reproductive Capacity of Plants.* London: Bell.

SIMPSON, G. G. (1953). *The Major Features of Evolution.* New York.

SPURWAY, H. (1953). Genetics of specific and subspecific differences in European newts. *Symp. Soc. Exp. Biol.* no. VII, Evolution.

WRIGHT, S. (1934). Physiological and evolutionary theories of dominance. *Amer. Nat.* **68**, 24–53.

ZEUNER, F. F. (1945). *The Pleistocene Period.* London: Ray Society Monograph.

318

POLYMORPHISM DUE TO SELECTION DEPENDING ON THE COMPOSITION OF A POPULATION

By J. B. S. HALDANE and S. D. JAYAKAR

Genetics and Biometry Laboratory, Government of Orissa, Bhubaneswar-3, Orissa, India

It has been frequently pointed out that if rarity confers selective advantage on a phenotype, and hence on a gene, this can be a cause of stable polymorphism. Thus mimicry becomes less and less advantageous as the ratio of palatable mimics to distasteful models rises. If a pathogen tends to adapt itself by selection of those genotypes which affect the commonest host genotypes, then rare host genotypes are favoured so long as they remain rare. The selective advantage or disadvantage of a gene responsible for an antigen causing immunization of a mother by the foetus is well known to vary with its frequency. More examples might be given. It may be thought advisable to describe such selection as non-Darwinian, reserving the term Darwinian for selection in which the advantage of belonging to a "favoured race", or better, favoured genotype, is independent of the frequency of that genotype in the population, or at least is never reversed by changes in that frequency. It is not suggested that Darwin was unaware of the existence of non-Darwinian selection. But as it is irrelevant to the large-scale evolution in which he was interested, he did not consider it in any detail.

We think most writers on this topic have assumed something like the following: "If genotype A is fitter than its alternative genotype B when its frequency in a population is below a certain value, and less fit when it exceeds it, there will be a stable equilibrium when the frequency is such as to equalise the fitnesses". This is not in fact true in theory, though it may be true in all or almost all cases which occur in nature. It is a well-known physical fact that if a system is brought back towards equilibrium too violently, it will overshoot the equilibrium and may go into undamped oscillation. Can this happen in a population under natural selection ?

Haploid Selection

As usual, the treatment of selection in a haploid, or a population consisting of two clones, is very simple. Suppose that generations are separate, and that the population consists, in generation n, of $(1-q_n)\,A+q_n\,B$, the population being so large that fluctuations may be neglected. Let the fitness of B relative to A be $1-\phi(q_n)$. Clearly there is an equilibrium when $\phi(q_n)=0$. This may theoretically be so for several values of q_n, but such cases, if they occur at all, must be very rare. Let $\phi(Q)=0$, and $q_n=Q+x_n$.

$$\cdot \quad q_{n+1}=\frac{q_n-q_n\,\phi(q_n)}{1-q_n\,\phi(q_n)}\,. \tag{1}$$

$$\text{So } x_{n+1}=\frac{-Q(1-Q)\,\phi(q_n)+x_n[1-(1-Q)\,\phi(q_n)]}{1-(Q+x_n)\,\phi(q_n)}\,.$$

But if ϕ is regular in the neighbourhood of Q,

$$\phi(q_n) = x_n \phi'(Q) + \tfrac{1}{2} x_n^2 \phi''(Q) + \cdots.$$

$$\text{So } x_{n+1} = \frac{[1-Q(1-Q)\phi'(Q)]\,x_n - (1-Q)\,[\phi'(Q)+\tfrac{1}{2}Q\phi''(Q)]\,x_n^2 + O(x_n^3)}{1-Q\phi'(Q)\,x_n}$$

$$= [1-Q(1-Q)\phi'(Q)]\,x_n - [(1-2Q)\phi'(Q) + Q^2(1-Q)\{\phi'(Q)\}^2 + \tfrac{1}{2}Q(1-Q)\phi''(Q)]\,x_n^2 + O(x_n^3). \tag{2}$$

When x_n is sufficiently small, x_{n+1} will be numerically smaller than x_n provided $1-Q(1-Q)\phi'(Q)$ lies between ± 1, that is to say

$$0 < Q(1-Q)\phi'(Q) < 2,$$

$$\text{or } 0 < \phi'(Q) < \frac{2}{Q(1-Q)}. \tag{3}$$

Since $Q(1-Q)$ reaches its maximum of $\frac{1}{4}$ when $Q = \frac{1}{2}$, $\dfrac{2}{Q(1-Q)} \geqslant 8$. So the equilibrium is stable to small displacements if $\phi'(Q)$ is positive and less than 8. It may be so for much higher values if Q or $1-Q$ is small.

If $0 < Q(1-Q)\phi'(Q)$, then, at least when x_n is sufficiently small, it does not change sign, that is to say the equilibrium is approached from above or below. If $Q(1-Q)\phi'(Q) = 1$, the equilibrium is approached very rapidly, x_{n+1} falling off with x_n^2. The details depend on the second term of (2). If $1 < Q(1-Q)\phi'(Q)$, then after some value of n, successive values of x_n have opposite signs, and the equilibrium is overshot in each generation, though it is approached more closely.

It is to be noted that for biologically plausible values of $\phi'(Q)$ the equilibrium is approached rather slowly. Thus if the fitness of B fell from 120% of that of A when $q=0$ to 100% when $q = Q = \cdot 4$ and 70% when $q=1$, while $\phi'(q)$ was constant, we should have $\phi'(Q) = \frac{1}{2}$, and $x_{n+1} = 0{\cdot}88 x_n$. The result of a disturbance of equilibrium would persist for a good many generations.

Whereas in most, if not all, cases so far considered by geneticists, the stability of an equilibrium calculated when generations are separate is not appreciably altered when they overlap, this is not true for non-Darwinian selection. Let us suppose that everything is as in the preceding paragraphs except that the population in year n is composed of $N(1-q_{n-1})\,b_1$ A individuals born in year $n-1$, $N(1-q_{n-2})b_2$ As born in year $n-2$, and so on, and similarly $N q_{n-r}[1-\phi(q_{n-r})]\,b_r$ B individuals born in year $n-r$. That is to say

$$q_n = \frac{\sum_r b_r q_{n-r}[1-\phi(q_{n-r})]}{1-\sum_r b_r q_{n-r}\phi(q_{n-r})}, \tag{4}$$

when summation is over all values of r, and $\sum_r b_r = 1$. This implies that selection is based on differences in infantile mortality, determined by the frequencies of the two types in the first year of life. This may often be an approximation to truth. Competition may be very intense between seedlings, but less intense between adults. Allowance for various types of competition in different years of life would lead to more complicated expressions, which would usually be compromises between (1) and (4). We have chosen a rather extreme but simple hypothesis to illustrate the stabilizing effect of overlap. We have assumed that all adults are equally fertile. Insofar as fertility is a function of age, this can be allowed for by adjustment of the values of b_r, and insofar as it is a function of genotype, by adjustment of that of $\phi(q)$. There is no difficulty in passing to the case where fertility is not concentrated in seasons; this involves integral equations.

Now if $\phi(Q)=0$ and $q_n=Q+x_n$, as before, (4) becomes

$$x_n=[1-Q(1-Q)\,\phi'(Q)]\,\sum_r b_r x_{n-r}+O(x_{n-r}^2).$$

If $k=Q\,(1-Q)\,\phi'(Q)$ this approximates to the linear recurrence equation

$$x_n=(1-k)\sum_{r=1}^{m} b_r\,x_{n-r} \qquad (5)$$

when x_n is small and m is the maximum age which any individual can attain. The corresponding integral equation is

$$x_t=(1-k)\int_0^{\infty} f(\tau)\,x_{t-\tau}d\tau,$$

where $f(\tau)$ is the probability of an A producing an offspring between ages τ and $\tau+\delta\tau$, and t is the time at which x is observed.

The solution of (5) is

$$x_n=\sum_{i=1}^{m} A_i\,\lambda_i^n$$

where $\lambda^m=(1-k)\sum_{r=1}^{m} b_r\,\lambda^{m-r}$,

λ_i is the i-th root of this equation, and A_i are parameters depending on initial conditions. The condition for stability is that every $\lambda_i<1$. It can be shown that if $0<k<1$ there is one real positive root less than unity and exceeding the moduli of all the other roots, which are complex or negative. Thus for $0<k\leqslant 1$ the situation is the same as in the case of separate generations. However when k exceeds unity the region of stability is often if not always increased. For example let $b_1=b$, $b_2=1-b$, $b_r=0$ $(r>2)$. Then

$$\lambda^2+(k-1)\,b\lambda+(k-1)\,(1-b)=0.$$

When $k=0$ the roots are 1 and $-(1-b)$.

When $0<k<1$ the positive root is smaller than 1, the negative exceeds $b-1$.

When $k=0$, both roots are zero.

When $k>1$, $\lambda=\frac{1}{2}\,(k-1)^{\frac{1}{2}}\,[\pm\{(k-1)b^2-4(1-b)\}^{\frac{1}{2}}-b(k-1)^{\frac{1}{2}}]$.

So when $k-1$ is small enough there are two complex roots, $\lambda = re^{\pm i\theta}$,

where $r^2 = (k-1)(1-b)$, $\cos 2\theta = \dfrac{b^2(k-1)}{2(1-b)} - 1$; when $k > 1 + \dfrac{4(1-b)}{b^2}$ the roots are real.

If $b < \frac{2}{3}$, the equilibrium becomes unstable when $k > 1 + \dfrac{1}{1-b}$; for example if $b = \frac{1}{3}$, when $k > 2\frac{1}{2}$, and if $b = \frac{1}{2}$, when $k > 3$. The system goes into undamped oscillations when k exceeds these values. If $b = \frac{2}{3}$, the system oscillates with $\lambda = -1$, and a period of one year when $k = 4$. It is unstable if $k > 4$. If $b > \frac{2}{3}$, the roots become real before k reaches its critical value, and the condition for instability is $k > 1 + \dfrac{1}{2b-1}$; for example if $b = \frac{3}{4}$, $k > 3$, if $b = \frac{7}{8}$, $k > 2\frac{1}{3}$. The critical values of k all lie between 2 and 4 inclusive, whereas if generations do not overlap the critical value is $k = 2$. Higher critical values can be obtained with larger numbers m of breeding seasons.

SELECTION IN DIPLOIDS

Consider a large random mating population, with separate generations, the nth generation being produced from gametes $(1-q_n)\,\mathbf{A} + q_n\,\mathbf{a}$, where $\mathbf{a}$ is recessive. Let the fitness of **aa** relative to **AA** and **Aa** be $1-\phi(q_n)$. Then

$$q_{n+1} = \frac{q_n - q_n^2\phi(q_n)}{1 - q_n^2\,\phi(q_n)}\,. \tag{6}$$

If, as before, $\phi(Q) = 0$, and $q_n = Q + x_n$, we find

$$\Delta x_n = \Delta q_n = -Q\,x_n\,[Q(1-Q)\,\phi'(Q) + \{(2-3Q)\,\phi'(Q) + \tfrac{1}{2}Q\,(1-Q)\,\phi''(Q) + Q^3(1-Q)\,[\phi'(Q)]^2\}\,x_n] + O(x_n^3). \tag{7}$$

Hence for stability $Q^2(1-Q)\ \phi'(Q)$ must be between 0 and 2. However it is more satisfactory to consider the fitness of the recessives as a function of their frequency $r_n = q_n^2$. If $f(r_n) = \phi(q_n)$ and $R = Q^2$, then $\phi'(Q) = 2Q\,f'(R)$. So the condition for stability is

$$0 < f'(R) < \frac{1}{Q^3(1-Q)}\,. \tag{8}$$

That is to say the relative fitness of the recessive or dominant must fall off as its frequency increases, but not too rapidly.

For $Q^3(1-Q)$ is maximal and equal to $\frac{27}{256}$ when $Q = \frac{3}{4}$, or $R = \frac{9}{16}$, so $f'(R) > \frac{256}{27} = 9{\cdot}481$ for instability. As before, the upper limit of stability may be found from equation (8) putting $k = Q^3(1-Q)\,f'(R)$. Stability is greatest when $f'(R) = \dfrac{1}{2Q^3(1-Q)}$.

The deviation x_n from equilibrium clearly diminishes approximately in a geometric progression whose common ratio is $1-k$. Even if $f'(R)$ has a value of $\frac{1}{2}$, which we consider improbably high, this ratio is likely to exceed 0·95; so progress to equilibrium will be slow, and, what is more important, deviations from it due to "random" events will only slowly be damped out.

There is no difficulty in finding results similar to (7) and (8) for more complicated hypotheses, or "models", for example one in which the fitness of **Aa** is intermediate between those of **AA** and **aa**.

For example if the fitnesses of **Aa** and **aa** relative to **AA** are $1-\psi(q_n)$ and $1-\phi(q_n)$, then

$$\Delta q_n = q_n(1-q_n)\,[(2q_n-1)\psi(q_n)-q_n\phi(q_n)] \tag{9}$$

approximately, and an equilibrium is possible when $q_n = Q$,
and $(2Q-1)\psi(Q)=Q\phi(Q)$. (10)

Then if $q_n = Q+x_n$,

$$\Delta x_n = (1-Q)\,[Q(2Q-1)\psi'(Q)-Q^2\phi'(Q)+\psi(Q)]\,x_n+O(x_n^2). \tag{11}$$

So the condition for stability is

$$0 < -\psi(Q)+Q^2\phi'(Q)+Q(1-2Q)\psi'(Q) < \frac{2}{1-Q}. \tag{12}$$

Similarly we may find conditions for stable equilibrium when more than two genes, at the same or different loci, are concerned. Inbreeding and assortative mating only have large effects on the composition of a population when the frequency of one of the genes concerned is fairly small. In the case here considered, either would give rise to conditions for stability intermediate between those found for haploids and diploids.

Discussion

The case discussed here is very simple. For a single pair of allelomorphs there are 9 different types of mating. Not merely may each have its own characteristic fertility, but for each of them there may be a characteristic pattern of prenatal and perinatal mortality as between the three genotypes. In fact a full treatment would involve the specification of 27 arbitrary parameters, or of 26 ratios of such parameters. A full specification of selective intensities at a locus such as *ABO* or *Rh* would be much more complicated.

However the analysis brings out two points. An equilibrium may be unstable because regulation is too intense. And the conditions for stability are widely different when generations overlap and when they are separate. Neither of these results is true for Darwinian selection.

On the other hand, in the cases considered, instability due to over-regulation is most unlikely to occur. From equation (9) we see that this would mean that a 1% increase in the frequency of recessives near the equilibrium would result in a fall of over 9·4% in their fitness. It is perhaps worth pointing out two conditions under which such a drop might conceivably occur. One such possibility is that the dominants or recessives, though fitter in other respects, should be liable to a severe epidemic disease when their frequency reaches a certain threshold. This threshold would not, of course, be definite, but in such a case large oscillations might occur. If, again, one form was a mimic, it is conceivable that the advantage of mimicry might fall off very rapidly when the ratio of mimics to models reached a critical level. Such a critical level would presumably depend on the details of learning or conditioning in a predator, and it is very unlikely that the critical ratio would be the same for different species of predators, or even for all members of a species.

Nevertheless in any consideration of equilibria of this kind, it is worth discussing the stability, and if possible, verifying it. It is likely that once such an equilibrium is approximately established, further selection will occur of modifiers which increases the fitness of the heterozygotes, and hence the equilibrium will be still further stabilized. It would of course be interesting to treat the hypotheses here considered stochastically, taking account of the finite number of a population. But it does not seem that this would greatly effect the conclusions.

SUMMARY

Polymorphism may be due to the fact that the fitness of a phenotype diminishes as its numbers increase. The stability of the equilibrium is discussed, and it is shown that under natural conditions instability is unlikely.

Addendum to

"Polymorphism due to selection depending on the composition of a population" by J. B. S. Haldane and S. D. Jayakar, *Journal of Genetics*, **58** (3), 318-323.

R. C. Lewontin (1958, *Genetics*, **43**, 419) had, unknown to us already proved that "stable equilibria may exist despite an inferiority of the heterozygote, provided that the adaptive values of the genotypes change properly with gene frequency", and for some of our conclusions we acknowledge his priority.

J. B. S. Haldane
S. D. Jayakar

3

SELECTION FOR A SINGLE PAIR OF ALLELOMORPHS WITH COMPLETE REPLACEMENT

By J. B. S. HALDANE AND S. D. JAYAKAR

Genetics and Biometry Laboratory, Government of Orissa, Bhubaneswar-3 Orissa, India

Introduction

Haldane (1924) discussed some simple cases of what he called familial selection, meaning selection with complete replacement within families or litters. Only a few of the possible cases were, however, considered, and it is now possible to produce a more general theory, though, as will be seen, the theory is far from complete even for the case of two allelomorphs.

Hull (1964) has obtained data on mice which are best explained by prenatal selection at one locus. There was evidence that this did not decrease the mean size of litters in which selection occurred. It emerged from a stimulating conversation between J.B.S.H. and Peter Hull and R.C. Lewontin that in such cases the algebra is unexpectedly easy.

We are of course aware that the hypothesis, or "model", is unduly simple. Nevertheless it covers cases where the relative fitness of foetal genotypes depends on the maternal genotype. If this is not the case, the number of parameters required in the autosomal case is reduced, but the algebra is not greatly simplified. We shall only deal here with the case of a single locus, a single pair of allelomorphs at it, and a large random mating population. The extensions to several allelomorphs, several loci, and inbred populations, are easy in principle, but complicate the algebra very considerably. The hypothesis that selective intensities are different in embryos of the two sexes clearly doubles the number of parameters required. It may be better to postpone such developments until the relatively simple cases here set out have been considered by others.

An Autosomal Gene Pair

We consider a pair of allelomorphs **G** and **g** at an autosomal locus. The use of a capital letter does not imply dominance. We suppose generations to be separate. Let the nth generation at fertilization consist of:

$$x_n\mathbf{GG}+2y_n\mathbf{Gg}+z_n\mathbf{gg}$$

where $x_n+2y_n+z_n=1$, $p_n=x_n+y_n$, $q_n=y_n+z_n$. Clearly p_n and q_n are the gene frequencies. The progeny of $\mathbf{GG}♀\times\mathbf{Gg}♂$ at fertilization are $x_ny_n\mathbf{GG}+x_ny_n\,\mathbf{Gg}$. We suppose that at birth (or later, if selection and replacement occur after birth within litters) they are $(1+a)\ x_ny_n\mathbf{GG}+(1-a)x_ny_n\,\mathbf{Gg}$. The total of progeny from such matings is unaltered, $1\geqslant a\geqslant -1$. We have six parameters such as a, and make the convention that they are given positive values when selection favours the maternal genotype. The progeny surviving to mate are shown in Table 1.

Table 1

Mother	Father	Mating frequency	Surviving progeny		
			GG	**Gg**	**gg**
GG	**GG**	x^2	x^2		
GG	**Gg**	$2xy$	$(1+a)xy$	$(1-a)xy$	
GG	**gg**	xz		xz	
Gg	**GG**	$2xy$	$(1-b)xy$	$(1+b)xy$	
Gg	**Gg**	$4y^2$	$(1-c)y^2$	$(2+c+\gamma)y^2$	$(1-\gamma)y^2$
Gg	**gg**	$2yz$		$(1+\beta)yz$	$(1-\beta)yz$
gg	**GG**	xz		xz	
gg	**Gg**	$2yz$		$(1-\alpha)yz$	$(1+\alpha)yz$
gg	**gg**	z^2			z^2

Explanation in text. x is written for x_n, and so on.

If selection were independent of maternal genotype we should have $a=-b$, $\alpha=-\beta$, and probably $c=b$, $\gamma=\beta$. However it is precisely in such cases as this that we may expect the relative viabilities of foetal genotypes to depend on the maternal genotype. This scheme may apply to selection in the human species at the ABO locus, but it cannot apply to selection at the Rh locus. For though the death of **Dd** offspring of **dd** mothers and **Dd** fathers may be compensated fully by replacement with **dd,** this cannot occur from the union of **DD**♂ and **dd**♀.

On adding the columns in Table 1 we have:

$$\left.\begin{aligned} x_{n+1}&=p_n^2+[(a-b)x_n-cy_n]y_n,\\ 2y_{n+1}&=2p_nq_n+[(-a+b)x_n+(c+\gamma)y_n+(-\alpha+\beta)z_n]y_n,\\ z_{n+1}&=q_n^2+[-\gamma y_n+(\alpha-\beta)z_n]y_n. \end{aligned}\right\} \qquad (1\cdot1)$$

If we put $a-b=d$, $\alpha-\beta=\delta$, this becomes

$$\left.\begin{aligned} x_{n+1}&=p_n^2+(dx_n-cy_n)y_n,\\ y_{n+1}&=p_nq_n+\tfrac{1}{2}[-dx_n+(c+\gamma)y_n-\delta z_n]y_n,\\ z_{n+1}&=q_n^2+(-\gamma y_n+\delta z_n). \end{aligned}\right\} \qquad (1\cdot2)$$

Thus we have reduced the parameters specifying selection to four.

Since $x_n = p_n - y_n$, $z_n = q_n - y_n$, we find:

$$p_{n+1} = p_n + \tfrac{1}{2}y_n\,[dp_n - \delta q_n + (\gamma + \delta - c - d)y_n], \tag{1·3}$$

$$y_{n+1} = p_n q_n + \tfrac{1}{2}y_n[-dp_n - \delta q_n + (c + d + \gamma + \delta)y_n], \tag{1·4}$$

with a similar equation for q_n. Clearly there are equilibria, stable or unstable, at $p=0$ and 1, and there may be equilibria at one or more intermediate values of p. When p_n is small, $y_n = p_n - O(p_n^2)$, while $q_n = 1 - p_n$. So from (1·3)

$$p_{n+1} = (1 - \tfrac{1}{2}\delta)p_n + O(p_n^2).$$

So the equilibrium at $p=0$ is stable if δ is positive, and p_n tends to zero with $(1-\frac{1}{2}\delta)^n$. If δ is negative this equilibrium is unstable. If $\delta = 0$, $p_{n+1} = p_n + \frac{1}{2}(\gamma - c)p_n^2 + O(p_n^3)$. So the equilibrium is stable if $c > \gamma$, though it is approached slowly, and unstable if $c < \gamma$. If $\delta = 0$ and $c = \gamma$: $p_{n+1} = p_n + \frac{1}{2}dx_n y_n$, so the equilibrium is stable if d is negative, unstable if d is positive. Similarly the equlilibrium at $p=1$ is stable if $d > 0$; if $d=0$ and $c<\gamma$; or if $d=0$, $c=\gamma$, $\delta<0$.

Let us now consider an equilibrium at $p_n = P$, where $1 > P > 0$. Let $P+Q=1$, and $y_n = Y$. Then from (1·3), since Y is not zero, $dP - \delta Q + (\gamma + \delta - c - d)Y = 0$, or

$$Y = \frac{dP - \delta Q}{c + d - \gamma - \delta}.$$ On substituting this value in (1·4) we find:

$$Y = PQ + Y\left[\frac{d(\gamma+\delta)P - \delta(c+d)Q}{c+d-\gamma-\delta}\right], \text{ or}$$

$$PQ = (c+d-\gamma-\delta)^{-2}(dP - \delta Q)\ \ [(c+d-\gamma-\delta-d\gamma-d\delta)P + (c+d-\gamma-\delta+c\delta+d\delta)Q],$$

whence

$$d(c+d-\gamma-\delta-d\gamma-d\delta)P^2 + [(\gamma-c)\,(c+d-\gamma-\delta) + d\delta(c+d+\gamma+\delta)]PQ$$
$$-\delta(c+d-\gamma-\delta+c\delta+d\delta)Q^2 = 0. \tag{1·5}$$

This is a quadratic equation for PQ^{-1}. The number of equilibria other than 0 and 1 is equal to the number of its real positive roots. However their number and stability can also, in many cases, be determined from the condition that stable and unstable roots must alternate. If d and δ are positive, i.e. $a > b$, $\alpha > \beta$, then there is one other unstable equilibrium, and (1·5) must have one negative root which is biologically meaningless. If d and δ are both negative, i.e. $a < b$, $\alpha < \beta$, then there is one stable equilibrium at an intermediate value, and again (1·5) has a negative root. If however d and δ have opposite signs, (1·5) may have two real positive roots, in which case one represents a stable, the other an unstable equilibrium. Or both roots may be negative or complex, in which case there is no equilibrium other than $p=0$ or 1.

We have to show that all these are actually possible. This is readily seen to be so when c, d, γ and δ are all numerically small when (1·5) reduces to

$$dP^2 + (\gamma - c)PQ - \delta Q^2 = 0, \text{ nearly}.$$

Hence $PQ^{-1} = \dfrac{c-\gamma \pm [(c-\gamma)^2 + 4d\delta]^{\frac{1}{2}}}{2d}$.

Since d and δ have opposite signs, $d\delta$ is negative. Both roots are complex if $(c-\gamma)^2 < -4d\delta$. In this case there is no intermediate equilibrium. We may suppose d to be positive, or $a>b$, without loss of generality. If $(c-\gamma)^2 > -4d\delta$ and $c>\gamma$ both roots are positive. If $(c-\gamma)^2 > -4d\delta$ and $c<\gamma$ then both roots are negative, and there is no intermediate equilibrium. Thus an intermediate equilibrium is only possible if $c-\gamma > 2(-d\delta)^{\frac{1}{2}}$. If $(c-\gamma)^2 + 4d\delta = 0$ the roots coincide, and yield an equilibrium which is effectively unstable, though change in its neighbourhood is very slow. Similar conditions can of course be derived from (1·5) when squares and products of the parameters are too large to be neglected.

In a small population drift will of course tend to fix the population at $p=0$ or 1, that is to say in homozygosity, if either is stable. On the other hand when d and δ are both negative, i.e. $a<b$, $a<\beta$, an intermediate equilibrium will alone be stable, and if drift leads temporarily to homozygosity in a small population, mutation or immigration will bring it back to the intermediate value. In all cases where an intermediate equilibrium is stable, $p_n - P$ falls off like a geometric series when it is sufficiently small.

The case where the only stable equilibrium involves the presence of both allelomorphs is perhaps the most interesting. The conditions for it are that $b>a$, $\beta>a$. Both these conditions mean that, on the whole, heterozygous embryos or foetus in heterozygous mothers are fitter than homozygous embryos or foetus in homozygous mothers. On the other hand if these conditions are not fulfilled c and γ may both be quite large and positive without stabilizing the intermediate equilibrium. That is to say greater fitness of heterozygotes carried by heterozygous mothers mated to heterozygous fathers is without influence; though the values of c and γ will, of course, influence the frequencies at an intermediate equilibrium. Thus a higher fitness of heterozygotes, averaged over all types of mother, is not a necessary or sufficient condition for a stable equilibrium. It is also perhaps worth noting that the case where both a stable and an unstable equilibrium occur with both genes present is not found for a single pair of allelomorphs whose fitnesses do not depend on the maternal genotype.

Selection at a Sex-linked Locus

We assume that the male sex is heterogametic or haploid. The adjustment to be made in the case of birds and Lepidoptera is obvious. Consider a pair of sex-linked allelomorphs **S** and **s**. Here selection of the kind considered can only operate in the progeny of heterozygous mothers, so the algebra is much simplified. The parameters b and β are taken as positive if the foetal genotype is that of the father. Since this very rarely if ever influences pre-natal fitness, $b+\beta=0$ as a general rule. Let ♀ genotypes in the nth generation occur in frequencies x_n**SS**, $2y_n$**Ss**, z_n**ss**, and ♂ genotypes in frequencies u_n**S**, v_n**s**. Let $p_n = x_n + y_n$, $q_n = y_n + z_n$. Clearly $u_n + v_n = p_n + q_n = 1$. The progeny surviving to mate are shown in Table 2.

Table 2

Mother	Father	Mating frequency	Surviving ♀ progeny SS	Ss	ss	Surviving ♂ progeny S	s
SS	S	ux	ux			ux	
SS	s	vx		vx		vx	
Ss	S	$2uy$	$(1-a)uy$	$(1+a)uy$		$(1+b)uy$	$(1-b)uy$
Ss	s	$2vy$		$(1+\alpha)vy$	$(1-\alpha)vy$	$(1-\beta)vy$	$(1+\beta)vy$
ss	S	uz		uz			uz
ss	s	vz			vz		vz

Here x means x_n, and so on.

On adding the progeny columns we find:

$$\left.\begin{aligned} u_{n+1}&=p_n+(bu_n-\beta v_n)y_n,\\ v_{n+1}&=q_n-(bu_n-\beta v_n)y_n,\\ x_{n+1}&=u_np_n-au_ny_n,\\ 2y_{n+1}&=u_nq_n+v_np_n+(au_n+\alpha v_n)y_n,\\ z_{n+1}&=v_nq_n-\alpha v_ny_n.\end{aligned}\right\} \qquad (2{\cdot}1)$$

Whence

$$\left.\begin{aligned} p_{n+1}&=\tfrac{1}{2}(p_n+u_n)+\tfrac{1}{2}(-au_n+\alpha v_n)y_n,\\ u_{n+1}&=p_n+(bu_n-\beta v_n)y_n,\\ y_{n+1}&=\tfrac{1}{2}(u_nq_n+v_np_n)+\tfrac{1}{2}(au_n+\alpha v_n)y_n,\end{aligned}\right\} \qquad (2{\cdot}2)$$

with similar equations for q_n and v_n. It is easily seen that there are equilibria when $p_n=u_n=y_n=0$, and $p_n=u_n=1$, $y_n=0$. There may also be an intermediate equilibrium. Equations (2·2) may be written:

$$\left.\begin{aligned} p_{n+1}&=\tfrac{1}{2}[p_n+u_n+\alpha y_n-(a+\alpha)u_ny_n],\\ u_{n+1}&=p_n+[-\beta+(b+\beta)u_n]y_n,\\ y_{n+1}&=\tfrac{1}{2}[p_n+u_n+\alpha y_n-2p_nu_n+(a-\alpha)u_ny_n].\end{aligned}\right\} \qquad (2{\cdot}3)$$

It is clear that when n is large and p_n, u_n and y_n are all small quantities of the same order,

$$p_{n+1}=\tfrac{1}{2}(p_n+u_n+\alpha y_n)+O(p_n^2),$$

$$u_{n+1}=p_n-\beta y_n+O(p_n^2),$$

$$y_{n+1}=\tfrac{1}{2}(p_n+u_n+\alpha y_n)+O(p_n^2).$$

Hence $y_n = p_n + O(p_n^2)$, and

$$p_{n+1} = \tfrac{1}{2}[(1+a)p_n + u_n] + O(p_n^2),$$
$$u_{n+1} = (1-\beta)p_n + O(p_n^2), \qquad (2\cdot4)$$

so that $2p_{n+2} - (1+a)p_{n+1} - (1-\beta)p_n = O(p_n^2)$.

Thus p_n tends to zero with the nth power of the numerically larger root of $2\lambda^2 - (1+a)\lambda - 1 + \beta = 0$, provided this root is less than unity. This is so if and only if $a < \beta$, in which case p_n tends to zero with λ^n, where

$$\lambda = \tfrac{1}{4}[(9+2a-8\beta+a^2)^{\frac{1}{2}} + 1 + a].$$

Thus if $a < \beta$ the equilibrium at $p_n = u_n = 0$ is stable, while if $a < b$ that at $p_n = u_n = 1$ is stable. In either case y_n tends to zero.

Let us now consider an intermediate equilibrium where $p_n = P$, $u_n = U$, $y_n = Y$. From (2·2),

$$\left.\begin{aligned} P &= U + (-aU + aV)Y, \\ U &= P + (bU - \beta V)Y. \end{aligned}\right\} \qquad (2\cdot5)$$

Hence $Y = 0$, or $(b-a)\;U + (a-\beta)V = 0$. Thus since $U + V = 1$,

$$U = \frac{a-\beta}{a-b+a-\beta}, \quad V = \frac{a-b}{a-b+a-\beta}. \qquad (2\cdot6)$$

These are positive if $a-b$ and $a-\beta$ have the same sign, that is to say in this case there is an intermediate equilibrium. It is clearly stable if $a > b$, and $a > \beta$, that is to say if the other two equilibria are unstable, and conversely. If one is stable and the other unstable, e.g. $a > b$, $a < \beta$, (2·6) gives one negative value and one exceeding unity. These have no biological meaning. Equations (2·3) and (2·6) give:

$$(a-b+a-\beta)P - (a\beta - ba)Y - a + \beta = 0,$$

$$(a-b-a+\beta)P - [2(a-b+a-\beta) - 2aa + a\beta + ba]Y + a - \beta = 0.$$

Whence

$$\left.\begin{aligned} P &= \frac{(a-\beta)\;[(a-b+a-\beta) - a(a-\beta)]}{(a-b+a-\beta)^2 - a(a-\beta)^2 - a(a-b)^2}, \\ Q &= \frac{(a-b)[(a-b+a-\beta) - a(a-b)]}{(a-b+a-\beta)^2 - a(a-\beta)^2 - a(a-b)^2}, \\ Y &= \frac{(a-b)\;(a-\beta)}{(a-b+a-\beta)^2 - a(a-\beta)^2 - a(a-b)^2}. \end{aligned}\right\} \qquad (2\cdot7)$$

Successive values of $p_n - P$ etc., when small, approximate to a geometric progression.

DISCUSSION

It is perhaps worth pointing out why the algebra in this case is relatively simple. Suppose that in the autosomal case the litter size, or total fertility, were different for different matings, we should require 14 parameters instead of 6 to specify selection in Table 1. And the equations analogous to (1·1) would all share a denominator, namely Wright's W, the mean fitness of the population, which is a quadratic function of x_n, y_n, and z_n. No doubt this is nearer to the truth than the hypothesis or "model" here studied. But the expressions for the stability of equilibria are very complicated, and numerical data do not exist and are unlikely to exist for many years.

We have found new conditions for stable polymorphism at a locus. Some do not involve a greater fitness of heterozygotes. Thus if in Table 2, b and β were zero, while a and α were negative, there would be stable polymorphism. It is difficult, but not impossible, to imagine mechanisms which would make a and α negative. They would perhaps, be more probable if the female sex were heterogametic, in which case this would mean that the female genotype differing from the mother's would be favoured. Since the mother's genotype as well as its own influences the characters of eggs and larvae in many cases in *Bombyx mori*, it seems likely that such effects might be found in Lepidoptera.

Overlap of generations will lead to the same equilibria, though the dynamics will require special treatment. Many variations on the theme are possible, but it would hardly be worth considering them all until a concrete case arises. The methods here used seem, however, to be fairly widely applicable.

SUMMARY

Recurrence equations are given for genotype frequencies at an autosomal or a sex-linked locus when selection is entirely prenatal, and all matings are equally fertile. In some cases stable polymorphism is possible. These do not necessarily require greater fitness of heterozygotes.

REFERENCES

HALDANE, J. B. S. (1924). A mathematical theory of natural and artificial selection, Part. I. *Trans. Camb. Phil. Soc.*, **23**, 19-41.

HULL, PETER (1964). Partial incompatibility not affecting total litter size in the mouse. *Genetics*, **50**, 563-570.

Mutation and Human Genetics

Haldane's contributions to human genetics, which at first began quite inadvertently because of his interest in genetic equilibria, were of great importance in laying the foundations of that science. Whether we consider the first estimation of human mutation rate (1932, 1935), pedigree analysis (1932), first estimation of linkage (1937), mutation damage in populations (1937), role of modifying genes (1941), gene-environment interaction (1946), or any other aspect of human genetics, we must consider Haldane's work first.

In his analysis of the effect of variation on fitness, Haldane (1937) showed that the impact of mutation on the fitness of a population is almost entirely dependent on the mutation rate but not on the deleteriousness of the individual mutations. This principle, which was later discovered independently by H.J. Muller, [1] was the basis for developing a theory of genetic loads by J.F. Crow [2] and had been applied to the analysis of genetic damage resulting from ionizing radiation.

During his last years in India (1957–64), he was deeply interested in the mating patterns and genetic consequences in the local populations. The last paper with S.D. Jayakar was written during that period and was quite deliberately designed as a bridge between anthropology and human genetics.

The papers included in this section contain novel concepts, methods, and suggestions that continue to influence the direction of human genetics today, though some younger workers may not be aware of the source of these ideas. This, as Haldane once said, is the greatest compliment one can pay to a scientist: to accept and incorporate his contributions so thoroughly that the need to mention his name seldom arises.

1. Muller, H.J., Our load of mutations. *Amer. J. Hum. Genet.*, 2: 111–176, 1950.
2. Crow, J.F., Genetic loads and the cost of natural selection . In: K. Kojima (Ed.), *Mathematical Topics in Population Genetics*. Berlin: Springer-Verlag.

[FROM JOURNAL OF GENETICS, VOL. XXV. NO. 2, pp. 251–255, FEBRUARY, 1932.]

A METHOD FOR INVESTIGATING RECESSIVE CHARACTERS IN MAN.

BY J. B. S. HALDANE.

(*John Innes Horticultural Institution, Merton.*)

HOGBEN (1931), who reviews the former literature, employs a method due to Lenz (1929) for investigating human characters which are believed to be recessive. Allowance is made for the fact that a number of families derived from unions of two heterozygotes are not included among the observed data because they contain no recessives. A value p is then found for the probability that (after making the necessary allowance) the child of two heterozygous parents should be recessive. Its standard error is determined by a method due to Hogben. If it differs from $\frac{1}{4}$ by less than several times its standard error, it is reasonable to assume that the character is recessive.

This method suffers from the defect that the calculation of p involves the expected value of $\frac{1}{4}$. The method here given does not involve this assumption, and leads to different values. The following theorem will be proved:

If a group of families derived from normal parents, each family containing at least one abnormal, consists of n_s families of size s, the values of s ranging from 1 to c, and contains R recessives in all, then the most likely value of q, the proportion of normals in a family (supposed constant), is the real root other than unity of the equation

$$\frac{R}{1-q} = \sum_{s=1}^{c} \frac{s \,.\, n_s}{1-q^s}, \qquad \text{......(1)}$$

and the standard error σ of q (and hence of $p = 1 - q$) is given by the equation

$$\sigma^{-2} = \frac{R}{q(1-q)^2} - \sum_{s=1}^{c} \frac{s^2 q^{s-2} n_s}{(1-q^s)^2}. \qquad \text{......(2)}$$

To prove this theorem, let the number of families of size s containing k abnormals be n_{sk}, so that

$$\sum_{k=1}^{s} n_{sk} = n_s.$$

Also the total number of abnormals in families of size s is given by

$$r_s = \sum_{k=1}^{s} k n_{sk}, \text{ and } R = \sum_{s=1}^{c} r_s.$$

We now apply Fisher's (1921) method of maximum likelihood. The probability that a family of s individuals will contain k abnormals is, as Lenz pointed out, ${}_sC_k\, p^k q^{s-k}$, provided we include the families containing no abnormals, the proportion of such families being q^s. Thus the probability that a family containing at least one abnormal will actually contain k is

$$\frac{{}_sC_k\, p^k\, q^{s-k}}{1 - q^s}.$$

The number of such families found is n_{sk}. Then the most likely value of q is found by making $L(q)$ a maximum, where

$$L(q) = \sum_{s=1}^{c} \sum_{k=1}^{s} n_{sk} \log \left(\frac{p^k q^{s-k}}{1 - q^s}\right).$$

The factor ${}_sC_k$, which is not a function of q, is omitted.

$$\therefore L(q) = \sum_{s=1}^{c} \sum_{k=1}^{s} n_{sk} \left[k \log (1 - q) + (s - k) \log q - \log (1 - q^s)\right].$$

The condition for this to be maximal is

$$0 = L'(q) = \sum_{s=1}^{c} \sum_{k=1}^{s} n_{sk} \left(\frac{k}{q - 1} + \frac{s - k}{q} + \frac{s q^{s-1}}{1 - q^s}\right)$$

$$= \sum_{s=1}^{c} \sum_{k=1}^{s} n_{sk} \left[\frac{s}{q(1 - q^s)} - \frac{k}{q(1 - q)}\right]$$

$$= \sum_{s=1}^{c} \left[\frac{s n_s}{q(1 - q^s)} - \frac{r_s}{q(1 - q)}\right]$$

$$= \sum_{s=1}^{c} \frac{s n_s}{q(1 - q^s)} - \frac{R}{q(1 - q)}.$$

$$\therefore \frac{R}{1 - q} = \sum_{s=1}^{c} \frac{s n_s}{1 - q^s},$$

since q is finite. This may be written

$$R = \sum_{s=1}^{c} \frac{s n_s}{1 + q + q^2 + \ldots q^{s-1}},$$

since $q \neq 1$, whence it is clear that the right-hand side decreases steadily from $\sum^{c} s n_s$ to $\sum^{c} n_s$, as q increases from 0 to 1, and as R lies between these values there is only one real positive root which is less than 1, if we disregard the solution $q = 1$. The standard deviation is given by

$$\sigma^{-2} = -L''(q) = \frac{\partial}{\partial q}\left[\frac{R}{q(1-q)} - \sum_{s=1}^{c} \frac{sn_s}{q(1-q^s)}\right],$$

where q is given the value determined by equation (1).

$$\therefore \sigma^{-2} = \sum_{s=1}^{c} \frac{(1 - sq^s - q^s)\,sn_s}{q^2(1-q^s)^2} - \frac{R(1-2q)}{q^2(1-q)^2}$$

$$= \frac{R}{q^2(1-q)} - \frac{R(1-2q)}{q^2(1-q)^2} - \sum_{s=1}^{c} \frac{s^2 q^s n_s}{q^2(1-q^s)^2}$$

$$= \frac{R}{q(1-q)^2} - \sum_{s=1}^{c} \frac{s^2 q^{s-2} n_s}{(1-q^s)^2}.$$

Let us apply this method to Sjögren's (1931) data on juvenile amaurotic family idiocy, as summarised by Hogben. We can clearly neglect the families where $s = 1$, since the terms due to them cancel out in both equations (1) and (2). Thus to find q we must solve the equation

$$\frac{6}{1+q} + \frac{21}{1+q+q^2} + \frac{40}{1+q+q^2+q^3} + \frac{35}{1+q+\dots q^4} + \frac{36}{1+q+\dots q^5}$$
$$+ \frac{49}{1+q+\dots q^6} + \frac{56}{1+q+\dots q^7} + \frac{18}{1+q+\dots q^8} + \frac{11}{1+q+\dots q^{10}}$$
$$+ \frac{12}{1+q+\dots q^{11}} + \frac{13}{1+q+\dots q^{12}} = 108.$$

Such equations are most easily solved by the method of trial and error. q is easily seen to be less than 0·75. $q = 0{\cdot}68$ makes the left-hand side $= 108{\cdot}72$, while $q = 0{\cdot}69$ makes it 106·39. $\therefore q = 0{\cdot}683$, $p = 0{\cdot}317$.

Putting $q = 0{\cdot}683$ in equation (2), we find

$$\sigma^{-2} = 995{\cdot}3.$$
$$\therefore \sigma = {\cdot}0317.$$

Hence p deviates from its expected value of 0·250 by 0·067, or 2·2 times its standard error. Such a deviation is almost certainly significant. Hogben finds $p = 0{\cdot}286$, and the standard deviation of this quantity calculated by his method is 0·015. The deviation is thus found to be 2·4 times the standard. The results obtained by the two methods do not diverge widely in this case, in so far as concerns the probability of so great a deviation from the expected value of $\frac{1}{4}$.

The relation between the two methods is as follows. Lenz solves the equation

$$\frac{R}{1-q} = \sum_{s=1}^{c} \frac{sn_s}{1-(\frac{3}{4})^s}.$$

If we call this value q_1 and proceed to solve the equation

$$\frac{R}{1-q} = \sum_{s=1}^{c} \frac{sn_s}{1-q_1^s},$$

we obtain a value q_2. Similarly by substituting q_2 on the right-hand side we obtain a value q_3 and so on. It can easily be shown that these values converge to the value of q given by equation (1). The approximation of q_1 is better, and the convergence quicker, the larger the average size of the families.

Another method of treating such data by the method of maximum likelihood is as follows. We can consider only the families of size s. Then for each such group of families we have

$$\frac{sn_s}{1-q^s} = \frac{r_s}{1-q}.$$

$$\therefore q^s r_s - qsn_s + sn_s - r_s = 0.$$

$$\therefore q = 1 - \frac{(1-q^s)\, r_s}{sn_s}.$$

This formula has been given by Bernstein (1931). We now substitute some value of q such as $\frac{3}{4}$ or $\frac{1}{2}$ on the right-hand side, and find q_1 on the left; we repeat until the values converge. This method has the great merit that mistakes in arithmetic are automatically corrected. Sjögren's data for $s = 4$ give the following successive approximations to q:

0·75, 0·6753, 0·62379, 0·59691, 0·58517, 0·58065, 0·57898, 0·57875.

We take 0·579 as the true value. The results for all Sjögren's data are given in Table I. It will be seen that the unexpectedly high value of p is wholly due to the small families. The high values in these seem to be significant. Thus for $s = 4$, the standard deviation of p is 0·093, the actual deviation 0·171. From data such as those of Table I it is possible to calculate the overall value of p, each individual value being weighted with the squared reciprocal of its standard error. But the result is rather inaccurate when the values of r_s are small.

TABLE I.

s	2	3	4	5	6	7	8	9	10	11	12	13
n_s	3	7	10	7	6	7	7	2	0	1	1	1
r_s	5	10	19	11	9	13	25	6	0	3	3	4
p	0·80	0·338	0·421	0·228	0·166	0·218	0·443	0·323	—	0·264	0·241	0·305

Several explanations are possible. In view of the extremely thorough nature of Sjögren's work it is hardly likely that any appreciable number of cases of juvenile amaurotic idiocy within the area studied were omitted. We may be dealing with a peculiar biological fact, but a psychological explanation is also possible. It may be that a number of parents, after producing one or two idiot children, voluntarily or involuntarily limited their families in future.

The method here given is certainly slower than that of Lenz and Hogben. But considering that Sjögren spent three years in his investigation, an expenditure of three hours on calculations concerning it is not excessive. It has two merits. In the first place it is free from any bias regarding the value of p, except that all values in the neighbourhood of that found are considered about equally likely, *a priori*. The exact assumption is given by Haldane (1932). In the second place it gives considerably better results if p deviates seriously from $\frac{1}{4}$. For example should double recessive characters exist, for which $p = \frac{1}{16}$, this value would not be given by the Lenz-Hogben method, if one started with the assumption that $q = \frac{3}{4}$. The method is obviously applicable to cases of sex linkage, where values of p in the neighbourhood of $\frac{1}{2}$ may be expected when all male offspring of normal parents in families containing at least one affected person are considered.

I have to thank Prof. Hogben for suggesting the investigation of this question, and for allowing me to see his paper in proof.

SUMMARY.

A method is given by which the true proportion of recessives may be calculated from human or other data on small families.

REFERENCES.

BERNSTEIN, F. (1931). "Ist die Weinbergsche Geschwistermethode neben der direkten Methode zu nutzen?" *Zeits. indukt. Abstamm. u. Vererb.* LVIII, 434.

FISHER, R. A. (1921). "On the mathematical foundations of theoretical statistics." *Phil. Trans. Roy. Soc.* A. CCXXII, 309.

HALDANE, J. B. S. (1932). "A note on inverse probability." *Proc. Camb. Phil. Soc.* (in the press).

HOGBEN, L. T. (1931). "The genetic analysis of familial traits. I. Single gene substitutions." *Journ. Genet.* XXV, 97.

LENZ, F. (1929). "Methoden der menschlichen Erblichkeitsforschung." *Handbuch der hygienischen Untersuchungsmethoden*, III, 700, Jena.

SJÖGREN, T. (1931). "Die juvenile amaurotische Idiotie—Klinische und erblichkeitsmedizinische Untersuchungen." *Hereditas*, XIV, 197.

THE
AMERICAN NATURALIST

Vol. LXVII January–February, 1933 No. 708

THE PART PLAYED BY RECURRENT MUTATION IN EVOLUTION

J. B. S. HALDANE
John Innes Horticultural Institution, Merton, London

The discovery that certain mutations occur with a measurable frequency has had a great influence on evolutionary speculation. It is the object of this paper to attempt to delimit the part which it may have played in evolution. The suggested effects have been primary and secondary. In the first place, it has been thought that as the result of recurrent mutation of a gene to its allelomorph, the new allelomorph has gradually spread through the population, displacing the original gene. In the second place, it has been pointed out that recurrent mutation of a gene would have secondary effects, even if the mutations were disadvantageous. Lethal genes, like parasites or predators, are part of the environment of the other genes. Fisher (1928) thought that the main secondary effect of disadvantageous mutations would be the accumulation of modifying genes tending to make the mutant type recessive. Some other secondary effects are suggested in this paper. Throughout I shall use the word "mutation" to denote a change in a single gene, and not with reference to such events as mutation in *Oenothera*, which generally depends on a rearrangement of the chromatin.

The evolutionary effects of mutation which will be considered are as follows:

(1) Evolution due to a mutation rate so large as to cause the spread of a disadvantageous character.

(2) Primary effects of the spread of genes nearly neutral from the point of view of natural selection: (a) Appearance of valueless but not harmful characters. (b) Disappearance of valueless but not harmful characters. (c) Disappearance of genes in the Y chromosome. (d) Disappearance of genes in the "complex" of permanently heterozygous species. (e) Disappearance of extra genes in polyploids and polysomics. (f) Primary increase of dominance.

(3) Secondary effects of frequent disadvantageous mutations: (a) Increase of dominance due to mutation of dominant allelomorphs. (b) Increase of dominance due to spread of modifying genes. (c) Selective value of polyploidy, polysomy, and duplication. (d) Male haploidy. (e) Heterogametism of male rather than female sex. (f) Concentration of mutable genes in the X chromosome. (g) Development of internal balance in the X chromosome.

In general, mutation is a necessary but not sufficient cause of evolution. Without mutation there would be no gene differences for natural selection to act upon. But the actual evolutionary trend would seem usually to be determined by selection, for the following reason.

A simple calculation shows that recurrent mutation (except of a gene so unstable as to be classifiable as multimutating) can not overcome selection of quite moderate intensity. Consider two phenotypes whose relative fitnesses are in the ratios 1 and $1-k$, that is to say, that on the average one leaves $(1-k)$ times as many progeny as the other. Then, if p is the probability that a gene mutates to a less fit allelomorph in the course of a life cycle, it has been shown (Haldane, 1932) that when k is small, the mutant gene will only spread through a small fraction of the population unless p is about as large as k or larger. This is true whether the gene is dominant or recessive.

Now p is usually small. The largest value found by Stadler (1929) in the case of 8 maize genes was 4×10^{-4}, the lowest being less than 10^{-6}. We may take 10^{-3} as an upper limit in ordinary cases. This means that a coefficient of selection k of 10^{-3} would prevent them from spreading very far. The best cases of repeated mutation of the same gene induced by abnormal environment are those of Goldschmidt (1929) and Jollos (1931). Unfortunately, the values of p can not be determined from their data, though it probably exceeded ·01. But the heat used by them on *Drosophila* larvae killed many, and sterilized many more, and it seems likely that such stringent environmental conditions would wipe a species out rather than force it into a particular evolutionary path.

Very high mutation rates due to heat may perhaps have played a part in evolution in two cases. It may have caused orthogenetic evolution of species near the tropical limit of their range, and thus may possibly be partly responsible for the greater diversity of species found in tropical as compared with temperate and arctic habitats. Again, the gonads of mammals and birds are permanently at a higher temperature than is usual in other organisms. It is possible that when this temperature was first evolved, it increased the mutation rate of their genes. At the same time many new ecological niches were open, and therefore many types of mutation possessed a selective advantage. These two facts may have played a part in the very rapid evolution of mammals during the Eocene. But no definite opinion on this question is called for till a population of *Drosophila* or some other form has been shown to evolve under the influence of high temperature. If this could be experimentally shown to occur, and not to be due to selection, such an experiment would be decisive.

There are other possible causes of a very rapid mutation rate. Natural radioactivity may have caused local outbursts of mutation, but a simple calculation dispels the attractive idea that the amount of radioactive substances near the earth's surface 10^9 years ago was sufficient even to double the present mutation rates. The evidence for mutation under chemical influences is at present inconclusive. Demereč (1929) has found that one gene may influence the mutability of another, and it is conceivable that such genes may have played a temporary part in evolution, being eliminated when a relative equilibrium was reached, and mutability ceased to be advantageous.

While, therefore, we can not deny the possibility that mutation frequency may occasionally have been large enough to counterbalance natural selection, and even to cause orthogenetic evolution of a disadvantageous character, such events must have been rare. I have pointed out elsewhere (Haldane, 1932) that many of the cases of orthogenesis ending in extinction can be explained on quite orthodox Darwinian lines. For the survival of the fittest individuals does not necessarily produce a fitter species, and competition based on such characters as embryonic or pollen tube growth rates may be expected in some cases to lead to monstrous adult forms. We must, therefore, expect that the main effects of recurrent mutation have been due to mutation rates of much less than one in a thousand per generation. It is to these that we now turn.

Where a number of allelomorphs seem to be of equal selective value, as in the case of those responsible for banding in snails and blood groups in man, their relative frequency in the population will be determined, not by the fitness of the genotypes, but by the stability of the genes. Diver (1929) has shown that the proportion of banded to unbanded *Cepaea* in England has not varied appreciably in the last few thousand years. k is therefore much less than one thousandth, and may be less than the mutation rate of one of the genes concerned. In this case, if the "banded" gene mutates less frequently than the "unbanded," it will spread until most British *Cepaea* are banded. Such cases are perhaps rare and their evolutionary importance slight, but they do seem to exist.

The main cases where mutation is a primary cause of evolution have in common the feature that mutations in one direction are weeded out by natural selection, those in the other being neutral. Consider the genetics of a useless organ such as the pelvis of a whale or the clavicle of a dog. Such organs must be practically neutral. The amount of extra calcium and phosphorus made available to a whale or dog by the complete disappearance of these bones would be extremely small, and neither whale nor dog, from the nature of their diets, can suffer from a shortage of these elements, where a small margin would be important. Of the genes affecting such vestigial organs a majority will probably affect other organs too, and be selected in accordance with these effects. A few genes will mainly affect the useless organ. Now the majority of mutations affecting an organ generally tend to bring about a reduction in its size. This is well seen in the case of the numerous genes affecting wings and bristles in *Drosophila*, and is intelligible on any biochemical theory of any gene action. The usual, though very slow, effect of mutations will thus be to diminish the size of vestiges. But as an organ becomes useless, genes which exaggerate it also become less harmful than before. For example, megalocornea would be of little harm to an animal living in complete darkness, and petalody of the stamens, though involving a slight waste of material, would not seriously handicap an apogamous plant. In spite of such occasional exceptions it is clear that the general trend will be towards the very slow progressive reduction of vestiges. As this will in some cases be due to the actual disappearance of genes, it may, in its later stages, be irreversible.

An important particular case of the disappearance by mutation of useless organs is the disappearance of the genes in the Y chromosome. There is strong reason to believe that the Y chromosome has been evolved from a chromosome with a normal complement of genes, originally homologous with the X. Such chromosomes appear still to exist in some dioecious plants, and in fish such as *Lebistes*. On this view the Y chromosome originally differed from the X only in respect of one gene. As soon as sex differences come to depend on more than one gene, crossing over must be suppressed in the heterogametic sex, or else the Y chromosome must differ so much from the X morphologically as to render crossing over rare.

Clearly, in so far as genes in the X chromosome are fully dominant, natural selection will not oppose recessive mutations of genes in the Y chromosome. And deficiencies, that is to say, complete disappearance of genes, are stabler than ordinary recessives, which may occasionally mutate back. Thus in the long run ordinary recessive genes will be replaced by deficiencies. In some cases where dominance is incomplete the relatively small disadvantage caused by heterozygosity will not be enough to weed out recessive mutations, and these will tend to accentuate the difference between the sexes. In other cases of incomplete dominance, dominance will evolve, as pointed out later, by the Fisher effect, until the Y gene can safely be lost.

On Darlington's (1932) theory of chromosome pairing it is necessary, if the X and Y chromosomes are to pass regularly to opposite poles, that a small length of both, in the neighborhood of the spindle fiber attachment, should remain homologous, and give rise to chiasmata. In this neighborhood a few genes are to be expected in the Y chromosome, and it was here that Stern (1929a) found the normal allelomorph of "bobbed."

A somewhat analogous case occurs in permanently heterozygous plants such as *Oenothera Lamarckiana*. Here, as Darlington points out, there is a certain section in many of the ring-forming chromosomes in which crossing over rarely if ever occurs. These sections appear to carry the genes of the Renner "complex." They should show a tendency to evolve in the same way as the Y chromosome. But this will be checked by the fact that the male gametophyte, and to a less extent the female gametophyte, is under the control of the genes carried by it, while the spermatozoon is not. This is probably one reason why the dioecious higher plants rarely show a marked dimorphism of X and Y, and these chromosomes pair regularly in prophase. Any general tendency of Y genes to mutate would be stopped by natural selection, as it would eliminate male-producing pollen. But in so far as the genes in the chromosome sections that do not cross over are indifferent to one at least of the gametophytes, there will be a tendency for a gene in one complex to disappear, while the corresponding gene in the other complex is unaltered or increases its dominance. Thus, although the degenerative process is never likely to go as far as in an animal Y chromosome, it is not surprising that many *Oenothera* species carry more lethals than are needed to produce a balanced system.

The next three processes on our list all have the same evolutionary effects, though due to rather different causes. The processes will therefore all be dealt with before the effects due to increase of dominance. When we consider any series of multiple allelomorphs we find that as regards any particular structure or function the phenotypes can be arranged in a certain order. Of course the consideration of another structure may give a different order, but there is usually a fair agreement. At one end of the series we usually find a dominant, at the other recessive forms. Thus in rodent color genetics we have the E series ranging from black through the wild gray and "Japanese" to yellow, the lightest form being recessive. On the other hand, the G (or A) series ranges from gray (in the mouse yellow) through "black and tan" to black. Here the darkest form is recessive. The wild type may be at one end of such a series or in the middle. But in the latter case we never find recessive genes on both sides. Thus in rodents we do not find two allelomorphs, one darker and one lighter than the wild form, and both recessive to it. As a general rule, however, the wild type is at one end of a series, usually the dominant end.

Goldschmidt's (1927) theory of dominance states that genes which catalyze a reaction rapidly are dominant over those which catalyze it slowly. But in many cases, *e.g.*, "bobbed" (Stern, 1929b) a limit is reached where further speeding up of the reaction or addition to the number of genes produces no further effect on the character studied. Where this is so, and the wild type is dominant, it is clear that *minus* mutations will give rise to recessive genotypes, and, if the wild type is fitter than these, the mutant genes will be eliminated by natural selection. On the other hand, *plus* mutations will have no effect on the adult genotype (at least as regards the character considered). There will, therefore, be a tendency for them to accumulate. In the absence of the secondary effects of mutation, we should expect to find in a given locus, first recessive genes and deficiencies in small numbers, constantly being produced by mutation and abolished by selection, and second a number of allelomorphs producing almost indistinguishable phenotypes, but some possessing a great deal more activity than the minimum required to produce the wild type. The proportion of these dominant allelomorphs, producing very similar genotypes, would depend on their relative mutation rates; in other words, on their relative stabilities.

Actually, however, the process of dominance evolution is probably supported by two secondary effects. Haldane (1930) pointed out that *plus* mutations in any locus may be favored by selection provided that the original gene is not completely dominant, since the original type of gene is at a disadvantage in heterozygotes, and the new gene is not. Fisher (1931) accepts this as a supplement to the mechanism of dominance evolution which he originally suggested, namely, the spread of modifying genes which increase dominance. Wright (1929) and Haldane (1930) have criticized Fisher's original theory, and it is far from certain which of the two secondary effects is likely to have the greatest effect in increasing dominance. It is to be noted that both the secondary causes of increased dominance are limited in their action, and cease when dominance is complete. Their intensity is proportional to the frequency of *minus* mutations in the locus concerned. If *plus* mutations are anything like equally common, the primary effect will be much more rapid than the secondary.

A particular case of the Fisher effect (secondary increase of dominance) is to be looked for in the case of sex-linked genes. The Y chromosome "empties" in the course of evolution, *i.e.*, genes borne by it disappear or at least pass into a recessive condition. This can be counteracted in two ways, by an increase of dominance of individual genes, or by the acquisition of intra-chromosomal balance. The former process would be favored if the genes in the Y chromosome disappeared one by one, the latter if they disappeared in blocks as the result of sectional deficiencies.

The evolutionary effects of increased dominance are, I think, more profound than Fisher has realized. On Goldschmidt's (1923) theory a dominant gene has a more extended sphere of action, both in space and time, than a recessive. So much of his theory may be accepted, even if we do not admit that it always contains more gene substance. Goldschmidt gives several examples from animal genetics, illustrating the wider spatial and temporal range of the more dominant gene, and they can be paralleled in plant genetics. Thus, in maize, a series of allelomorphs, not unlike the scute-achaete series in *Drosophila*, governs the distribution of anthocyanin over the cobs, silk, husks and grain, the form with the widest distribution being dominant (Anderson, 1924). In *Primula sinensis* de Winton and Haldane (1932) find that JJ flowers are fully colored, jj open white, but later assume a pale color, while Jj open white or pale, but later color up so as to overlap JJ. Thus two "doses" of J produce their effect quicker than one.

Now consider an organism in which a number of genes are just sufficient, in the homozygous condition, to produce the most advantageous adult phenotype. The result of increased dominance will be to strengthen their action so that, where possible, its range both in space and time is increased. But however much the latter is extended, there will always, on Goldschmidt's view, be a period when the homozygote is more advanced towards the adult condition than the heterozygote, even if both are quite alike in the final stage. Thus in so far as developmental abnormality is disadvantageous, the Fisher effect will always be tending to increase the activity of the genes.

This tendency may be held up on biochemical grounds, or by natural selection if such extension of activity is disadvantageous. But it will be the normal tendency. Thus, where the embryo is sheltered by an eggshell or uterus, its form has very little survival value, and the time of action of genes originally active only in the adult will tend to extend progressively back into the life cycle. Whatever be the embryonic form at any stage, there will in general be an advantage in keeping to the normal schedule of development, and thus a disadvantage in the incomplete dominance which, on Goldschmidt's theory, all heterozygotes must show in their early stages.

We thus have a sound explanation, in terms of mutation and natural selection, for the phenomena of tachygenesis and recapitulation. Genes will at first come into action rather late, but gradually extend their sphere of action in time, and on the whole the genes responsible for the phylogenetically older characters of the adult will come into action earliest. But these phenomena are of course far less likely to occur where there is an unsheltered larva in which form and function have strong survival values. We need not be surprised, for example, that limb buds appear at an earlier stage in the development of the body as a whole in Amniota than in Amphibia.

Similar arguments hold good concerning neoteny. Genes which originally determined temporary embryonic or larval characters will tend to extend their action forward into adult life. The preservation in the adult of the embryonic cranial flexure, which has been an orthogenetic trend in the evolution of the Primates, culminating in the human head, has not only been of advantage to the adults when they become climbers and later bipeds, besides permitting hypertrophy of the neopallium. It has also been a result of mutation pressure by the genes responsible for cranial flexure in the foetus; and if Fisher is right, it has been encouraged by their tendency to develop a "factor of safety" protecting them against mutant genes which would otherwise have been dangerous in the heterozygous condition.

We can thus restate, in modern terminology, Weissmann's theory of the "Kampf der Theile." Every gene tends to increase its activity, and the process continues until natural selection or the increased activity of other genes puts a stop to it. The process is extremely slow, simply because mutation is rather infrequent, but it will account for otherwise obscure orthogenetic tendencies.

Another tendency quite similar to that pointed out by Fisher is as follows. If a zygote contains four genes of a kind instead of two, the possibilities of harmful mutation are reduced. Thus Stadler (1929) found it much harder to produce mutations by x-rays in polyploid than diploid cereals. Duplication affecting only a few genes would confer a relatively slight advantage. But duplication of a large section, polysomy of a whole chromosome, or polyploidy, might confer a considerable advantage, provided it caused neither unbalance nor sterility. Whether this advantage is sufficient to be of evolutionary importance is not clear, but the possibility exists. In any case such an evolutionary step, on whatever grounds the new type may survive, leaves such of the doubled genes as are fully dominant at the mercy of mutation, provided meiosis is so regular that each chromosomal locus finds a definite mate. For recessive genes will only be eliminated if recessive mutations occur both in the original locus and the duplication, and all four of the recessive genes occur in one zygote. While the duplication or polyploidy may be preserved because it protects against mutations in some thousands of loci at once, the single genes will tend to disappear one at a time because they only protect one locus apiece. The final result will be that most of the genes will return to the diploid condition, but their spatial relations will have been greatly altered. The process is therefore probably cyclical.

We now come to a group of secondary effects connected with the cytology of sex. Consider an organism such as the bee, in which the male is haploid. Recessive lethal and semi-lethal gene mutations presumably occur, and kill off a certain number of males. But they can never kill a female (or diploid neuter) unless they are sex-limited in their incidence. As there appears to be an excess of drones over the minimum number needed, such lethal mutations, provided they are fully recessive, are of no disadvantage, and indeed of some slight advantage, to the species. If, on the other hand, the male were diploid and the female haploid, lethals would diminish the number of females, and thus be disadvantageous. There may well be sound physiological reasons why haploid animals are never female, but the above argument furnishes an additional reason for this fact.

The same argument applies, with less force, to sex-linked genes in general. When once the majority of the genes in the Y chromosome have become inactive, recessive lethal mutations in the X chromosome will only kill off males. So in any species where more males exist than are needed to secure the fertilization of all females, it is advantageous that the male should be the heterogametic sex. We should therefore expect to find female heterogametism mainly developed in groups where monogamy is the rule. In such a case the killing off of males would have as serious an effect on fertility as the killing off of females. Actually monogamy is the usual condition in birds, and in Lepidoptera it is rather uncommon for one male to fertilize several females. These are, of course, the two principal groups in which the female is heterogametic.

In a species where the male is heterogametic and males are produced in excess, there will clearly be a small advantage in any rearrangement of the genes by which those that frequently give rise to lethal mutations come to lie in the X chromosome. Such unstable genes will then only kill males. Owing to the greater ease of detecting sex-linked lethals, as compared with autosomal lethals, the evidence from *Drosophila* which at first sight suggests the truth of this deduction is of course worthless. But the human evidence points in this direction. Sex-linked recessives, such as haemophilia and Leber's disease, which would be semi-lethal in a state of nature, are fairly common. If loci giving lethal mutants were equally common in all chromosomes such defects should only be about one twenty-third as frequent as autosomal recessives recognizable by their causing congenital abnormalities in several members of a family. This is almost certainly not the case. And the fact is not surprising. In a stage of social evolution where a number of young males can get no mates and may be a nuisance to the herd, a few sex-linked lethals may be a positive advantage to the species, as is the presence of genes conducing to cancer, which kills off superfluous old men and women, at the present day.

A probably still more important influence on gene arrangement is the tendency discovered by Muller (1930) for internal balance to develop in the X chromosome, thus minimizing the differences between XX and XY individuals. This tendency must be at work in all zygotes of at least one sex, while the former is only operative in those carrying a lethal or semi-lethal gene. The tendency to balance may, however, be regarded as a secondary effect of the accumulation of recessive lethals in the Y chromosome. Indeed this accumulation can only proceed as the X develops internal balance.

It is noteworthy that the zygote of higher plants is to a large extent automatically protected against lethals by the fact that many genes are active in the male gametophyte. The majority of the zygotic lethals known in plants kill by suppressing the formation of chlorophyll, which is of course irrelevant to the gametophyte. Those which interfere with other fundamental cell functions will usually kill pollen tubes, and never attain homozygosity in a zygote. Moreover, they will rapidly be eliminated, even in the heterozygous condition, the number being halved in each generation. In so far as this is true we may expect that recurrent lethal mutation has been less important as a factor in the evolution of higher plants than of animals. Certainly there is rather little evidence for tachygenesis in plant evolution or recapitulation in plant development.

It must at once be admitted that much of this paper is frankly speculative, and that some of the speculations may prove groundless. As Wright (1929) has pointed out, the effects of recurrent mutation are at best extremely slow. Many of them may prove as unimportant in organic evolution as the tides raised by the planets on the sun have been in cosmic evolution. Others may turn out to have had as marked effects as have the tides in the evolution of the earth-moon system. Only careful and quantitative work will decide. Such effects, if they exist on a sufficient scale, will explain certain orthogenetic phenomena which have seemed to demand a vital urge, racial memory, and so on. But just because the theories here put forward are in some degree intellectually satisfying, it is important that they should not be accepted without stringent examination.

SUMMARY

Recurrent mutations not only provide the material for selection to act upon. They may give rise to primary and secondary effects, the former due to the accumulation of mutant genes, the latter to the selective value of conditions which protect the organism against lethal genes.

Among the phenomena which can be accounted for by these phenomena are the disappearance of useless organs, recapitulation and the fact that the heterogametic sex is usually male.

LITERATURE CITED

E. G. Anderson
1924. "Pericarp Studies in Maize, II. The Allelomorphism of a Series of Factors for Pericarp Color," *Genetics*, 9: 442–453.

C. D. Darlington
1932. "Recent Advances in Cytology," London.

M. Demereč
1929. "Genetic Factors Stimulating Mutability of the Miniature-gamma Wing Character of *Drosophila virilis*," *Proc. Nat. Acad. Sci.*, 15: 834–838.

C. Diver
1929. "Fossil Records of Mendelian Mutants," *Nature*, 124: 183.

R. A. Fisher
1928. "The Possible Modification of the Response of the Wild Type to Recurrent Mutations," AMER. NAT., 62: 115–126.
1931. "The Evolution of Dominance," *Biol. Rev.*, 6: 345–368.

R. Goldschmidt
1927. "Physiologische Theorie der Vererbung," Berlin.
1929. "Experimentelle Mutation und das Problem der sogenannten Parallelinduktion. Versuche an Drosophila," *Biol. Zbl.*, 49: 437–448.

J. B. S. Haldane
1930. "Note on Fisher's Theory of Dominance, and on a Correlation between Dominance and Linkage," AMER. NAT., 64: 385–406.
1932. "The Causes of Evolution," London and New York.

V. Jollos
1930. "Studien zum Evolutionsproblem, I. Über die experimentelle Hervorrufung und Steigerung von Mutationen bei Drosophila melanogaster," *Biol. Zbl.*, 50: 541–554.

H. J. Muller
1930. "Types of Visible Variations Induced by X-rays in Drosophila," *J. Genet.*, 22: 299–334.

L. J. Stadler
1929. "Chromosome Number and the Mutation Rate in Avena and Triticum," *Proc. Nat. Acad. Sci.*, 15: 876–881.

D. De Winton and J. B. S. Haldane
1932. "Genetics of *Primula sinensis*, II," *J. Genet.* (in press).

C. Stern
1929a. "Untersuchungen über Aberrationen des Y-Chromosoms von *Drosophila melanogaster*," *Z. I. A. V.*, 51: 253–353.
1929b. "Über die additive Wirkung multipler Allele.," *Biol. Zbl.*, 49: 261–290.

S. Wright
1929. "Fisher's Theory of Dominance," AMER. NAT., 63: 274–279.

VOLUME XXXI OCTOBER, 1935 No. 3

THE RATE OF SPONTANEOUS MUTATION OF A HUMAN GENE.

BY J. B. S. HALDANE.

SATISFACTORY data on rates of spontaneous mutation exist for *Zea* and *Drosophila*, but not for vertebrates. However, such data may be determined for man by indirect methods. Clearly the rate at which new autosomal genes recessive to the normal type appear can only be accurately estimated where either inbreeding or very extensive back-crossing to recessives is possible. But under ordinary conditions new dominants or sex-linked recessives can be detected more readily.

The sex-linked recessive condition haemophilia has been known for over a century. Since only a small minority of haemophilics live long enough to breed, and (as will be seen) over one-third of all haemophilia genes in new-born babies are in the *X*-chromosome of males, the condition would rapidly disappear unless new haemophilia genes arose by mutation. The only alternatives would be that heterozygous females were more fertile than normal, or that in their meiosis the normal allelomorph of haemophilia was preferentially extruded into a polar body. Neither of these alternatives seems likely.

It is, moreover, certain that new haemophilia genes sometimes arise by mutation. In the Gross family investigated by C. V. Green (Davenport, 1930) a woman (III, 7) had two haemophilic sons with normal colour vision, and two colour-blind sons with normal blood, besides a daughter who transmitted haemophilia to two sons. The mother therefore carried the gene for colour blindness in one *X*-chromosome and that for haemophilia in the other. As she had a colour-blind brother, maternal uncle and maternal aunt, but no haemophilic relatives, she must have received the *X*-chromosome carrying colour blindness from her mother, and that carrying haemophilia from her father. But her father was tested for haemophilia, and found to be normal. (Through error in Davenport's paper he is referred to as II, 3 in the pedigree, as II, 6 in the text.) Hence a mutation must have occurred in the *X*-chromosome received from the father. Davenport suggests that it occurred in the ovary of III, 7. But as all her sons were colour blind or haemophilic it seems more likely that it occurred in the testis of her father, or during her early embryonic life.

Gettings' case (Fig. 603 in Bulloch and Fildes, 1912) is also good evidence for mutation. A woman had one normal and five haemophilic sons. Her father and maternal grandfather were normal. She had three normal brothers and three normal sisters who bore normal sons. Her mother's brothers and the male descendants of her mother's sisters were also normal. Hence her haemophilia gene probably, although not certainly, arose by mutation. There are a number of similar cases in the literature.

We now assume, and will later attempt to show, that most large human populations are in approximate equilibrium as regards haemophilia, selection being balanced by mutation.

If x be the proportion of haemophilic males in the population, and f their effective fertility, that is to say their chance, compared with a normal male, of producing offspring, then in a large population of $2N$, $(1-f)\,xN$ haemophilia genes are effectively wiped out per generation. The same number must be replaced by mutation. But as each of the N females has two X-chromosomes per cell, and each of the N males one, the mean mutation rate per X-chromosome per generation is $\frac{1}{3}(1-f)\,x$, or if f is small, a little less than $\frac{1}{3}x$. Hence we have only to determine the frequency of haemophilia in males to arrive at the approximate mutation rate.

This simple calculation is confirmed, and some other data arrived at, by a more formal treatment. Let **h** represent the gene for haemophilia. **H** its normal allelomorph, so that men are **H** or **h**, women **HH**, **Hh** or possibly **hh**. Homozygous haemophilic women are certainly very rare, and may not exist.

Let eggs be formed in the ratio 1 **H** : x**h**, and spermatozoa in the ratio 1 **H** : y**h**. Then if mating is at random the zygotes are formed in the proportions 1 **HH** : $(x+y)$ **Hh** : xy **hh** ♀, and 1 **H** : x **h** ♂. Inbreeding on the scale found in human populations would only serve to increase the proportion of **hh** females, which is in any case negligible. x and y are clearly small numbers.

Let f be the relative effective fertility of haemophilic males, f' that of haemophilic females. f means the number of children ultimately begotten by 1000 haemophilic males, divided by the number begotten by 1000 normal males. As many haemophilics die young and others do not marry, this number is a small fraction. Pearson pointed out to Bulloch and Fildes (1912) that the marriage rate of male bleeders is 9·6 per cent., that of females in the same families being 36·8 per cent. Further, a larger proportion of such males than of normal males presumably die while their wives are still potentially fertile.

So we may take f as 0·25 or less, though probably exceeding 0·1. It is likely that several allelomorphs of haemophilia exist. In Hay's case (408 of Bulloch and Fildes' collection) only four out of twenty-one affected males died of the disease, and four begot children. This family has now apparently been lost sight of, or haemophilia has died out in it. However, another family in the United States, the Molyneux of Pennsylvania, exhibits the same phenomenon. Green (Davenport, 1930) investigated branches of it, including nineteen haemophilics, besides other haemophilic families. Dr Green writes of one of them: "His does not seem to be a very severe case of haemophilia, but it is by far the most severe of any of the Molyneux." In the case of others haemophilia was not discovered until the age of five or ten years. Several of the boys play football, though suffering abnormally from bruises. There is no doubt that the character is a sex-linked recessive. As it has preserved its distinctive character of mildness in a number of different families, it cannot be due to the ordinary haemophilia gene along with modifiers in other chromosomes. There is strong reason to suspect that we are dealing with a distinct gene. If it is not allelomorphic with the ordinary gene we have the surprising, but not impossible, situation of two genes with very similar effects in the same one out of twenty-four chromosomes. It seems more likely that we are dealing with a relatively harmless allelomorph.

Whereas the normal allelomorph is at best very dangerous, there is no recorded death from haemophilia among Green's nineteen cases, and many have married and begotten children. Clearly the effective fertility of these "minor haemophilics" is not greatly depressed, and f probably exceeds $\frac{1}{2}$. If the two allelomorphs arose by mutation with equal frequency, the milder form would clearly be much more frequent. We therefore conclude that mutation to the major form is more frequent. This is quite in keeping with what is known elsewhere. In *Drosophila* mutations of the eye-colour to white are more frequent than to all its allelomorphs (eosin, apricot, etc.) together.

The value of f' for **hh** females is conjectural. Perhaps no such female has ever been observed. It may be that $f' = 0$, the condition being lethal, as Davenport suggests, or that $f' = 1$, the disease being sex-limited as well as sex-linked. However, the value of f' does not affect our calculations.

In their total of reliable families containing haemophilics, Bulloch and Fildes found a large excess of males over females and of haemophilic over normal males. In the forty pedigrees collected in the first part of their Table II, which they regard as the most satisfactory, there are 189 sibships containing 406 male bleeders, two doubtful males, 236 normal

21-2

males, 464 females, and fifty-six whose sex is not stated. Eleven of the females were said to be bleeders. Now no family is included unless it contains at least one bleeder. The above total therefore does not give a fair sample of the progeny of heterozygous mothers, but it does give us the sibs of all the haemophilic males in these pedigrees, provided that we subtract one male haemophilic from each family, that is to say 189 from the total. We then get 217 bleeders, two doubtful, and 236 normal among the males, and 455 males, fifty-six doubtful, and 464 females for the sex distribution. Both are very satisfactory approximations to equality, and there is no reason whatever to doubt that segregation, both as regards sex and haemophilia, is perfectly normal. Hogben (1931), using different data and methods, found 28·5 per cent. of haemophilics in the progeny of haemophilic females, or quite a small deviation from the expected 25·5 per cent.

Bulloch and Fildes also find a rather high fertility among the mothers of haemophilics. In a group of forty pedigrees which they regard as their most reliable, they find that the average size of a family containing at least one haemophilic male is 6·1. This large size is partly an expression of bias in selection. For suppose we have in a population n heterozygous women who have had families of s children. The chance that any particular child is haemophilic is approximately $\frac{1}{4}$. So the chance that a family of size s will contain no haemophilic member is $1-(\frac{3}{4})^s$. Hence the number of such families actually recorded will be $n'=n\,[1-(\frac{3}{4})^s]$. Hence when in a collection of families we find n' of size s containing $n's$ children, these represent $\frac{n'}{1-(\frac{3}{4})^s}$ families from **Hh** mothers, containing $\frac{n's}{1-(\frac{3}{4})^s}$ children. For example Bulloch and Fildes' collection (in Table II, part I) includes seven families of one child and twenty-two of two children. These figures should be raised to twenty-eight and 50·386 respectively. Applying the correction we find that the average fertility of **Hh** women in Bulloch and Fildes' data is reduced from their figure of 6·1 to 5·0. This figure is still rather high, but a glance at the Tenna and Mampel pedigrees shows that the homozygous women in them were also very fertile.

In a sample of the collected haemophilia pedigrees much more than half of those sisters of haemophilics who are recorded as having had sons had at least one haemophilic son. I do not regard this as significant. For a pedigree generally begins with a fairly young male. It is then discovered that he had haemophilic uncles and cousins. Hence the uncles in the pedigree are assured of at least one heterozygous sister. Also the progeny of haemophilics' sisters are likely to be included in the pedigree if they include haemophilic sons, but not otherwise. Until further data are available it seems best to assume that haemophilia obeys the same laws as the large majority of sex-linked characters in other animals.

Let μ be the frequency of mutation of the normal allelomorph **H** to the abnormal **h** per generation in women, ν in men. That is to say μ is the probability of finding, in any particular gamete of a woman, an X-chromosome now carrying **h**, although it carried **H** when she was conceived, and similarly with ν.

Then the effective breeding population is in the proportions

$$1\ \mathbf{HH} : (x+y)\ \mathbf{Hh} : f'xy\ \mathbf{hh}\ ♀, \text{ and } 1\ \mathbf{H} : fx\ \mathbf{h}.$$

So apart from mutation they would produce eggs in the ratio $1\ \mathbf{H} : x'\ \mathbf{h}$, and spermatozoa in the ratio $1\ \mathbf{H} : y'\ \mathbf{h}$, where $x' = \frac{x+y+2f'xy}{2+x+y} = \frac{1}{2}(x+y)$ very nearly, and $y' = fx$.

As a result of mutation these numbers must be equal to x and y respectively. Hence $x = \frac{1}{2}(x+y) + \mu$, $y = fx + \nu$. So

$$x = \frac{2\mu+\nu}{1-f}, \quad y = \frac{2f\mu+\nu}{1-f},$$

and the mean mutation rate is $\frac{1}{3}(2\mu+\nu) = \frac{1}{3}(1-f)\,x$ as found above.

Before attempting to assess x, a few other calculations may be made. The ratio of heterozygous females to haemophilic males is $1 + \frac{2f\mu+\nu}{2\mu+\nu}$, a quantity lying between $1+f$ and 2. This is the ratio at birth. In the actual population, owing to the high death-rate of the haemophilics, there may well be over twice as many heterozygotes as haemophilics.

In a population of N females and N males at fertilisation there are $3N$ X-chromosomes, of which a total $\frac{(4\mu+2f\mu+3\nu)\,N}{1-f}$ carry **h**. The number of new **h** genes arising by mutation is $(2\mu+\nu)\,N$, and the same number must die out, in a stationary population. Hence in such a population the mean life of a haemophilic gene in generations is

$$\frac{(4+2f)\,\mu+3\nu}{(1-f)\,(2\mu+\nu)}, \text{ or } \frac{3}{1-f} - \frac{2\mu}{2\mu+\nu}.$$

The first term certainly exceeds 3 and is probably less than 4; the second lies between 0 and 1, and is equal to $\frac{2}{3}$ if $\mu = \nu$. Hence the mean life of a haemophilia gene in a stationary population, *i.e.* the number of individuals in whom it appears, lies between two and four generations, and is probably about three. In these calculations we neglect genes which only affect a single cell or a group of cells, and do not determine the genotype of an individual. In a phase of rapid population growth, such as is now closing in Western Europe and North America, the mean life is much longer. Thus if a population increases by 50 per cent. in each generation, the fact that one-third of the **h** genes are destroyed in each generation does not diminish the number of "old" **h** genes.

If the above analysis is correct the number of sporadic cases of haemophilia must be far larger than a study of pedigrees would suggest. This may well be the case, since it is unlikely that pedigrees containing single isolated cases would be published. Of all cases of haemophilia a fraction $\frac{(1-f)\,\mu}{2\mu+\nu}$ should be sons of homozygous mothers and wholly isolated. A further fraction $\frac{(1-f)\,(\mu+\nu)}{2\mu+\nu}$ should be sons of heterozygous mothers who had arisen by mutation, and should therefore have no haemophilic relatives except brothers, and other descendants of their mothers. An adequate survey of a whole population for haemophilia would allow of a verification or disproof of these predictions, and an estimate of the difference, if any, of mutation rate in the two sexes. The figures quoted above are all derived from a study of large pedigrees, so the proportion of haemophilic males was only slightly below a half.

We must now attempt to determine x, the fraction of all males born who develop haemophilia. No really satisfactory data exist. Bulloch and Fildes found only two haemophilics out of 137,676 consecutive admissions to the London Hospital (sex ratio not given). On the other hand Manson (1928) found three cases among 25,500 consecutive examined English recruits during the war.

Dr Julia Bell has records of thirty-four certain and seven doubtful cases at present living in Greater London, supplied by seven London hospitals. I find it difficult to suppose that this number represents as much as half the living cases in Greater London, or less than one-tenth. The number of cases among the four million or so males of London would thus be 70–350. If the expectation of life in haemophilics were normal, these numbers would probably be at least doubled. So a rough estimate of the proportion of haemophilics among male births in London is 35–175 per million. Thus x quite certainly exceeds 10^{-5}, and probably lies between 0·00004 and 0·00017. The population of London is drawn from many different areas, and this figure is likely to give a fairer idea of the frequency in England as a whole than would a figure based on a similar population in northern England.

Now $1-f$ is at least 0·75 and probably larger. The mutation rate, $\frac{1}{3}(1-f)x$, is therefore certainly greater than 1 in 400,000, probably lying between 1 in 100,000 and 1 in 20,000. We may take 1 in 50,000 as a plausible figure.

This estimate is very little affected by the value of f, provided this lies between 0 and $\frac{1}{4}$, which is undoubtedly true. It has been assumed that the population is in approximate equilibrium. Let us suppose that this is not the case, but that f, μ and ν are constant. Let x_n be the value of x in the nth generation, and let $x_n = z_n + \dfrac{2\mu+\nu}{1-f}$. Then

$$x_{n+2} - \tfrac{1}{2}x_{n+1} - \tfrac{1}{2}fx_n = \mu + \tfrac{1}{2}\nu.$$

Whence $$z_{n+2} - \tfrac{1}{2}z_{n+1} - \tfrac{1}{2}fz_n = 0,\ z_n = a\lambda^n + b\kappa^n,$$

where $$\lambda = \tfrac{1}{4}(1+\sqrt{8f+1}),\quad \kappa = \tfrac{1}{4}(1-\sqrt{8f+1}),$$

and a and b are constants determined by the earlier state of the population. After a few generations the second term becomes negligible, and

$$x_n = \frac{2\mu+\nu}{1-f} + a\lambda^n.$$

λ lies between 0·5 for $f=0$ and 0·683 for $f=0·25$. So any departures from equilibrium diminish in geometric progression. How rapidly they do so may be seen by examining the hypothesis that all existing haemophilics are derived from haemophilics or heterozygotes in an earlier population, and that mutation does not occur. In that case the frequency of haemophilia thirty generations ago, if $f=0·25$, the least favourable hypothesis for the mutation theory, would have been 100,000 times as great as at present, in other words all Englishmen at the time of the Norman conquest would have been haemophilics!

Hence the existing population must be close to equilibrium unless the mutation rate has recently changed. If this is so our estimate lies between the present value and the value a few generations ago. The only alternatives to accepting a mutation rate of the order calculated seem to be the postulation of a fertility in heterozygous females of $\dfrac{2}{1+f}$, or over 1·6 times the normal, or a correspondingly great abnormality in their segregation. But in the male sex segregation is entirely normal. So if the females are more likely to receive a haemophilic than a normal gene, while males are not, we must assume selective fertilisation. Unless some such unjustifiable assumption is made, it must be accepted that the mutation rate is of the order of magnitude here given.

Discussion.

The figure arrived at, of about one spontaneous mutation in about 50,000 life cycles, is within the limits found for other organisms. Thus in *Zea* Stadler (1932) found rates from just over 1 per 1000 to less than 1 per 1,000,000 for seven colour genes. In *Drosophila melanogaster* Muller (1928) found a rate of nearly 1 in 100 for the appearance of lethal genes at a particular locus in the second chromosome. These, however, may have been deficiencies, as they occurred near the end of an inversion in a balanced lethal stock. On the other hand Patterson and Muller (1930) estimate the rate of mutation at the white locus as 1 in 400,000 to white, and 1 in 600,000 to other allelomorphs. A few other loci showed a rate of the same order. These rates can be increased about 100 times by X-rays.

Thus expressed in frequency per life cycle the rate of mutation at the haemophilia locus is higher than any well-authenticated mutation rate in *Drosophila*. The same is probably true if we consider frequency per cell generation, since the number per life cycle in man is only about twice that in *Drosophila*. On the other hand the rate per year is very much larger in *Drosophila* than in man. Taking the mean lengths of a generation as 14 days and 30 years, the human mutation rate corresponds to a rate of 1 in 40,000,000 per *Drosophila* generation, and less if spontaneous mutation rate is a function of temperature. A gene appearing with this rate, if obvious in its manifestation, would probably have been detected once or twice if sex-linked, and not at all if autosomal.

Penrose's (1934) data on epiloia, a rare human autosomal dominant which does not often survive for more than two or three generations before it is extinguished by selection, suggest a mutation rate of the same order of magnitude as that here found for haemophilia.

Bulloch and Fildes, from a survey of the literature, think that haemophilia is a good deal commoner in northern than southern Europe. The data collected by Komai (1934) show that it is not very rare in Japan. If differences exist they are almost certainly due to differences in the mutation rate rather than the effective fertility. These in turn may be due to genetical or environmental differences between the peoples concerned. It is clear that this question, like that of the exact value of the mutation rate, can only be solved when an adequate biological survey of several human populations of a million or more have been made.

Similar calculations may be made for other rare lethal or sublethal human abnormalities. Haldane (1927) showed that for a rare dominant or an autosomal recessive of frequency x the mutation rate required to preserve equilibrium in a random mating population is $(1-f)\,x$. This is equally true for any other mating system. For in a population of N, $2N(1-f)\,x$ abnormal recessive genes are eliminated by selection in each generation, and the same number must be furnished anew by mutation. This argument is unassailable for dominants or sex-linked recessives, but must be applied with great care to autosomal recessives. For if a recessive character has a frequency of 1 per 1,000,000, then in a random mating population there are 2000 heterozygotes per 1,000,000. If the gene is lethal, an increased effective fertility of 0·05 per cent. in the heterozygotes would be enough to counteract the selection of the homozygotes. It is quite possible that heterozygosis for amaurotic idiocy may decrease the intelligence quotient by 1 per cent. This would probably cause an increased fertility under existing social conditions.

Moreover, in the case of autosomal recessives, after any disturbance, such as might be produced by a change in the amount of inbreeding or by several other causes, the equilibrium between selection and mutation is only re-established with extreme slowness, whereas in other cases the process is very rapid. Hence the frequency of occurrence of lethal and sublethal recessive abnormalities does not do more than suggest the order of magnitude of the mutation rates of the genes concerned.

Besides haemophilia and epiloia a number of other sublethal dominant or sex-linked conditions are known. Thus cleidocranial dysostosis, neuro-fibromatosis, and blue sclerotics associated with bone fragility are dominants, while anidrotic ectodermal dysplasia can be a sex-linked recessive, or sex-linked with occasional dominance in females. These diseases are not very uncommon, and Cockayne (1933) points out that neurofibromatosis often arises by mutation, while his data show that the effective fertility is quite low. In these cases we must assume a mutation rate of over 1 per 1,000,000, and the same is probably true for lethal and sublethal recessives such as the amaurotic idiocies and xeroderma pigmentosum. If the above arguments are correct it would seem that, taking the generation as the unit of time, man is a rather more mutable species than *Drosophila*.

SUMMARY.

The rate of mutation at which the gene for haemophilia appears in the population of London is estimated at about once in 50,000 human life cycles. There are probably two distinct allelomorphs at the same locus, the milder type arising less frequently by mutation than the severe type.

I have to thank Dr Julia Bell and Dr C. V. Green for most generously placing at my disposal data collected on behalf of the Medical Research Council and the Research Committee of the American Medical Association.

REFERENCES.

BULLOCH, W. and FILDES, P. (1912). *Treasury of Human Inheritance*, **1**, 169.

COCKAYNE, E. A. (1933). *Inherited Abnormalities of the Skin and Appendages.* Oxford.

DAVENPORT, C. B. (1930). "Sex linkage in man." *Genetics*, **15**, 401.

HALDANE, J. B. S. (1927). "A mathematical theory of natural and artificial selection. Part V." *Proc. Camb. phil. Soc.* **23**, 838.

HOGBEN, L. T. (1931). *Genetic Principles in Medicine and Social Science.* London.

KOMAI, T. (1934). *Pedigrees of Hereditary Diseases and Abnormalities found in the Japanese Race.* Kyoto.

MANSON, J. S. (1928). *Observations on Human Heredity.* London.

MULLER, H. J. (1928). "The measurement of gene mutation rate in *Drosophila*, its high variability, and its dependence upon temperature." *Genetics*, **13**, 279.

PATTERSON, J. T. and MULLER, H. J. (1930). "Are 'progressive' mutations produced by X-rays?" *Ibid.* **15**. 495.

PENROSE, L. S. (1934). *The Influence of Heredity on Disease.* London.

STADLER, L. J. (1932). "On the genetic nature of induced mutations in plants." *Proc. 6th Int. Cong. Genet.* Menasha, Wis.

THE
AMERICAN NATURALIST

VOL. LXXI July–August, 1937 No. 735

THE EFFECT OF VARIATION ON FITNESS

DR. J. B. S. HALDANE
JOHN INNES HORTICULTURAL INSTITUTION

THERE is good reason to believe, with Darwin, that natural selection has played a very important part in evolution. The great interest of the evolutionary process has tended to divert attention from the action of natural selection in stabilizing species in their existing monomorphic or polymorphic facies. Yet this latter phenomenon is easily observable.

On the other hand, the evolutionary process is exceedingly slow. Forms usually change little in 100,000 years. Now Haldane (1924) showed that a dominant character causing an increase of 0.1 per cent. in the fitness of its carriers would increase from a frequency of .001 per cent. to one of 99 per cent. in a random mating population in 23,400 generations, and somewhat more rapidly in an inbred population; in fact, on a geological time scale, almost explosively. But a difference of fitness of this magnitude could not be detected. In order that an observed viability difference of 0.1 per cent. should exceed twice its standard error, we should have to observe at least sixteen million individuals. To detect so small a difference in fertility we should have to count their progeny.

It may be possible to observe evolution by natural selection in a species which is adapting itself to a new environment. In other cases we can very rarely hope to notice evolutionary changes within a human lifetime. From the standpoint of an individual human observer species may be regarded as almost in equilibrium. Our only reason to hope for observable evolution is that owing to glaciation, agriculture, fishing and industry, the balance of nature has recently been upset in a manner probably without precedent in our planet's history; and hence on the Darwinian theory we should expect that evolution was proceeding with extreme and abnormal speed.

However, in what follows we shall deal entirely with populations in equilibrium. Every species observed with sufficient care has been found to include members less fit than the average and whose lack of fitness is heritable. Their number in a sufficiently large population is approximately constant, and in spite of selection does not diminish, either because the genes or chromosomal abnormalities responsible for them are continually being replenished as the result of mutation, or because they are advantageous in a different combination. We shall here discuss the effect of such deleterious genes on the fitness of the species.

We must first define fitness. This is easiest in a hermaphrodite organism. We can say that the fitness of any particular genotype (or group of genotypes) is half the mean number of progeny left by an individual of that genotype. Progeny due to self-fertilization are counted twice over. Certain conventions are necessary. Obviously, individuals must be counted at the same stage of the life-cycle, *e.g.*, at birth or maturity. Also when determining our average fitness we must take arithmetic means in space, but geometric means in time. Thus if two organisms have 18 and 2 progeny, respectively, their mean fitness is 5, not 3. And in an organism with two generations per year, the autumn generation being 5 times as numerous as the spring population, the mean fitness of the spring population is 5, of the autumn population 1/5, their mean being unity, the geometric mean, not 2.6, the arithmetic mean.

If we take the generation as our unit of time, the natural logarithm of the fitness is the Malthusian parameter as defined by Fisher (1930). Fisher took the year as his unit; and where generations are not sharply defined an astronomical unit is preferable to a biological. In such a case the precise mathematical theory (Norton 1928, Haldane 1926) is rather complicated. However, our general conclusions are unaffected by the complications.

In a bisexual organism a correction must be made for the sex-ratio. And in a polymorphic population with several exogamous genotypes (*e.g.*, a plant with trimorphic heterostylism) the matter is further complicated. An example of the necessary computations is given by Fisher (1935) in the case of *Lythrum Salicaria*. However, unless a mutant gene or chromosomal abnormality affects the sex-ratio no complications of this type occur in the case of animals.

It must be emphasized that high fitness of a particular genotype as here defined does not ensure its increase, even in the absence of back mutation. Thus a type carrying an extra chromosome fragment may be both more viable and more fertile than the normal but may nevertheless tend to die out because the fragment is contributed to less than half the viable gametes. Or a gene advantageous to the zygotes may be handicapped in pollen-tube competition with an allelomorph. However, most characters are determined by genes. And since as a result of normal mendelian segregation genes do not increase or diminish in number in a population, increase of fitness will cause a spread of the genes which determine it, other things being equal. Finally, fitness as defined above may be a function of the mating system in the population considered, and will be altered by changes in the degree either of inbreeding or of assortative mating, as well as by Darwinian sexual selection. For example, the fitness of an unfit type is generally lowered by inbreeding, because it is more likely to find an unfit mate than in an outbred population.

It is clear that the mean fitness of all members of a species must always be very close to unity, if we average over any length of time. If the fitness were 1.01 the population would increase 20,959 times in 1,000 generations. In almost all species the mean fitness over 1,000 generations must vary from unity by far less than one per cent. But in any species some genotypes have a fitness less than unity, ranging to zero in the case of lethal genes and genes causing complete sterility. So it is clear that the fitness of the standard type containing no deleterious genes must exceed unity. A population composed of such a type would of course increase until, owing to its pressure on the means of subsistence, the fitness was again reduced to unity.

At any gene locus in a population there are a number of possible conditions which may be listed as follows:

1. *Equilibrium*
   a. Equilibrium between genes whose effect on fitness is of the order of their mutation rates or smaller.
   b. Equilibrium due to greater fitness of heterozygotes than homozygotes.
   c. Equilibrium due to the constant production by mutation of genes lowering fitness and thus eliminated by selection.
   d. Equilibrium due to exogamy.
   e. Equilibrium due to inhomogeneous environment, etc.
2. *States of Change*
   a. Decrease in frequency of a gene lowering fitness.
   b. Increase in frequency of a gene lowering fitness.

There will also be equilibrium due to a combination of causes. *E.g.*, heterozygous forms such as the thrum primrose which are kept in existence by exogamy may also be *per se* fitter than homozygotes. And equilibrium 1(a) shades off into 1(b) and 1(c) imperceptibly.

Equilibria of types a, b, d and e may give rise to polymorphism. Type c will give a number of abnormalities, each much rarer than the normal type, but the population as a whole will be monomorphic, except for sexuality and results of equilibrium due to other causes. We shall now investigate equilibria due to this cause.

New genes constantly arise by mutation. It is well known that most mutant types are less fit than the normal in the wild state, even if they are more so in abnormal conditions such as domestication. It is *a priori* obvious that this must be so. For a gene with any appreciable mutation frequency must have appeared many times in the past (except perhaps in species such as the elephants or *Sequoia gigantea* with very few individuals). Hence if it produced an increase of fitness, it would already have spread through the population.

It is, however, hardly justifiable to describe such abnormal genes as pathological in all cases, although they may be so. In the first place, they may lead to increased fitness in a different environment. Thus Sax (1926) found that bean plants from recessive white seeds were more fertile than their sisters from colored seeds in good years, less so in bad years when the environment was presumably more like that of wild plants. Secondly, several abnormal genes together may increase fitness, as Haldane (1931) and Wright (1931) have pointed out. If so the standard or normal type is not the fittest type in the population. Nevertheless, the fittest type will not spread, since the abnormal genes generally occur one at a time, thus lowering fitness, and only rarely all together.

It is at once clear that in equilibrium such abnormal genes are wiped out by natural selection at exactly the same rate as they are produced by mutation. It does not matter whether the gene is lethal or almost harmless. In the first case, every individual carrying it, or if it is recessive, every individual homozygous for it, is wiped out. In the second the viability or fertility of such individuals may only be reduced by one-thousandth. In either case, however, the loss of fitness to the species depends entirely on the mutation rate and not at all on the effect of the gene upon the fitness of the individual carrying it, provided this is large enough to keep the gene rare. This conclusion will be proved in detail for the four individual cases.

Dominant Autosomal Abnormal Genes

Consider a normal gene which mutates to a dominant allelomorph with frequency μ per locus per generation. The situation is precisely the same with regard to a cytological abnormality, such as duplication, deficiency or inversion, provided it lowers the fitness in the heterozygous condition and exhibits mendelian inheritance. If the dominant gene lowers the fitness appreciably it will be rare, like most human dominant abnormalities, and homozygotes will be so rare as to be negligible. Let N be the number of the population, x the frequency of the mutant type and f its fitness. f is of course an average value and must be less than unity, even if the mutant gene increases fitness in certain genetic combinations or in certain environments.

Then in each generation the number of abnormal genes is increased by $(2 - x)\mu N$ as the result of mutation. It is diminished by $x(1 - f)N$ as the result of selection. As there is equilibrium $(2 - x)\mu N = x(1 - f)N$, so

$$x = \frac{2\mu}{1 - f - \mu}$$

Since μ is generally a small quantity of the order of 10^{-6} or less, $x = \frac{2\mu}{1 - f}$ approximately. Thus if $\mu = 10^{-6}$ and $f = 0$, $x = 2 \times 10^{-6}$. If $f = .999$, $x = 2 \times 10^{-3}$. The gene remains rare until $1 - f$ is nearly as small as μ. The loss of fitness to the species due to the gene is $x(1 - f)$, $= 2\mu - \frac{2\mu^2}{1 - f - \mu}$, or 2μ very approximately. This is independent of the value of f.

When a species is highly inbred, even a rare dominant will often appear in the homozygous condition. This will be particularly the case in a species which is predominantly self-fertilized. Let us suppose that the fitnesses of the heterozygote and homozygote are f_1 and f_2, respectively, their frequencies y and x, respectively. Then from the conditions of equilibrium

$$y = 2\mu(1 - y - x) - \mu y - \tfrac{1}{2} f_1 y$$
$$x = \mu y - f_2 x - \tfrac{1}{4} f_1 y$$

Hence, neglecting small quantities,

$$x = \frac{f_1 \mu}{(2 - f_1)(1 - f_2)} \qquad y = \frac{4\mu}{2 - f_1}$$

And the loss of fitness to the species is $(1 - f_1)y -$

$(1 - f_2)x$, or $\frac{(4 - 3f_1)\mu}{2 - f_1}$ which lies between μ and 2μ, as is otherwise obvious. Similar expressions can be obtained for less intense degrees of inbreeding.

Sex-linked Abnormal Genes

Again let the frequency of mutation be μ, the frequency of the gene in the population x, and the fitness in females (supposed to be homogametic as in mammals) f_1, in males f_2. Assuming a sex-ratio of equality, there are $\frac{3}{2}N$ loci in the whole population. Of the $\frac{3}{2}Nx$ abnormal genes Nx will be in females, $\frac{1}{2}Nx$ in males. Hence the mutation rate $(\frac{3}{2} - x)\mu N$ must be equal to the selection rate Nx $\left(\frac{1 - 2f_1 - f_2}{3}\right)$

Hence

$$x = \frac{3\mu}{2\left(\frac{1 - 2f_1 + f_2}{3}\right)}$$

The loss of fitness is

$$x\left(\frac{1 - 2f_1 - f_2}{3}\right)$$

or $\frac{3}{2}\mu$. This is true whether the gene is dominant, recessive or intermediate, provided only that f_1 or f_2 is large enough in comparison with μ to keep it rare. A fuller treatment of this question has been given by Haldane (1935) in a discussion of the origin of haemophilia by mutation.

Of course the actual state of affairs in the population depends on the degree of dominance of the gene. A recessive gene will manifest itself in males only. A dominant gene will appear in about twice as many females as males. A gene of intermediate dominance will appear in some members of each sex. But so long as it remains so rare that homozygous females are not found, one gene is destroyed for each individual eliminated by natural selection, just as with a rare autosomal dominant.

Recessive Autosomal Genes

Here let μ, f and x have their former values, and let $2y$ be the frequency of heterozygotes. Then the number of abnormal genes produced per generation is $2(1 - x - y)\mu N$, the number eliminated $2x(1 - f) N$. The factor 2 arises in the latter case because the destruction of a homozygote involves that of two abnormal genes. Provided that x and y are small, $x = \frac{\mu}{1 - f}$ and the loss of fitness to the species is μ. In a random mating population, if p be the frequency of the recessive gene, $x = p^2$, $y = 2p$, so $(1 - p)\mu = p^2(1 - f)$, and

$$x = \frac{\mu}{2(1-f)^2}\left[2(1-f) - \mu - \sqrt{4(1-f)\mu - \mu^2}\right]$$

For small values of μ this approximates very closely to $\frac{\mu}{1 - f}$ provided f differs appreciably from unity. Thus if $\mu = 10^{-6}$, $f = .99$, the value of x is only 2 per cent. below $\frac{\mu}{1 - f}$, a correction entirely negligible in view of our slight knowledge of mutation-rates.

The correction is still smaller in the case of a partially inbred population, where y is smaller for a given value of x.

If we take the members of wild populations which are fairly outbred, for example, *Drosophila melanogaster*, *D. obscura* and *D. sub-obscura*, *Trifolium pratense*, *Lolium perenne* and so on, we find that on inbreeding very large numbers of autosomal recessive genes more or less injurious in their effects are disclosed. Data and references to former work are given by Gordon (1936). These genes are not of course a fair sample of the mutants which appear in the species. They do not include dominants or sex-linked genes, which are not at all or only partially protected from selection by their normal allelomorphs. They also do not include incompletely recessive genes, which cause an appreciable loss of fitness in the heterozygous condition.

For consider a gene of frequency p in a random mating population, whose heterozygotes have a frequency $2p(1-p)$ and fitness f_1, the homozygotes a frequency p^2 and frequency f_2. The gene appears at a rate $2(1-p)\mu$ and is eliminated at a rate $2p(1-p)(1-f_1) - 2p^2(1-f_2)$. When these rates are equal,

$$p = \frac{k_1 + \mu - \sqrt{(k_1 - \mu)^2 + 4k_2\mu}}{2k_1 - 2k_2} \quad \text{where } k_1 = 1 - f_1, \quad k_2 = 1 - f_2$$

If μ is small compared with k_1 and k_2 this approximates closely to $\frac{\mu}{k_1}$ or $\frac{\mu}{1-f_1}$. In other words, the frequency of homozygous mutants is almost the same as with a rare dominant, *i.e.* negligible. The fraction of the total loss of fitness μ which is due to the homozygote is $\frac{k_2\mu}{2k_1^2}$, which is negligible unless $(1-f_2)\mu$ is of the order of $(1-f_1)^2$. In this case the loss of fitness to the species lies between μ and 2μ.

It is also clear that incompletely sex-linked genes (Haldane, 1936) will behave like autosomals, and that sex-limitation, incomplete manifestation and other like complications will not affect our results.

Since different genes mutate independently, they will be distributed independently in the population, even when linked. Hence if F be the fitness of the standard type, which is necessarily greater than unity, we have

$$F = \prod (1 - m)^{-1}$$

where the multiplication is taken over all loci: and for any autosomal locus, m is the sum of the mutation rates of recessive allelomorphs, and twice those of dominant allelomorphs. For a sex-linked locus m is $\frac{3}{2}$ times the sum of all mutation rates.

$$\begin{aligned} \log_e F &= -\Sigma \log_e (1 - m) \\ &= \Sigma m + \tfrac{1}{2}\Sigma m^2 + \tfrac{1}{3}\Sigma m^3 + \cdots \end{aligned}$$

But since every value of m is small, we have very approximately

$$\log_e F = \Sigma m$$

In other words the Malthusian parameter of the normal genotype is equal to the sum of the mutation rates of all deleterious genes and aberrations, multiplied by the factors 2 and $\frac{3}{2}$ in certain cases. If Σm is small, F approximates to $1 + \Sigma m$ and the loss of fitness due to mutation is Σm.

We must next consider other equilibria. Haldane (1927) showed that if the mutation rates of A to a and a to A are μ and ν, respectively, if $1 - k$ be the fitness of aa when those of AA and Aa are unity, and if p be the frequency of the gene a in a random mating population, then if μ, ν and k (or $1 - f$) are all small,

$$kp^3 - kp^2 - (\mu + \nu)p + \mu = 0$$

This equation has one or three real positive roots between 0 and 1. In the former case there is one stable equilibrium, in the latter two stable and one unstable. Here the loss of fitness to the whole population is kp^2, or $\mu - \frac{\nu p}{1 - p}$. This is less than μ, the value where k is large compared with μ and ν, but is of the same order, and always positive. Thus if $\mu = .00007$, $\nu = .00018$, $k = .00016$, then $p = \frac{1}{4}$, $\frac{1}{16}$ of the population are recessives, and the loss of fitness is .00001, whereas if ν were zero, $\frac{7}{16}$ of the population would be recessives, and the loss of fitness .00007 or equal to μ.

Next consider the case where the heterozygote Aa is fitter than either homozygote AA or aa. Let the fitnesses of the three types be in the ratios $\alpha\, AA : 1\, Aa : \beta\, aa$. Let the actual fitnesses be $(1 - k)AA$, $(1 - h)Aa$, $(1 - l)aa$. And let the frequency of the gene a be p, that of A q. We can neglect mutation, provided $1 - \alpha$ and $1 - \beta$ are much larger than the mutation rates. We find from the conditions of equilibrium

$$p = \frac{h - k}{2h - k - l} \qquad q = \frac{h - l}{2h - k - l}$$

From the condition that the mean fitness should be unity,

$$p^2 l + q^2 k = 2hpq.$$

Whence

$$h^2 = kl.$$

Also

$$\alpha = \frac{1-k}{1+h}, \quad \beta = \frac{1-l}{1+h}$$

Whence

$$h = \frac{(1-\alpha)(1-\beta)}{1-\alpha\beta}, \quad k = \frac{(1-\alpha)^2}{1-\alpha\beta}, \quad l = \frac{(1-\beta)^2}{1-\alpha\beta}$$

The total loss of fitness to the species is $(h+k)q^2 + (h+l)p^2 = h$, as is otherwise obvious. Hence, for example, if $\alpha = .99$, $\beta = .9$, that is to say if the two homozygous forms are 1 per cent. and 10 per cent. less fit than the heterozygous form, the loss of fitness is 0.92 per cent. for the species as a whole. In general $\dfrac{(1-\alpha)(1-\beta)}{1-\alpha\beta}$ is of the order of magnitude of the loss of fitness which would be caused if the whole species consisted of the fitter type of homozygote.

We see then that a single pair of genes causing increased fitness in the heterozygote has a far greater effect in lowering the fitness of the species than any gene which causes unfitness of a more serious character, provided that the heterozygote is not fitter than either homozygote. Hence there will be very strong selective influence in favor of any method by which the whole species may approximate to the phenotype of *Aa*. This may occur in at least four ways. By a mechanism of the *Oenothera* type the species may be kept in permanent heterozygosis. An allelomorph may appear which has intermediate effects between *A* and *a*, and which thus approximates to the phenotype of *Aa* when homozygous. If *A* and *a* are antimorphic a duplication may give a homozygote with *AA* in one pair of loci, and *aa* in another. Finally other genes may modify *AA* or *aa* towards the phenotype of *Aa*. In each of the last three cases the species will again become approximately homozygous.

In the type of equilibrium first discussed the Fisher effect will arise. That is to say, dominants will tend to become recessive, and recessives to disappear, owing to the presence of modifiers. If the spread of the modifiers is so slow that the species may always be considered in equilibrium for the main gene, it follows that the intensity of selection as measured by the loss of fitness will be unchanged throughout this process.

It remains to give some sort of estimate of the loss of fitness caused by mutation in a species. In *Drosophila melanogaster* the mean rate of mutation of sex-linked lethals per chromosome per generation is about .003, of autosomal lethals in the second chromosome .004, according to Muller (1928). According to Timofeeff-Ressovsky (1935) we may expect genes with no visible effect, but lowering fitness, to be about twice as frequent. The third chromosome probably behaves like the second. The total loss of fitness to the species is thus about $3(.003 \times \frac{3}{2} - .004 \times 2)$ or about 4 per cent. This may be taken as a rough estimate of the price which the species pays for the variability which is probably a prerequisite for evolution. The mutation rates of two human genes seem to be rather higher than those found in *Drosophila* (Haldane 1935, Penrose and Gunther 1935) if measured per generation, though not per year, so the figure for man is probably of the same order, though a little higher. In other words, if we could achieve the aim of negative eugenics and abolish all genes (including autosomal recessives, most of which can not even be detected at present) which seriously lower fitness in our present environments, we might expect a gain in fitness of the order of 10 per cent., though this might lower our capacity for evolution in a changed environment.

Summary

In a species in equilibrium variation is mainly due to two causes. Some deleterious genes are being weeded out by selection at the same rate as they are produced by mutation. Others are preserved because the heterozygous form is fitter than either homozygote. In the former case the loss of fitness in the species is roughly equal to the sum of all mutation rates and is probably of the order of 5 per cent. It is suggested that this loss of fitness is the price paid by a species for its capacity for further evolution.

REFERENCES

Fisher, R. A.

1930. "The Genetical Theory of Natural Selection." Oxford.

1935. *Jour. Genet.*, 30: 369–382.

Gordon, C.

1936. *Jour. Genet.*, 33: 25–60.

Gunther, M., and Penrose, L. S.

1935. *Jour. Genet.*, 31: 413–30.

Haldane, J. B. S.

1924. *Trans. Camb. Phil. Soc.*, 23: 19–41.

1926. *Proc. Camb. Phil. Soc.*, 23: 607–15.

1927. *Proc. Camb. Phil. Soc.*, 23: 838–44.

1931. *Proc. Camb. Phil. Soc.*, 27: 137–142.

1935. *Jour. Genet.*, 31: 317–326

1936. *Ann. Eugen.*, 7: 28–57.

Muller, H. J.

1928. *Genetics*, 13: 280–357.

Norton, H. P. J.

1928. *Proc. Lond. Math. Soc.*, 28: 1–45.

Sax, K.

1926. *Bot. Gaz.*, 82: 223–7.

Timofeeff-Ressowsky, N. W.

1935. *Gott. Nachricht. Math.-Phys. Klasse*, N. F., 1: 163–80.

Wright, S.

1931. *Genetics*, 16: 97–159.

575.116 : 612.115.4 575.116 : 612.845.5/6

The Linkage between the Genes for Colour-blindness and Haemophilia in Man

By Julia Bell and J. B. S. Haldane, F.R.S.
Galton Laboratory and Department of Genetics, University College, London

(*Received* 18 *December* 1936)

It is well established that colour-blindness and haemophilia are due to sex-linked genes. These genes appear to manifest themselves in all males who carry them. In women the gene for haemophilia is probably always recessive, the cases of alleged haemophilia in heterozygous women being very doubtful. On the other hand, colour-blind women whose putative fathers are not colour-blind occur too frequently to be explained by illegitimacy (Bell 1926). So colour-blindness is probably not always recessive. On the other hand, women homozygous for the gene appear always to be colour-blind. No cases of incomplete recessiveness occur in the new pedigrees here presented. It will be assumed that a woman who is not colour-blind is not homozygous for the gene for colour-blindness.

There are two distinct forms of colour-blindness, namely protanopia ("red-blindness") and deuteranopia ("green-blindness"). According to Waaler (1927) the genes determining them form a series of five allelomorphs with the normal gene, and those for protanomalia and deuteranomalia. Haldane (1935) suggested that there are at least two different allelomorphic genes for haemophilia.

Morgan (1910) showed that in *Drosophila melanogaster* genes which are sex linked, and therefore completely linked in spermatogenesis, are partially linked in oogenesis. This principle has since been extended to other species of *Drosophila*, and *mutatis mutandis* to pigeons (Cole and Kelley 1919), to poultry and other organisms; and on the basis of the data so obtained the chromosomes have been mapped.

It is important to demonstrate that the principles of linkage which have been worked out for other animals also hold good for man. The choice of colour-blindness for one of the two genes whose linkage was to be investigated is obvious. Over 2 % of human males are colour-blind, and a distinctly larger fraction are anomalous trichromats. Of the remaining sex-linked abnormalities some are very rare, whilst others affect the eyes and would thus lead to confusion, or at best difficulty, in the detection of colour-blindness. Haemophilia is not excessively uncommon, and could have no effect on the detection of colour-blindness. Moreover, certain physicians specialize in its treatment, and thus considerable numbers of cases are available. It was decided to seek for haemophilics, to test their colour vision and that of their non-haemophilic brothers, and to follow up the family history if both conditions were found in the same family.

Addresses of haemophilics were kindly sent to us by a number of physicians, including Dr. Macfarlane of St Bartholomew's Hospital, Dr. Cockayne of Great Ormond Street Hospital, Dr. Miller of St Mary's Hospital, and Professor Bulloch of the London Hospital. Dr. W. D. Wright of the Royal College of Science, South Kensington, undertook to test the colour vision of these patients and their brothers for us.

The cases which emerged from this preliminary enquiry were seventeen haemophilics and thirteen unaffected brothers of haemophilics. Among these Dr. Wright found deuteranopia in two haemophilics of different families. The other members of these families were then followed up as far as possible, and examinations of colour vision were made on all available members who were liable to inherit the defect, and occasionally on others. For this purpose Ishihara's tests were used. In no case was the diagnosis in doubt. We have to acknowledge with gratitude a grant from the Medical Research Council for the expenses involved in this work.

We owe two other pedigrees to the courtesy of colleagues, Dr. W. J. B. Riddell of Glasgow and Dr. C. L. Birch of Chicago. In each case the investigation is still incomplete and full accounts will be published elsewhere. They have, however, permitted us to publish the parts of their pedigrees which are relevant to our enquiry. Finally, Dr. Madlener of Kempten (Germany) most kindly gave us further information concerning members of the family previously published by him (Madlener 1928) in which the first evidence of linkage between the two genes was obtained. Thus with the pedigree published by Davenport (1930) we have information concerning six families in which these two conditions occur. The information is sufficient to leave no doubt as to the existence of linkage, but its intensity is not yet established with accuracy.

Description of New Pedigrees

The pedigree A, fig. 1, including the colour-blind haemophilic IV 9, had already been investigated with regard to haemophilia, and was given to us by IV 9, a patient of Dr. Macfarlane's discovered by Dr. Wright to be deuteranopic. We examined the colour vision in eight more members of this family, and found the pedigree, so far as we were able to verify it, correct in all particulars amongst the descendants of II 1 and II 2. The haemophilics are limited to one branch of the family, namely the descendants of III 2.

IV 9 is an intelligent and co-operative man, and personally arranged for the examination of his cousins and nephews. Unfortunately a family quarrel prevented our testing the vision of the non-haemophilic brother, IV 2, who wrote that "though I bear at present the name of *X*... I consider myself of no blood relationship to that family and no useful purpose would be served by visiting me". We called in order to try if persuasive methods could secure a valuable addition to our knowledge, but were not admitted to his house. III 2 has two living brothers who are not haemophilic, but we were unable to examine their colour vision.

The most interesting point in this pedigree is the limitation of the haemophilia to one branch of the family. The two normal nephews of IV 9, who had a chance of being haemophilic and colour-blind, were actually neither. Thus no crossing-over had occurred in the family, the absence of haemophilia in the cousins of IV 9 being explicable by mutation. The information regarding linkage is, however, meagre.

The pedigree B, fig. 2, provides a much better illustration of linkage.

V 1 and V 2 are cases of haemophilia under the care of Dr. Macfarlane. They appear to be typical examples of the disease, with a history of repeated haemorrhages into their joints; V 2 has recently been away from work for more than 11 weeks following a slight injury; the bleeding was so severe as to soak through his mattress and drip on to the floor.

Starting from these men, who combined haemophilia and deuteranopia, the family was followed, and seven further males who, from their relationship to V 1, were potentially haemophilic or colour-blind, were examined. The family is somewhat scattered, one member living in Devonshire.

V 3 died in early infancy having shown no symptoms of haemophilia.

V 6 died in infancy from haemorrhage following circumcision. The parents were told at hospital that, had the family history been known, this operation would not have been performed. It is believed, probably correctly, by the family that this child had haemophilia.

III 1 is said to have been a very severe case of haemophilia. One of his sisters reports that he had a stiff leg from the age of 20, the result of repeated haemorrhages into the joints. He died at about 32. III 1 was the only haemophilic child of his mother. Her six sons by a different father were all healthy. We were able to see three of these and the children of two of

K 2

them. III 5 is aged about 78. The remaining three brothers, III 2, are dead or inaccessible, but have shown no signs of haemophilia. Information concerning this branch of the family was given by V 1 and V 2. They are intelligent young men, ready to co-operate; they took very considerable trouble to seek out their relations, many of whom they had never seen before, and to arrange for us to see them and test their colour vision. These brothers also put us in touch with III 18 of another branch of the family.

III 18, aged 60, is a frail-looking intelligent little shoemaker. He was married late and had lived at home with his mother and his three affected brothers for a long period of years, when he says the endless topic of conversation was the presence and source of haemophilia in the family. He volunteered the information that members of the family had the disease either severely or not at all, and said there could not be the slightest doubt with regard to who was, or was not, affected in his family. He described the disease in his brothers and uncle. According to him his mother had had four or more brothers, some of whom were certainly haemophilic; perhaps all had the disease, but he cannot be quite sure of this; he also can only be sure with regard to one affected brother of his maternal grandmother. He says that they have never been able to trace the transmission of the disease through a male in this family, except in the case of III 1. He knew of the affection of III 1, but only heard through our visit of the affection of his grandsons, V 1, V 2 and V 6.

III 18 was a little uncertain with regard to the children of II 6; he was assured that all members of her family, except a daughter, had died in infancy; he believed that all her sons were haemophilic. He had lost touch with the family of his sister, III 14, who died many years ago, but fortunately a letter to the old address brought an immediate response from IV 20, who was still living there.

IV 20 gave an account of his sibship agreeing in each particular with his uncle's, thus showing the reliability of the latter's statements. He brought with him a medical certificate affirming his haemophilia, and has evidently suffered severely from the disease.

We have thus found that all the four living haemophilics in this pedigree are colour-blind. On the other hand, four non-haemophilic brothers and one non-haemophilic son of a haemophilic's sister are not colour-blind. Thus in this family the linkage between haemophilia and colour-blindness has been complete.

The pedigree described in fig. 3, which we owe to Dr. Riddell, contains an example, so far unique, of two brothers, both of whom are colour-blind but only one haemophilic. The haemophilia in this family is confined to one sibship whose mother, II 4, has three brothers and seven sister's sons, none of whom has shown symptoms of haemophilia. Their colour vision has not yet been investigated.

With regard to the pedigree of fig. 4, Dr. Birch states that there is a tradition in the family concerned that individuals with haemophilia have normal colour vision, while males who are not haemophilic are colour-blind. She has only been able so far to test the validity of this tradition in two cases. Her patient III 1, a haemophilic, was found to have normal colour vision, while III 3, one of his non-haemophilic brothers, was found to be colour-blind, apparently deuteranopic. II 4 and III 4 are reported by their relatives to be colour-blind, while III 2 is believed to have had normal colour vision. Dr. Birch hopes to test the colour vision of II 3, II 4, II 5, III 4 and IV 4, and to publish the full results in a forthcoming memoir on the subject of haemophilia.

Mutation

Haldane (1935) pointed out that haemophilia would be rapidly extinguished by natural selection if the gene did not constantly arise anew by mutation. He estimated the frequency of this event in the population of London at about 2×10^{-5} per X-chromosome per generation. A communication by Dr. Birch as to its frequency in Illinois suggests a distinctly higher value, of the order of 10^{-4}, for that population.

The pedigrees of figs. 1 and 3 are most readily interpreted on the hypothesis of mutation. III 2 of fig. 1 has borne three haemophilics and one normal son; she is therefore either heterozyous $\left(\frac{+}{\mathbf{h}}\right)$ or a mixture of homozygous and heterozygous tissue $\left(\frac{+}{+} \text{ and } \frac{+}{\mathbf{h}}\right)$.

Now suppose that the gene **h** present in the haemophilic descendants of III 2 did not originate by mutation in any member of the pedigree shown, it follows that I 2, II 2, and III 2 were heterozygous for it, since I 1 and II 1 were normal. In view of the accuracy of the statements of III 2 and IV 9 where they could be verified, and their openness in discussing the problem, we think that their statements as to the absence of haemophilia in this part of the pedigree may be accepted.

We can now ask, what is the probability that two heterozygous women, I 2 and II 2, should have had no haemophilic sons, and that their daughters, other than III 2, should have been equally fortunate? It must be stated that II 3 represents three sons, all of whom survived long enough to marry. Of the two daughters, II 4, one had two sons surviving infancy, and a daughter with two sons; the other had one son, and two daughters with one and three sons respectively. We shall neglect III 3 who died in infancy.

First consider the probability apart from the information supplied by linkage. The probability that the two mothers should have had five normal sons is 2^{-5}. The probability that the daughter of a heterozygous woman should have n normal sons is $\frac{2^n+1}{2^{n+1}}$. The values of n for the seven daughters, II 2, III 2, III 5, III 7, III 8, III 11 and III 13 are 2, 1, 1, 4, 1, 1 and 3. The probability is therefore $3^6 \times 5 \times 17 \times 2^{-25}$, or 0·00185. This would be slightly lessened if we considered the further information provided by daughter's daughters' sons.

It can be considerably diminished in view of the evidence as to the linkage between the genes **c** and **h**, presented later. In the sons of III 7, III 8 and III 13 colour-blindness appears without haemophilia, while in IV 9 both are combined. Hence in the oogenesis of either II 2 or III 2 the genes must have crossed over. The probability of this event is about $2x$, where x is the small frequency of crossing-over. Taking x as 0·05, the probability is reduced to 0·0002 approximately.

In Riddell's pedigree, fig. 3, either mutation occurred, or I 2 was heterozygous. As she had three normal sons and her two daughters, II 6 and II 7, had four and three sons respectively, the probability of this is $9 \times 17 \times 2^{-12}$, or 0·037. So here the evidence for mutation is strong, but by no means conclusive.

In Green's case, Davenport (1930) and Haldane (1935) have pointed out that there is very strong evidence for mutation, based on relatives not shown in fig. 6. The probability is $5 \times 2^{-10}x$, or about 0·00025.

Thus out of six pedigrees chosen because colour-blindness occurred in them, three show evidence of mutation varying from strong to almost conclusive. This is a much higher proportion than occurs in the bulk of the published material. The reason is, we think, obvious. Accounts of sporadic cases are less likely to be published than of families containing many haemophilics. In the investigation of haemophilia the stress has so far been laid on its heredity rather than on its origin.

Terminology

The genes for colour-blindness and haemophilia will be represented by the letters **c** and **h**. The fact that the latter probably and the former certainly has several allelomorphs is irrelevant. Their normal allelomorphs will be represented, using Morgan's symbolism, by +. Thus a man is either

$++$ (normal), **c**$+$ (colour-blind), $+$**h** (haemophilic), or **ch** (colour-blind haemophilic). A woman, being diploid for these genes, is $\frac{++}{++}$, $\frac{++}{c+}$, $\frac{++}{+h}$, $\frac{++}{c\,h}$ or $\frac{+h}{c+}$, if phaenotypically normal. The latter two genotypes will differ in their progeny. The sons of $\frac{++}{c\,h}$ women will be mainly normal or colour-blind haemophilic. Those of $\frac{+h}{c+}$ women will be mainly haemophilic or colour-blind, but rarely both or neither. The other possible female genotypes are $\frac{c+}{c+}$, $\frac{c+}{c\,h}$, $\frac{+h}{+h}$, $\frac{+h}{c\,h}$ and $\frac{ch}{ch}$. It is possible that the $\frac{h}{h}$ genotypes are inviable. In any case they are very rare indeed.

Besides these types others may possibly exist. The gene for haemophilia appears to arise anew by mutation. If the mutation only occurs at meiosis, the above list is complete. If, however, it arises at a somatic division, mosaics may exist. Such mosaics, if male, would probably not be haemophilic. If haemophilia is due to a lack of some substance in the plasma, this would be supplied by the non-haemophilic tissues of a mosaic man. Such a man might transmit the gene to all, some, or none of his daughters according as all, some, or none of his testicular tissue carried the gene. A mosaic woman would not be haemophilic, but might transmit haemophilia to less than half of her sons. It is possible that III 2 in fig. 1 and II 4 in fig. 3 were of this type.

The Detection and Estimation of Linkage

Let x be the frequency of recombination between the loci of **c** and **h** so that the cross-over percentage is $100x$. Let $y = 1-x$.

It is our task to obtain as much information as possible from the data about the frequency x of crossing-over between the loci of the genes **c** and **h**. We have on the one hand to find out whether its estimated value departs significantly from $\frac{1}{2}$, its value in the absence of linkage, and on the other to obtain the best estimate of its true value. Our task is complicated by four considerations:

1. The gene **h** may arise by mutation. While this is a rare event in the population as a whole, it is frequent among the immediate ancestors of haemophilics, since, as has been shown by Haldane (1935), the frequency of mutation is about one-quarter of the frequency of the disease.
2. The gene **c** is not very rare in the population. It is excessively unlikely,

in the absence of close inbreeding, that haemophilia should arise from two different sources in one pedigree. Protanopia or deuteranopia might do so with a probability which is by no means negligible.

3. The estimation of x by any of the classical inverse probability methods involves the presupposition that all values of x in the neighbourhood of that found are equally probably *a priori*. We shall see that this is not so.

4. The sample observed is still so small that the probability distribution of x about its estimated value is far from normal. We cannot, therefore, speak of the probable or standard error of our estimate without further qualifications.

The method adopted is as follows: we estimate the frequency p of the gene **c** in the general population. We make out a pedigree showing the descent of the gene **h** in each pedigree, without reference to our knowledge concerning **c**. In doing so we have assumed that III 2 of fig. 1 and II 4 of fig. 3 were $\frac{+}{\mathbf{h}}$, and not mosaic. As they had seven haemophilic and only two normal sons, this seems to be justified. We have also neglected the possibility of illegitimacy. This would only be relevant in considering the daughters of a haemophilic man. Only two such occur in our pedigrees, and both proved their legitimacy by bearing haemophilic sons. Mutation at the **c** locus, if it occurs at all, is certainly too rare to be of any importance. So is non-disjunction.

Taking the pedigree of haemophilia as given, we determine:

1. $P(x, p)$. The probability, as a function of x and p, that, given that the first observed colour-blind man in the pedigree was actually colour-blind, all other relevant males in the pedigree possessed the type of colour vision which they actually did.

2. $P(\frac{1}{2}, p)$. The same probability for $x = \frac{1}{2}$, that is to say the probability of obtaining the observed result in the absence of linkage. If there have been no cross-overs, this is sufficient. If there have been, we must further calculate $P'(\frac{1}{2}, p)$, the probability of obtaining a result as favourable or more favourable to the hypothesis of linkage, in the absence of linkage.

3. $P(x, 0)$. The same probability for $p = 0$, i.e. neglecting the possibility that colour-blindness could have had a double origin.

4. $P(\frac{1}{2}, 0)$. The same possibility for $x = \frac{1}{2}$, $p = 0$, and $P'(\frac{1}{2}, 0)$ in case crossing-over has occurred.

The last is the easiest to calculate, and the first the hardest, but in practice it will be found that $P(x, 0)$ and $P'(\frac{1}{2}, 0)$ are sufficiently accurate. We shall see that all the values of $P(x, p)$ approximate very closely to $x^k(1-x)^{n-k}$, where n and k are not necessarily integers. We may say that we have tested

n ova and found k cross-overs. This simplified statement is sufficiently accurate for our data, but would not be so in general.

On multiplying the values of P for the six pedigrees we obtain a cumulative value. The cumulative value of $P'(\frac{1}{2}, p)$ gives us the probability that the data which appear to prove the linkage could really be due to sampling error. The assumption is involved that colour-blindness shows Mendelian segregation. Hogben (1932) has shown that this is very approximately true.

The cumulative value of $P(x, p)$ enables us to estimate x. The estimate is, however, as we shall see, extremely rough.

The Frequency of Deuteranopia in the General Population

The colour-blindness in all six pedigrees here considered is deuteranopia. Data as to the frequency of protanopia and deuteranopia are given by Waaler (1927) for Oslo, v. Planta (1928) for Basle, Schmidt (1936) for Berlin, and Wright (unpublished) for London. Dr. Wright, who most kindly permits us to use his results, suspects that they may be a little high, as some of them were obtained from volunteers who may have had special reasons for desiring to be tested. The London value of $1{\cdot}20 \pm 0{\cdot}30$ % is well within the limits of sampling error of the overall value of $1{\cdot}42 \pm 0{\cdot}097$ %, and we shall take $p = 0{\cdot}0142$. It will be seen that the correction for p is actually negligible, but it will not always be so if the work begun in this paper is carried on.

Table I—Percentage Frequency of Colour-blindness in Males

	Waaler	v. Planta	Schmidt	Wright	Total
Number tested	9049	2000	6863	1338	19,250
Protanopes	0·88	1·60	1·09	1·27	1·01
Deuteranopes	1·03	1·50	1·97	1·20	1·42

Pedigree A (fig. 1)

We assume that III 2 is heterozygous, though she is possibly a mosaic. If so, less weight is to be attached to the fact that V 5 is not a deuteranope: how much less weight is uncertain. We also know that IV 8 is heterozygous for haemophilia, since she had a haemophilic son, but we do not know the genotype of IV 7. We have now to determine P, given that IV 9 is a deuteranope, and that neither V 5 nor V 8 are deuteranopes.

It is at once clear that $P(\frac{1}{2}, 0) = \frac{9}{16}$. For if no information is derivable from linkage the probability that a deuteranope's sister is herself $\frac{+}{c}$ is $\frac{1}{2}$,

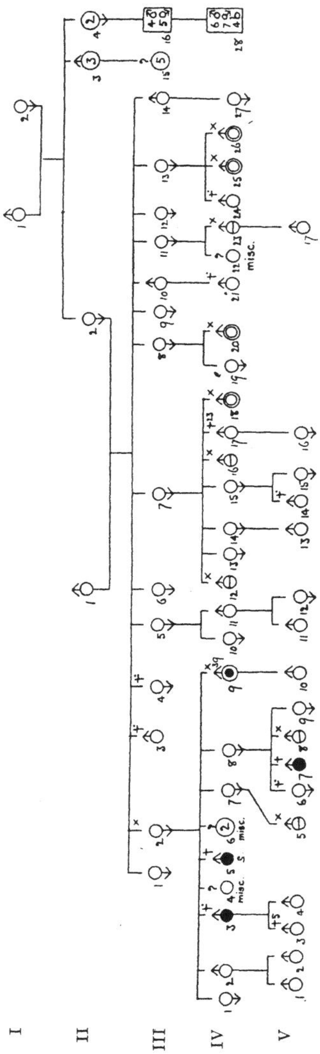

Fig. 1—Pedigree A. ⊙ haemophilic deuteranope; ● haemophilic; ◎ deuteranopic; ⊖ normal colour vision; × seen; + died in infancy.

and hence the probability that her only son, or only observed son, is a deuteranope is $\frac{1}{4}$. The probability that two such sons are not deuteranopes is therefore $(\frac{3}{4})^2$.

To calculate $P(x, 0)$ we note that III 2 is either $\frac{+\,+}{\mathbf{c}\ \mathbf{h}}$ or $\frac{+\,\mathbf{h}}{\mathbf{c}\,+}$. The respective probabilities of these two genotypes are clearly y and x. If she was $\frac{+\,+}{\mathbf{c}\ \mathbf{h}}$ the further probability that IV 8 is $\frac{+\,+}{\mathbf{c}\ \mathbf{h}}$ is y, for she is known to be $\frac{+}{\mathbf{h}}$, and the further probability that her non-haemophilic son is a non-deuteranope is y, making a cumulative probability of y^3 for this, the most probable causal nexus between IV 9 and V 8.

TABLE II—PROBABILITIES OF DIFFERENT CONNEXIONS OF V 8 AND V 5 WITH IV 9 (EXPLANATION IN TEXT)

V 8(+ +)	IV 8		III 2		IV 7		V 5(+ +)
					$\frac{+\,+}{+\,+}$	$\frac{1}{2}y$	1
y	$\frac{+\,+}{\mathbf{c}\ \mathbf{h}}$	y			$\frac{+\,+}{+\,\mathbf{h}}$	$\frac{1}{2}x$	1
			$\frac{+\,+}{\mathbf{c}\ \mathbf{h}}$	y			
1	$\frac{+\,+}{+\,\mathbf{h}}$	x			$\frac{+\,+}{\mathbf{c}\,+}$	$\frac{1}{2}x$	$\frac{1}{2}$
					$\frac{+\,+}{\mathbf{c}\ \mathbf{h}}$	$\frac{1}{2}y$	y
					$\frac{+\,+}{+\,+}$	$\frac{1}{2}x$	1
y	$\frac{+\,+}{\mathbf{c}\ \mathbf{h}}$	x			$\frac{+\,+}{+\,\mathbf{h}}$	$\frac{1}{2}y$	1
			$\frac{+\,\mathbf{h}}{\mathbf{c}\,+}$	x			
1	$\frac{+\,+}{+\,\mathbf{h}}$	y			$\frac{+\,+}{\mathbf{c}\,+}$	$\frac{1}{2}y$	$\frac{1}{2}$
					$\frac{+\,+}{\mathbf{c}\ \mathbf{h}}$	$\frac{1}{2}x$	y

The various possibilities are scheduled in Table II. The first and last columns give the probability that two sons should have been born of mothers of the genotype given in the adjacent column. The second and fourth columns give the probability that a woman of the genotype considered should have been born of a mother of the genotype given in the central column. The central column gives the probability that a woman of that genotype should have been the mother of IV 9. Thus if III 2 is $\frac{+\,\mathbf{h}}{\mathbf{c}\,+}$ which has a probability x, then IV 7 is $\frac{+\ +}{+\ \text{c}}$ with a further probability $\frac{1}{2}y$, and V 5 is + + with a further probability $\frac{1}{2}$.

Hence we find:

$$P(x,\ 0) = (y^2+x)\,y(\tfrac{1}{2}y+\tfrac{1}{2}x+\tfrac{1}{4}x+\tfrac{1}{2}y^2)+(y+xy)\,x(\tfrac{1}{2}x+\tfrac{1}{2}y+\tfrac{1}{4}y+\tfrac{1}{2}xy)$$
$$= \tfrac{1}{4}(4y^4+8xy^3+17x^2y^2+7x^3y)$$
$$= y^2+\tfrac{7}{4}x^2y+\tfrac{3}{2}x^2y^2$$
$$= y^2\left(1+\frac{13x^2}{4y^2}-\frac{19x^3}{4y^3}+\frac{25x^4}{4y^4}\dots\right).$$

Hence the leading term is y^2, and $n = 2$, $k = 0$.

To calculate $P(\frac{1}{2},\ p)$ we note that the only possible second source of deuteranopia is the husband of III 2. The probability that he was normal is $1-p$. If so the value of P is $\frac{9}{16}$, as found above. The probability that he was a deuteranope is p. If so his daughters are equally likely to be $\frac{+}{\text{c}}$ or $\frac{\text{c}}{\text{c}}$. Hence the probability that V 5 is a deuteranope is $\frac{3}{4}$, and similarly for V 8. The probability that neither is a deuteranope is $\frac{1}{16}$. Hence

$$P'(\tfrac{1}{2},p) = P(\tfrac{1}{2},p) = \tfrac{9}{16}(1-p)+\tfrac{1}{16}p$$
$$= \frac{9-8p}{16}$$
$$= \left(1-\frac{8p}{9}\right)P(\tfrac{1}{2},\ 0).$$

Thus in this case the allowance for a secondary source diminishes $P(\frac{1}{2},\ x)$ and thus increases the evidence for linkage. In other pedigrees it has the opposite effect. No further evidence would have been gained had the colour vision of IV 7 and IV 8 been examined, for, since each produced a son with normal vision, neither can have been $\frac{\text{c}}{\text{c}}$. An examination of IV 1 would, however, have given a little more information.

To calculate $P(x,\ p)$ we note that if the husband of III 2 was normal the analysis of Table II holds good. If he was deuteranopic the corresponding probabilities are given in Table III.

In this case the term contributed to $P(x,\ p)$ is

$$p[x^2y(\tfrac{1}{4}y+\tfrac{1}{2}x^2)+x^2y(\tfrac{1}{4}x+\tfrac{1}{2}xy)] = \tfrac{1}{4}px^2y(3x+y).$$

So $P(x, p) = \frac{1}{4}(1-p)(4y^4+8xy^3+17x^2y^2+7x^3y)+\frac{1}{4}p(x^2y^2+3x^3y)$

$$= \tfrac{1}{4}(4y^4+8xy^3+17x^2y^2+7x^3y)-p(y^4+2xy^3+4x^2y^2+x^3y)$$

$$= y^2+\tfrac{7}{4}x^2y+\tfrac{3}{2}x^2y^2-p(y^2+x^2y+2x^2y^2)$$

$$= (1-p)\left(y^2+\frac{7-4p}{4-4p}x^2y+\frac{3-4p}{2-2p}x^2y^2\right).$$

TABLE III—PROBABILITIES OF DIFFERENT CONNEXIONS OF V 8 AND V 5 WITH IV 9 IF III 2'S HUSBAND WAS A DEUTERANOPE

V 8(+ +)	IV 8		III 2		IV 7		V 5(+ +)
					c+ / ++	$\frac{1}{2}y$	$\frac{1}{2}$
0	c+ / ch	y	++ / ch	y	c+ / +h	$\frac{1}{2}x$	x
x	c+ / +h	x			c+ / c+	$\frac{1}{2}x$	0
					c+ / ch	$\frac{1}{2}y$	0
					c+ / ++	$\frac{1}{2}x$	$\frac{1}{2}$
0	c+ / ch	x	+h / c+	x	c+ / +h	$\frac{1}{2}y$	x
x	c+ / +h	y			c+ / c+	$\frac{1}{2}y$	0
					c+ / ch	$\frac{1}{2}x$	0

Hence the values of n and k are unaltered. Since the multiplication of $P(x, p)$ by a quantity independent of x does not affect the estimation of x, the sole effect of not neglecting p is to multiply the coefficient of x^2 by $1+\frac{3p}{7(1-p)}$ or 1·006, and that of x^2y^2 by $1-\frac{p}{3(1-p)}$ or 0·995. These corrections are quite negligible.

However, had V 5 been a deuteranope, the leading terms in $P(x, p)$ would have been $xy-py^2$. Since, as we shall see, x is a small quantity of the same order as p, though probably about three times as large, the correction would have been very important. If enough pedigrees are investigated such a case will probably arise, and a method has therefore been devised which is capable of dealing with it.

It is obvious that, in this case, we could calculate $P(x, p)$ directly, and derive the other three values of P by substitution. However, their direct evaluation is instructive, and also furnishes a useful check.

If III 2 was a mosaic we can readily obtain maximal values for P. Completely neglecting IV 7 and V 5, we find

$$P(x,\ 0) = y + 2x^2y,$$

$$P(\tfrac{1}{2},\ 0) = \tfrac{3}{4}.$$

If III 2 is a mosaic, the true values lie between these and those found earlier.

Pedigree B (fig. 2)

To avoid circumlocution we have redrawn the relevant parts of pedigree B, and inserted some additional individuals in fig. 2*a*. Given the pedigree of haemophilia and the fact that M is a deuteranope, we have to calculate the probability P that I, L and N are deuteranopes, while E, F, G, H and K are not. Since α, β, γ, ζ and η all had haemophilic sons, it is clear that they are, or were $\frac{+}{\mathbf{h}}$, whilst ϵ may have been so. It may be remarked that the value of P is the same, from whichever of the haemophilic deuteranopes we start our calculation.

To calculate $P(x, p)$ we note that if there was only one source of deuteranopia, D must have been a deuteranope. Hence η is $\frac{+\ +}{\mathbf{c}\ \mathbf{h}}$ which has a probability y, and the further probability that N is a deuteranope is also y, giving a cumulative probability y^2. Since D was a deuteranope, the probability that β was $\frac{+\ +}{\mathbf{c}\ \mathbf{h}}$ is y, the probability that she was $\frac{+\ \mathbf{h}}{\mathbf{c}\ +}$ is x. The cumulative probabilities of these two contingencies are thus y^3 and xy^2.

If β was $\frac{+\ +}{\mathbf{c}\ \mathbf{h}}$, the probability that her three sons E, F and G are non-deuteranopes is y^3, the same probability for K being $\frac{1}{4}(4y^2 + 5xy + 3x^2)$ as found in the similar case in pedigree A. Further, β must have received both **c** and **h** from α. The probability that α was $\frac{+\ +}{\mathbf{c}\ \mathbf{h}}$ is therefore y, the probability that she was $\frac{+\ \mathbf{h}}{\mathbf{c}\ +}$ is x. Since γ is known to have been $\frac{+}{\mathbf{h}}$, the further probability that she was $\frac{+\ +}{\mathbf{c}\ \mathbf{h}}$ is $y^2 + x^2$. (She cannot have been $\frac{+\ \mathbf{h}}{\mathbf{c}\ +}$ if β was $\frac{+\ +}{\mathbf{c}\ \mathbf{h}}$.) Given that γ was $\frac{+\ +}{\mathbf{c}\ \mathbf{h}}$, the further probability that H and I were as found

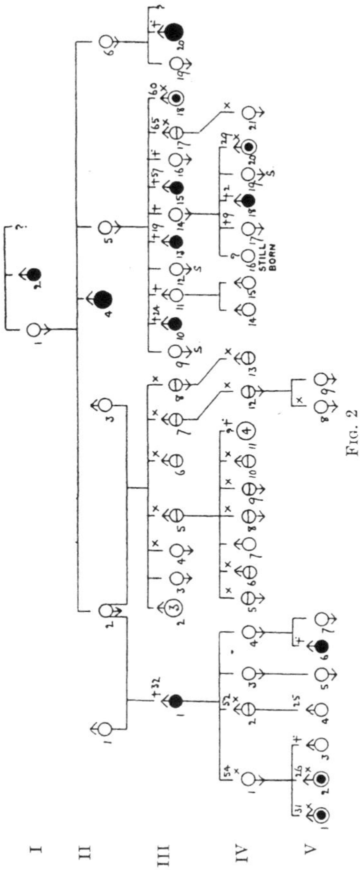

FIG. 2

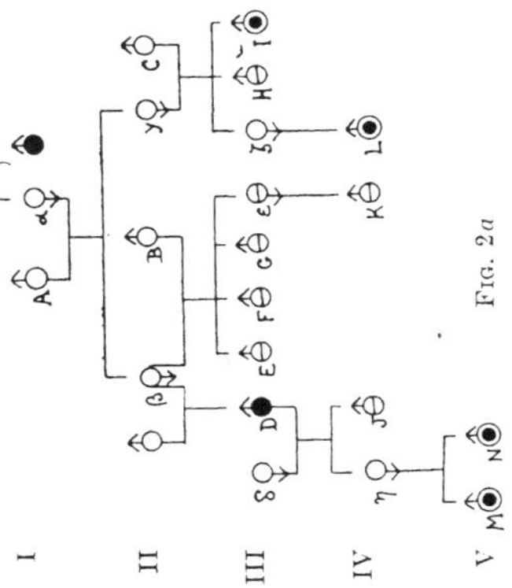

FIG. 2*a*

FIG. 2—Pedigree B. ● haemophilic; ⊙ haemophilic deuteranope; ⊖ normal colour vision; × seen; + died in infancy.

is y^2. The probability that L is a deuteranope is also y^2. Thus the cumulative probability from β onwards is

$$\tfrac{1}{4}y^7(4y^2+5xy+3x^2)(y^2+x^2),$$

and the contribution to $P(x, 0)$ corresponding to the contingency that β was $\frac{+\;+}{\mathbf{c}\;\mathbf{h}}$ is

$$\tfrac{1}{4}y^{10}(4y^2+5xy+3x^2)(y^2+x^2).$$

If, however, β was $\frac{+\;\mathbf{h}}{\mathbf{c}\;+}$, the probability that E, F and G were as found is x^3. The further probability that K was as found is $\frac{1}{4}(3y^2+7xy+2x^2)$, the proof being as in pedigree A. Further, since β received **c** and **h** from different parents, A must have been **c**+ and α $\frac{+\;+}{+\;\mathbf{h}}$. Hence γ was $\frac{+\;\mathbf{h}}{\mathbf{c}\;+}$. The probability that H and I were as found is x^2, the probability that L was as found xy. For ζ must have been $\frac{+\;+}{\mathbf{c}\;\mathbf{h}}$, as she was heterozygous for both genes. Hence the cumulative probability from β onwards is $\frac{1}{4}x^6y(3y^2+7xy+2x^2)$, and the contribution to $P(x, 0)$ is

$$\tfrac{1}{4}x^7y^3(3y^2+7xy+2x^2)(y+x)^2,$$

the last term being added for the sake of homogeneity. Hence

$$\begin{aligned}
P(x, 0) &= \tfrac{1}{4}y^{10}(4y^2+5xy+3x^2)(y^2+x^2)+\tfrac{1}{4}x^7y^3(3y^2+7xy+2x^2)(y+x)^2 \\
&= \tfrac{1}{4}(4y^{14}+5xy^{13}+7x^2y^{12}+5x^3y^{11}+3x^4y^{10}+3x^7y^7+13x^8y^6 \\
&\qquad\qquad +19x^9y^5+11x^{10}y^4+2x^{11}y^3) \\
&= 1-\tfrac{51}{4}x+\tfrac{153}{2}x^2-\tfrac{1145}{4}x^3+\dots \\
&= y^{\frac{51}{4}}\left(1+\frac{51x^2}{32y^2}-\frac{45x^3}{64y^3}+\dots\right),
\end{aligned}$$

$$n = 12\tfrac{3}{4},\; k = 0.$$

$$P(\tfrac{1}{2}, 0) = 3^2\times 2^{-13}.$$

It is to be noted that $y^{\frac{51}{4}}$ is a far better approximation than $1-\frac{51}{4}x$. Since $n = 12\frac{3}{4}$ we may say that the genes **c** and **h** have had $12\frac{3}{4}$ opportunities of separating, and have taken none of them. The steps in the pedigree, each of which contributes unity to n, are:

Mη, ηN, Dβ, βE, βF, βG, βx, $\alpha\gamma$, γH, γI, $\gamma\zeta$ and ζL.

The two steps $\beta\epsilon$, ϵK contribute $\frac{3}{4}$ between them. We can at once apply this simple method to any given pedigree, and thus evaluate n and k. The residual terms such as $\frac{51}{32}x^2y^{43}$ represent contingencies involving crossing-over on two or more occasions. They are negligible when x is small, but essential for the calculation of $P(\frac{1}{2}, 0)$. In a large pedigree it may therefore be most convenient to calculate n and $P(\frac{1}{2}, 0)$ separately.

The calculation of $P(\frac{1}{2}, p)$ and $P(x, p)$ is somewhat more complicated, and the extra accuracy obtained turns out to be negligible. It is, however, necessary to demonstrate this fact, and the method demonstrated will be applicable in cases where the correction can no longer be neglected. Five contingencies would give a second source of deuteranopia in the pedigree:

1. δ produced a **c** + gamete from which η was formed.
2. B was **c** +.
3. A was **c** + and α was $\frac{+}{\mathbf{c}}\left(\text{either } \frac{+\ +}{\mathbf{c\ h}} \text{ or } \frac{+\ \mathbf{h}}{\mathbf{c}\ +}\right)$.
4. α was $\frac{\mathbf{c}\ +}{\mathbf{c\ h}}$.
5. C was **c** +.

Each of these contingencies has an *a priori* probability p. Further, any two or more of them may be true simultaneously, except (3) and (4). These are excluded because β and γ had sons with normal vision and were therefore not $\frac{\mathbf{c}}{\mathbf{c}}$. We shall neglect these multiple contingencies, which contribute to the coefficient of p^2 in the expansion of P. Since p^2 is much smaller than the standard error of p, this is clearly justifiable.

It is most convenient to calculate $P(\frac{1}{2}, p)$ and $P(x, p)$ separately, since we are only interested in the leading terms in the expansion of the latter. To calculate $P(\frac{1}{2}, p)$ we multiply $P(\frac{1}{2}, 0)$ by $(1-5p)$ and add terms corresponding to each of the five contingencies. These are as follows:

1. Since J is not colour-blind, the probability must be halved. For if δ had been $\frac{+}{\mathbf{c}}$, the chance of his being so would be $\frac{1}{2}$. On this hypothesis it is no longer sure that D was colour-blind, and it is best to begin the calculation at the other end of the pedigree, that is to say to ask "Given that I is colour-blind, and that δ contributed a **c** + gamete to η, what is the probability that the various individuals had the type of colour vision found, neglecting the information supplied by the pedigree of haemophilia?" On this hypothesis the value of $P(\frac{1}{2}, 0)$ would be calculated as follows: γ was $\frac{+}{\mathbf{c}}$. Hence the probability that H and L are as found is 2^{-3}. The probability that

β was $\frac{+}{+}$ is 2^{-2}, the probability that she was $\frac{+}{\mathrm{c}}$ is 3×2^{-2}. If β was $\frac{+}{+}$, the probability that E, F, G and K are as found is 1. And since D was $+$, the probability that M and N were colour-blind is 2^{-2}. If however β was $\frac{+}{\mathrm{c}}$ the probability that E, F, G and K are normal is 3×2^{-5}. The further probabilities that D was $+$ and c are each $\frac{1}{2}$. If D was $+$, the probability that M and N are colour-blind is $\frac{1}{4}$. If D was c, the probability is 1. Hence on this hypothesis

$$P(\tfrac{1}{2}, 0) = 2^{-3}[2^{-2} \times 2^{-2} + 3 \times 2^{-2} \times 3 \times 2^{-5} \times 2^{-2}(2^{-2}+1)]$$
$$= 173 \times 2^{-14}.$$

So the contribution to $P(\frac{1}{2}, p)$ on this contingency is $173 \times 2^{-15}p$.

2. The probability that a colour-blind man B and his heterozygous wife β should have a normal daughter whose only son is normal is $\frac{1}{4}$, as opposed to $\frac{3}{4}$ if B was normal. The contribution is therefore $3 \times 2^{-13}p$.

3. The probability that β and γ were both heterozygous is now $\frac{1}{4}$ instead of $\frac{3}{4}$, so the contribution is $3 \times 2^{-13}p$.

4. The probability that γ was heterozygous is now 1 instead of $\frac{3}{4}$, and the contribution is therefore $3 \times 2^{-11}p$.

5. The probability, given that γ was heterozygous, that L is colour-blind is now $\frac{3}{4}$ instead of $\frac{1}{4}$, so the contribution is $3^3 \times 2^{-13}p$.

Hence $P(\frac{1}{2}, p)$

$$= (1-5p)\, 9 \times 2^{-13} + p(173 \times 2^{-15} + 3 \times 2^{-13} + 3 \times 2^{-13} + 3 \times 2^{-11} + 27 \times 2^{-13})$$
$$= 9 \times 2^{-13} + 173 \times 2^{-15}p$$
$$= 9 \times 2^{-13}\left(1 + \frac{173p}{36}\right).$$

Thus $P(\frac{1}{2}, 0)$ must be multiplied by 1·0673.

In calculating $P(x, p)$ we need only consider the changes in the first three terms, namely $y^{14} + \frac{5}{4}xy^{13} + \frac{7}{4}x^2y^{12}$, in the homogeneous expansion of $P(x, 0)$, since it will be shown later that the third term and *a fortiori* later terms are negligible. As above, each contingency contributes a term to be added to $(1-5p)\,P(x, 0)$.

1. Since J is $+\,+$, the term must be multiplied by $\frac{1}{2}$. If η is $\frac{\mathrm{c}\,+}{\mathrm{c}\,\mathrm{h}}$, M and N must have been deuteranopes. The probability is $y^{-2}P(x, 0)$. If η was $\frac{\mathrm{c}\,+}{+\,\mathrm{h}}$, the probability that M and N are deuteranopes is x^2. Further, D was not a deuteranope, which involves a further probability of x if β was $\frac{+\,+}{\mathrm{c}\,\mathrm{h}}$,

and a power of x if she was $\frac{+\ \mathbf{h}}{\mathbf{c}\ +}$. Hence the probability that η was $\frac{\mathbf{c}\ +}{+\ \mathbf{h}}$ is negligible, and the contribution is $\frac{1}{2}y^{-2}\,P(x,\,0)\,p$ or

$$\tfrac{1}{2}(y^{12}+\tfrac{5}{4}xy^{11}+\tfrac{7}{4}x^2y^{10}+\dots)\,p.$$

Multiplying by $(y+x)^2$ for the sake of homogeneity, this becomes

$$(\tfrac{1}{2}y^{14}+\tfrac{13}{8}xy^{13}+\tfrac{21}{8}x^2y^{12}+\dots)\,p.$$

2. If β was $\frac{+\ \mathbf{h}}{\mathbf{c}\ +}$, the probability has a leading term x^7y^7 and is negligible. If β was $\frac{+\ +}{\mathbf{c}\ \mathbf{h}}$, the probability that ϵ and K have normal vision is $\frac{1}{4}(y^2+xy+2x^2)$ instead of $\frac{1}{4}(4y^2+5xy+3x^2)$. So the contribution to $P(x,\,p)$ is

$$(\tfrac{1}{4}y^{14}+\tfrac{1}{4}xy^{13}+\tfrac{3}{4}x^2y^{12}+\dots)\,p.$$

3. If A was $\mathbf{c}\,+$, then, since β and γ were not $\frac{\mathbf{c}\ +}{\mathbf{c}\ \mathbf{h}}$, they must have been $\frac{\mathbf{c}\ +}{+\ \mathbf{h}}$. As shown above the probability has a leading term x^7y^7 and is negligible.

4. β must have been $\frac{+\ +}{\mathbf{c}\ \mathbf{h}}$, so must γ. That is to say the probability that γ was $\frac{+\ +}{\mathbf{c}\ \mathbf{h}}$ is raised from y^2+x^2 to unity. So we must substitute $(y+x)^2$ for y^2+x^2 in the expression for P. The contribution is thus

$$(y^{14}+\tfrac{13}{4}xy^{13}+\tfrac{17}{4}x^2y^{12}+\dots)\,p.$$

5. Assuming that γ was $\frac{+\ +}{\mathbf{c}\ \mathbf{h}}$ and C was $\mathbf{c}\,+$, the probability that L is a deuteranope is raised from y^2 to y^2+xy+x^2. The probability that γ was $\frac{+\ \mathbf{h}}{\mathbf{c}\ +}$ is negligible. So the contribution is

$$(y^{14}+\tfrac{9}{4}xy^{13}+4x^2y^{12}+\dots)\,p.$$

Hence

$$P(x,p)=(1-5p)\,(y^{14}+\tfrac{5}{4}xy^{13}+\tfrac{7}{4}x^2y^{12}+\dots)+p(\tfrac{11}{4}y^{14}+\tfrac{59}{8}xy^{13}+\tfrac{93}{8}x^2y^{12}+\dots)$$

$$=\frac{4-9p}{4}\left(y^{14}+\frac{10+9p}{8-18p}xy^{13}+\frac{14+23p}{8-18p}\,x^2y^{12}+\dots\right)$$

$$=\left(1-\frac{9p}{4}\right)y^{14-\frac{10+9p}{8-18p}}\left[1+\frac{204-558p-1171p^2}{8(4-9p)^2}\frac{x^2}{y^2}+\dots\right]$$

or, neglecting powers of p,

$$=\left(1-\frac{9p}{4}\right)y^{\frac{51}{4}-\frac{63p}{16}}\left(1+\frac{51+115p}{32}\frac{x^2}{y^2}+\dots\right).$$

L 2

Hence n is decreased from 12·75 to 12·695. It will be seen later that this has a negligible effect on the estimate of x.

Riddell's Pedigree

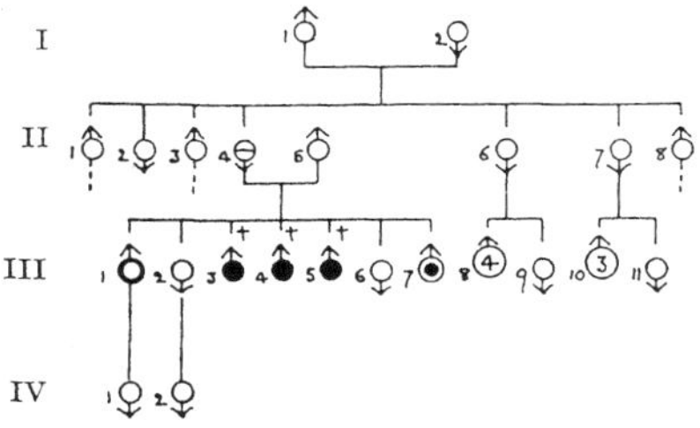

Fig. 3—Riddell's Pedigree. ● haemophilic; ⊙ colour-blind haemophilic; ◎ colour-blind; ⊖ normal colour vision.

Here we have the only case of crossing-over in our material. If II 4 is $\frac{+}{\mathbf{h}}$, then, whether she is $\frac{+\ +}{\mathbf{c\ h}}$ or $\frac{+\ \mathbf{h}}{\mathbf{c}\ +}$, the value of $P(x, 0)$ that is to say, the probability, given that III 7 is colour-blind, that III 1 should also be colour-blind is $2xy$. There is no correction for a second source of colour-blindness, since II 4 is not colour-blind. So

$$P(x, p) = 2xy,$$

$$P(\tfrac{1}{2}, p) = \tfrac{1}{2},$$

$$n = 2, \quad k = 1.$$

In this case, however, the appropriate function is $P'(\frac{1}{2}, p)$, the probability that a result as favourable to the hypothesis of linkage, or more so, should arise from random sampling. As the observed result is as unfavourable as possible, it follows that

$$P'(\tfrac{1}{2}, p) = 1.$$

Unfortunately there is, at least in the present state of our knowledge, the possibility that II 4 is a mosaic who was originally $\frac{+\ +}{\mathbf{c}\ +}$ but of whom a portion has mutated to $\frac{+\ +}{\mathbf{c\ h}}$, or $\frac{+\ \mathbf{h}}{\mathbf{c}\ +}$. Both types of tissue would be represented in her ovaries. We consider such a possibility unlikely, but to neglect it would be intellectually dishonest. Hence an alternative explanation, though not, we think, a probable one, can be given for the apparent case of crossing-over. Crossing-over will not be conclusively demonstrated until it occurs in the gametes of a woman who could not be a mosaic.

BIRCH'S PEDIGREE

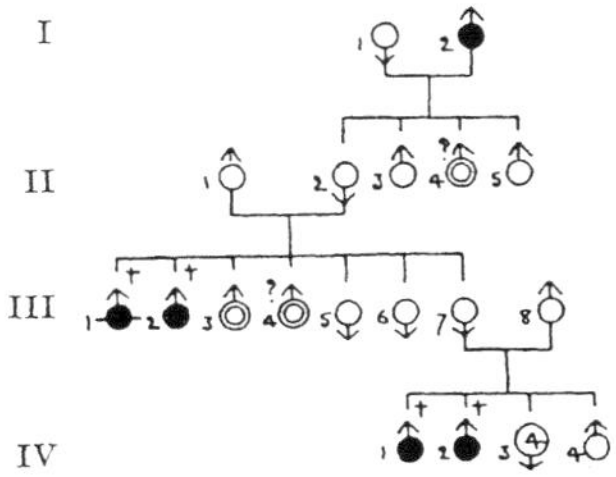

FIG. 4—Birch's Pedigree. ● haemophilic; ◎ colour-blind; -●- haemophilic, normal colour vision.

Here our only certain information regarding vision concerns III 1 and III 3. $P(x, 0)$ is calculated as follows: given that III 3 is colour-blind, the probability that II 2 is $\frac{+\ +}{\mathbf{c}\ \mathbf{h}}$ is y, the probability that she is $\frac{+\ \mathbf{h}}{\mathbf{c}\ +}$ is x. Hence the probability that III 1 was not colour-blind is y^2+x^2. So

$$P(x,\ 0) = y^2+x^2,$$

$$P(\tfrac{1}{2},\ 0) = \tfrac{1}{2}.$$

If and when it is established that III 4 is colour-blind, these values will be diminished to y^3+x^3 and $\frac{1}{4}$. If II 4 is colour-blind, I 1 must have been $\frac{+\ +}{\mathbf{c}\ +}$; so II 2 was $\frac{+\ \mathbf{h}}{\mathbf{c}\ +}$ and $P(x, 0) = y^2$ or y^3. There is here no correction for a second source of colour-blindness, since II 2 had both colour-blind and normal sons and must be heterozygous for **c**. We therefore find

$$P(x,\ p) = y^2+x^2,$$

$$P(\tfrac{1}{2},\ p) = \tfrac{1}{2},$$

$$n = 2,\ \ k = 0,$$

with the proviso that the values of P will probably be reduced by further information.

Madlener's Pedigree

Madlener (1928) published the first pedigree in which linkage between colour-blindness and haemophilia is probable. He has kindly supplemented it by further information. The relevant part of this pedigree is given in fig. 5. I 1 had a number of haemophilic relatives. I 1, III 2, and III 4 are described as colour-blind (*rot-grünblind*, presumably deuteranopic) in Madlener's paper, and the latter two were tested at the time when it was written. IV 3 was at that time too young to test.

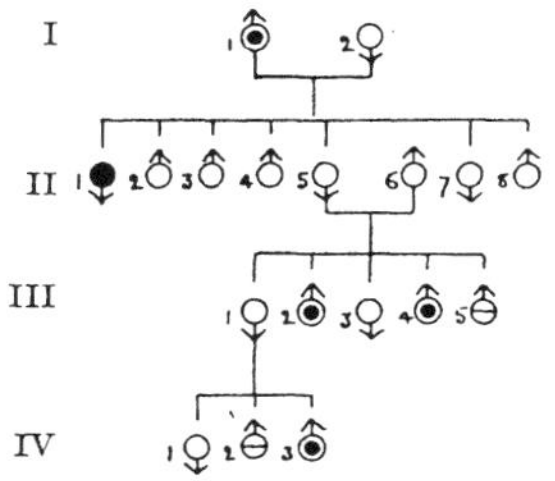

Fig. 5—Madlener's Pedigree. ⊙ Colour-blind haemophilic; ⊖ normal colour vision; ● haemophilic.

In answer to our enquiry Madlener consulted III 1, whom he describes as having great *Familiensinn*. She gave him the following further information. III 5 and IV 2 have normal colour vision, and IV 3, who is still alive and has had no severe haemorrhage since 1928, is definitely colour-blind. She knows of no colour-blind members of the family other than the haemophilics. While her information does not carry so much weight as that concerning III 2 and III 4 who are known to have been examined by a colleague of Dr. Madlener's, we see no reason to reject it.

The most remarkable feature of the pedigree is the haemophilic girl II 1, whose case is carefully discussed by Madlener. Unfortunately he had not personally examined her. He concluded that she was a genuine haemophilic. Now her mother, I 2, had four normal sons and three normal brothers. Further, her father, maternal grandfather, two maternal uncles, and five sons of two sisters were normal. The probability of this, if she was heterozygous for haemophilia, is $5{\cdot}9 \times 2^{-15}$, or 0·00009. If she was homozygous, the chance that she produced an **h** gamete is about 0·00002. Lenz suggested to Madlener that she was a pseudo-hermaphrodite, and really a male. This involves the fantastically unlikely coincidence of the transference of haemophilia from father to son with gross anatomical abnormality in the son. It seems safest to conclude either that **h** is here dominant over its normal allelomorph, or that the case was incorrectly diagnosed.

$P(x, 0)$ is calculated as follows: II 5 was $\frac{+\ +}{\mathbf{c}\ \mathbf{h}}$. The probability that III 2, III 4, and III 5 were as found is y^3. Further III 1, since she transmitted both **c** and **h**, and could only have got them from her mother, must be $\frac{+\ +}{\mathbf{c}\ \mathbf{h}}$. This has a further probability y. The further probability that her two sons IV 2 and IV 3 are as found is y^2. Thus

$$P(x, 0) = y^6,$$

$$P(\tfrac{1}{2}, 0) = 2^{-6}.$$

The expressions are very simple when, as in this case, we have exact information about the common ancestor. The two possible secondary sources of colour-blindness are I 2 and II 6. If I 2 had contributed a **c**+ gamete to II 5, II 5 would have been $\frac{\mathbf{c}\,+}{\mathbf{c}\,\mathbf{h}}$, and III 5 would have been colour-blind. Hence the effect of considering I 2 is to multiply P by $(1-p)$. If II 6 was colour-blind, III 1, who is known to be $\frac{+}{\mathbf{h}}$ and $\frac{+}{\mathbf{c}}$, must be $\frac{\mathbf{c}\,+}{+\,\mathbf{h}}$, which has a probability x, since II 5 was $\frac{+\ +}{\mathbf{c}\ \mathbf{h}}$. The further probability that IV 2 and IV 3 are as found is x^2.

So
$$P(x, p) = (1-p)[(1-p)y^6 + px^3y^3]$$

$$= (1-p)^2 y^6 \left[1 + \frac{px^3}{(1-p)y^3}\right],$$

$$n = 6,\quad k = 0,$$

and
$$P(\tfrac{1}{2}, p) = (1-p)\,2^{-6}.$$

Green's Pedigree

I have to thank the late Dr. C. V. Green for full information about this pedigree, which was compiled by him and published by Davenport (1930). The relevant part is given in fig. 6. I 2, who is III 7 of Davenport's pedigree, had a colour-blind brother, two colour-blind maternal uncles, and other colour-blind relatives, but no haemophilic relatives other than those shown. The colour-blindness appears to be deuteranopia. Let us first assume that I 2 was a double heterozygote, and not a mosaic. If so, since she was almost certainly $\frac{+\mathbf{h}}{\mathbf{c}+}$, she derived the gene **h** from a mutated paternal gamete, since her father was not haemophilic, and her colour-blindness came from her mother.

In this pedigree **c** and **h** are repelled. We ask, given the pedigree of haemophilia and the fact that II 3 is colour-blind, what is the probability that II 4, II 6, III 1 and III 5 are as found? Since I 1 and II 1 are not colour-blind a second source is excluded, and $P(x, p) = P(x, 0)$.

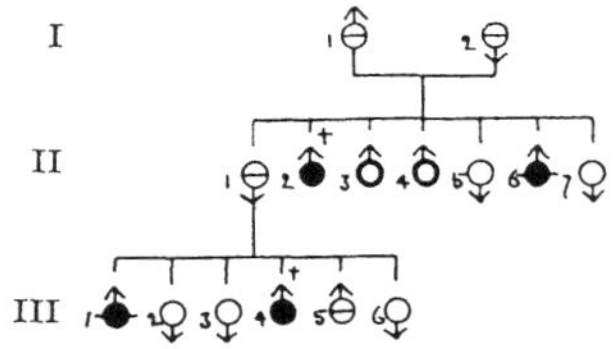

FIG. 6—Green's Pedigree. ◎ colour-blind; ● haemophilic; ⊖ normal colour vision; ⊖● haemophilic, normal colour vision.

The probability that I 2 is $\frac{+\mathbf{h}}{\mathbf{c}+}$ is y, the probability that she is $\frac{+\ +}{\mathbf{c}\ \mathbf{h}}$ is x. Hence the probability that II 4 and II 6 are as found is y^3 in the first case, x^3 in the second. If I 2 is $\frac{+\mathbf{h}}{\mathbf{c}+}$, the probability that II 1 is $\frac{+\ +}{+\ \mathbf{h}}$ is y, in which case III 1 and III 5 were certainly non-deuteranopic. The probability that II 1 is $\frac{+\ +}{\mathbf{c}\ \mathbf{h}}$ is x, and the further probability that III 1 and III 5 are not deuteranopic is xy. So if I 2 is $\frac{+\mathbf{h}}{\mathbf{c}+}$, the probability that III 1 and III 5 are as found is $y+x^2y$.

If on the other hand I 2 is $\frac{+\ +}{\mathbf{c}\ \mathbf{h}}$, the probabilities that II 1 is $\frac{+\ +}{\mathbf{c}\ \mathbf{h}}$ and $\frac{+\ +}{+\ \mathbf{h}}$ are y and x respectively, and the probability that III 1 and III 5 are non-deuteranopes is $x+xy^2$.

Hence
$$P(x, p) = P(x, 0) = y^3(y+x^2y)+x^3(x+xy^2)$$
$$= y^4+x^2y^4+x^4(1+y^2)$$
$$= y^4\left(1+\frac{x^2}{y^2}-\frac{2x^3}{y^3}+\ldots\right)$$
and
$$n = 4, \quad k = 0,$$
$$P(\tfrac{1}{2}, p) = P(\tfrac{1}{2}, 0) = 5\times 2^{-5}.$$

Let us suppose that I 2 is a mosaic of $\frac{+\ +}{\mathbf{c}\ +}$ and $\frac{+\mathbf{h}}{\mathbf{c}+}$ $\left(\text{or possibly } \frac{+\ +}{\mathbf{c}\ \mathbf{h}}\right)$. We cannot be sure that II 3 and II 4 were derived from the latter. Hence our value of P must be based on II 6, III 1 and III 5, though II 3 and II 4 give us the information that I 2 is heterozygous for **c**. In this case

$$\begin{aligned} P(x,\,p) &= y(y+x^2y)+x(x+xy^2) \\ &= y^4+2xy^3+4x^2y^2+2x^3y+x^4 \\ &= y^2+3x^2y^2+2x^3y+x^4, \end{aligned}$$

for $P(\tfrac{1}{2},\,p) = 5\times 2^{-3}$, $n = 2$, $k = 0$. However, the former hypothesis seems much more probable.

Significance of the Data

Assuming that all doubtful cases were heterozygotes and not mosaics, the product of the five values of $P(\tfrac{1}{2},\,0)$ and one of $P'(\tfrac{1}{2},\,0)$ is $3^4\times 5\times 2^{-29}$, or $7{\cdot}54\times 10^{-7}$. The product of the values of $P(\tfrac{1}{2},p)$ is this number multiplied by approximately $1+\frac{35p}{12}$ or 1·041, that is to say $7{\cdot}84\times 10^{-7}$. This number would be appreciably modified if the segregation of **c** in heterozygous mothers were abnormal. But it could hardly exceed 10^{-5}.

Let us next assume that all the doubtful women were mosaics; and, further, that all their non-haemophilic sons were derived from their non-mutated sectors. Both these hypotheses are most unlikely. But, even so, the product of the $P(\tfrac{1}{2},\,0)$ values is $3^3\times 5\times 2^{-25}$, or $4{\cdot}04\times 10^{-6}$. The true value lies somewhere between this and $7{\cdot}84\times 10^{-7}$, a good deal closer to the latter.

In other words, the probability that our finding of linkage is an error due to a run of luck is about one in a million. It is, moreover, difficult to frame any hypothesis other than linkage which will account for the results. In three pedigrees, A, B and Madlener's, the two genes are coupled; in two pedigrees, those of Birch and Green, they are repelled. This fact at once negates any theory as to a physiological connexion between the two diseases. It is, however, exactly what would be expected from analogy with animal genetics.

Estimation of the Frequency of Crossing-over

We shall now consider the estimation of x on the hypothesis that all small positive values have an equal *a priori* probability. We first assume that the three doubtful women were not mosaics. The product of the leading terms in the product of the six values of $P(x, p)$ is

$$x^{\Sigma k}(1-x)^{\Sigma(n-k)} = x(1-x)^{27\cdot 75}.$$

If this is plotted against x we get a very skew frequency curve giving the probability that x lies between given limits. The modal or maximum likelihood value is $x = \frac{1}{28\cdot 75} = 0\cdot 035$. This result may, however, be rather misleading. The mean value is

$$\frac{\int_0^1 Pxdx}{\int_0^1 Pdx} = 0\cdot 065.$$

This is the estimated probability that the next son of a doubly heterozygous woman to be examined will be the product of crossing-over. The median X is given by

$$\int_0^X Pdx = \tfrac{1}{2}\int_0^1 Pdx$$

and is equal to 0·057. That is to say, the frequency of recombination based on a large sample is as likely to exceed 5·7 % as to fall below it. The quartile values are 0·032 and 0·088, so this estimate is very uncertain.

We have next to determine the corrections due to including the terms in the expansion of P involving x^3 on the one hand, and p on the other. The product of the values of $P(x, 0)$ is

$$xy^{27\cdot 75} + \tfrac{219}{32}x^3y^{25\cdot 75} + \ldots.$$

The mean is therefore increased from 0·0650 to 0·0685, with similar slight effects on the mode and median.

The correction for secondary sources is still more negligible. The estimation of x is not affected by the constant terms by which P is multiplied. Σn is reduced from 28·75 to 28·695. This raises the mean from 0·0650 to 0·0651. There is also a very slight change in the correction for x^3. It must however be remembered that in future work it may not be possible to neglect one or both of these corrections.

If all the three doubtful women were mosaics, and further if all their non-haemophilic sons were derived from non-mutated tissue, we should have $n = 23\cdot 75$, $k = 0$. The modal value of x would be zero, the mean 3·88 %, and the median 2·76 %, with quartiles at 1·16 % and 5·45 %. It must, however, be remembered that somatic mosaics in man are very rare.

Cockayne (1933) records three only for conditions affecting the skin, and these were very probably due to chromosome elimination rather than gene mutation. Finally, even if all the women in question were mosaics, it is unlikely that all their non-haemophilic sons were derived from mutated tissue. There is therefore very little reason for lowering our estimates of x.

THE *A PRIORI* PROBABILITY

The calculations so far made other than the estimate based on maximum likelihood would be true if, and only if, the *a priori* probability of all small values of x were equally great. This is certainly not so. First consider a chromosome of genetical length l, that is to say in which the sum of the probabilities of crossing-over between a series of genes at short distances along the chromosome is l. Further, suppose that both genes and probabilities of crossing-over are evenly distributed along it. Then the distribution of x, the distance between two genes taken at random (which for small values, such as exclude double crossing-over, is equal to the distance between the genes), is

$$df = \frac{2(l-x)}{l^2}\,dx.$$

If l is of the order of unity, which is probably the case for the human X-chromosome, this will entail a correction equivalent to adding unity to the value of n, and the median estimate will be reduced from 0·057 to 0·053.

But actually the correction is probably larger, though its magnitude is unknown. If we consider the existing data on linkage in animals, we find that there are two fairly sharply contrasted types. The common type, illustrated by the female *Drosophila*, the mouse, rabbit, hen, etc., shows cross-over values ranging from nearly zero to about 50 %, and possibly exceeding this value in rare cases. In the other type, which is characteristic of the male *Drosophila*, and of both sexes in such polymorphic species as *Lebistes reticulatus* and *Paratettix texanus*, all, or almost all, cross-over values are less than 10 %. The evidence brought forward by Haldane (1936) suggests that man belongs to the first class, as do the four rodents which are the only other mammals in which linkage has been studied.

Now the chiasmata, whose genetical effect is crossing-over, always seem to be somewhat localized. That is to say, crossing-over is relatively rare in some regions of a chromosome. The genes may or may not be evenly distributed, but regions are generally found where genes are common, and crossing-over rare. Thus in the distal or "left-hand" end of the X-chromosome and the proximal regions of the autosomes of *Drosophila melanogaster* many genes are located, but crossing-over is very infrequent. And if two genes are taken at random, there is a considerable probability that both will lie in such a region. Hence cross-over values between pairs of genes taken at random show a peculiar distribution. There is a sharp maximum in the neighbourhood of zero, and another maximum somewhere between 45 and 50 % due to genes at considerable distances from one another. The curve then drops again to zero near 50 %, but this part of the curve is difficult to map, owing to large errors, due both to sampling and to differential viability.

Fig. 7 represents the distribution of 3828 map distances between 88 genes located in the X-chromosome of *Drosophila melanogaster*. It was kindly plotted for us by Mr. F. Minns from data given in Drosophila Information Service, corrected for unpublished results obtained by Dr. H. Grüneberg on the location of *roughest*. The distances were grouped by units. The drop between 1 and 2 units is perhaps accidental. The data for the autosomes, though less numerous, yield similar results.

Since cross-over values are very approximately equal to map distances for values less than 0·15, but do not exceed 0·50 when the map distance does so, it follows that the maximum in the neighbourhood of zero is correctly represented, while the second maximum is not. If $df = f(x)\,dx$ be the frequency distribution of cross-over values, and $P(x)$ is defined as above, we can answer the following question: "If the human data here given referred to *Drosophila melanogaster*, what would be the median cross-over value to be expected?"

The median value X is given by

$$\int_0^X P(x)f(x)\,dx = \tfrac{1}{2}\int_0^1 P(x)f(x)\,dx.$$

We obtain a value of $f(x)$ by smoothing. Mr. Minns has fitted a quintic to the points between $x = 0{\cdot}005$ and $0{\cdot}355$ on fig. 7.

If $z = 100x - 17{\cdot}5$, its equation is

$$f(z) = 72{\cdot}618 - 1{\cdot}7756z - 0{\cdot}17326z^2 + 0{\cdot}01634z^3 + 0{\cdot}0009737z^4 - 0{\cdot}00007408z^5.$$

The values given by the equation were used up to $x = 0{\cdot}15$. For higher values $f(x)$ was taken as constant, since as the result of double crossing-over it exceeds the value deducible from fig. 7. The inaccuracy so introduced is slight, as the area of the tail of the curve for $P(x)\,f(x)$ beyond $x = 0{\cdot}15$ is only 5·0 % of the total.

The modal value of x is about 2·5 %. The median is 4·7 %, with quartiles at 2·5 and 8·1 %. The curve is rendered skewer by the correction, and the estimates of x are all lowered. However, the change is less than the probable error. It is clear that the correction for *a priori* probability will become

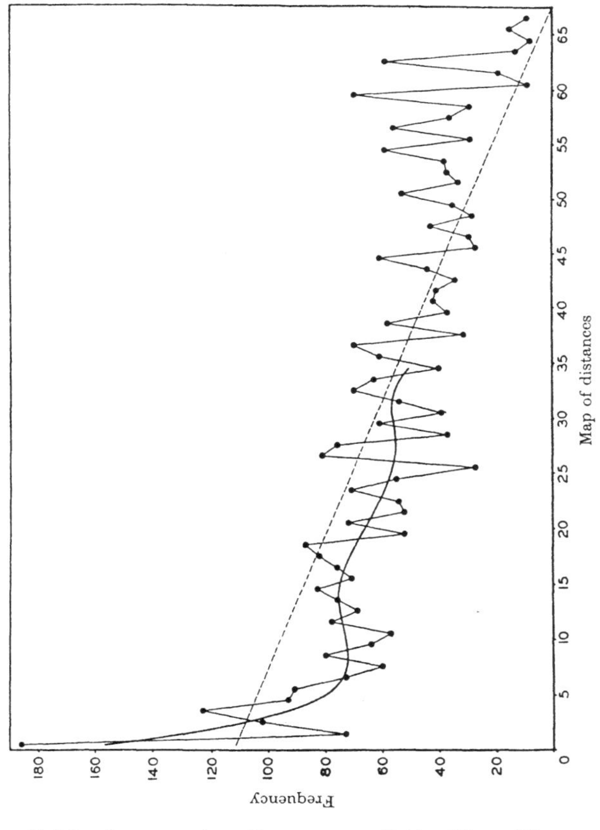

FIG. 7—Frequencies of map distances between pairs of genes in the X-chromosome of *Drosophila melanogaster*. Dotted line, frequency distribution if genes were evenly distributed on the genetical map. Curve, quintic giving best fit.

negligible when enough pedigrees are available. Meanwhile we may take 5 % as a reasonable median value.

The correction for *a priori* probability is considerably larger if we neglect the possibly mosaic women, taking $n = 23{\cdot}75$, $k = 0$. For in this case the sharp maximum of $f(x)$ when x is zero is of much greater importance. The mode is zero, the median 1·9 %, or half its former value.

Discussion

The linkage here investigated is so close that on quite a small amount of material it has been possible to demonstrate its existence without leaving grounds for reasonable doubt. If such close linkage is typical of the human species, the search for further cases will be an easier task than appeared probable at first sight, and its results will be of considerable practical value.

The present case has no prognostic application, since haemophilia can be detected before colour-blindness. If, however, to take a possible example, an equally close linkage were found between the genes determining blood group membership and that determining Huntington's chorea, we should be able, in many cases, to predict which children of an affected person would develop this disease, and to advise on the desirability or otherwise of their marriage.

Meanwhile, as a means to the mapping of the X-chromosome, it is desirable that all persons suffering from any disease showing sex-linked inheritance, and their brothers, should be examined for colour-blindness and, if possible, for anomalous trichromatism. Since about 8 % of males in north-western Europe show one or other of these defects, the search should be fruitful.

This research should lead, within a few years, to a determination of the approximate map distances of the loci of these genes from that of colour-blindness. Mapping would not be possible until another common sex-linked, or incompletely sex-linked, gene substitution has been discovered. The search for new immunological characters may be expected to reveal such a gene within the next generation.

Should Haldane's (1936) claim to have discovered a group of incompletely sex-linked genes be confirmed, it is also desirable that male cases of xeroderma pigmentosum, recessive epidermolysis bullosa dystrophica, etc., and their brothers should be similarly examined.

The theoretical method used in this paper has been unduly cumbrous. It has, however, been given in full for three reasons. In the first place it was necessary to show that certain conditions could be neglected. Secondly, the correction for a second source of colour-blindness will become important when a colour-blind man of an unexpected type as regards blood coagulation is discovered, and it is uncertain whether he is due to crossing-over or to a second source of colour-blindness. In Riddell's pedigree this uncertainty was avoided by testing the colour vision of the mother. Finally, the later terms in the expansion of $P(x, 0)$ will become important if, in the case of another sex-linked character, x turns out to be larger. Thus if there were 20 % of crossing-over between the loci of the genes for colour-blindness and anidrosis, $\frac{x^2}{y^2}$ would be 0·0625 instead of 0·0028, and would no longer be negligible.

The following simplified method may be used for the further investigation of the linkage between colour-blindness and haemophilia:

1. The pedigrees of haemophilia and colour-blindness are determined. In each case crossing-over is assumed not to have occurred unless there is evidence that it has occurred. A single source only of each abnormality is assumed.

2. A number, n, of gametes tested is determined by the following conventions: for each relationship between a doubly heterozygous mother and a child whose genotype is observed or deduced, n is increased by unity. The amount by which n is to be increased for daughters of double heterozygotes whose genotype is not inferable with certainty is a matter for calculation in individual cases. Examples occur in three of the pedigrees here considered.

3. A number, k_1, of undoubted cross-over gametes is similarly calculated. If there are cases which could be explained either by crossing-over or a second source of colour-blindness, numbers k_2, k_3, etc., of facultative cross-overs are calculated.

4. If k_2, k_3, etc. $= 0$, the probabilities regarding x are as if we had observed k_1 cross-overs in a sample of n. The estimate $\frac{k_1}{n}$ is therefore a modal value, and so long as k_1 is small will differ appreciably from the mean $\frac{k_1+1}{n+2}$, and the median.

5. If some of the apparent cross-overs are colour-blind, and a second source is possible, the likelihood of a given value of x is an expression of the form

$$P = (1-x)^{n-k_1-k_2-k_3\cdots}\, x^{k_1}\,(x-p)^{k_2}\,(x-\tfrac{1}{2}p)^{k_3}\ldots.$$

An example of the manner in which these latter terms might arise is given on p. 131. The estimates of x are to be obtained by determining the mode, mean, and median of this function.

6. Until more is known as to the circumstances in which haemophilia arises by mutation it is desirable to estimate x on two different samples. The first would include the progeny of all women who are certainly heterozygous. The second would exclude all persons who might have arisen from

a homozygous portion of the ovaries of a woman who was possibly a mosaic due to somatic mutation. If these two samples differ significantly, the second must be used for our estimation. Until such a difference is proved we can see no good reason to correct for the rather remote possibility of mosaicism.

7. Until n is of the order of 100 the estimates of x will be appreciably too high, owing to the fact that small values of x have a greater *a priori* probability than large.

Summary

Four new pedigrees are described in which cases both of colour-blindness and of haemophilia occur. The two pedigrees already published are considered, and the information concerning one of them is supplemented. In three of the six pedigrees haemophilia appears to have arisen afresh by mutation.

The genes for colour-blindness and haemophilia are closely linked. The probability that the results attributed to linkage could have arisen by sampling is less than 4×10^{-6}. So far only one case of crossing-over has occurred, and even this is not absolutely certain, as the mother of the man in question may possibly be a mosaic due to somatic mutation. It is estimated that the frequency of crossing-over is as likely to lie below 5 % as above it.

References

Bell, J. 1926 Colour blindness. *Treasury of Human Inheritance*, **2**, pt 2.
Cockayne, E. A. 1933 "Inherited Abnormalities of the Skin and its Appendages." Oxford Univ. Press.
Cole, L. J. and Kelly, F. J. 1919 *J. Genet.* **4**, 183–203.
Davenport, C. B. 1930 *J. Genet.* **15**, 401–44.
Haldane, J. B. S. 1935 *J. Genet.* **31**, 317–326.
— 1936 *Ann. Eugen.* **7**, 28–57.
Hogben, L. 1932 *J. Genet.* **25**, 108–9, 302–6.
Madlener, M. 1928 *Arch. Rass.- u. GesBiol.* **20**, 390–4.
Morgan, T. H. 1910 *Science*, N.S. **32**, 120–2.
v. Planta, P. 1928 *Arch. Ophtal.* **120**, 253–81.
Schmidt, J. 1936 *Z. Bahnärzt.* **2**.
Waaler, G. H. M. 1927 *Z. indukt. Abstamm.- u. VererbLehre*, **45**, 279–333.

THE RELATIVE IMPORTANCE OF PRINCIPAL AND MODIFYING GENES IN DETERMINING SOME HUMAN DISEASES

By J. B. S. HALDANE, F.R.S.

(With One Text-figure)

A VAST amount of rather speculative theories have been produced regarding natural selection in man. It is probable that in modern civilized communities reproductive selection, that is to say, selection on a basis of fertility, is more important than strictly Darwinian selection on the basis of survival. But the opposite was probably the case through most of man's career. Moreover, what little exact genetical knowledge we possess relates wholly to selection on the basis of survival.

A number of genes are known which diminish the expectation of human life, but yet allow long enough life to permit of reproduction by many individuals. Bell (1939) has shown that in a number of such cases the period between the onset of the disease and death is almost independent of the age of onset. Thus the age of onset is a valuable index of the selective disadvantage of the gene.

With the discovery of modifying genes there has been a tendency in some quarters to postulate their existence and importance on a very wide scale, while other writers have stressed the importance of environment. Among a group of persons affected with a given disease, whose genetical basis is roughly known, we can examine the relative importance in determining the age of onset, of:

(1) Differences in the main gene itself. That is to say, there may be two or more different main genes, each giving a characteristic mean age of onset, with some variation round it.

(2) Differences in modifying genes, which, while not causing the disease, may favour early or late onset if a main gene is present.

(3) Differences in environment, which again may favour early or late onset.

The recent work of Bell (1934, 1935, 1939) enables us, for the first time, to answer this fundamental question in certain cases. Bell takes a large group of patients, and finds the correlation between age of onset in pairs of sibs (and sometimes also in parents and offspring). Let us see what we should expect on various extreme hypotheses. It is not suggested that any one is ever exactly true, but one or other may prove a good approximation to the truth in a particular case.

If the age of onset were determined wholly by the main gene, and if there were only one main gene, we should expect to find the age of onset exactly the same in all cases, say 7 years. But if there were several different genes we should expect to find several different ages of onset, say one group at 4 years, another at 12, and another at 30. If there were several different recessive allelomorphs, some ages of onset would characterize homozygotes, and these would almost invariably be found where the parents were related. Where they were unrelated we should sometimes find heterozygous "compound" recessive types, probably with intermediate ages of onset. In every case of dominance parent and offspring would be affected by the same gene, and have the same age of onset. Thus the correlation would be unity. Two sibs would always have the same pair of recessive main genes except where one parent was affected, and happened to be a heterozygous compound. Thus the correlation between sibs would be very close to unity.

Next suppose that only one main gene were present in the population, but that there were also a number of modifying genes which affected the age of onset. For example, glaucoma is due to abnormally high pressure within the eye. We might expect the gene or genes which are responsible for high arterial pressure to accelerate its onset. If there were only one main gene and a considerable number of modifiers we should expect to find the same situation as with characters such as stature, which appears to be controlled by many genes. The correlation coefficients would be about 0·5, probably a little higher for sibs, and a little lower for parents and offspring. In the case of a dominant gene, the normal parent would, on the average, be responsible for just as much modification as the affected parent, though we should in general have no clue as to the nature of the modifiers to be found in a normal individual.

If there were one main gene and no modifiers, but environment played a large part in determining the age of onset, we should expect to find some correlation, but its value would be low and uncertain. It would be much higher between sibs than between parent and offspring. For sibs are generally brought up in a similar environment, but the family environment may change a great deal within a generation. It would also be higher in a disease manifesting itself in childhood than later in life, since sibs are brought up in the same home and may separate later on. If environment were important in determining the age of onset we might expect to find this fact recognized, and there might be large occupational and sex differences, as there are with cancer, which undoubtedly has a genetical basis in many instances. The influence of the environment is recognized in the case of the congenital photosensitivities, such as haematoporphyria and xeroderma pigmentosum. If there were no genetical basis for correlation, we should expect to find coefficients well below 0·5 in most cases.

Bell's findings are summarized in Table 1. In no case except the first is there any marked sex difference in frequency or in age of onset.

Table 1. *Correlation coefficients of ages of onset (after Bell)*

		Pairs of siblings		Parent and offspring	
Disease	Type	n	r	n	r
Optic atrophy (males only)	S.L. Rec.	812	0·510	—	—
Glaucoma	Dom.	256	0·897	113	0·813
Huntington's chorea	Dom.	442	0·465	153	0·593
Peroneal atrophy	Dom.	164	0·803	0·8	0·764
	Rec.*	108	0·840	—	—
Friedreich's ataxia	Dom.	144	0·925	—	—
	Rec.	500	0·694	—	—
Spastic ataxia	Dom.	198	0·812	—	—
	Rec.	164	0·845	—	—
Spastic paraplegia	Dom.	154	0·884	—	—
	Rec.	218	0·852	—	—
Grouped ataxias and paraplegia	Dom.	—	—	135	0·743

* Includes a few sex-linked cases.

The last line refers to grouped cases of dominant Friedreich's ataxia, spastic ataxia, and spastic paraplegia, which in Bell's opinion, though not in my own, may be manifestations of the same fundamental inherited abnormality. The precise value to be attached to the significance of these coefficients is rather uncertain, because except in the case of Huntington's chorea, the distribution of ages of onset is highly asymmetrical, and the theory of normal correlation does not apply. However, there is little doubt that in most cases the values are significantly above 0·5. Thus in the case of recessive Friedreich's ataxia, the value of Fisher's (1938) transformed coefficient z is $0{\cdot}856 \pm 0{\cdot}045$. This differs from $z = 0{\cdot}549$, the value corresponding with $r = 0{\cdot}5$, by nearly seven times its standard error. In the case of dominant peroneal atrophy, when parents and offspring are compared, $z = 0{\cdot}996 \pm 0{\cdot}109$, and the difference from 0·549 is over four times its standard error. On the other hand, the difference between the transformed fraternal and parental correlations for Huntington's chorea is about 1·9 times its standard error, and therefore not quite significant.

Actually these coefficients are, if anything, underestimated. Bell points out that in the case of the ataxias and spastic paraplegia the age of onset is, on an average, earlier in younger than elder sibs, perhaps because the parents are on the look-out for signs of the disease. Thus the coefficient of correlation is slightly raised if the table is made asymmetrical, age of onset being correlated in elder against younger sibs.

She has kindly calculated the effect of this in the case of recessive Friedreich's ataxia, and finds that it is raised from 0·694 to 0·711. Further, she has separated the dominant and recessive forms of the same disease which cannot be distinguished clinically. The ages of onset in the two groups overlap, but it is much later on the average in the dominants. If this had not been done, the correlations would be much higher. Thus the coefficient for dominant and recessive spastic ataxia combined is 0·890.

The calculation of the correlations between age of onset in sibs may be regarded as an analysis of variance, the variance within sibships being small compared with that between sibships when r is high. Thus in the case of dominant Friedreich's ataxia, $0{\cdot}925^2$ or 85·6% of the variance is between sibships, only 14·4% being within them.

I think that there is no escape from the conclusion that several different main genes are concerned in the causation of the diseases other than optic atrophy and Huntington's chorea. On no other hypothesis could the correlation coefficients be so large. The argument is particularly clear in the case of parent-offspring correlation. When the age of onset of glaucoma in a parent is known we have eliminated a fraction $1-r^2$, or 0·661 of the variance in the ages of onset in the offspring. Suppose that both parents influence this age by contributing modifiers, this fraction would be expected to be about $\frac{1}{4}$, since half the modifiers from each parent are lost by segregation. Even if we neglect segregation, there is not enough variance left over for the normal parent's modifiers to produce unless we postulate assortative mating so intense as to give rise to a correlation coefficient of over 0·5 for the modifying genes in the parents.

If we could distinguish the different main genes we could reduce the correlation coefficients to more normal values. Thus by dividing up the genes responsible for spastic ataxia into a dominant and recessive class, Bell was able to reduce a coefficient of 0·890 to two of 0·845 and 0·812. If we divide the pedigrees of dominant spastic ataxia into two groups, in one of which the age of onset is always under 50, in the other always over, we obtain two correlation tables, with $n = 162$, $r = 0{\cdot}562$, and $n = 36$,

$r = 0{\cdot}027$. It is not of course suggested that this represents a real genetical division, but it happens that in this particular table all sibships can be divided into those with ages of onset over or under 50.

In the same way we can divide her correlation table for dominant Friedreich's ataxia into three parts. She considered seventy-two pairs of sibs, so there were 144 entries in the table. In the forty cases where the age of onset in one sib was under 5, it was invariably so in the other. In the twelve cases where it was between 35 and 39 in one sib, it was also so in the other.

The argument for the existence of numerous genes is made all the more plausible because Bell has already shown that in the last four diseases of Table 1 there is a dominant and a recessive form. Besides these there is a sex-linked recessive form of peroneal atrophy, and in one pedigree (490) spastic paraplegia behaves as a sex-linked recessive. If then three different genes may be responsible for a group of cases which are indistinguishable clinically, why not five or six? The different genes may in some cases be allelomorphic. The demonstration of this must await linkage tests. If the argument of Haldane (1940*a*) is accepted, recessive spastic paraplegia is due to a group of partially sex-linked genes, and their allelomorphism is highly probable. The dominant form is due to autosomal genes.

Pedigree 464 (due to Fry) suggests an interesting possibility. It is shown in Fig. 1. The grandfather of the three affected children was healthy up to 65, when his gait became uncertain. At 86 he had marked

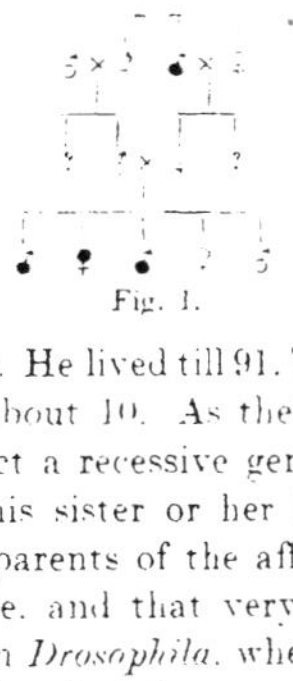

Fig. 1.

ataxia and other symptoms. He lived till 91. The grandchildren developed the disease at the age of about 10. As their parents were double first cousins we naturally suspect a recessive gene. It seems likely that the affected grandfather and his sister or her husband were both heterozygous for it, as were the parents of the affected sibs, but that it only showed in one heterozygote, and that very late in life. Examples can be quoted, particularly from *Drosophila*, where a gene generally behaves as a recessive, but occasionally shows up as a "weak" dominant.

Similarly, in case 499, a woman who had married her uncle had a spastic paretic gait at the age of 72, but except for one attack in middle life, could walk without sticks till 62. Three daughters developed symptoms at about 40, and were severely crippled at 50. Several other cases, for example 385, where there is no inbreeding, are nevertheless suggestive of the same possibility, namely, that some of the genes concerned are incompletely recessive.

No doubt, even in the cases of high correlation, modifying genes may play a part. Bell's correlation tables show a few striking outliers. Thus in the case of recessive Friedreich's ataxia there were three cases out of 250 where the age of onset in sibs differed by over 25 years. If these were omitted from the table, the coefficient of correlation would be raised from 0·694 to 0·802. There is a strong suggestion that about 1% of the population may carry modifying genes which markedly delay the onset of this disease if the main gene is present.

Dr Bell has kindly permitted me to use a table prepared by her of the differences in age of onset of the disease in pairs of sibs. Besides calculating the mean difference we may proceed as follows. If each family were large enough there would be a mean age of onset in affected members, and a distribution round this mean. We can readily determine the even cumulants of this distribution.

These cumulants are half those of the differences, if we count each difference both as positive and negative, and make Sheppard's correction. Thus if ν_2 and ν_4 are the mean values of the squares and fourth powers of the differences, we have, for the distribution about the family mean,

$$\sigma^2 = \tfrac{1}{2}\nu_2 - \tfrac{1}{12}, \quad \gamma_2 = \beta_2 - 3 = \frac{2\nu_4 - 6\nu_2^2 + \frac{1}{30}}{(\nu_2 - \frac{1}{6})^2} = \frac{2(\nu_4 - \nu_2 + \frac{1}{10})}{(\nu_2 - \frac{1}{6})^2} - 6.$$

The unit of grouping is taken as a year. Actually it is larger in a fraction of the cases. Thus the true value of σ is slightly smaller than that given, the true value of γ_2 slightly larger. However, as Sheppard's correction never amounts to 2%, the further correction to be made is small. The results of this calculation are shown in Table 2.

Table 2. *Differences of age of onset within sibships*

Disease	Type	Mean	S.D.	γ_2
Friedreich's ataxia	Dom.	2·61	3·10	+ 6·52
	Rec.	2·47	3·38	+ 39·6
Spastic ataxia	Dom.	6·03	6·04	+ 2·47
	Rec.	3·51	6·14	+ 21·2
Spastic paraplegia	Dom.	3·99	5·01	+ 12·5
	Rec.	3·01	5·91	+ 26·5

A somewhat more accurate value of γ_2 could be obtained from the complete data. The standard deviation round the family mean varies between 3 and 6 years, and the values of γ_2 are all positive, and are large in the case of recessives. This means that there are fewer small and more large deviations than in a normal distribution with the same standard deviation, particularly in the case of recessives. This is what we should expect if there were a few modifying genes with considerable effect, but in most families there was very little modification. It is, however, curious that modifiers for recessives seem to be more frequent or more effective than those for dominants.

There is some evidence for the existence of modifying genes in the case of Huntington's chorea. Bell found that of 385 affected males 60·3% had affected fathers, and of 336 affected females 51·5% had affected mothers. If we consider grandparents also we have the results of Table 3.

Table 3. *Huntington's chorea*

	Affected		Normal		
Affected ancestors	Males	Females	Males	Females	q
Mother and grandmother	36	47	29	24	0·559
Mother and grandfather	43	59	32	32	0·548
Father and grandmother	36	36	24	41	0·438
Father and grandfather	92	55	53	77	0·394

In this table normals are not included unless they appear to have reached the age of 30. q is the frequency of affected females plus normal males. These results are consistent with the theory (Haldane, 1936) that some of the genes which modify the age of onset are sex-limited in their effect. Thus if there are modifiers in a family increasing the age of onset in females there will be an excess of males among the affected and of females among the normal. This will account for the results tabulated. The differences between q values are not all significant, but their order is as expected.

Discussion

This paper is of course of a preliminary nature. Data for ages of onset must exist for a number of diseases. Ages of death would in some cases be equally valuable or more so, since here there is no subjective element. Any other measurable character of the disease would be equally valuable, provided it is fairly definite. Thus in pedigrees of myopia we could use the strength in dioptres at some standard age, in dwarfism the height, and so on. But a very variable character, such as the coagulation time in haemophilia, would be useless.

Differences in age of onset in man probably correspond with differences in penetrance in *Drosophila* or other insects. If we imagine all cases in a pedigree to be examined at the age of 25 only, late age of onset would appear as low penetrance. On Goldschmidt's theory genes act by determining the rates of processes. In man a morbid process may lead to manifest disease at any age. In an insect an abnormal developmental process will not produce any visible effect on the morphology unless it does so before the imago is fully formed. Thus a study of ages of onset can tell us a good deal more than a study of penetrance for equal numbers studied.

So far as concerns the question of evolution, Huntington's chorea seems to agree with the conditions postulated by Fisher (1931) in his theory of the evolution of dominance. Modifiers are presumably being selected which delay the age of onset. Perhaps Huntington's chorea was a disease of infancy in *Sinanthropus*. And if eugenic measures are not taken against it, it may be confined to old age in our remote descendants, in which case the main gene will spread, and homozygotes appear, so that it will be, in effect, a recessive disease. But in the case of the other conditions (except Leber's disease, which is either sex-linked or cytoplasmic) the main effect of selection will be to weed out those main genes which produce an early onset, particularly where the disease is dominant.

This is discussed in detail elsewhere (Haldane, 1940*b*). As pointed out by Bell, selection causes the dominant forms to be less severe than the recessives. Modifying genes may exist, but where the average difference in age of onset between sibs is only 2 or 3 years, they cannot be very important, and must be selected very slowly. A great deal more work will be required before we can judge whether the presence of modifiers in accordance with Fisher's theory is common or rare in the human species.

Summary

Bell's data on the age of onset of some human hereditary diseases are discussed. In glaucoma, peroneal atrophy, Friedreich's ataxia, spastic ataxia, and spastic paraplegia, the age of onset in all affected members of a pedigree is nearly the same, while different pedigress differ widely. Thus a number of different main genes must be responsible for the clinically indistinguishable diseases in different families. In optic atrophy and Huntington's chorea the differences of age of onset within a pedigree are nearly as large as those between different pedigrees. So the same main gene may be responsible for all cases, while modifying genes account for much of the difference in age of onset. The bearing of these facts on evolutionary theories is discussed.

REFERENCES

BELL, S. (1934). "Huntington's chorea." *Trans. Hum. Inher.* **4**, 1.

—— (1935). "On the peroneal type of progressive muscular atrophy." *Trans. Hum. Inher.* **4**, 69.

—— (1939). "On hereditary ataxia and spastic paraplegia." *Trans. Hum. Inher.* **4**, 141.

FISHER, R. A. (1931). "The evolution of dominance." *Biol. Rev.* **6**, 345.

—— (1938). *Statistical Methods for Research Workers*, 6th ed. Edinburgh: Oliver and Boyd.

HALDANE, J. B. S. (1936). "A search for incomplete sex-linkage in man." *Ann. Eugen., Lond.*, **7**, 28.

—— (1940*a*). "The partial sex-linkage of recessive spastic paraplegia." *J. Genet.* (in the Press).

—— (1940*b*). "The conflict between selection and mutation of harmful recessive genes." *Ann. Eugen., Lond.* (in the Press).

SELECTION AGAINST HETEROZYGOSIS IN MAN

By J. B. S. HALDANE, F.R.S.

From the Department of Biometry, University College, London

INTRODUCTION

Landsteiner & Wiener (1941) described a new human gene pair. Rabbits, or better guinea-pigs, injected with blood from the monkey, *Macacus rhesus*, develop an antibody which agglutinates the corpuscles of many human beings. The agglutinogen, or **Rh**+ property, was found on the red corpuscles of 1380 or 86·5 % of 1596 Americans. (The majority were tested by Levine *et al.*, their colour not being stated.) It was present in 84·6 % of 448 whites, and 92·04 % of 113 coloured people, the difference not being quite significant ($\chi^2 = 3{\cdot}59$, $P = 0{\cdot}06$). It was shown to be due to a single autosomal dominant gene, which may be called **Rh** without ambiguity.

Levine, Vogel, Katzin & Burnham (1941) followed up earlier work, which they summarized, on the causation of *erythroblastosis fetalis*. This phrase is now generally used in the United States to replace the former less precise term *icterus gravis neonatorum*. The onset of the disease is before birth or within a few days after. It is characterized by anaemia, jaundice, and production of immature erythrocytes. It is almost invariably fatal unless treated by blood transfusion. It is far from rare. Darrow (1938) recorded eleven cases among 4358 births. It is familial, in the sense that several cases often occur in a sibship, but it is not known to occur in related sibships with unusual frequency. Nor is it hereditary, since so far few if any affected individuals have survived to transmit it. A good deal more information as to its genetics should be available when treated survivors have had children. The true incidence seems to be well above 1 in 400 conceptions. Levine, Katzin & Burnham (1941) report on thirty-six pregnancies of mothers whose immune reactions (as described later) threatened erythroblastosis to their children. They found that ten babies were normal, six had erythroblastosis, three had died neonatally, five were stillborn, ten were abortions or miscarriages, and two unknown. Thus the total number of deaths was four times the number of cases actually diagnosed. If in general it is only double, the total death-rate must be about 0·5 % of all conceptions.

Among 111 cases of foetal erythroblastosis Levine, Vogel, Katzin & Burnham found that in 90 % the mother was **rh rh**, and the baby **Rh rh**. When investigated, the mother was usually found to have developed anti-**Rh** agglutinin. Such women may succumb to a transfusion from a member of their own blood group who possess the **Rh** agglutinogen. It appears that the foetal antigen passes through the placenta into the mother, and the maternal antibody passes back into the foetus, damaging the red blood corpuscles and causing haemolytic jaundice. The erythroblastosis is due to the regenerative activity of the foetal marrow and perhaps other haematopoietic organs, which flood the circulation with immature erythrocytes. In the 10 % of cases where the mother was not **rh rh**, Levine and his colleagues believe that other antigens, perhaps similarly inherited, are responsible.

However, in the 90 % of cases where the mother was **rh rh** and the baby **Rh rh**, another causal agent besides **Rh** must have been concerned. Among white Americans, assuming random mating, 36·9 % are **Rh Rh**, 47·7 % **Rh rh**, and 15·4 % **rh rh**. Thus 0·154 (0·369 + 0·477), or 9·36 % of all conceptions are **Rh rh** babies carried by **rh rh** mothers. If the figures given above for frequency are representative, only 2·5–10 %, say about 5 %, of these babies develop the disease. These patients are not distributed at random among the potential mothers. If they were so, it would be rare to find several affected sibs in one family, whereas actually more than half are often affected. It seems clear that some women, though fortunately a minority, habitually develop placentae which allow the passage of the antigen and antibody in question. The passage of an antibody from mother to child is not, of course, abnormal, and accounts for passive immunity to several diseases during the first months of life. The passage of an antigen from child to mother is abnormal. Since the abnormal permeability persists through the reproductive period, and the mothers of jaundiced babies are said generally to be healthy unless given a blood transfusion, it seems likely that the abnormal permeability is not generally due to infection, deficiency, poisoning, or other environmental influences, but is at least often genetically determined. Only further research will decide this question. Very little is known as to the variability of the placental permeability within a species. Dienst (1905) perfused the still attached placentae of 160 women through the umbilical vessels with a methylene blue solution under slight pressure, and found the dye in the urine of thirty-two, or 20 % of them. This may of course have been due to the rupture of vessels before birth. However, in view of the very great differences of permeability between mammalian species, we should expect, on Darwinian principles, to find appreciable intraspecific differences.

The possibility of a sharp difference in permeability between the placentae of different mothers is in agreement with the well-known innate difference in the capacity for excreting the blood-group antigens in saliva and other secretions. The genes responsible cannot be the same in the two cases, since group-antigen secretion is much commoner than high placental permeability. The excretion of the antigen in either case may be due rather to its active production by certain cells than to its passive permeation from the blood plasma. The matter is the more doubtful because the **Rh** antigen is thought to be restricted to the red corpuscles, instead of being found in all cells. Another possible cause for individual differences would be differences in the molecular weight of the antigen or antibody. Kabat (1939) has observed the production of antibodies of unusually low molecular weight in horses immunized over prolonged periods, but I know of no similar observations regarding antigens. In what follows I shall assume that the second factor involved in the disease is abnormally high placental permeability, while leaving the question open whether this is due to abnormality in maternal or foetal tissues, or in both. If the abnormality is innate in the foetus, it might still be true that about half the children of a given marriage would display it if one did so, and thus develop erythroblastosis if the mother was **rh rh** and the baby **Rh rh**.

Theory of selection against heterozygotes

We must now calculate the selective effects of the death of a fraction k of the order of 0·05, of the **Rh rh** children of **rh rh** mothers. Consider a population in which generations are separate, and the survivors from one generation occur with the frequencies:

$$z\ \mathbf{Rh\,Rh},\quad 2y\ \mathbf{Rh\,rh},\quad x\ \mathbf{rh\,rh}.$$

Let mating be at random. The frequency of **Rh rh** children from **rh rh**♀ × **Rh Rh**♂ is xz, that of **Rh rh** children from **rh rh**♀ × **Rh rh**♂ is xy, totalling $x(y+z)$. Of these a fraction k dies. Thus the survivors in the succeeding generation will be in the ratios:

$$(y+z)^2\ \mathbf{Rh\,Rh} : (y+z)(2x+2y-kx)\ \mathbf{Rh\,rh} : (x+y)^2\ \mathbf{rh\,rh}.$$

If x', $2y'$, z' be the frequencies of the genotypes in the succeeding generation, then:

$$z' = \frac{(y+z)^2}{1-kx(y+z)}, \quad y' = \frac{(x+y)(y+z) - \frac{1}{2}kx(y+z)}{1-kx(y-z)}, \quad x' = \frac{(x+y)^2}{1-kx(y+z)}. \tag{1}$$

Now let $p = x+y$, the frequency of **rh** gametes. Then $x = \dfrac{p^2}{1-kx(1-p)}$, and $p' = \dfrac{p - \frac{1}{2}kx(1-p)}{1-kx(1-p)}$, whence $\Delta p = \dfrac{kx(1-p)(p-\frac{1}{2})}{1-kx(1-p)}$. It follows that p increases if it exceeds $\frac{1}{2}$, and diminishes if it is less than $\frac{1}{2}$. Thus $p = \frac{1}{2}$ is a position of unstable equilibrium, whilst $p = 0$ or $p = 1$ (homozygosis) are stable equilibria. If k is small, x approximates to p^2, and $\Delta p = kp^2(1-p)(p-\frac{1}{2}) + O(k^2)$.

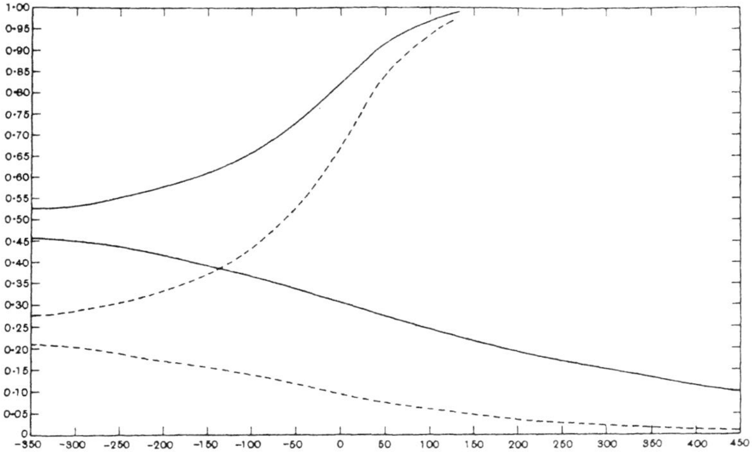

Fig. 1. Abscissa: time in generations. Ordinate of plain curve: frequency p of the **rh** gene. Ordinate of dotted curve: frequency x of the **rhrh** phenotype. Selection against **rh**. $k = 0{\cdot}05$.

Treating this as a differential equation, i.e. putting dp/dt for Δp, the unit of time being a generation, we find

$$kt = \int \frac{dp}{p^2(1-p)(p-\frac{1}{2})},$$

whence
$$\tfrac{1}{2}kt + C = \frac{1}{p} + \log_e\left[\frac{(p-\frac{1}{2})^4}{p^3(1-p)}\right] = \frac{1}{p} + 4\log_e\left|\frac{1}{2p} - 1\right| - \log_e\left(\frac{1}{p} - 1\right). \tag{2}$$

The frequency x of recessives is approximately p^2, so

$$\tfrac{1}{2}kt + C = \frac{1}{\sqrt{x}} + 4\log_e\left|\frac{1}{2\sqrt{x}} - 1\right| - \log_e\left(\frac{1}{\sqrt{x}} - 1\right). \tag{3}$$

The graphs showing p and x as functions of t are given in Fig. 1. The zero of time is taken arbitrarily so that the inflexions on the (p, t) curves occur when $t = 0$, and $p = \dfrac{9 \pm \sqrt{17}}{16}$, i.e. $0{\cdot}8202$ or $0{\cdot}3048$.

The equations (1) can of course also be used for step-by-step calculation when k is not small. They may then be treated as recurrence equations, writing x_n for x, x_{n+1} for x', and so on. It is convenient to put $r_n = \frac{1}{2p_n - 1}$, whence

$$r_{n+2} - r_{n+1} = \frac{k(1-r_{n+1})(1+r_n)^2}{8r_{n+1}r_n}, \quad p_n = \frac{1-r_n}{2r_n}, \quad x_n = \frac{2(r_{n+1}-r_n)}{k(1-r_n)}. \tag{4}$$

However, until k is accurately known, equations (2) and (3) are quite sufficiently accurate. Nor need the slight effects of such inbreeding as occurs in human populations nor of overlap between generations be considered.

Evolutionary consequences

If $k = 0{\cdot}05$, as we saw reason to suggest, it would take 619 generations to reduce x from 13·9 %, the mean for Americans, to 1 %. This is only about 15,000 years, a very short time in human evolution. If, as we also saw reason to suspect, the value of k is at least in part genetically determined, it would doubtless also change during this period. However, apart from possible future results of medical or eugenic practice, it would probably tend to increase rather than to diminish. For at the present time the good effects of high placental permeability in improving foetal respiration, nutrition, and excretion, are presumably balanced by the disadvantages of antigen and perhaps antibody permeation. As **rh** was eliminated, the latter disadvantages would diminish, so k might increase, and evolution be speeded up. For these reasons, it would seem that the American population, and presumably those of Europe, are at present in a very unstable situation.

One of three alternatives must, I think, be true:

(1) Recent environmental changes have led to a sharp increase in placental permeability.

(2) Selection against heterozygotes is balanced by counter-selection.

(3) The present genetical situation is of recent origin, and probably due to racial mixture.

If the first were true, we should expect that permeability to the antigen and antibody in question would frequently appear and disappear during the life of a mother, and that striking differences in the incidence of the disease would be observed between town and country, or between different social classes. Neither seems to be the case. The balancing influence could be either heterosis giving an advantage to **Rh rh** over both homozygotes, or an advantage to **rh rh** homozygotes. If the fitness of the heterozygotes is $1 + K$ times that of the homozygotes, we should have for equilibrium

$$(1+K)(y+z)(2x+2y-kx) = 2(x+y)(y+z).$$

Hence
$$K = \frac{kx}{2(x+y)-kx} = \tfrac{1}{2}kp \text{ approximately}.$$

Thus K is about 0·009. On this hypothesis $p = 1$ and $p = \frac{2K}{k}$ are stable equilibria, $p = \frac{1}{2}$ and $p = 0$ unstable. It would be very surprising if the first gene for a human agglutinogen found to have a lethal effect had also a heterosis effect of the same order. For if there is any heterosis effect in the case of the blood-group genes, it is certainly far less than this. If the recessive homozygote has an advantage measured by $1 + K$, K must be about 0·004. It would be surprising, on this hypothesis, that the **Rh** gene had not disappeared altogether, since the elimination of dominant genes lowering fitness is fairly rapid. So large an advantage for an agglutinogen would also be surprising.

On the third hypothesis the present unstable situation is due to racial mixture in the not very remote past. In the absence of counter-selection any human community left to itself must ultimately become homozygous for **Rh** or **rh** by the joint effects of selection and random survival, save for very rare exceptions due to mutation. However, the final stage of the elimination of **rh** would be slow except in the case of a small and therefore inbred group. But selection is sufficiently weak to allow mutation and random survival occasionally to swing a small population over from one type of homozygosis to the other. It is possible that the European races have arisen through the crossing of peoples homozygous for **Rh** with smaller numbers of peoples homozygous for **rh**. The difference between the white and coloured Americans is not quite significant, but taking it at its face value, the gene frequency p is 39·0 % for the whites and 29·2 % for the coloured. This

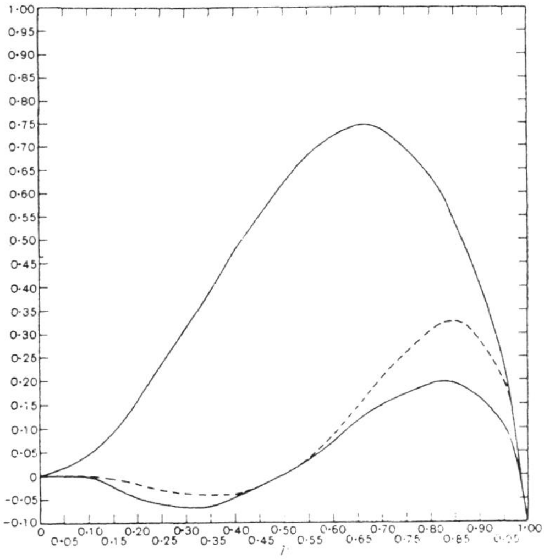

Fig. 2. Abscissa: frequency p of the **rh** gene. Ordinate of upper curve: percentage mortality. Ordinate of dotted curve: percentage effect on gene frequency p per generation. Ordinate of lower curve: percentage effect on recessive frequency x per generation. Selection against **Rhrh**. $k = 0{\cdot}05$.

would be intelligible had **rh** been fairly rare among the pure negro ancestors of the coloured people. Thus a survey of races for the frequencies of **Rh** is likely to be of peculiar interest.*

The death-rate from erythroblastosis is $kx(y+z)$, or approximately $kp^2(1-p)$. This is maximal when $p = \frac{2}{3}$, or $x = 0{\cdot}4$. Whereas we saw the effect of selection on the gene frequency is

$$dp/dt = kp^2(1-p)(p-\tfrac{1}{2}),$$

which reaches its maximum value $2^{-13}(107+51\sqrt{17})k$, or $+0{\cdot}0265k$ when $p = 0{\cdot}8202$, and its minimum value of $2^{-13}(107-51\sqrt{17})k$ or $-0{\cdot}01265k$ when $p = 0{\cdot}3048$. The effect on zygotic frequency reaches its maximum of $24(117+62\sqrt{6})\,10^{-5}k$, or $+0{\cdot}06453k$, when $p = 0{\cdot}8449$, and its minimum of $24(117-62\sqrt{6})\,10^{-5}k$, or $-0{\cdot}008368k$, when $p = 0{\cdot}3551$. The situation is illustrated in Fig. 2. From the point of view of Darwinism as generally expounded, it is somewhat paradoxical

* Landsteiner, Wiener and Matson (*J. Exp. Med.* 76, p. 73, 1942) have since found that only one out of 120 American Indians was **rh rh**.

that the evolutionary effect of natural selection is so little related to the elimination of the unfit, as shown by the death-rate. Indeed, when $p = \frac{1}{2}$, there is no evolutionary effect, yet the unfit are being eliminated at 84·375 % of the maximum rate. There is a similar lack of parallelism during the elimination of an autosomal recessive, though not of an autosomal dominant.

It is possible that the facts discovered by the American workers have a bearing on mammalian evolution in general, and particularly the origin of mammalian species. Placental permeability varies very greatly between different species. Needham (1931, vol. **3**) has reviewed the literature. He concludes that ungulates and carnivores form less permeable placentae than women, while mice, rats, and perhaps rabbits, form more permeable placentae. The placentae of other primates, insectivores, and bats are about as permeable as the human. The permeability in mice and rats is so great that they have been able to dispense with those important foetal excretory organs, the allantois and mesonephros.

Thus while selection of the type here considered is unlikely in ungulates and carnivores, it is quite possible that all rodent placentae would be permeable to **Rh** and its antibody. But since genetically determined antigenic differences occur in mice (Gorer, 1936) without any lethal effect, the antigens in question presumably do not permeate the placenta, any more than do the blood-group antigens in man.

Consider a species including a race A of **RR** zygotes, and a race B of **rr** zygotes, where **R** is a gene responsible for an antigen with properties similar to those of **Rh**, and permeating all placentae. Clearly all zygotes from B♀ × A♂ would develop erythroblastosis, and generally perish. On the other hand, the F_1 and F_2 from A♀ × B♂ would be unaffected, though one-eighth of the F_3 would be affected. Thus crossing between the varieties would be prevented in one direction only. If, however, race A were $\mathbf{R_1R_1r_2r_2}$, and race B $\mathbf{r_1r_1R_2R_2}$, where $\mathbf{R_1}$ and $\mathbf{R_2}$ determine antigens of the type considered, then all F_1 zygotes would be damaged, and the races would in effect be separate species, though genes might pass for one species to the other through $\mathbf{R_1R_1R_2R_2}$ or $\mathbf{r_1r_1r_2r_2}$ races, if such existed. It is at least possible that some cases of interspecific sterility are determined in this way.

Selection against an inversion

A somewhat different type of selection against heterozygosis also probably occurs in man. Inversions within a chromosome are probably not very rare. A few may influence gene action by a position effect, thus having a selective advantage or disadvantage when homozygous. In this case selection will cause one gene order to spread through the species or a race. However, position effects of inversions are not very common in *Drosophila* and almost unknown elsewhere. Where an inversion has no somatic effect, it may still give rise to defective chromosomes by single crossing-over within the inversion. In *Drosophila* Beadle & Sturtevant (1935) showed that, at least where the inversion does not include the centromere, such defective gametes are eliminated in the polar bodies during oogenesis, and hence inversion heterozygotes do not give rise to defective eggs. And since there is no crossing-over in the male, they do not give rise to defective spermatozoa. On the other hand, in man, even if defective chromosomes are eliminated in the polar bodies, they are likely to pass into spermatozoa which, though viable, give rise to inviable or defective zygotes. Koller (1937) described abnormal meioses in human testes which he attributed to an inversion, and which would probably have led to this effect. If so the effective fertility of inversion heterozygotes is reduced. Although the effective reduction is probably different in the two sexes, very little inaccuracy is involved if, in the case of an autosomal inversion, we take the mean value, and suppose that the effective fertility in both sexes is reduced to $1 - k'$ of the normal.

If p is the frequency of an inversion in the gametes forming one generation, the effective parents of the next generation are in the ratios

$$p^2 AA : 2(1-k')p(1-p)\,Aa : (1-p)^2\,aa,$$

where A and a represent the two chromosomal sequences. Thus in the next generation

$$p' = \frac{p - k'p(1-p)}{1-2k'p(1-p)}, \quad \Delta p = \frac{k'(2p-1)p(1-p)}{1-2k'p(1-p)} = 2k'p(1-p)(p-\tfrac{1}{2}) \text{ approximately.}$$

If $dp/dt = 2k'p(1-p)(p-\frac{1}{2})$, then

$$k't = \log_e\left(\frac{1}{4p(1-p)} - 1\right) + C, \quad p = \frac{1}{2}\left[1 \pm \frac{1}{\sqrt{\{1+e^{k'(t_0-t)}\}}}\right].$$

Thus, as in the case of **Rh**, $p = \frac{1}{2}$ is an unstable equilibrium, and if p is plotted against t, the curve consists of two branches with a common asymptote $p = \frac{1}{2}$, and asymptotes $p = 1$ and $p = 0$ representing stable equilibria. In the case of an inversion, however, the curves are symmetrical about $p = \frac{1}{2}$. The selection due to an inversion is far more efficient than that due to an antigen in the neighbourhood of $p = 0$. That is to say the antigenic difference has a selective effect of the same order as that of an inversion for most gene frequencies, but if far less effective in eliminating the last few recessives.

As with an antigenic difference, a rare inversion, advantageous when homozygous, might yet be eliminated by this selective effect, though it would spread through a population once it had reached a certain frequency.

Eugenic and hygienic considerations

From the point of view of practical eugenics it is obviously futile to urge that all **rh rh** women, some 14 % of the total, should be prevented or even dissuaded from marrying the **Rh Rh** and **Rh rh** men who make up the remaining 86 %. Nor can **rh rh** be regarded as a character to be eliminated by sterilization or otherwise. And yet the effects of the **Rh**-**rh** gene difference certainly account for more human deaths than any other gene difference so far known, and very possibly for more than all other known gene differences together. Hence eugenists cannot neglect it. Research on the etiology of high placental permeability is an urgent problem which is doubtless already being tackled. If it is largely due to a particular gene substitution, the gene in question must be much rarer than **rh**, and therefore a more suitable target for negative eugenics. Even if no systematic attempt were made to eradicate such a gene, there would be a strong case for dissuading **rh rh** women, known also to be so constituted as to be destined to form permeable placentae, from marrying **Rh Rh** or **Rh rh** men, and at least an arguable case for compulsion. Such women occur with a frequency of 0·7 % or perhaps less.

Even the strongest opponent of negative eugenics might well approve of the testing of pregnant women for the presence or absence of the **Rh** antigens, and further testing of **rh rh** women for the development of anti-**Rh** agglutinin. If this were present not only would it be necessary to avoid giving them transfusions from a donor carrying **Rh**, but their babies could be tested for erythroblastosis at birth, and treated, if possible, before the disease was fully developed. If the **Rh** haptene can be isolated from its protein carrier, it might be possible to inject it into pregnant women in such amounts as to neutralize their anti-**Rh** agglutinins, and thus prevent erythroblastosis.

Finally, it is important to emphasize that a familial but rarely hereditary disease has been traced to a genetic cause other than a recessive gene. Another possible cause of this type of disease incidence is of course a balanced translocation in one parent. It is quite possible that antigenic differences of a similar kind may account for a number of congenital conditions which have been ascribed in the past to recessive genes on the one hand, or to ill-defined bad prenatal conditions on the other. The object of this paper is not merely to discuss the mathematical, evolutionary, and eugenical consequences of the remarkable discoveries of Levine, Vogel, Katzin, Burnham, Landsteiner, and Wiener, but to point out their very great interest to every student of eugenics.

SUMMARY

The discovery by American workers, that erythroblastosis fetalis, a severe disease of unborn and newborn babies, is due to an innate antigenic difference between mother and child, is described. It is pointed out that this leads to selection against heterozygotes, and the consequences of this selection are calculated. The bearings of this discovery on human evolution, on the origin of species, and on practical eugenics, are discussed.

REFERENCES

G. W. Beadle & A. H. Sturtevant (1935). *X*-chromosome inversions and meiosis in *Drosophila melanogaster*. *Proc. Nat. Acad. Sci., Wash.*, **21**, 384.

R. R. Darrow (1938). Icterus gravis (erythroblastosis) neonatorum. An examination of etiologic considerations. *Arch. Path.* **25**, 378.

A. Dienst (1905). Das Eklampsiegift; vorläufige Mitteilung. *Zbl. Gynäk.* **29**, 353.

P. A. Gorer (1936). The detection of antigenic differences in mouse erythrocytes by the employment of immune sera. *Brit. J. Exp. Path.* **17**, 42.

E. A. Kabat (1939). The molecular weight of antibodies. *J. Exp. Med.* **69**, 103.

P. Koller (1937). The genetical and mechanical properties of sex chromosomes. III. Man. *Proc. Roy. Soc. Edinb.*, **57**, 194.

K. Landsteiner & A. S. Wiener (1941). Studies on an agglutinogen (**Rh**) in human blood reacting with anti-rhesus sera and with human iso-antibodies. *J. Exp. Med.* **74**, 309.

P. Levine, E. M. Katzin & L. Burnham (1941). Isoimmunization in pregnancy. Its possible bearing on the etiology of erythroblastosis fetalis. *J. Amer. Med. Ass.* **116**, 825.

P. Levine, O. Vogel, E. M. Katzin & L. Burnham (1941). Pathogenesis of erythroblastosis fetalis: statistical evidence. *Science*, **94**, 371.

J. Needham (1931). *Chemical Embryology*. Cambridge.

THE INTERACTION OF NATURE AND NURTURE

By J. B. S. HALDANE

The interaction of nature and nurture is one of the central problems of genetics. We can only determine the differences between two different genotypes by putting each of them into a number of different environments. We compare two pure lines of mice not only as regards colour, hair form, and other characters which are little affected by nurture, but for such characters as resistance to different bacterial and virus infections, each of which must be tested by appropriate changes of environment. We may require a wheat to be resistant to each of a number of unfavourable conditions, such as drought, frost, and attacks by several different varieties of rust. The line must be exposed to each of these separately.

The problem is, of course, exceedingly complex, but certain facts about it are so simple that they are apparently never stated. As they are matters of logic rather than experiment, I first put them forward (Haldane, 1936) at a congress mainly composed of philosophers, though in a rudimentary form which is here expanded.

Suppose that we have two genetically different populations A and B, and two different environments X and Y. The results will be clearest if A and B are clones or pure lines, and X and Y constant in all measurable respects. But this need not be the case. For example, A and B may be subspecies or even species, and X and Y geographical localities. Suppose also that the individuals show a character which can be measured, such as length of tail or life, number of eggs laid in two years, or mean butter-fat percentage; or a character which can be graded, such as colour intensity, dominance in combats, or intelligence as estimated by a battery of tests. The differences between all, some, or none of the combinations may be statistically significant.

First suppose that all four experiments give results which differ significantly, so that they can be placed in an order, as in Fig. 1. Arrangement 1*a* means that race A in environment X did

Type 1*a*

	X	Y
A	1	2
B	3	4

Type 1*b*

	X	Y
A	1	3
B	2	4

Type 2

	X	Y
A	1	4
B	2	3

Type 3

	X	Y
A	1	2
B	4	3.

Type 4*a*

	X	Y
A	1	3
B	4	2

Type 4*b*

	X	Y
A	1	4
B	3	2

Fig. 1.

'best', i.e. had the highest mean weight, milk yield, colour intensity, etc., while race A in environment Y did 'second best' and so on. Of course, with a different criterion the order might be different. Now there are just twenty-four ways of arranging the numbers 1, 2, 3, 4 in a square; and if we choose A and X so that AX is the best combination, there are just six ways, which are shown in Fig. 1.

If we reverse the order, e.g. grade the lightest colour instead of the darkest as number 1, the six types are unchanged. For example, type 1 a becomes

	X	Y			Y	X
A	4	3	or	B	1	2
B	2	1		A	3	4

as before.

Each represents a type of interaction. In interactions of type 1, A does better than B in each environment, and X is superior to Y for each race. Types 1 a and 1 b do not differ essentially, for if the difference between X and Y is diminished sufficiently, 1 b passes over into 1 a. Eugenists claim that interaction of type 1 a is the most important for our own species. Environmentalists stress the importance of type 1 b, even when they differ as to whether the 'best' environment X is socialism, free-for-all competition, or life in accordance with their own religious beliefs. But both are apt to forget the existence of the four other types of interaction. Numerous examples of both types 1 a and 1 b are to be found in the literature. For example, if A are white recruits, B negro recruits to the U.S. army in 1917–18, and the criterion the median score in the army Alpha test, then if X is New York and Y Tennessee we find an interaction of type 1 a; if X is New York and Y Arkansas, we find one of type 1 b, according to the data of Yerkes (1921). The median values were;

	New York	Tennessee	Arkansas
Whites	58·3	44·0	35·6
Coloured	38·6	29·7	16·1

It is clear that, whichever pair of states is compared, the interaction is of the same kind. The fact that the Tennessee whites did a little better, and the Arkansas whites a little worse than the New York coloured people, does not alter its character. Of course, on the above facts it is quite impossible to decide whether if the whites and negroes had been placed in identical environments from birth (or better, as a result of ovarian transplantation, from conception) there would have been any significant differences between the white and coloured people. The possession of a pigmented skin was a handicap to a person born in the U.S.A. about 1900. Whether a part of this handicap was due to congenital intellectual inferiority is quite unknown. It is only certain that much of it was due to other causes.

The second type of interaction is highly characteristic of domesticated plants and animals. A specialized race A gives a higher yield than a race B which is nearer to the wild type, in a favourable but highly artificial environment. But in more primitive conditions it does worse. Consider two of the Scottish breeds of beef cattle, A the Aberdeen Angus, and B the Galloway. Under optimal conditions X, A produces more beef. The mean weight of show steers with an average age of 1 yr. 10 months at Smithfield from 1902 to 1911 was 1737 lb. for A and 1224 lb. for B. The Galloways, to quote *British Breeds of Livestock* (1920), 'will thrive and put on flesh on very poor grazing, and are admirably suited to cold, wet, climatic conditions'. But they 'bear heavy feeding very well'. Thus if Y represents a poor pasture and cold wet climate, the Galloway B does not do badly, but it does better on good pasture X. The hill farmers who breed Galloways would breed Aberdeen Angus if it paid them. But in environment Y, the breed A is not so good an economic proposition as B. It would probably have a high death-rate, and the survivors would not thrive. Unfortunately, I can find no figures comparing the performance of these breeds in poor environmental conditions. Cases are, however, available in plants, where, for example, wheat A does better than B when sparsely sown, and worse when densely sown. In fact it would be more accurate to say that our domestic animals and plants have been selected for variable response to their environment than for a consistently favourable response. It has been suggested that the highest human types only excel in a favourable environment, and fail completely in an adverse one which had a less disastrous effect on the average individual. I doubt if this is generally true, but it may well be true for some genotypes.

With interactions of types 3 and 4 the change of environment from X to Y affects the two genotypes in opposite directions. This situation is very common. Bridges & Brehme (1944) and others list responses of mutant types in *Drosophila melanogaster* to temperature which are summarized in Table 1. It will be seen that abnormalities of many different types are enhanced by heat, and a slightly but not significantly greater number enhanced by cold.

Table 1

Eye colour	Eye size	Eye surface	Venation	Wing size	Wing shape	Bristles	Mis llaneous
doughnut +	Bar +	morula +	Abruptex +	Beadex^r −	balloon −	bobbed −	bithorax +
light +	Deformed −	pebbled +	bifid +	Crimp +	bent +	condensed +	cloven thorax −
maroon-like −	eyeless +	sparkling −	Cell +	Clipped +	blistered −	Dichaete +	cut (bead effect) −
mottled of	Lobe +	...	cubitus	dumpy +	Curly +	hook +	pentagon (body colour) −
In (2LR) 40*d* −	scutenick −	...	interruptus −	fringed +	fluted −	morula +	reduplicated (legs) −
mottled-28 −	welt +	...	heavy vein −	jagged +	jaunty +	Notopleural −	sable (body colour) −
white-buff −	...	...	knot −	narrow −	pleated −	polychaetoid −	scutenick (scutellum) +
white-blood +	...	...	Plexate −	roughish −	Pufdi +	polychaetous +	staroid (pleiotropic) +
			suppressor of	vestigial −	pupal −	scabrous +	short-wing (pleiotropic) +
			veinlet −				tetraltera −
			thick veins −	...	Stubble rec[2] −	...	
					vesiculated −	...	...

\+ Abnormality increased by heat.
− Abnormality increased by cold.

Suppose A is fringed[2], B vestigial, X is 19° C., Y 30° C., and the flies are graded by wing area. AX is slightly scalloped, AY more deeply so, BY a narrow strap, and BX a mere scale. Another example of type 3 interaction may be taken from our own species. Let A be a group of normal children, B a group of mild mental defectives. Let X be an ordinary school. Y a special school for defectives. A will beat B on educational tests in either environment, but A will be better adjusted in the ordinary school, B in the special school.

In type 4 interaction each genotype does best in an environment to which it is adapted. One cannot say that either race or either environment is superior. The adaptation may be to climate or other physical conditions, or to parasites. Thus Europeans have a longer expectation of life than negroes in European cities, partly owing to their comparative immunity to tuberculosis. But in many parts of West Africa the negroes probably have the advantage. largely through their greater resistance to yellow fever.

Quite analogous 'pre-adaptations' are found among the *D. melanogaster* mutants. Thus polychaetous and polychaetoid are autosomal recessives in chromosomes 2 and 3 respectively, both producing extra bristles. Polychaetous overlaps the wild type at 19° C., but gives a good crop of extra bristles at 28–30° C. Polychaetoid overlaps the wild type at 25° C. and higher temperatures, but is clearly distinguishable at 19° C.

Many of the published results on photoperiodicity give excellent quantitative examples of type 4 interaction. For example, Hawkes (1943) obtained the following results for mean weight of tubers from two clones of *Solanum andigenum* in long and short days respectively over three years. The short days were 8½ hr., the long varied from 13 to 16 hr.

	Short	Long
Clone 1108	134	37
Clone 1068	91	131

In selection of stocks for agricultural purposes in different districts one is only concerned with interactions of types 2 and 4, in which each race is superior in a particular environment. Where the demand is heavy and transport is an important item in the costs, a crop will be grown or a stock raised in comparatively unfavourable environments. Interaction of type 2 may then be important. Where demand is less urgent or transport costs small, interaction of type 4 is more likely. Thus in Britain we find a place for tough but slow-growing breeds of sheep and cattle in our mountainous districts, but in peacetime we do not grow wheat unless a pretty high yield per acre is obtainable. So for sheep and cattle interactions of type 2 are fairly common, whereas type 4 is probably commoner with wheat so far as Britain is concerned. We require somewhat different types of wheat for the dry chalk uplands and the fens. For the planet as a whole this is probably not so. The spring wheats grown near the northern limit of cultivation give a poor yield per acre, but winter wheats would give less. The interaction is thus of type 2.

To obtain a further insight into the relation between the different types of interaction, let us suppose that the difference between the two environments X and Y is made very small. This is always possible when the difference is one of a single factor such as temperature, humidity, or length of day. It is not necessarily possible for differences of locality, since all the above, besides differences in soil, biological environment, and so on, may be important, and they may interact in a complex manner. If X and Y are very similar, then AX and AY can differ little. Similarly, BX and BY can differ little. Thus the interaction is of type 1*a* if the change of environment affects the two genotypes in the same way, and of type 3 if it affects them in opposite ways.

Next consider what occurs if X and Y differ considerably, but A and B are very similar. This can, of course, be achieved if for B we substitute a mixture of 99 % A and 1 % B, the organisms being kept separate (e.g. mice in individual cages) to avoid biological interactions such as infection or crossing. But we cannot, in general, find a single genotype intermediate between two others in all respects, any more than we can find a locality. In particular, alleles in a multiple series which are intermediate in one respect are not necessarily so in another. If, however, A and B are very similar the interaction is of type 1*b* if the genetic change has the same effect in both environments, of type 2 if it has the opposite effect. For example, if A is superior to B in both environments we get type 1*b* interaction. But if, for example, B is slightly tougher but less specialized than A we may expect an interaction of type 2 if X is a more favourable environment than Y.

It follows that if A is very similar to B, and X to Y, we can only get an interaction of type 1. Type 1 may, in fact, be regarded as the limiting type when differences are small. And type 4 is only likely to come into operation when both A and B and X and Y differ markedly. But in almost all species the range of environments and genotypes is so large that interactions of this type must occur. Professor Penrose has pointed out to me that it is important that the performance measured or graded in all four tests should be exactly the same. Thus at first sight it might seem legitimate to say that a group A of children proved more intelligent than group B when confronted with a verbal test X, and less so when confronted with a maze test Y. But in such a case we cannot really compare the performance of A in respect to X and Y. Suppose that A are English and B foreign children, it is probable that the test scores will have been standardized so that a representative group of English children scores about 100. If so the only possible types of results are as follows (X and Y being interchanged if necessary):

	X	Y				X	Y	
A	102	97	(1a)	or	A	102	97	(3)
B	90	81			B	81	90	

if the English children are consistently superior. If they are consistently inferior we get the same two types. If, however, the English children do better on one test, but worse on the other, we get:

	X	Y				X	Y	
A	102	97	(2)	or	A	97	102	(4a)
B	117	84			B	117	84	

Interactions of types 1b and 4b with significant differences cannot be obtained. This is, however, possible if the different types of performance can be compared by some objective standard, for example, the economic value of milk or beef produced. If so it is of course clear that the order may alter with a change in prices or transport conditions, and it is clearly very hard to make such comparisons in the case of men.

In many practical cases the differences between two or more of the four measured characters are not significant. If this is so it may or may not be possible to specify the type of interaction. There are two types of indetermination. First of all two or three of the characters may be indistinguishable, though significantly different from the other or others. Thus if environment X is sterile, and Y infected, then AX and BX will probably give no deaths, and AY will not do so if A is immune to the disease in question, whereas BY will do so if B is susceptible. Secondly, two characters may differ significantly. But another may lie between them without differing significantly from either. Thus if each measurement were based on a fairly large sample, we might get such a result as AX $9{\cdot}0 \pm 0{\cdot}5$, BX $8{\cdot}2 \pm 0{\cdot}6$, AY $7{\cdot}5 \pm 0{\cdot}4$. Here AX and AY differ by 2·34 times the standard error of their difference. But AX and BX only differ by 1·02 times this quantity, BX and AY by 0·97 times.

Type 1a or 1b

	X	Y
A	1	2
B	2	4

Type 1a or 3

	X	Y		X	Y		X	Y		X	Y
A	1	2	A	1	1	A	1	1	A	1	1
B	4	4	B	3	4	B	4	3	B	3	3

Type 1b or 2

	X	Y		X	Y		X	Y		X	Y
A	1	3	A	1	4	A	1	3	A	1	4
B	1	4	B	1	3	B	1	3	B	2	4

Type 2 or 4b

	X	Y
A	1	4
B	2	2

Type 3 or 4a

	X	Y
A	1	2
B	4	2

Type 4a or 4b

	X	Y		X	Y		X	Y		X	Y
A	1	3	A	1	4	A	1	4	A	1	3
B	4	1	B	3	1	B	4	2	B	3	1

Fig. 2.

Fig. 2 deals with the first case. The top left-hand square means that AX had the highest score, AY and BX equal second, and BY fourth. The other possible results give no information about the type of interaction. For example, if A was an immune variety, B susceptible to a disease, X a sterile environment, Y an infected one, we might get

	X	Y
A	1	1
B	1	4

if all individuals survived the experiment except some of the infected B population. If, however, the experiment lasted longer it could turn out that, in environment X, A was longer-lived or shorter-lived than B. It could also turn out that the infection slightly shortened A's expectation of life. But it might however lengthen it. Some bacteria are useful symbionts, for example, those which produce vitamin K in the human gut. But when their ancestors first invaded the guts of our ancestors, they may well have killed off some genotypes. Thus all six types of interaction are possible.

Where one score lies between two others without differing significantly from either, things are more complicated. Thus consider the situation

	X	Y
A	1	(2)
B	3	4

in which AX and BY differ significantly, but AY does not differ significantly from either. If the experiment were repeated on a larger scale we might get a result:

	X	Y	Type 1a
A	1	2	
B	3	4	

	X	Y	Type 3
A	2	1	
B	3	4	

or

	X	Y	Type 1b
A	1	3	
B	2	4	

In any given case it is easy to work out the possibilities.

In practice we generally have to consider a large number of genotypes and environments, and the number of possible types of interaction is very great. Thus if we have m genotypes and n environments, but can rearrange the order of the genotypes and environments after the experiment is completed, we have $\frac{(mn)!}{m!\,n!}$ possible types of interaction; for example, if $m = n = 10$, there are $7{\cdot}09 \times 10^{144}$ types. Even for the simplest case but one, of two genotypes in three environments or three genotypes in two environments, there are sixty types of interaction. Similarly, if we classify our environments in several different ways, e.g. hot and cold, dry and moist, there are, in the simplest case of a $2 \times 2 \times 2$-fold table, 5040 types of interaction; for a (2^n)-fold table $(2^n - 1)!$ types. If, on the other hand, we choose several different criteria of performance, e.g. milk yield, beef yield, and capacity for ploughing, there are seventy-two different types of interaction in the simplest case of two genotypes, two environments, and two criteria, and in general for m genotypes, n environments, and k criteria, $\frac{(mn!)^k}{m!\,n!\,k!}$ types of interaction. Clearly there would be no advantage in attempting to generalize our classification. One point is, however, worth making.

Of the $\frac{(mn)!}{m!\,n!}$ types of interaction of m genotypes and n environments, only $\frac{(mn!)}{(m!)^n n!}$ are such that the order of merit of the m genotypes is the same in every environment, and only $\frac{(mn)!}{m!\,(n!)^m}$

are such that the order of merit of the n environments is the same for every genotype. This can readily be seen by considering the number of ways in which an order of this rare type can be deranged. For example, three races in three environments have 10,080 types of interaction. In only 280 of these is the order of the three races the same in each environment. It is much harder to calculate the number of types of interaction in which the order of merit of the genotypes is the same in every environment, and the order of merit of environments the same for every genotype. This number is 1 (type $1a$) for $m = n = 2$, and 5 for $m = 3$, $n = 2$, or $m = 2$, $n = 3$.

A few words may be said about the application of the ideas hêre developed to agriculture and to eugenics. The agricultural problem is enormously simpler because there is comparatively little crossing between stocks of the same species, and these stocks are homozygous for many of the genes responsible for the differences between them. But our own species is not so divided up, and even if extreme eugenical principles were accepted by a people or practised by a dynasty of tyrants, many centuries would elapse before races or classes attained the degree of genetical homogeneity of the average breed of cattle. Still more important, each domestic plant or animal breed is judged in the main by a single economic criterion. No doubt the criterion is biologically complicated. Thus besides milk yield and quality, fertility, rate of maturing, resistance to disease, and meat production by male castrates, are all of some importance in a breed of dairy cattle. And within a whole domestic species, only a few types of performance are required. Thus sheep are bred with a view to meat production, and also to that of several types of wool, of fleeces for coat linings and the like, and of several types of ornamental fur. In a few countries they are used for milk production and transport. But the division of labour in a modern society, quite apart from any question of cultural or spiritual excellence, demands many different human abilities, each of which may give a different ranking order.

At first sight it might be regarded as a sound agricultural policy to select the genotypes which give the best performances in each of a fairly large series of typical environments. Unfortunately in current practice far too much attention is paid to performance in highly favourable environments, and there is a tendency to lose sight of type 2 interactions. In consequence a breed of cattle may be 'graded up' so as to give a high milk production under optimal conditions. But it may actually give a lower one under poorer conditions, particularly when allowance is made for deaths. It may also turn out that the highest ranking genotype is a heterozygote, perhaps a multiple heterozygote. This is certainly true for some fancy breeds, and for economically valuable breeds such as Dexter cattle. If so one or both of the homozygous forms must be kept as breeders, though their actual performance may be relatively low. In sheep-breeding it is a common practice to cross certain breeds, the hybrids not being used for further breeding. Thus Scottish Blackfaced ewes are commonly crossed with Border Leicester rams. This practice is sometimes carried so far that a breed is mainly valued for its performance as a parent. Thus to quote *British Breeds of Livestock*, 'now practically all the purebred flocks of Cotswolds are maintained to provide rams for crossing purposes'. In the United States maize for agricultural purposes is largely grown from crosses of homozygous lines of comparatively low yield. Finally, first crosses between poultry of different breeds are reared on a large scale not mainly on account of hybrid vigour but because their sex can be determined on hatching.

In our own species we know little as to the good or bad results of interracial crosses, since race mixture is always complicated by culture mixture. But it is a curious commentary on human racial theories that if we could argue from animal breeding to human breeding, the first cross between different races would probably often be more vigorous than either pure race, whatever might happen in later generations. So a dictator who combined the ruthlessness of one lately deceased with a greater knowledge of biology might have encouraged racial crossing, whilst preventing the further breeding of the hybrids; and a far-sighted human biologist, while not recommending widespread interracial crossing in the present state of our ignorance, might favour the preservation of pure stocks of even the least progressive races, not merely for their possible future performance, but for their possible value in hybridization at a later date.

It might, however, be thought a sound agricultural policy to discard all stocks other than those which give the best performance in one or other of a well-chosen series of environments, and those which may be needed for breeding heterozygous types. This view is based on the false assumption that the environment will not change greatly. The following are among the obvious changes which may occur:

(1) Emergence of new diseases.

(2) Changes in agricultural technique, e.g. introduction of machinery, the use of new types of fertilizer, the use of hormones, vernalization, and so forth.

(3) Changes in demand, causing, e.g. a great increase in the area under a given crop.

(4) Changes in environment due to export.

The first of these is a fundamental reason for preserving considerable genetical diversity. It is particularly important with clonally grown plants, where a very high degree of homogeneity is obtained. A striking example occurred in the banana. Large areas of Central America and the West Indies were grown with the triploid clone called Gros Michel. This is particularly susceptible to the fungus *Fusarium cubense*, causing Panama disease, and the spread of this disease has therefore had serious effects on the banana industry, and greatly stimulated genetical work intended to produce other sterile clones. Similar dangers are to be expected if a single pure line of wheat is grown over wide areas. Since the evolutionary steps by which a parasite may adapt itself to a new host cannot be foreseen, much less prevented, such events can only be guarded against by the maintenance of a high level of genetical diversity. All that we can be sure of is that the biological environment will change.

Similarly, the possibility of changes in agricultural technique call for a large reserve of genotypes. Vernalization permits the use of autumn wheats in cold climates where only spring wheats could formerly be grown. But it is unlikely that the varieties of autumn wheat which give the best results when vernalized are those which give the best results when sown in autumn in a warmer climate. Similarly the variety of sheep which will give the highest yield of wool in a given area when their fertility is increased by hormone injections is not necessarily that which will give the highest yield when not so treated.

In fact the type of classification here adopted is not really adequate for the practical problems of agriculture because it does not take time, and particularly environmental change, into consideration. If the environment X is liable to change into environment Y we need, besides our A stock, a B stock in reserve which will give an interaction of type 2 or type 4. As we do not know the nature of Y beforehand this means that we should have a considerable number of stocks in reserve, including even definitely inferior stocks which, though they are not themselves likely to be of value, may carry valuable genes.

An increased area is likely to call for interactions of type 2, since the organism in question will have to be grown in less favourable environments than before. Export, for example of British cattle to tropical countries, calls for interactions of type 4, though probably type 2 is more likely to be achieved in practice.

The same arguments apply to eugenic policy. We are not justified in condemning a genotype absolutely unless we are sure that some other genotype exists which would excel it by all possible criteria in all possible environments. We can only be reasonably sure of this in the case of the grosser types of congenital mental and physical defect. A moderate degree of mental dullness may be a desideratum for certain types of monotonous but at present necessary work, even if in most or all existing nations there may turn out to be far too many people so qualified.

In a society which was perfect from the eugenical point of view there would be no interactions of types 1 or 3; genotypes of consistently inferior performance would have been eliminated. Similarly, in a society which was optimal from the point of view of environment there would be no interactions of types 1 or 2. People would not be placed in environments where they could not do their best, at least in some respect. It follows that interactions of type 4 are the ideal at which we should aim. That is to say in the ideal society there would be a diversity of social functions and of human endowments, but no social function could be dispensed with without damage to the society, and no individual could exercise a different function without performing it less efficiently and happily than those who were actually doing so. This ideal is obviously remote and probably never fully attainable, but it is perhaps worth stating. Meanwhile our efforts should be mainly concentrated on the elimination of interactions of type 1, that is to say the elimination of environments which are unfavourable to all genotypes, and of genotypes which are inferior in all environments.

SUMMARY

A simple classification of the possible types of interaction between two stocks and two environments is given. This classification is applied to a number of concrete cases arising in genetics, agriculture and eugenics.

I should like to acknowledge my debt to Dr J. M. Rendel for many of the ideas here put forward concerning breeds of livestock, while acquitting him of any erroneous views of which I may have been guilty.

REFERENCES

C. B. BRIDGES & K. S. BREHME (1944). The mutants of *Drosophila melanogaster*. *Publ. Carneg. Instn*, no. 552.

British Breeds of Livestock (1920). H.M. Stationery Office. London.

J. B. S. HALDANE (1936). Some principles of causal analysis in genetics. *Erkenntnis*, 6, 346.

G. HAWKES (1943). *Photoperiodism in the Potato*. Cambridge: Imp. Bur. Plant Breeding and Genetics.

R. M. YERKES (1921). Psychological examining in the U.S. army. *Mem. Nat. Acad. Sci.* 15, 689.

THE MUTATION RATE OF THE GENE FOR HAEMOPHILIA, AND ITS SEGREGATION RATIOS IN MALES AND FEMALES

By J. B. S. HALDANE, F.R.S.

THE MEAN MUTATION RATE

Haldane (1935), on rather rough data, estimated the mutation rate for haemophilia, that is to say, the frequency per X-chromosome per generation with which this gene appears, as being between 10^{-5} and 5×10^{-5}, probably about 2×10^{-5}. Haldane & Philip (1939) investigated Birch's (1937) pedigrees, and found that, when the necessary corrections for the bias due to ascertainment had been made, daughters of haemophilics bore 15 normal, 14 haemophilic, and 1 doubtful sons, while $55{\cdot}9 \pm 8{\cdot}3$ % of the sisters of haemophilics were heterozygous. Giving the maximum weight to doubtful cases in each direction, they found 60·5 and 47·0 % heterozygotes.

Andreassen (1943) has published a collection of 63 pedigrees of haemophilia in Denmark. Owing to the small and relatively immobile population studied, his material is superior to Birch's and *a fortiori* to that of previous workers, in two respects. It covers every case in Denmark during 15 years, so the frequency in the population is known, and there are better medical records of early cases. He also states the propositus, or proband, in each pedigree, though he omits certain details which Birch has given. His estimate of the mutation rate is certainly more accurate than that of Haldane (1935).

However, I believe his calculated value of $1{\cdot}9 \times 10^{-5}$ is distinctly too low, for the following reason. Haldane (1935) showed that if μ and ν are the rates per generation at which the normal allelomorph mutates to the gene for haemophilia in females and males respectively, if x is the frequency of haemophilia among males in the population at birth, and f the fitness of haemophilic males as a fraction of that of normals, then

$$2\mu + \nu = (1-f)\,x,$$

so that the mean mutation rate is $\frac{1}{3}(1-f)\,x$. Andreassen accepts this calculation. He finds that in 1943 there were 81 haemophilics among 1,820,000 Danish males. He also finds that the mean life of a haemophilic between 1860 and 1925 was 18 years, that of Danish males in 1905 being 55 years. He therefore takes x as $\frac{81 \times 3}{1{,}820{,}000}$ or $1{\cdot}33 \times 10^{-4}$. But he calculated f, the mean fitness, or effective fertility, as follows. The 205 haemophilics in his pedigrees had 110 children. Their 145 healthy brothers had 138 children. Thus the mean fitness (or effective fertility) of the haemophilics was $\frac{110 \times 145}{205 \times 130}$, or 0·564 (his figure is 0·57). I believe that this estimate is far too high for the following reasons. Each pedigree is based on a propositus, a haemophilic who was alive in Denmark between 1928 and 1943. Since many were quite young, the propositi have had rather few children. A large fraction of the children are contributed by their grandparents. One great-grandparent of a propositus, and 9 grandparents, were haemophilics. Among them they had 57 children. In particular, the haemophilic grandparent of the propositus in pedigree 39 had 10 children and 9 haemophilic grandchildren, with 2 haemophilic great-grandchildren, a truly remarkable dysgenic performance. It is obvious that the pedigrees include all the few very fertile haemophilics who lived in Denmark in the nineteenth century. The ten men in question were born between 1828 and 1883. If they were omitted we should be left with 195 haemophilics and only 53 children. The value of f would then be $\frac{53 \times 145}{195 \times 138}$, or 0·286. I believe that this is a much better estimate of f. If we take cognizance of the fact that the fertility of brothers is correlated by subtracting the 19 normal brothers of the 10 haemophilic ancestors and their 29 children from the total of controls, we get $f = \frac{53 \times 126}{195 \times 109} = 0{\cdot}314$. However, in this case we might have weighted the bias in the other direction, since the haemophilic ancestors had 7 haemophilic brothers with 5 children. Subtracting these also, we get $f = \frac{46 \times 126}{190 \times 109} = 0{\cdot}280$. I shall adopt the value 0·286.

The following considerations show that it is plausible. According to Andreassen's Fig. 5 (only graphical data are given) 64 % of haemophilics died before the age of 20, 19 % between 20 and 30, and 6 % between the ages of 30 and 40, whereas only 17 % of normals died before 20, and another 9 % between 20 and 40. Thus the number of haemophilics reaching the age of 20 is only 0·41 that of normals, the number reaching the age of 40 being 0·15. The net fertility, or fitness, is just half-way between these two figures, as was to be expected.

Taking $x = 1{\cdot}33 \times 10^{-4}$ and $f = 0{\cdot}286$, we find a mean mutation rate of

$$\tfrac{1}{3}(1 - 0{\cdot}286) \times 1{\cdot}33 \times 10^{-4} = 3{\cdot}16 \times 10^{-5}.$$

This is distinctly higher than Andreassen's value of $1{\cdot}9 \times 10^{-5}$, but I believe it to be sounder. Quite comparable fallacies are extremely common in the literature of human genetics. Thus an unduly high fertility has been attributed to the mothers of haemophilics, and to persons carrying several autosomal dominants, simply because those who appear in the early generations of a pedigree are highly selected for fertility. The phenomenon of anticipation, by which a disease appears earlier in the lifetime of the later members of a pedigree, is usually, and perhaps always, due to a similar unconscious selection.

Prof. Penrose has suggested to me that a number of cases of haemophilia dying at birth or in the first week of life may have been missed, especially if they were sporadic. He points out that sporadic cases of a dominant abnormality tend to be severer than inherited cases, as those individuals who survive to breed will tend to carry genes diminishing the severity of the condition (Penrose, 1936). The same must be true, though in much lesser degree, for a sex-linked recessive. If this is so the true mutation rate is even higher than my estimate, and the fitness f is lower.

Segregation

Making the same corrections as Haldane & Philip (1939) Andreassen found 21 normal and 18 haemophilic sons of the daughters of haemophilics, giving, with their data, a total of 36 normal, 32 haemophilic, and 1 doubtful, in excellent agreement with the equality expected.

He did not, however, make any calculation concerning the segregation of the gene in females, as evidenced by the frequency of heterozygosis, among the sisters of haemophilics. This seems worth doing, since the segregation is both of genetical interest, and of importance for eugenical prognosis. I have therefore tabulated all sisters of haemophilics in the pedigrees, except those who appear in them because they were ancestresses of propositi. The reason for this omission was explained by Haldane & Philip. The symbol 1 III 2 in Table 1 denotes the second member (reading from the left) of the third generation of pedigree 1, and so on. Where a symbol for several children occurs in a pedigree, I count it as a unit for the purpose of denoting other members of the same generation. The asterisks denote women each of whose brothers was the only haemophilic in his pedigree, and therefore possibly a sporadic mutant. I have also added the corresponding cases from Haldane & Philip's Table III, omitting the sisters of possible sporadic mutants. The value $1-k$ is the probability that a heterozygous woman should have so many normal sons. When calculating k on the basis of grandchildren, it is assumed that the frequency p of heterozygosis among the daughters of heterozygotes is $\frac{1}{2}$. The argument is circular, since we are trying to determine p. But Haldane & Philip showed that the error involved altered their estimate of p from 0·559 to 0·560. It will therefore be neglected. In general k is not the probability that a woman of the class in question should be homozygous. So we cannot add the numbers in each class of Table 2 multiplied by their appropriate k values. Instead, Haldane & Philip showed that the maximum likelihood estimate of p, the frequency of heterozygotes, is obtained as follows. Let a be the number of certainly heterozygous women. Let b_k be the number of possibly homozygous women who had a number of male descendants giving the probability k.

Then, by their equations (1) and (2).

$$p\Sigma\frac{kb_k}{1-kp}=a,\quad \sigma_p^{-2}=\frac{1}{p}\Sigma\frac{kb_k}{(1-kp)^2},$$

the summations being made over all the classes of Table 2. On the basis of the pooled data of Tables 1 and 2 we have, if we omit the sisters of the sporadic cases,

$$\begin{aligned}\frac{49}{p}&=\frac{40}{2-p}+\frac{19}{\frac{4}{3}-p}+\frac{9}{\frac{8}{7}-p}+\frac{3}{\frac{16}{15}-p}+\frac{2}{\frac{32}{21}-p}+\frac{2}{\frac{64}{63}-p}+\frac{1}{4-p}+\frac{2}{\frac{8}{3}-p}\\&\quad+\frac{1}{\frac{16}{7}-p}+\frac{2}{\frac{8}{5}-p}+\frac{1}{\frac{16}{13}-p}+\frac{1}{\frac{64}{49}-p}+\frac{1}{\frac{512}{491}-p}\qquad(1)\\&=\frac{40}{1+q}+\frac{57}{1+3q}+\frac{63}{1+7q}+\frac{45}{1+15q}+\frac{62}{1+31q}+\frac{126}{1+63q}+\frac{1}{3+q}+\frac{6}{5+3q}\\&\quad+\frac{7}{9+7q}+\frac{10}{3+5q}+\frac{13}{3+13q}+\frac{49}{15+49q}+\frac{491}{21+491q},\quad\text{where } p+q=1.\end{aligned}$$

Hence $p=0{\cdot}547\pm0{\cdot}059$.

The agreement with the theoretical value of 0·50 is thus very satisfactory, and slightly better than on the earlier data.

It will be shown later that the sporadic cases are mostly the sons of heterozygous mothers, and not the products of individual mutation. If we assume that they are all the sons of heterozygotes, we must include in Table 2 the women marked by asterisks, and three similar cases from Haldane & Philip's Table III. Equation (1) now becomes

$$\frac{49}{p}=\frac{43}{2-p}+\frac{22}{\frac{4}{3}-p}+\frac{9}{\frac{8}{7}-p}+\text{etc.},\qquad(2)$$

the remaining terms being unaffected. This gives $p=0{\cdot}527\pm0{\cdot}059$. The fit is even better than before.

It may be hoped that in future it will be possible to determine the frequency of heterozygotes directly. For Andreassen finds that the coagulation time of their blood by Bürker's (1913) method is slower than normal. Unfortunately, with the technique which he uses, he states (p. 86) that one of 31 known heterozygotes had a coagulation time 'within the limits of the normal range'. Actually a comparison with his Fig. 10 shows that although the time when coagulation began was shorter than that of some (?4) of 81 normal women, as is occasionally the case with mild haemophilics, the time when coagulation ended was $10\frac{1}{2}$ min., whereas the maximum time among the 81 normals was 10 min. It would seem that he is, if anything, unduly modest as to the efficacy of his technique, which is likely to err in less than 3 % of cases, and is clearly of very great eugenic value.

He has applied this technique to 1 III 1, and finds her to be a heterozygote, but does not report on any other members of Table 2.

Table 1. *Ancestresses of one or more haemophilic males*

1 III 2, 2 III 6, 4 II 1, 8 III 1, 13 III 6, 14 IV 4, 16 III 11, 21 III 2, 22 III 1, 22 IV 9, 22 V 3, 30 III 3, 31 III 3, 35 III 9, 39 II 6, 39 IV 1, 39 IV 15, 39 IV 21, 39 IV 23, 40 III 10, 41 III 4, 50 III 1, 51 III 4. Total 23, plus 26 from Haldane & Philip's Table II.

Table 2. *Ancestresses of normal males only*

(*a*) One son. 1 III 1, 4 II 3, 4 II 8, 8 III 6, 8 IV 3, 10 II 9*, 15 III 18, 16 III 6, 17 II 8, 17 III 8, 17 III 9, 18 II 11, 22 VII 3, 23 II 11, 23 II 12, 35 III 10, 36 III 3, 36 III 3, 36 III 4, 37 III 5, 39 II 5, 39 IV 17, 41 III 3, 41 III 5, 43 II 4, 51 III 5. Total 24, plus 16 from Haldane & Philip's Table III. $k = \frac{1}{2}$.

(*b*) Two sons. 2 III 1, 5 III 1, 15 III 17, 22 V 12, 26 III 5, 37 II 4, 40 IV 6, 55 III 8*, 57 III 4*. Total 7, plus 12 from Haldane & Philip's Table III. $k = \frac{3}{4}$.

(*c*) Three sons. 15 III 13, 37 III 7, 40 III 15, 40 III 20, 49 IV 10. Total 5, plus 4 from Haldane & Philip's Table III. $k = \frac{7}{8}$.

(*d*) Four sons. 45 III 4. Total 1, plus 2 from Haldane & Philip's Table III. $k = \frac{15}{16}$.

(*e*) Five sons. Nil, plus 2 from Haldane & Philip's Table III. $k = \frac{31}{32}$.

(*f*) Six sons. 31 III 2. Total 1, plus 1 from Haldane & Philip's Table III. $k = \frac{63}{64}$.

(*g*) No sons, one daughter's son. One from Haldane & Philip's Table III. $k = \frac{1}{4}$.

(*h*) No sons, two sons of one daughter. 5 III 6. Total 1, plus 1 from Haldane & Philip's Table III. $k = \frac{3}{8}$.

(*i*) No sons, three sons of one daughter. 50 II 5. Total 1. $k = \frac{7}{16}$.

(*j*) One son, one daughter's son. 13 III 4. Total 1, plus 1 from Haldane & Philip's Table III. $k = \frac{5}{8}$.

(*k*) Two sons, one daughter's son. One from Haldane & Philip's Table III. $k = \frac{13}{16}$.

(*l*) One son, one son of one daughter, two of another. 17 II 2. Total 1. $k = \frac{49}{64}$.

(*m*) Four sons, three sons of one daughter, one son of another daughter. 48 II 1. Total 1. $k = \frac{491}{512}$.

* Sisters of possible mutants.

Sex difference in mutation rates

This method for the detection of heterozygotes also makes possible the exact solution of a very interesting question, which I had intended at a later date to attack by statistical methods. This is the question whether the rate at which the normal allelomorph mutates to haemophilia is the same in the two sexes. If μ is the rate of mutation in female X-chromosomes, ν in male X-chromosomes, **h** the gene for haemophilia, we suppose that the frequencies of the haemophilic gene in female and male gametes are $x/(1+x)$ and $y/(1+y)$, so that the effective breeding population is in the ratios

$$1\,\mathbf{HH} : (x+y)\,\mathbf{Hh} : f'xy\,\mathbf{hh} \text{ female, and } 1\,\mathbf{H} : fx \text{ male,}$$

where f is the fitness of haemophilic males, and f' that of haemophilic females, if they exist. Then Haldane showed that if mutation is balanced by selection, $x = \dfrac{2\mu+\nu}{1-f}$, $y = \dfrac{2f\mu+\nu}{1-f}$, and that of all haemophilic males a fraction $\frac{(1-f)\mu}{2\mu+\nu}$ are the sons of homozygous mothers. Let us call this fraction m. Of Andreassen's 63 propositi, the pedigrees show that 43 were the sons of heterozygous mothers, either because the mother had haemophilic relatives other than her sons, or because she had several haemophilic sons. This leaves 20 pedigrees each including only one haemophilic. In 5 of these (10, 11, 28, 29 and 42) Andreassen found that the haemophilic's mother, sister, or both, had a coagulation time so slow that she was classed as heterozygous. In the remaining 15 pedigrees (7, 12, 19, 20, 27, 33, 38, 46, 47, 55, 57, 58, 59, 60 and 63) no such tests were made. The mother was doubtless heterozygous in some of these. So $m < \frac{15}{63}$, and $\mu/(2\mu+\nu) < 0{\cdot}333$. Thus $\mu < 1{\cdot}001\,\nu$. We can obtain a very rough estimate of it as follows. In 8 pedigrees (7, 12, 19, 27, 33, 46, 59 and 63) the haemophilic had no brothers. In 4 pedigrees (38, 47, 58 and 60) he had 1 normal brother, in 2 (20 and 57) 4 normal brothers, and in 1 (55) 5 normal brothers.

A mother may be heterozygous on physiological evidence, that is to say on her coagulation time, or on genetical evidence. If she had a haemophilic descendant, and also a haemophilic relative other than a descendant, the genetic evidence is conclusive. If, however, she had more than one haemophilic son, one haemophilic son and one or more haemophilic grandsons or great grandsons through a daughter, or haemophilic grandsons or great grandsons through several daughters, she is probably heterozygous, but there is another possibility. The gene for haemophilia may have arisen by mutation in a part of her body, including the ovaries in whole or part. In such a mosaic individual the gene in question would be present in half or less of the female pronuclei of the ova. On the other hand, the blood would probably be normal, the substance necessary for coagulation and absent in haemophilics being supplied by the normal tissues in adequate amounts. At worst we should expect such mosaics often to fall within the normal range, since heterozygotes almost overlap it.

The mothers of Andreassen's 63 propositi can be classified as follows:

A. Certainly heterozygous on genetical grounds, 24 (nos. 2, 3, 6, 8, 14, 17, 18, 22, 23, 24, 26, 31, 34, 35, 37, 39, 40, 43, 45, 48, 49, 50, 52, 56).

B. Probably heterozygous on genetical grounds, 19 (nos. 1, 4, 5, 9, 13, 15, 16, 21, 25, 30, 32, 36, 41, 44, 51, 53, 54, 61, 62).

C. Probably heterozygous on physiological grounds, 4 (nos. 11, 28, 29, 42).

D. Probably heterozygous on physiological and genetical grounds, 1 (no. 10).

E. Possibly homozygous, 15 (nos. 7, 12, 19, 20, 27, 33, 38, 46, 47, 55, 57, 58, 59, 60, 63).

Group A had haemophilic descendants and other relatives. Group B had several haemophilic sons, or a haemophilic son and a haemophilic daughter's son. Group C had one haemophilic son and a delayed coagulation time. The mother of no. 42 also had a daughter with delayed coagulation. Group E had one haemophilic son each, and their coagulation time was not tested. Among the 37 women with delayed coagulation time were 12 mothers of group A, and 3 of group B, besides all of group C. Thus no cases were found suggesting mosaicism, though 7 possible cases were tested. If such a condition occurs, it is probably rare.

We have seen that μ is probably less than ν. However, the following argument suggests that it is much smaller. Of the 20 mothers of sporadic haemophilics 4 were directly proved to be heterozygous, and one to be heterozygous or conceivably mosaic, by blood tests. The sister of the 21st sporadic case bore a haemophilic son during the investigation. Now if the mothers of 20 p of the 20 single cases were homozygous, the probability that all the 5 mothers examined were heterozygous is $(1-p)^5$. Thus the median value of p is given by $(1-p)^5 = \frac{1}{2}$, whence $p = 0{\cdot}1294$, and $20\,p = 2{\cdot}59$. Thus it is plausible that about 2·59 of the 63 propositi had homozygous mothers. So $m = \frac{2{\cdot}59}{63}$, whence $\frac{\mu}{\nu} = \frac{1}{(1-f)/m - 2} = 0{\cdot}065$ approximately.

Thus the mutation rate in the X-chromosome of females is probably less than one-tenth of that in males, i.e. $\mu < 10^{-5}$, $\nu = 10^{-4}$. Let us estimate the probability that all 5 mothers would have been found heterozygous had μ been equal to ν. In this case $m = \frac{1}{3}(1-f) = 0{\cdot}238$ The probability that n mothers of propositi were homozygous is $m^n(1-m)^{63-n}\frac{63}{n!(63-n)!}$. If n of the 20 mothers of single haemophilics were homozygous, the probability that the first 5 tested should all be heterozygous is $\frac{(20-n)(19-n)\ldots(16-n)}{20.19.18.17.16}$, or $\frac{(20-n)!\,15!}{20!(15-n)!}$. So the probability required is

$$\sum_{n=0}^{15}\left[m^n(1-m)^{63-n}\frac{63!(20-n)!\,15!}{n!(63-n)!\,20!(15-n)!}\right] = 0{\cdot}0083.$$

Thus it is almost certain that the mutation rate per gene is less in women than in men.

This conclusion is so important, if true, that it seems worth while to show that it is supported by evidence other than the investigation of the coagulation times of the mothers of haemophilics, though only the latter will enable a valid estimate to be made. If all, or almost all, the mothers of haemophilics are heterozygous, then if we take all the sibships in which the propositus was the only haemophilic, we should find the same frequency of normal brothers whether or not the mother was proved to be heterozygous on genetical evidence. We therefore take all sibships from groups A and B in which the propositus was the only haemophilic, and compare them with those of groups C + D and E, in which by definition there was only one haemophilic. The result is shown in Table 3.

Table 3. *Fraternities containing one haemophilic*

Group	Total fraternities	Number of normal brothers						Total normal brothers	Mean normal brothers	
		0	1	2	3	4	5			
A	14	4	8	1	1	0	0	13	0·93	0·94
B	4	1	2	1	0	0	0	4	1·00	
C + D	5	2	1	1	1	0	0	6	1·20	1·15
E	15	8	4	0	0	2	1	17	1·13	

In group E, where the mother could be homozygous, there were 17 normal sons in 15 fraternities, in the other groups 23 in 23 fraternities. The excess of 2 sons is not significant. If we supposed that the mothers of 4 and 5 normal sons were homozygotes who had borne mutants, this would leave only 4 normal sons for the other 13 mothers, or well below expectation. This argument therefore supports the figure reached above, of 2 or 3 homozygotes only in group E.

A study of Birch's (1937) and Hoogvliet's (1942) pedigrees leads to a similar result. We regard the first numbered patient in each of Birch's pedigrees, and the haemophilic whose colour vision is first described in Hoogvliet's, as the propositus. 23 of Birch's 73 propositi, namely, 7, 9, 12, 16, 18, 23, 24, 28, 29, 35, 38, 39, 40, 41, 43, 47, 55, 57, 65, 71, 78, 92 and 98, had no haemophilic brothers, but could not have been mutants. 21 of them, namely, 1, 2, 17, 21, 30, 32, 44, 46, 49, 50, 52, 62,

66, 69, 70, 73, 74, 76, 87, 88 and 93, had no haemophilic relatives, and could have been mutants, except that 74 had a haemophilic monozygotic twin, who counts with him as a single zygote.

Two, 68 and 91, are omitted as doubtful: 68 had perhaps a haemophilic brother and 91 a possibly haemophilic grandfather and 2 normal brothers. The propositus of Hoogvliet's pedigree I could not have been a mutant, those of B, E and F may have been. Clearly for comparison we must combine Andreassen's groups A and B and groups C, D and E. We then have the result of Table 4.

Table 4. *Fraternities containing one haemophilic*

		Total fraternities	No. of normal brothers						Total normal brothers
			0	1	2	3	4	5	
Not mutants	Andreassen	18	5	10	2	1	0	0	17
	Birch	23	17	2	3	0	1	0	12
	Hoogvliet	1	0	1	0	0	0	0	1
	Total	42	22	13	5	1	1	0	30
Possibly mutants	Andreassen	20	10	5	1	1	2	1	23
	Birch	21	9	10	0	1	0	1	18
	Hoogvliet	3	1	1	1	0	0	0	3
	Total	44	20	16	2	2	2	2	44

If the two populations were strictly comparable we should expect only 31·4 normal brothers of the possible mutants. Probably several mothers of large fraternities were homozygous, though the difference is not quite significant. We should expect 5·7 out of the 44 to have been so. It is extremely unlikely that as many as half were.

In any case, if we accept the results of investigation of the blood of females, only 39 out of 146 propositi, or 26·7 %, could have been mutants. It follows that $\frac{\mu}{2\mu+\nu} < \frac{39}{146(1-f)}$ or $\mu < 1{\cdot}49\nu$. This is a much weaker result than that obtained before, because Birch and Hoogvliet made no physiological tests for heterozygosity. However, it agrees with the earlier result.

Discussion

The order of magnitude of five human mutation rates is now roughly known (Haldane, 1947). That of haemophilia averaged over the chromosomes is about equal to that of chondrodystrophy. If it is much greater in males than females, the rate in men is the highest yet found. Sirks (1937) ascribed the sporadic appearance of haemophilia to crossing over between the X- and Y-chromosomes. He suggested that the latter normally contains the gene for haemophilia. On this hypothesis the mother of a haemophilic must always be heterozygous. Andreassen found that the 5 mothers of sporadic haemophilics whom he examined were so, as would be expected on Sirks's view.

On the other hand, Table 4 suggests that the mothers of sporadic and hereditary haemophilics differ to some extent, which would not be the case on Sirks's theory. However, the difference is not fully significant. If an appreciable fraction of the mothers of sporadic haemophilics have normal coagulation time it will be possible to dismiss Sirks's theory. If not, it will have to be considered very seriously, though it has several difficulties (Haldane, 1938). For example, some Y-chromosomes must carry the normal allelomorph of haemophilia, and hence the daughter or sister of a haemophilic should occasionally transmit the gene through a normal son to a son's daughter, who would be haemophilic. In Fig. 1 X represents a normal X-chromosome, X' one carrying the gene for haemophilia, Y a normal Y-chromosome, $\bar{Y}$ one carrying the normal allelomorph of haemophilia.

No pedigree like that of Fig. 1 is certainly known, though there is a case of apparent transmission through a healthy male in the Tenna pedigree (Bulloch & Fildes, 1912, Fig. 373). However, the man in question, Christian Bueler (III 25) died in 1789, and in a small village community may well have married a relative, even if he was not a mild haemophilic. Moreover, a further point may now be made against Sirks. If sporadic haemophilia is due to crossing over, it is very surprising that its apparent mutation rate falls among those of four autosomal loci.

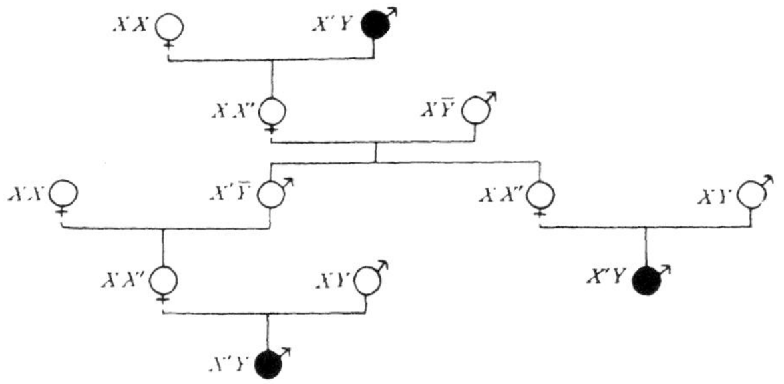

♂ Normal male. ● Haemophilic male.

Fig. 1. Hypothetical pedigree of haemophilia if Y-chromosomes sometimes carry its normal allelomorph.

If the difference between the sexes is due to mutation rather than crossing over, many explanations could be suggested. The primordial oocytes are mostly if not all formed at birth, whereas spermatogonia go on dividing throughout the sexual life of a male. So if mutation is due to faulty copying of genes at a nuclear division, we might expect it to be commoner in males than females. Again the chromosomes in human oocytes appear to pass most of their time in the pachytene stage. If this is relatively invulnerable to radiation and other influences, the difference is explicable. On either of these hypotheses we should expect higher mutability in the male to be a general property of human and perhaps other vertebrate genes. It is difficult to see how this could be proved or disproved for many years to come.

Both on scientific and eugenical grounds it is of the greatest importance to examine the coagulation time of the female relatives of haemophilics. If almost all turn out to have an abnormally long coagulation time it will be necessary to adopt either Sirks's theory or that of different rates in the two sexes. It will also follow that if a woman has had a haemophilic son, half her subsequent sons are likely to be haemophilic, even if she has no other haemophilic relatives. This is not the case with chondrodystrophy (Mørch, 1941). It will also be possible to test the sisters and other female relatives of haemophilics. If this were done, and all heterozygotes, as well as haemophilic men, refrained from breeding, the frequency of haemophilia could be greatly reduced.

For consider a population in equilibrium in which the sex ratio is unity, and the probability that a new born baby will live to be the parent of n sons is the coefficient of t^n in the expansion of e^{t-1} (Fisher, 1922). Consider a female heterozygous for haemophilia. Let P be the probability that at least one of her male descendants will be a haemophilic. The probability that she will have no haemophilic son is easily seen to be $e^{-\frac{1}{2}}$.

On an average she will have $\frac{1}{2}$ a heterozygous daughter. Hence

$$P = 1 - e^{-\frac{1}{2}} + e^{-\frac{1}{2}}\tfrac{1}{2}P = \frac{e^{\frac{1}{2}} - 1}{e^{\frac{1}{2}} - \frac{1}{2}} = 0{\cdot}565.$$

Thus only just over half the mutations occurring in males ever lead to the birth of a haemophilic, whilst those which do so lead to the birth of 1·8 haemophilics on an average. In an expanding population P is of course somewhat larger, in a declining one somewhat smaller. Now at equilibrium the frequency of haemophilics when no eugenic measures are taken is $\nu/(1-f)$ if μ can be neglected in comparison with ν. If only one male were allowed to appear in each pedigree the frequency would be reduced to $P\nu$, that is to say to a fraction $(1-f)P$, or 41 %, of the present frequency. If μ is not negligible, the frequency would be reduced from $\dfrac{2\mu+\nu}{1-f}$ to $\mu + P(\mu+\nu)$, that is to say to a fraction $(1-f)\left[P + \dfrac{(1-P)\mu}{2\mu+\nu}\right]$, which is under 57 % if μ is less than ν.

Thus a very substantial reduction is possible, even though the supply of haemophilics is kept up by mutation; and the detection of heterozygous women is an important eugenic measure. But it is to be noted that, even in a community where sterilization on eugenical grounds was legal, it could not be applied to haemophilics, since it would often be fatal; and since 52 % of heterozygous women have an increased tendency to bleed, and 14 % a fairly severe one, this operation would be appreciably more dangerous to them than to women in general. Hence continence or contraception appears, in this case at least, to be preferable to sterilization.

Summary

Andreassen's data on haemophilia give the following results:

1. The mean mutation rate to haemophilia per chromosome per generation is $3{\cdot}2 \times 10^{-5}$, somewhat higher than the value of $1{\cdot}9 \times 10^{-5}$ calculated by him.

2. The mutation rate is much higher, and possibly ten times higher, in male than in female X-chromosomes.

3. Combining his data with those of Birch, 31 + 1 doubtful out of 69 sons of the daughters of haemophilics were themselves haemophilic, and $52{\cdot}7 \pm 5{\cdot}9$ % of the sisters of haemophilics were heterozygous.

REFERENCES

M. Andreassen (1943). Haemofili i Danmark. *Opera ex domo biologiae hereditariae humanae Universitatis Hafniensis*, **6** (Copenhagen).

C. L. Birch (1937). Haemophilia. Clinical and genetic aspects. *Illinois Med. Dent. Monogr.* **1**, **4** (Urbana, Ill.).

K. Bürker (1913). Vereinfachte Methode der Bestimmung der Blutgerinnungszeit. *Pflug. Arch. ges. Physiol.* **149**, 318.

W. Bulloch & P. Fildes (1912). *Treas. Hum. Inher.* **1**, 256.

R. A. Fisher (1922). On the dominance ratio. *Proc. Roy. Soc. Edinb.* **42**, 321.

J. B. S. Haldane (1935). The rate of spontaneous mutation of a human gene. *J. Genet.* **31**, 317–26.

J. B. S. Haldane (1938). The location of the gene for haemophilia. *Genetica*, **20**, 423–30.

J. B. S. Haldane (1947). The formal genetics of man. *Proc. Roy. Soc.* B (in the Press).

J. B. S. Haldane & U. Philip (1939). The daughters and sisters of haemophilics. *J. Genet.* **38**, 193–200.

B. Hoogvliet (1942). Genetische en klinische beschouingen naar aanleiding van bloederziekte en kleurenblindheid in dezelvde familie. *Genetica*, **23**, 93–209.

E. T. Mørch (1941). *Chondrodystrophic dwarfs in Denmark*. Copenhagen.

L. S. Penrose (1936). Autosomal mutation and modification in man with special reference to mental defect. *Ann. Eugen., Lond.*, **7**, 1–16.

M. J. Sirks (1937). Haemophilia as a proof for mutation in man. *Genetica*, **19**, 417–22.

Croonian Lecture

The formal genetics of man

By J. B. S. Haldane, F.R.S.

(*Delivered 7 November 1946—Received 18 December 1947*)

Man has obvious disadvantages as an object of genetical study. The advantages are that very large populations are available, and that many serological differences and congenital abnormalities have been intensively investigated.

Some characters are found to obey Mendel's laws with great exactitude. In others the deviations are such as to suggest the existence of a considerable selective mortality, perhaps prenatal. In yet other cases the observations are biased because we only know that we are investigating the progeny of two heterozygotes when the family includes at least one recessive. Statistical methods which eliminate this bias are described.

Still more complex methods are needed for the detection and estimation of linkage. Several such cases have been detected with greater or less certainty, and the frequency of recombination between the loci of the genes for colour-blindness and haemophilia is now estimated at 10 ± 4 %. If the theory of partial sex-linkage be accepted, it is possible to make a provisional map of a segment of the human sex chromosome.

When a gene is sublethal, as are those for haemophilia and achondroplasic dwarfism, its elimination by natural selection is in approximate equilibrium with its appearance by mutation, and the frequency of the latter process can be estimated. The mutation rates at five human gene loci lie between 4×10^{-5} and 4×10^{-6} per locus per generation. These are the only estimates available for vertebrates. The rates per generation are rather higher than those in *Drosophila*, but those per day are so small that much, or even all, human mutation may be due to natural radiations and particles of high energy.

In 1906 Bateson delivered a lecture to the Neurological Society on 'Mendelian heredity and its application to man' in which he described the genetics of brachydactyly and congenital cataract, which are dominant to the normal (the word is used loosely, since the abnormal homozygote is unknown). He suggested that albinism and alcaptonuria were recessive, and he described the laws of inheritance of haemophilia and colour-blindness, though he did not, of course, give the explanation of these laws which is now accepted.

In the ensuing 40 years a very large number of pedigrees have been collected, unfortunately with very variable standards of accuracy. These show that more than a hundred different human abnormalities are certainly due to single gene substitutions, and that several hundred more are probably so. For example, Cockayne (1933) listed eighty abnormalities of the skin, hair, nails, and teeth which are probably due to dominant autosomal genes, eighteen to autosomal recessives, and thirteen to sex-linked genes. In over half the cases the evidence is adequate.

On the other hand the genetical analysis of the normal polymorphism of a race such as our own for colour, size, and shape has not gone far. The genetics of eye colour, for example, are far more complex than was originally thought, and stature is undoubtedly determined by a large number of genes, as well as by environmental influences. Still less progress has been made in the analysis of the genetics of those differences in skin colour and hair shape which exist between the major human races. However, immunology has revealed a polymorphism existing in all races which was wholly unexpected when Bateson wrote. Its genetical basis is exceedingly simple; perhaps because antigens are direct products of gene action, while pigments are the end products of complex chains of metabolic processes in which many, if not all, of the steps are controlled by different genes: and the processes of morphogenesis are even more complicated. Meanwhile, genetics have developed along many lines, of which three are especially important. It has been shown that genes are material structures located at definite points in the chromosomes. If we can homologize the genes of organisms which conjugate and the 'transforming principles' of bacteria, which can apparently transfer them to one another without conjugation, just as they carry out a communal metabolism, the work of Avery, MacLeod & MacCarty (1944) suggests that genes, at least in some phases of their life cycles, may consist wholly of desoxy-ribose nucleic acid.

We have learned a good deal about the causal chain between a gene and its manifestation. Goldschmidt was a pioneer in this work. You, Mr President, played an important part in the analysis of the genetical control of anthocyanin production in flowers. Beadle, Tatum and others were able to specify the stages in the production of arginine and other essential metabolites controlled by different genes in *Neurospora*. In this country, Grüneberg, in the mouse, and Waddington, in *Drosophila*, investigated the genic control of morphological development.

Finally, a number of workers, notably Dobzhansky, Dubinin, Fisher, Haldane, Teissier & l'Heritier, Tsetverikov, and Wright have investigated the genetics of populations both practically and theoretically, and they and others have discussed the bearing of their results on the problem of evolution.

All these methods are applicable to our own species. There is, however, a widespread belief that what I may call formal genetics, that is to say the study of heredity and variation, based on the description and counting of individuals, has ceased to be important, and that in future genetics will consist mainly of the study of biochemical and morphogenetic processes controlled by genes, and of evolutionary changes in populations; while the mere enumeration of the results obtained from various matings, and deductions drawn from such enumeration, are no longer of great interest. As I propose to devote this lecture to the pure or formal genetics of man, I may perhaps be pardoned if I state what seem to me to be the legitimate aims of human genetics, and so to justify what some will regard as a reactionary standpoint.

The final aim, perhaps asymptotic, should be the enumeration and location of all the genes found in normal human beings, the function of each being deduced from the variations occurring when the said gene is altered by mutation, or when several allelomorphs of it exist in normal men and women. In addition, information would be gathered on the effect of changes involving sections of chromosomes, such as inversions, translocations, deficiencies, and duplications.

The number of genes in a human nucleus almost certainly runs into thousands, possibly tens of thousands. Each has, so far as one can judge, a highly specific biochemical function. The end result of such a genetical study as I have adumbrated would be an anatomy and physiology of the human nucleus, which would be incomparably more detailed than the anatomy and physiology of the whole body as known at present. This end will perhaps be achieved in part by non-genetical methods, such as ultramicroscopic operations on the nuclei of human cells in tissue culture.

No doubt one result of such a study will be the possibility of a scientific eugenics, which may bear the same relation to the practices now or recently in vogue in certain countries as chemotherapy bears to the bleedings and purgations of early medicine. But other results may be more important. A knowledge of the human nucleus may give us the same powers for good or evil over ourselves as the knowledge of the atomic nucleus has given us over parts of the external world.

In this lecture I shall be largely concerned with the localization of genes in human chromosomes. A simple example will show why this is important. One of the common causes of blindness is retinitis pigmentosa. Ten years ago it could be said that in some pedigrees this disease was transmitted as a dominant, in others as a recessive of the ordinary type, occasionally as a sex-linked recessive. In 1936 I argued that some pedigrees showed partial sex-linkage, a phenomenon which I shall describe later. We can now say tentatively that one of the genes, the abnormality of which causes this condition, is carried in that segment of the sex chromosomes of which women possess two, and men only one; another, which may give dominant or recessive mutants, in that segment of the same chromosomes of which both sexes possess two; while other such genes, how many we do not know, are carried in the other chromosomes. It is reasonably sure that they control different processes. And this is borne out by the fact that the partially sex-linked recessive type is never associated with deafness, while one of the autosomal recessives is so associated.

Pathologists will have to work out the aetiology of the different genetical types. They can hardly hope to do so until they are distinguished, if, as seems probable, each gene controls a different process. And just as the methods for the cure of bacillary and amoebic dysentery are very different, so it is unlikely that the same therapeutic measures will succeed against diseases, however similar in their symptoms, which are due to different genes. They certainly do not do so in *Drosophila melanogaster*. In that species at least four different recessives give eye colours which are scarlet because they lack a yellow pigment found in the normal eye, which is a derivative of tryptophane. The eye colour of the mutant *vermilion* can be made normal by injecting the larvae with kynurenine, for the gene present in normal flies but inactive in *vermilion* flies is concerned in the oxidation of tryptophane to kynurenine. But *cinnabar* flies are not cured, because they cannot catalyze a further stage in the pigment formation; and *cardinal* and *scarlet* flies are not cured because their eye rudiments cannot take up the pigment precursor (Ephrussi 1942). The four genes in question are carried at different loci in three chromosomes.

The first step in formal genetics is to establish that certain characters are inherited in accordance with Mendel's laws, and in particular that segregation occurs in Mendelian ratios.

This is certainly true in many cases where large numbers have been studied. Thus according to theory a member of blood group *AB* produces equal numbers of *A* and *B* gametes. Table 1* shows that this is the case, the deviation from theory being less than the standard error of sampling. In the mating *A* × *AB* the *A* children are derived from *A* gametes of the *AB* parent, the *B* and *AB* children from *B* gametes; and so on. Such an agreement implies not only that the two types of gamete are

TABLE 1

parents	children in group: *O*	*A*	*B*	*AB*	total
O × *AB*	8 !	633	646	3 !	1290
A × *AB*	0	533	247	312	1092
B × *AB*	2 !	183	406	232	823
AB × *AB*	0	28	36	65	129

total *A* gametes 1609
total *B* gametes 1647 } $(d-1)\,n^{-\frac{1}{2}} = 0{\cdot}648$.
total homozygotes from *AB* × *AB* 64.
total heterozygotes from *AB* × *AB* 65.

* From Wiener (1943), p. 190. This includes all data published since 1931. Before this date only groups of over 250 children are included. This criterion omits three children of *AB* mother assigned to group *O* by two workers who had tested seven and nine children of such mothers, and whose findings have perhaps received undue attention.

formed in equal numbers, but that there is no marked selective mortality of either type of zygote. Thirteen children occur in unexpected groups. These represent the combined effects of illegitimacy, technical errors, and conceivably mutation or abnormal segregation of chromosomes. Clearly these causes combined will produce results smaller than sampling error.

In the case of the pair of allelomorphic genes which respectively produce the *M* and *N* agglutinogens, there is at least prima facie evidence for very abnormal segregation. Where such cases have been investigated in animals, they have so far almost always been found to be due to selective mortality, or in fact natural selection, one genotype having a higher deathrate in the early stages of life than another. Taylor & Prior (1939*a*) found that the progeny from the marriages of heterozygotes which they had examined included a considerable excess of heterozygotes. They were convinced that this was not due to technical errors, and found a similar excess in the pooled data of other workers, giving 54·85 % of heterozygous children, the excess being 3·08 times its standard error. Wiener (1943) believes the excess to be an artefact due to the use of incompletely absorbed testing fluids, and that no such excess occurs where this error is avoided. Now if the sera used give too many *MN* children they should also give too many *MN* parents. Taylor & Prior (1939*b*) showed that in most series of data the square of the number of *MN* individuals approximates to four times the product of the numbers of *M* and *N*, while a few show a great excess. I have therefore applied their test to all the series in Wiener's table 46, and eliminated cases where χ^2 exceeds four for the parents.† I have also omitted two small series containing 40 children between them, and two Japanese and one German series which were not available in English libraries, and have inserted one German series. The results are shown in table 2. The values of χ are calculated by Taylor & Prior's method, a positive value denoting an excess of *MN* over expectation among the parents. It will be seen that there are 54·85 % of heterozygotes. The excess is 3·16 times its standard error. The probability of so large an excess or defect by sampling error is 0·0016. If it were due to the systematic use of incompletely absorbed testing fluids, we should expect to find a lower percentage of heterozygotes in those series where χ is negative. The value found is 56·77 %, which is slightly, but not significantly higher. The excess of *M* over *N* children is just below twice its standard sampling error, and not statistically significant.

If the numbers of heterozygotes (*MN*) and homozygotes (*M* + *N*) in the different groups are compared, we find $\chi^2 = 17{\cdot}21$ for 11 degrees of freedom. Thus $P = 0{\cdot}10$, and the data are not significantly heterogeneous, as they would probably be if some workers had used faulty methods.

Table 3 shows the totals found for all types of marriage by the twelve authors cited in table 2. Illegitimacy, technical errors, and mutation clearly account for

† Wiener gives the reasons for excluding Lattes & Garrasi's (1932) data. The other relevant values of χ are: Dahr (1940) + 4·51, Hirzfeld & Kostuch (1938) + 2·16, Landsteiner & Wiener (1941) + 2·002, Wiener & Sonn (1943) − 2·20. The last three values may well all be due to sampling error.

1-2

very few unexpected classifications. In the case of the $MN \times M$ and $MN \times N$ marriages, the differences between the classes where equality is expected are less than twice their standard errors. It will be seen that the mean number of children examined per $MN \times MN$ marriage was decidedly less than that in the other groups. The figure 2·73 is not of course the mean fertility per marriage, as sterile marriages were excluded, it was not always possible to examine all the living children, and

TABLE 2

authors	number of families	χ	children M	MN	N
Landsteiner & Levine	11	+0·017	17	31	7
Wiener & Vaisberg	25	−0·006	29	58	29
Schiff	33	+1·808	18	48	22
Crome	9	+0·083	4	10	4
Clausen	70	−0·777	38	74	28
Blaurock	23	+1·002	25	40	25
Moureau	53	+0·444	45	102	41
Hyman	32	+0·906	10	41	16
Matta*	{20 {20	−0·781} −1·741}	9	45	10
Dahr & Bussmann	30	−0·514	38	70	18
Taylor & Prior (a)	56	−0·349	10	38	8
Holford	34	+1·185	24	37	14
total	416	—	267	594	222

* One group in Egypt, one in Glasgow.

TABLE 3. PROGENY OF DIFFERENT MARRIAGES INVOLVING M AND N

parents	number of families	M	MN	N	total	mean children per family
$M \times M$	147	425	3 !	0	428	2·91
$M \times N$	151	1 !	477	2 !	480	3·18
$N \times N$	74	0	0	232	232	3·13
$MN \times M$	397	597	662	4 !	1263	3·18
$MN \times N$	292	2 !	428	483	913	3·13
$MN \times MN$	396	267	594	222	1083	2·73
total	1457	—	—	—	4399	3·02

investigators tend to choose large families. Nevertheless, it suggests that such marriages are less fertile than the average. The shortage of total children and of homozygotes can both be explained if homozygotes have a higher deathrate (probably prenatal) than heterozygotes. The prenatal and infantile fitness of the homozygotes is about 82 % of that of the heterozygotes, so at least 18 % of them must die at an early stage. If there had been 594 homozygotes instead of 489, the mean family size would have been 3·00. The hypothesis of selective death implies that 105, or 2·3 % of a group of 4504, human zygotes were eliminated, probably before birth. If the $MN \times MN$ marriages had been as fertile as the rest, we should have expected 155 more children from them, making a total of 4659, of whom 3·4 % were eliminated.

This is a substantial fraction of all conceptions, and it would seem that if a scientific study of the problem of human population is to be undertaken, it would be desirable to investigate a group of say 5000 married couples (including sterile couples) serologically, in order to discover whether certain types are less fertile than others, and whether certain human genotypes are eliminated prenatally. It would be essential, in such a study, to tabulate the results of reciprocal unions such as $MN♀ \times M♂$, and $M♀ \times MN♂$, separately. Unfortunately, many of the authors cited did not do so. It is of course possible that Wiener's hypothesis is correct. Nevertheless, the matter seems sufficiently important to warrant further study.

In the case of the *Rh* group of genes it is known that certain classes of offspring are killed off because they immunize their mother, and their blood corpuscles are destroyed by her antibodies. Such a mechanism will not explain the results found with *M* and *N*. Moreover, the elimination of homozygous offspring of two heterozygous parents would make the equilibrium between the two genes unstable, whereas in fact their frequencies in different peoples are much less variable than those of other genes responsible for serological differences.

Whatever may be the final answer to these questions, I hope I have shown that the exact investigation of the segregation of common genes is not a matter of merely academic interest.

I must pass on to the methods which are used in the investigation of the segregation of rare genes. When the rare gene is a dominant there are no statistical difficulties provided the gene manifests itself in all heterozygotes, and early in life. We cannot possibly expect to find Mendelian ratios for such a character as Huntington's chorea, whose mean age of appearance is about 35 years. We should expect to find good results in the case of hereditary skin diseases, which are easily and accurately diagnosed, and mostly manifested at an early age. Table 4 shows the children from unions of affected and normal persons in the sixteen diseases inherited as dominants of which Cockayne (1933) in his classical treatise was able to collect records of over 100 such children. A few of my numbers differ slightly from his totals through the exclusion of doubtful pedigrees. As a result of sampling error we should expect a normal distribution about zero with unit variance of the values of $(d-1)n^{-\frac{1}{2}}$, when d is the number of affected minus that of normal, and n is their sum. There are three aberrant values. The low incidence of neurofibromatosis may possibly be accounted for by its variable age of onset and sublethal character. Some individuals carrying the gene may have died prenatally, others may not yet have developed it when observed. Hypoplasia of the enamel is due to genes in at least two different chromosomes (Haldane 1937) and therefore presents complications. Tylosis, which is an abnormal thickening of the skin of the palms and soles, generally develops in the first year of life. It seems to present a definite exception to the usual rules, and demands further investigation. The similar anomalous cases which occur in the literature of dominant abnormalities of other organs are easier to explain by faulty diagnosis. There seems no reason to doubt that the segregation of most human dominant abnormalities follows Mendel's laws.

The ratios in which a gene pair segregates cannot be obtained so simply when one allelomorph is fully recessive. This is due to the fact that the compilation of a pedigree introduced a certain bias. The bias may be of a very simple kind. Birch (1937) in Chicago and Andreassen (1943) in Copenhagen collected 146 pedigrees of haemophilia, a sex-linked recessive condition, transmitted to and from males

TABLE 4. PROGENY OF INDIVIDUALS AFFECTED WITH DOMINANT ABNORMALITIES OF THE SKIN, HAIR, NAILS, AND TEETH

abnormality	affected	normal	$(d-1)\,n^{-\frac{1}{2}}$
piebaldness	133	118	+ 0·88
cutaneous xanthomatosis	98	111	− 0·83
telangiectasis	320	302	+ 0·43
epidermolysis bullosa simplex	193	163	+ 1·54
epidermolysis bullosa dystrophica	147	181	− 1·82
monilethrix	92	89	+ 0·15
porokeratosis	70	91	− 1·58
tylosis plantaris et palmaris	594	483	+ 3·35
ichthyosis vulgaris	86	98	− 0·81
alopecia congenita	130	118	+ 0·70
onychogryphosis	242	253	− 0·45
hypoplasia of enamel	84	50	+ 2·81
neurofibromatosis	115	160	− 2·61
naevus aplasticus	53	61	− 0·66
fistula auris	63	60	+ 0·18
angioneurotic oedema	182	206	− 1·17
total	2602	2544	+ 0·79

TABLE 5. SONS OF HAEMOPHILICS' DAUGHTERS

	families	normal sons	haemophilic sons
mothers of patients	17	11	26 (− 17)
other mothers	26	25	23 + 1?
total	43	36	49 + 1?(− 17) = 32 + 1?

through females. Each pedigree began with a patient whose relatives were then traced. In order to verify that the condition is due to a single gene we must show, among other things, that the daughters of haemophilics bear equal numbers of normal and haemophilic sons. If we study the daughters of haemophilics in the pedigrees we find a considerable excess of haemophilic sons. However, a further analysis (table 5) shows that this excess is confined to the mothers of the patients from whom the compilation of the pedigree started.

The reason is simple. The mothers of patients were investigated because the patient was discovered to be haemophilic. Hence at least one of their sons must have been haemophilic. The other daughters of haemophilics may have borne no haemophilic sons, indeed one was fortunate enough to bear three normal sons and no haemophilic. We can allow for this bias by subtracting one haemophilic from each family including a patient. The total then becomes 36 normal sons, with 32 haemophilics and one doubtful, a very good approximation to equality. A similar but more complicated analysis shows that about half the sisters of haemophilics transmit the disease. A neglect of this elementary point has led to the most remarkable conclusions as to the fertility of human stocks afflicted with hereditary disease. For if a character is passed on to half the children of an afflicted person, it will not be recognized as hereditary unless at least one child possesses it. We shall thus exclude all families of no children, half the families with only one child, a quarter of those with two, and so on, thus giving a wholly false impression of the fertility of such stocks. Where, on an average, the character only appears in one-quarter of the children, the exaggeration is still greater.

Unfortunately, the very simple type of correction which was applicable to the pedigrees of haemophilia cannot always be applied.

Consider a recessive character such as albinism or amaurotic idiocy which, by analogy with animals, is to be expected in one-quarter of the progeny of unions between two heterozygotes of normal appearance. We have in general no evidence that a pair of parents is heterozygous, except that they have produced at least one recessive. We cannot therefore study the progeny of a number of pairs of known heterozygotes, as we can in animal experiments. We can only study the progeny of those pairs which have produced at least one recessive.

Clearly the frequency of recessives in such sibships* is greater that the expected quarter. For it is 100 % in sibship of one, and over 50 % in sibships of two. The method for assessing the frequency p which would be found in a very large sibship from data on small ones depends on how the data are collected.

Let a_{rs} be the number of sibships of s members, of which r are abnormal.

Let $t_s = \sum_r a_{rs}$, i.e. the total number of sibships of s members.

Let $N = \sum_{r,s} a_{rs}$, i.e. the total number of sibships.

Let $R = \sum_{r,s} (ra_{rs})$, i.e. the total number of abnormals.

Let $S = \sum_{r,s} (sa_{rs})$, i.e. the total number of sibs.

Let $q = 1-p$.

Now consider two ideal cases. In the first case a whole population is surveyed, and all sibships containing at least one abnormal are tabulated. This is possible in a small European country. Thus Sjögren (1931) probably tabulated over 90 % of the Swedish families in which a case of juvenile amaurotic idiocy had occurred in the twentieth century. In this case the estimate of p is given by:

$$\frac{R}{p} = \sum_s \left[\frac{st_s}{1-q^s}\right],$$

* The word sibship means a set of siblings, that is to say brothers and/or sisters.

and its standard error is given by:

$$\sigma_p^{-2} = \frac{R}{p^2 q} - \frac{1}{q^2}\sum_s \left[\frac{s q^s t_s}{(1-q^s)^2}\right].$$

Unfortunately, this cumbrous equation, due to Haldane (1938), can be shown to yield a result with a smaller standard error than a simpler one due to Weinberg. Perhaps a quicker but equally efficient method may be devised.

In the second ideal case all children leaving school in a certain year, or better all children born in a certain 6 months, are examined. The sibs of all abnormal children are tabulated. Clearly if a sibship contains three abnormals, it is three times as likely to be tabulated as if it contains only one, and so on, apart from an obvious correction for twins. In this case the estimate of p is

$$p = \frac{R-N}{T-N}, \quad \text{and} \quad \sigma_p^2 = \frac{(T-R)(R-N)}{(T-N)^3},$$

an elegant result due to Weinberg (1927).

Applying these methods to Pearson, Nettleship & Usher's (1913) collection of 411 sibships from normal parents including at least one albino, 864 out of 2435, or 35·48 %, were albinos.

Applying the first correction

$$p_1 = 0{\cdot}3082 \pm 0{\cdot}0107,$$

applying the second $\quad p_2 = 0{\cdot}2238 \pm 0{\cdot}0092.$

The Mendelian value of $\frac{1}{4}$ lies between these two estimates, and there is reason to think that if an exact correction were possible, the Mendelian ratio would be found. A simple example will show the need for other corrections. According to Andreassen (1943), in the year 1941 there were 1,820,000 males in Denmark, of whom 81 were haemophilic. Almost all their families were investigated, and valuable results were obtained. However, haemophilics have a much shorter average life than ordinary males (about 18 years in Denmark). So a large fraction, probably the majority, of the haemophilics born between 1910 and 1930 were dead by 1942. A family into which three haemophilics were born in that time was more likely to contain a living haemophilic in 1942 than one into which only one was born. But it was not exactly three times as likely. If half the haemophilics had died, and there was no correlation in the age of death between haemophilic sibs, it was 1·75 times as likely. Hence the true value of p would lie somewhere between the two extreme estimates. Special methods could and should be developed for such cases.

They are important because they offer a possibility of investigating selective prenatal death, of verifying the general applicability of genetical principles to man, and of developing, in comparatively simple cases, the quite peculiar statistical methods which are required when the genotypes of parents must be deduced from the phenotype of the children, with an accuracy which increases with the size of the sibship. These methods may be said to play the same part in human genetics that standard culture methods play in animal and plant genetics. Without them qualitative conclusions may be drawn, but quantitative work is impossible in the case of many genes.

We now pass to the methods for the location of genes on the human chromosomes. A serious beginning has been made with the mapping of two sections. One is the segment of the *X* chromosome which is responsible for sex determination, in which the ordinary sex-linked genes are located. The other is the segment common to the *X* and *Y* chromosomes. With regard to the remaining twenty-three there is fairly good, but never conclusive, evidence, for the compresence in one chromosome of two genes. For each type of location appropriate statistical methods have been developed.

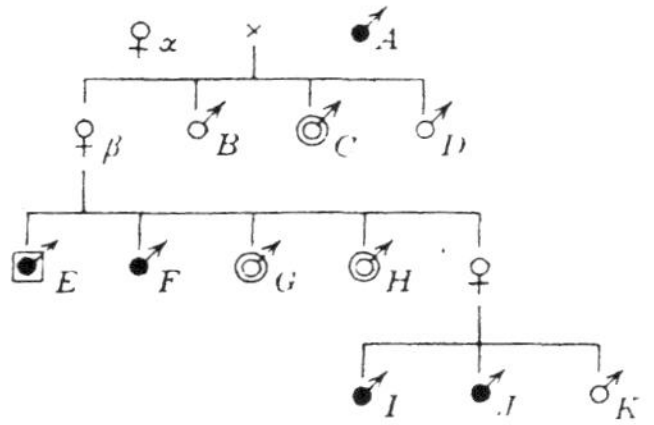

FIGURE 1. ♂, normal male; deuteranopic male, not haemophilic; haemophilic male, vision untested; haemophilic trichromatic male.

Let us begin with the differential segment of the *X*. A large number of sex-linked recessive genes have been located there. The mode of inheritance of the characters determined by them is highly characteristic. The abnormality determined by any one of them is far commoner in men than women. It is not transmitted from a father to his son. But it occurs in about half the sons of heterozygous women, who include the daughters of affected men. The *X* chromosomes of *Drosophila* species have been mapped by studying the segregation of genes in the progeny of mothers who are heterozygous for two or more pairs of sex-linked allelomorphs.

Cytological studies have shown that the maps so obtained depict real material structures, as X-ray diffraction and reflexion have shown that the structural formulae of the organic chemist depict real objects.

At one locus in the human *X* chromosome abnormalities are very common. About 8 % of all men are colour-blind or anomalous colour-matchers. Hence if we wish to estimate the percentage of recombination between the loci of haemophilia and colour-blindness we must search for colour-blindness among haemophilics and their brothers. Seventeen pedigrees are known in which both abnormalities are found. Of the total information available from them, about a third was collected by Bell & Haldane (1936), another third by the Dutch physician Hoogvliet (1942) and the remainder by five others.

The method employed can be illustrated by two simple examples. Figure 1 shows a pedigree in which A was a haemophilic, while α carried the gene for colour-blindness in one of her two X chromosomes. She also gave it to β, who had two colour-blind sons. So β had the genes for these two defects in different chromosomes (in the *trans* position, if we like a metaphor from organic chemistry, or in repulsion in Bateson & Punnett's terminology). Of β's three surviving sons, one was a haemophilic trichromat; two were colour-blind, but had normal blood. Now if x is the frequency of recombination between the two loci concerned, the probability of β producing just these three sons is $(1-x)^3$, given that she had one haemophilic and two non-haemophilics. If one of the non-haemophilics had had normal vision it would have been $x(1-x)^2$, and so on. On this pedigree taken alone the best estimate of x is clearly zero.

Figure 2, which is part of Bell & Haldane's (1937) pedigree A, of 98 members, raises a rather more subtle problem.

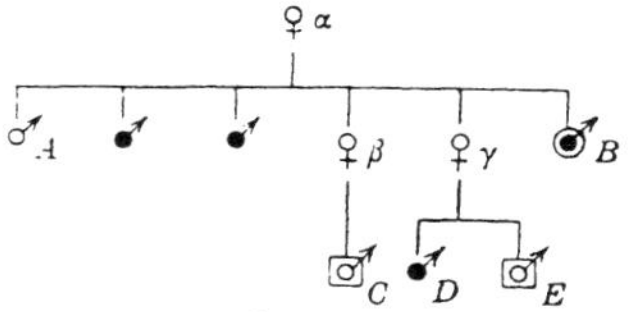

FIGURE 2. ♂, normal male; ♂, haemophilic male, vision untested; ♂, trichromatic male, not haemophilic; ♂, haemophilic deuteranopic male.

This was solved approximately by Bell & Haldane (1936), but my colleague Dr Smith has produced a more accurate method (Haldane & Smith 1947). We ask what is the probability that seven persons related in the manner shown should have just these phenotypes. If p_c and p_h are the frequencies of the genes **c** and **h** for colour-blindness and haemophilia, we ask what is the probability that α should have been heterozygous for both of them. Clearly it is $4p_c(1-p_c)p_h(1-p_h)$. If α was doubly heterozygous and her husband normal, there are eight possible sets of events in the formation of ova by α, β, and γ which could have given the observed results. They are shown in figure 3 and the probability of each is given, putting $y = 1-x$. It is the product of five factors representing the probabilities of the formation of five different eggs. These are shown in each case. Since γ had a haemophilic son who died in infancy we know that she received the gene **h** from her mother. This excludes sixteen other possibilities whose probability is zero. It does not exhaust the possibilities. For though we can be sure that neither α nor her husband was haemophilic, we cannot be sure that one or both of them was not colour-blind. So the total probability has two more terms, each containing p_c^2. It is

$$\tfrac{1}{8}p_c p_h[3(1-p_c)(1-2x+4x^2-4x^3+x^4)+p_c(x^2-x^4)].$$

Since p_c is of the order of 0·01 it can in practice be neglected in this case, but not in all cases.

The corresponding expression for the pedigree of figure 1 is

$$2^{-11} p_c p_h (1-x)^3.$$

These probabilities are of course small, partly because the genes in question are rare, partly because the particular pattern of segregation found is one of a vast number which are possible, like the 635,013,559,600 equiprobable bridge hands. However, each is maximal for some value of x between 0 and 1 inclusive: in the cases considered, for $x = 0$. In other pedigrees a cross-over has occurred, i.e. the genes **c** and **h** have entered a woman in one gamete and left her in different ones or vice versa. In these the polynomial is maximal for some other value of x. The product of the seventeen polynomials derived from the different pedigrees is maximal when $x = 0{\cdot}098$, and we may estimate the frequency of recombination between the two loci as $9{\cdot}8 \pm 4{\cdot}2$ %.

White (1940) found $64{\cdot}8 \pm 12{\cdot}7$ % of recombination between the loci of colour-blindness and of myopia with nystagmus, so the genetical map of the human X chromosome is likely to be as long as that of *Drosophila melanogaster*, though probably shorter than that of *Gallus domesticus*.

Ten years ago I accounted for the peculiar inheritance of certain characters on the hypothesis that the genes concerned in their determination were located in that segment of the sex chromosomes which is common to the X and Y, and may be exchanged between them (Haldane 1936). Such genes are said to be partially sex-linked.

At that time I put forward the hypothesis with considerable misgiving, but it has been generally accepted, and I shall therefore state it with comparative confidence. Penrose (1946*b*) has recently given an alternative explanation for some cases which appear to conform to it, but he does not think that this will explain all the cases. First, consider a dominant gene in this segment. If a woman has it, necessarily in an X chromosome, she will transmit it, on an average, to half her children, regardless of sex. If a man has it in his Y, he has inherited it from his father, and will probably transmit it to most of his sons but a few of his daughters. If he has it in his X he has inherited it from his mother, and will transmit it to most of his daughters but a few of his sons. Thus the sex of the affected children of affected males will generally be the same as that of the affected paternal grandparent. The fewer the exceptions, the nearer the locus to the differential segments containing the sex determiners, and (in the X) the loci of such genes as haemophilia.

Only one such partially sex-linked dominant is known, namely retinitis pigmentosa in some pedigrees. Penrose (1946*b*) has, I think disproved Pipkin & Pipkin's (1945) claim to have found a second such, zygodactyly, or webbing of the toes. It is possible that my own claim in the case of retinitis pigmentosa will equally be disproved.

The location of partially sex-linked recessives is not so simple, but I think some of its results are more certain. Where the parents are first cousins, the sex of the affected offspring is usually the same as that of the paternal grandparent through whom the parents are related. For if this grandparent was a male the father carries the gene in his Y chromosome, and will transmit it predominantly to his sons, as in figure 4. If she was a female they will mostly be daughters. If the parents are not known to be related, we can only say that in any particular sibship the affected members will be predominantly of one sex, though in all sibships together no such predominance is to be expected, except in the case of very rare conditions where the parents are mostly consanguineous.

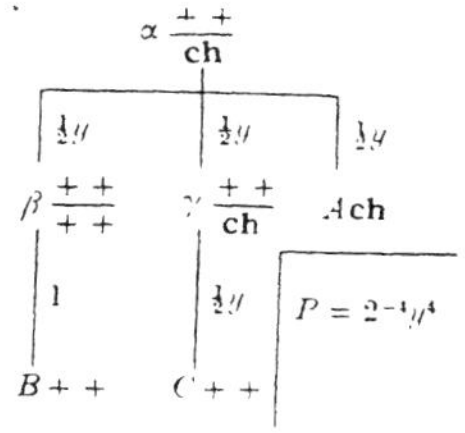

1.

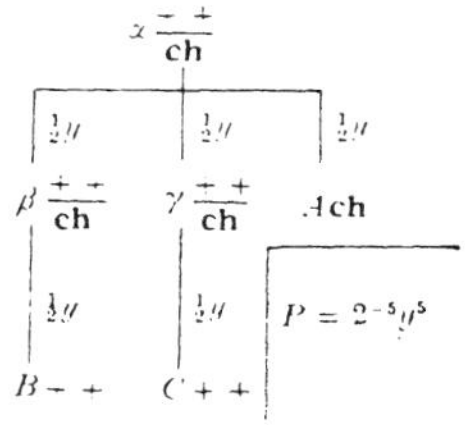

2.

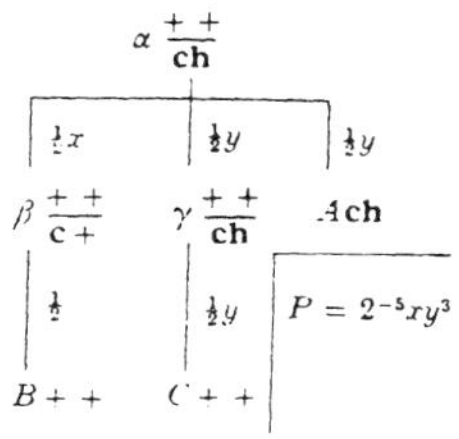

3.

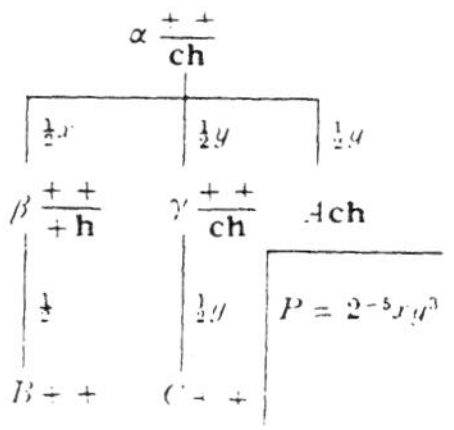

4.

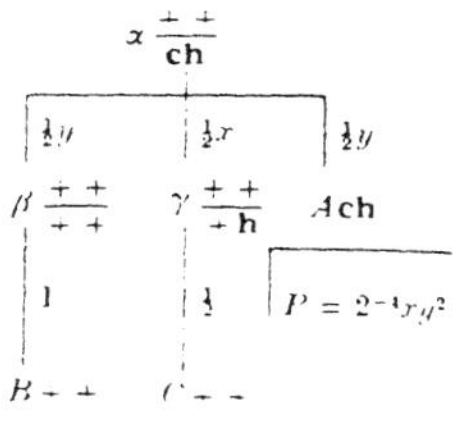

5.

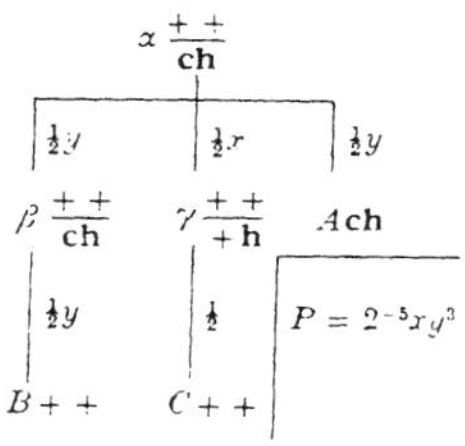

6.

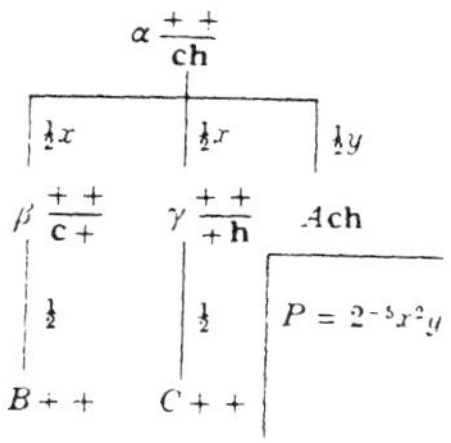

7.

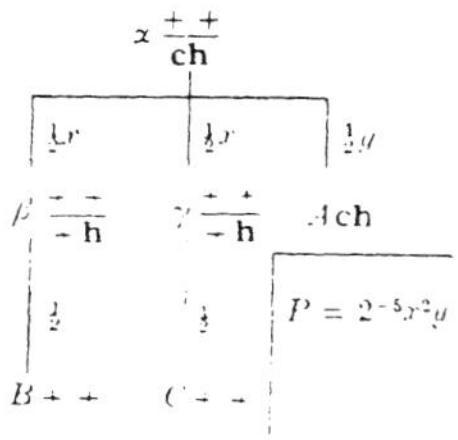

8.

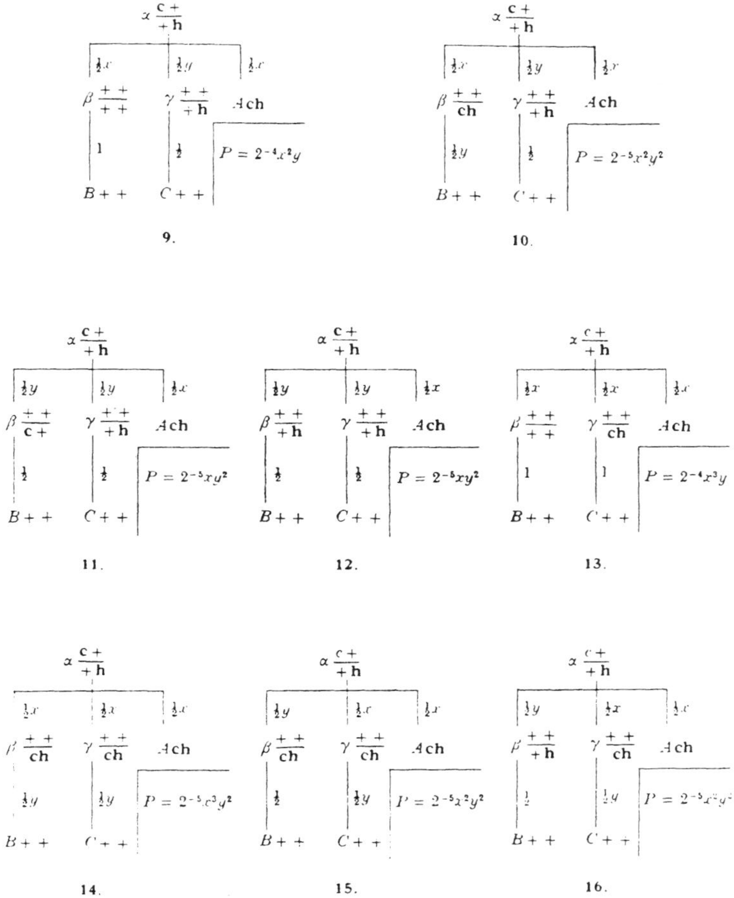

FIGURE 3. Sixteen possible explanations of the pedigree of figure 2. In each case the probability of the five different steps is given, together with their product. The overall probability is the sum of these products, multiplied by the probability that **c** and **h** should be compresent in α.

Fisher (1936) developed a most elegant method for the detection of partial sex-linkage in such cases. Suppose a sibship consists of N normal females, n normal males, A affected females, a affected males, and that

$$u = (N - n - 3A + 3a)^2 - (N + n + 9A + 9a),$$

then in the absence of partial sex-linkage the expected value of u is zero, in its presence it is $\frac{1}{9}k(1 - 2x)^2$, where $k = (N + n + 9A + 9a)^2 - (N + n - 81A + 81a)$, and x is the frequency of recombination. Thus if the sum of a large number of u values is significantly positive partial sex-linkage can be inferred, and its intensity estimated.

I have since shown (Haldane 1948) that if we calculate a polynomial for each sibship on the lines developed for the investigation of linkage between sex-linked genes, its logarithm can be expressed as a series in ascending powers of $(1 - 2x)^2$. The coefficient of $(1 - 2x)^2$ is Fisher's u. Thus the sum of Fisher's u scores gives a perfect test for the presence of linkage, though not a quite unbiased estimate of its intensity. There is, however, a further complication. In the absence of linkage the sampling distribution of Σu is not normal, but positively skew. So a high positive value gives a rather exaggerated estimate of the significance of the evidence for linkage. When allowance is made for this (Haldane 1946) most, but not quite all, of the data formerly regarded as significant remain so.

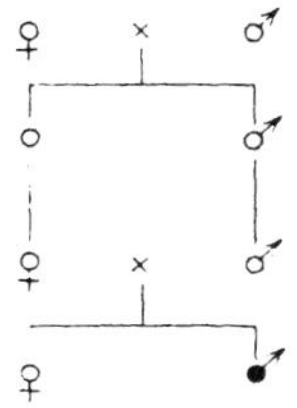

FIGURE 4. ♂, male homozygous for a partially sex-linked recessive. The sex of his maternal grandparent is irrelevant.

The Croonian Lecture was originally intended to be on 'local motion', and I shall therefore illustrate recessive partial sex-linkage by discussing spastic paraplegia, a disease in which the tonus of the limb muscles gradually increases until walking becomes impossible. Bell (1939) collected forty-four pedigrees in which one or more children of normal parents were affected with this disease.

Applying Fisher's method we have $\Sigma u = 1256 \pm 231$, and the estimated frequency of recombination is $17 \cdot 5\,\%$. The significance is not as high as it appears, since the sampling distribution in the absence of linkage is very skew positively. But it is not in doubt. It is wholly possible that while most of the families are segregating for a partially sex-linked gene, others are segregating for an autosomal one. To determine whether this is so, about five times the present number of families would be required, and it would be necessary to devise new statistical methods. There is also a suggestion, both from the results of the direct method applied to the progeny of cousin marriages, and the indirect method based on Fisher's 'u' scores, that a few cases diagnosed as spastic ataxia, and perhaps even as Friedreich's ataxia, may be due to partially sex-linked genes. The large majority are not (Haldane 1941 a).

On the basis of such statistical work I located seven genes on this segment. The standard errors of their distances are so large that I do not think that a map is worth publishing. However, the loci of dominant and recessive genes for retinitis pigmentosa, probably allelomorphs, lie about 30 units from the sex-determining or differential segment, while the loci of five other genes, namely those for achromatopsia, epidermolysis bullosa, xeroderma pigmentosum, spastic paraplegia, and Oguchi's disease, seem to lie between 21 and 44 units from it. In addition a lethal gene for convulsive seizures with mental deterioration is probably located in this segment (Snyder & Palmer 1943) while a gene concerned in some cases of hare-lip and cleft-palate may be so (Philip & Mather 1940).

The next step in this investigation will perhaps be the discovery of families in which colour-blindness is segregating along with a partially sex-linked gene such as those for spastic paraplegia or xeroderma pigmentosum. In the latter case in particular we should be able to detect linkage in doubly heterozygous females between genes in the two segments of the *X*, and thus to produce a unified map. Even more valuable would be the discovery of a gene as common as those for colour-blindness and anomalous matching, in either section of the *X* chromosome. The most hopeful field for such a discovery is among the antigens.

I have deliberately restricted my own work on human linkage to the sex chromosomes, because in every satisfactory pedigree sex as well as abnormality is recorded. Other workers more industrious than myself have looked for linkage between autosomal genes. Since man has twenty-three pairs of autosomes, the probability that a particular pair of loci will lie in the same chromosome is of the order of $\frac{1}{23}$, though rather more, because the chromosomes are of unequal size. On the other hand a recombination value of over 25 % is unlikely to be detected until data accumulate in very considerable quantity.

Two genes are very possibly linked with those for the blood-group antigens. These are the recessive gene for phenylketonuria (Penrose 1946*a*) and the partially dominant gene for allergy (Finney 1940; see also Finney 1941, 1942). A phenylketonuric apparently lacks some enzyme concerned in the metabolism of phenylalanine, and consequently excretes up to 1 g./day of phenylpyruvic acid. As a further consequence there is a shortage of material for melanin formation, and the hair is of a lighter colour than that of other members of the family. Far more important, thought is impossible. Phenylketonurics are usually idiots or imbeciles, at best feeble-minded.

Penrose (1946*a*) has developed a statistical method for dealing with such cases, when the children in a family can be examined, but the parents cannot. Consider a series of sibships in which some members are normal, others are phenylketonurics, some have the *B* antigen, i.e. belong to group *B* or *AB*, others belong to other groups. Consider what is to be expected if the loci concerned are on the same chromosome. In some sibships the recessive genes for phenylketonuria and absence of *B* antigen have been in the same chromosome in both parents. In these, the sibs who are phenylketonurics will probably not possess antigen *B*, or more accurately, will be less likely than normals to possess it. If the genes are in different chromosomes in one or both parents, those who are phenylketonurics will probably possess antigen *B*. Over a group of sibships there will be no association between the two characters, but in any particular sibship they will be positively or negatively associated.

Now if we observe any pair of sibs, they must fall into one of the nine categories of table 6.

TABLE 6. THE NINE POSSIBLE TYPES OF SIB-PAIRS IN A SIBSHIP SEGREGATING FOR THE B ANTIGEN AND PHENYLKETONURIA. EXPLANATION IN TEXT

	BB	Bb	bb	total
NN	$a_{11}+$	$a_{12}-$	$a_{13}+$	c_1
NP	$a_{21}-$	$a_{22}+$	$a_{23}-$	c_2
PP	$a_{31}+$	$a_{32}-$	$a_{33}+$	c_3
total	b_1	b_2	b_3	1

Here N and P denote normality and phenylketonuria B and b the presence and absence of the B antigen. Thus a pair of sibs of whom one is normal and one phenylketonuric, but both belong to group O, falls into the category $NP.bb$. If the two gene pairs are located in different chromosomes the expected number E_{23} of sib-pairs in this category will be the product of the numbers of NP pairs and bb pairs, divided by the total, that is to say $b_3 c_2 s$. If they are in the same chromosome it will be less. In general, linkage will increase the numbers in the categories labelled + in table 6, and diminish it in the remainder. Penrose (1946*a*) found the figures of table 7.

TABLE 7. NUMBERS OF SIB-PAIR TYPES FOUND BY PENROSE, WITH EXPECTATIONS IN THE ABSENCE OF LINKAGE

	BB		Bb		bb		total
NN	17	(9·125)	11	(16·947)	89	(90·928)	117
NP	10	(15·365)	34	(28·535)	153	(153·100)	197
PP	1	(3·510)	7	(6·518)	37	(34·972)	45
total	28		52		279		359

In this table the bracketed numbers are the expectations in the absence of linkage. Thus $9{\cdot}125 = \dfrac{117 \times 28}{359}$. In the absence of linkage, Penrose finds that

$$\xi = \left[\frac{a_{11}}{E_{11}} + \frac{a_{13}}{E_{13}} + \frac{a_{31}}{E_{31}} + \frac{a_{33}}{E_{33}} + \frac{4a_{22}}{E_{22}} - \frac{2a_{12}}{E_{12}} - \frac{2a_{21}}{E_{21}} - \frac{2a_{23}}{E_{23}} - \frac{2a_{32}}{E_{32}}\right] \div \left[s\left(\frac{1}{b_1} + \frac{4}{b_2} + \frac{1}{b_3}\right)\left(\frac{1}{c_1} + \frac{4}{c_2} + \frac{1}{c_3}\right)\right]^{\frac{1}{2}}$$

is normally distributed with mean zero and unit variance. A positive value indicates linkage. In this case the value is $-1{\cdot}51$ which is not in itself significant. But Penrose informed me that when the O antigen and the two forms of the A antigen are also taken into consideration, the value rises to 1·78. Since this is in the direction expected on theoretical grounds, the probability of obtaining so large a value by chance is 0·046 or one in twenty-two. Such a value is usually taken as on the borderline of significance A few more families may well establish this linkage conclusively.

Finney (1940) used modifications of Fisher's *u* statistics, and concluded from Zieve, Wiener & Fries' (1936) data that the gene for allergy was linked with those for the blood groups. However, it must be emphasized that the genetics of allergy are not so simple as those of phenylketonuria. The probability of obtaining so large a deviation in the expected direction is 0·04, after correcting for skewness. His result and Penrose's are weaker evidence for linkage than appears at first sight because man has twenty-three pairs of autosomes, so the *a priori* probability of linkage is only about 0·04. This means that considerably stronger evidence for linkage is required than in *Drosophila melanogaster* where the *a priori* probability is about 0·5.

Burks (1939) published preliminary results which very strongly suggest linkage between genes for hair colour and defective teeth. Unfortunately only a statistical summary was given, and as I have pointed out elsewhere (Haldane 1941*b*) other explanations besides linkage are possible, though perhaps not very likely. She also obtained evidence of linkage between genes for myopia and eye colour. Penrose (1935) and Rife (1941) obtained suggestions of linkage between blood groups and hair colour, and interdigital pattern and left-handedness respectively.

Finally, Kloepfer (1946) has made a most comprehensive study involving nineteen characters, and obtained evidence suggesting a number of linkages. The most impressive are those between eye colour and flare (or projection) of the ears, and between ability to taste phenyl-thio-urea and ear size. Unfortunately nothing is yet known as to the genetics of ear size and structure.

Finally, there is massive negative evidence showing that various genes, notably those for blood groups, blood types (*M* and *N*), and ability to taste phenyl-thio-urea, are not linked with one another nor with sex. Such work is inevitably tedious, but it is striking how long a time elapsed before linkage was discovered in poultry or peas, and how rapidly knowledge accumulated once the first linkages were discovered.

Up till now we have considered the behaviour of genes in so far as they reproduce their like (or perhaps better, are copied exactly) at each nuclear division. When this does not happen, a new type of gene arises which generally, but by no means always, reduces the fitness of the organism either (*a*) at once, if it is a dominant; (*b*) when it appears in a male, if it is a sex-linked recessive; or (*c*) when two genes of the new type are contributed by different parents to the same zygote, if it is an autosomal recessive. This process of change is called mutation. Clearly it may be due to a failure of the copying process, or to a change induced in the model between copyings by physical means such as X-rays or chemical means such as $\beta\beta'$-dichlorethyl disulphide. Mutation occurs spontaneously, that is to say under normal conditions, in all organisms so far studied; but as it is a rare process, it can only be measured when vast numbers are available. The rate was first measured in *Drosophila melanogaster*, then in *Zea Mays*, and finally by Gunther & Penrose (1935) and Haldane (1935) in man. More exact estimates, fully confirming these figures, have been made in Denmark in the last 6 years.

The rate can be measured directly, as was done by Mørch (1941) for achondroplasia, or chondrodystrophy. This is the condition found in the familiar short-legged type of dwarf. In 1938 there were eighty-six such dwarfs in Denmark among 3,800,000 people. They have a very low fertility, but when they breed, about half their offspring are similar dwarfs. The large majority of dwarfs, however, are the offspring of normal parents with no dwarfs in their families. It is clear that the gene for dwarfism arises sporadically by mutation. Out of 132,761 children born of normal parents in hospitals in Copenhagen and Lund over a period of 21 years, eleven were dwarfs of this type. This gives a mutation rate of $4{\cdot}1 \times 10^{-5} \pm 1{\cdot}2 \times 10^{-5}$ per normal gene per generation, or about $1{\cdot}2 \times 10^{-6}$ per year, since the mean age of normal parents is 35 years. The probability that the true value should be as low as 10^{-5} per generation is 0·0011, the probability that it should be as high as 10^{-4} is 0·0001, so the order of magnitude is certain.

Mørch also estimated the mutation frequency indirectly. Most such dwarfs die at or within 2 days of birth, and a number more in the first year of life, but after this their expectation of life is normal. If 80 % die in the first year, which is his estimate, there would be 415 such dwarfs in Denmark but for this mortality, or a frequency of $1{\cdot}09 \times 10^{-4}$. Now 108 dwarfs had 27 children, and their 457 normal sibs had 582, thus their fitness from a Darwinian point of view is $\frac{27}{108} \times \frac{457}{582}$, or $f = 0{\cdot}204$. That is to say in each generation natural selection effectively eliminates 80 % of the dominant genes, and but for mutation there would be no dwarfs left on earth within seven generations, or say two centuries, if Danish figures are typical. However, the two processes are in approximate equilibrium. So if x is the frequency at birth, the mutation rate $\mu = \frac{1}{2}(1-f)x = 4{\cdot}3 \times 10^{-5}$. The factor $\frac{1}{2}$ arises because we are dealing with a population of chromosomes equal to twice the population of human beings. The two estimates agree very well, but the second is much less accurate, since it depends on the figure for the infant mortality. Mørch, using a rather different argument, gets $4{\cdot}8 \times 10^{-5}$.

Professor Penrose has pointed out to me that Mørch's data are open to three criticisms. In some pedigrees, though not in any of those which he collected, there is evidence that the gene for achondroplasia can fail to manifest itself, as in Richsbieth's (1912) pedigree 608. The cases where two normal parents had more than one achondroplasic child may be due to this cause or to a mutation at an early stage in the development of a gonad. A correction for this possibility makes very little difference to the estimate of the mutation rate, since the gene is detected on its first appearance, even if this be occasionally delayed. Secondly, Mørch did not personally examine all the infants, and it is possible that some may have been wrongly diagnosed. This is plausible, since he himself failed to confirm the diagnosis of achondroplasia made by another worker in a Norwegian family. Finally, the frequency increases with parental age to an extent inexplicable if all the dwarfs born of normal parents are mutants, but explicable if some of them are due to bad prenatal conditions, as with mongoloid imbeciles. It may therefore well be that Mørch's figure is too high. But the true value is almost certainly above 10^{-5}.

For most diseases only the indirect method is available. Andreassen (1943) has applied it to haemophilia in Denmark. However, I believe (Haldane 1947b) that his calculations give rather too low a result. Haemophilia is due to a sex-linked recessive gene. Hence only about one-third of the genes for haemophilia in a population are exposed to natural selection at any moment. More accurately, if μ and ν are the mutation rate in the female and male sexes respectively,

$$2\mu + \nu = (1 - f)x,$$

where x is the frequency in males at birth. Now there were just eighty-one haemophilics alive in Denmark in 1941, and their mean life is 18 years compared with 55 for Danes in general. So $x = 1{\cdot}33 \times 10^{-4}$. The fitness f, that is to say the mean number of progeny, compared with that of the population in general, appears to be 0·28. I have criticized Andreassen's much higher figure, $f = 0{\cdot}59$. It follows that $2\mu + \nu = 9{\cdot}6 \times 10^{-4}$, or a mean mutation rate of $3{\cdot}2 \times 10^{-4}$. Now if the mutation rates were equal in the two sexes, i.e. $\mu = \nu$, nearly a third of all haemophilics would be single cases due to mutation in homozygous mothers. Andreassen has shown that the gene for haemophilia is not completely recessive. Heterozygous women sometimes bleed abnormally, but always have an abnormally long coagulation time, by which they can be detected. Using this technique he has not yet found a case where the mother of a haemophilic was homozygous. Doubtless such a case will be found. But it can be concluded that ν is much larger than μ, very likely ten times as large. If this is correct we should have, very roughly, $\nu = 8 \times 10^{-5}$, and $\mu = 8 \times 10^{-6}$.

Similar estimates are available for three other conditions. Gunther & Penrose (1935) found $4\text{–}8 \times 10^{-6}$ for epiloia, Philip & Sorsby (unpublished) found $1{\cdot}4 \times 10^{-5}$ for retinoblastoma, and Møllenbach (according to Kemp 1944) finds $5\text{–}10 \times 10^{-6}$ for aniridia (Kemp's figure of double this value appears to be the mutation rate per zygote, not per gene). The median rate is about 10^{-5}. Unfortunately, this method cannot be applied to autosomal recessive conditions.

Pätau & Nachtsheim (1946) have estimated the mutation rate of the autosomal dominant gene *Pg* which is responsible for the Pelger anomaly, a failure of segmentation of the nuclei of polymorphonuclear leucocytes. *Pg* + individuals are thought to be less resistant to disease than $+/+$, whilst by analogy with rabbits, it is suggested that *Pg*/*Pg* is a lethal genotype. However, too little is known as to the viability of heterozygotes to allow an indirect estimate of the mutation frequency. The authors estimated the frequency of the condition as 0·001, and found that out of twelve persons showing the Pelger anomaly, and both of whose parents could be examined, one parent was affected in ten cases, neither in two cases. This gives a mutation rate of $\frac{1}{2} \times 10^{-3} \times \frac{2}{12}$, or 8×10^{-5}. Even if the frequency were accurately known, and if 120 cases had been examined instead of twelve, this estimate would be somewhat high, simply because the cases with both parents living are a selected group, and include a higher fraction of cases with normal parents than of those with one affected. However, the order of magnitude agrees well with the figures given above, and is unlikely to be incorrect by a power of ten.

It is certain that these figures are not representative. Consider a well-known and unmistakable dominant such as lobster claw. Five families with this gene are known

11-2

in England. They are quite fertile, but presumably their fitness, or net fertility, is a little below the average, or the condition would be commoner. Lewis & Embleton's (1908) pedigree goes back to a son of allegedly normal parents born in 1793. In the case of such a conspicuous abnormality mutation is a far likelier explanation than adultery. But it is extremely doubtful whether the mutation occurs in Britain once in 10 years. Five isolated cases were described in Britain between 1895 and 1918. That is to say its mutation frequency is of the order of 10^{-7} per generation. This is probably a much more representative figure than those of 10^{-5} or over. Unfortunately, the indirect method becomes quite unreliable when, as in this case, the fitness is near unity. Finally, we have such cases as that of the 'porcupine men' of the Lambert family (literature, see Cockayne 1933), a most striking dominant mutation, perhaps a translocation, carried by the *Y* chromosome. This has only been recorded once, and would have stood a good chance of being recorded in any civilized country, in the last 2000 years. It was twice described in the *Philosophical Transactions* of this Society. The mutation rate is probably below 10^{-10}.

A man or woman consists of about 2^{48} cells, that is to say a representative cell is separated from the fertilized ovum by about fifty mitoses. The primordial ova are all formed at birth, and do not undergo further mitoses. A man may produce 2^{40} spermatozoa in a lifetime, so the mean number of mitoses is somewhat greater in the male than the female germ-line, but probably not over 100 in the former.

Thus a mutation rate even of the order of 10^{-4} means that the gene-copying process, at worst, goes wrong about once in a million times, whether as the result of a failure of copying, or of a change in between two copying processes. A similar degree of accuracy in crystal growth would give a crystal with under ten flaws per millimetre, and 10^{10} successive flawless layers would give a perfect crystal several metres in length. The living substance of our bodies is clearly far more accurately copied than the successive layers of a crystal.

In *Drosophila* the natural mutation rate is of the order of 10^{-6} to 10^{-5} per generation for the more mutable loci, such as that whose mutation produces a white eye, and considerably lower for the stabler genes. Natural mutation is increased about threefold by a rise of 10° C, and is therefore largely due to a chemical reaction. As a generation in *Drosophila melanogaster* takes about 10 days and a fly contains about 2^{23} cells, while the mutation rate of the more labile genes is about one-fifth of that of man per generation, it follows that human mutation rates are about twice those of *Drosophila* per nuclear division, and about one two-hundredth of those of *Drosophila* per day, though the body temperature is about 13° higher. It has been calculated that natural radiations and particles of high energy will account for only 0·001 of the mutations in *Drosophila*. It is clear that if so they may account for about a fifth of those in man, and in view of the uncertainty of our knowledge as to the efficiency of particles from K^{40} and cosmic rays in producing mutations, and the different radiosensitivity of different genes, it is quite possible that radiation may account for most human mutation. Mørch found that the rate of mutation to achondroplasia increased with age, but it was not clear whether maternal or paternal age was most important. If this finding is confirmed it suggests a cumulative effect, either of radiation, or of successive nuclear divisions, during a lifetime. The apparently higher rate in males suggests that the number of nuclear divisions may be an important factor in human mutation. To sum up, there are three possible known causes of mutation, a chemical reaction with a temperature coefficient, radiation, and imperfections of copying, which might have a positive or negative temperature coefficient. The first predominates in *Drosophila*, the second or third probably does so in man. There must be about a thousand achondroplasic dwarfs in Britain. If the ages of their parents at their births were determined, it would be possible to decide between these alternatives, since the egg of a woman of 45 has undergone no more nuclear divisions than that of a girl of 15. It is worth remarking that it is quite practicable to obtain data of this kind on populations of 40 million human beings, and wholly impracticable to do so on 40 million of any other mammal.

The mutation rate is probably more or less adaptive. Too high a mutation rate would flood a species with undesirable mutations, too low a one would probably slow down evolution. Man and *Drosophila melanogaster* have about the same rate per generation, and this could not be increased ten times without a very great loss of fitness (Haldane 1937). Other species such as five species of *Sciara* (Metz 1938) have far lower rates per generation though not necessarily less than the human rate per day. But it is doubtful whether the human rate could be lowered much further, since a substantial fraction of it is due to natural radiation. In fact a very great prolongation of human life, or at any rate of the reproductive period, might be incompatible with the survival of the human species.

I hope that, in this brief survey, I have shown that human genetics has reached the stage when it can claim to be a branch of biology with its own peculiar problems and methods. I have only dealt with a few of them. This lecture could equally well have been devoted to the human antigenic structure, to human prenatal physiology, or to variation in human sensory and intellectual capacity, all of which a human geneticist must study. If I have confined myself to the more quantitative aspects, my excuse must be that in dealing with a branch of science where erroneous views may have important political consequences, in such a lecture as this it is desirable to concentrate on those problems where political or social bias is least likely to be effective, and where we may hope to raise a solid theoretical structure by methods like those which have been fruitful in the other branches of science.

References

Andreassen, M. 1943 Haemofili i Danmark. *Opera ex domo biologiae hereditariae humanae Universitatis Hafniensis*, **6** (Copenhagen).

Avery, O. T., Macleod, C. M. & MacCarty, M. 1944 *J. Exp. Med.* **79**, 137–157.

Bateson, W. 1906 *Brain*, pt. 2, pp. 157–179.

Bell, J. & Haldane, J. B. S. 1936 *Proc. Roy. Soc.* B, **123**, 119–150.

Bell, J. 1939 *Treas. Hum. Inher.* **4**, pt. 3.

Birch, C. L. 1937 *Illinois Med. Dent. Monogr.* **1**, 4.

Burks, B. 1939 *Proc. Nat. Acad. Sci., Wash.*, **24**, 512–514.

Bläurock, G. 1932 *Münch. Med. Wschr.* **74**, 1552–1556.

Clausen, J. 1932 *Hospitalstidende*, **75**, 196–206.

Cockayne, F. A. 1933 *Inherited abnormalities of the skin and its appendages.* Oxford: University Press.

Crome, W. 1933 *Dtsch. Z. ges. gerichtl. Med.* **21**, 435–450.

Dahr, P. & Bussmann, R. 1938 *Dtsch. Med. Wschr.* **64**, 818–821.

Dahr, P. 1940 *Z. ImmunForsch.* **97**, 168–188.

Ephrussi, B. 1942 *Cold Spring Harbor Symp.* **10**, 40–48.

Finney, D. J. 1940 *Ann. Eugen.* **10**, 171–214.

Finney, D. J. 1941 *Ann. Eugen.* **11**, 10–30, 115–135.

Finney, D. J. 1942 *Ann. Eugen.* **11**, 224–244.

Fisher, R. A. 1936 *Ann. Eugen.* **7**, 87–104.

Gunther, E. R. & Penrose, L. S. 1935 *J. Genet.* **31**, 413–430.

Haldane, J. B. S. 1935 *J. Genet.* **31**, 317–326.

Haldane, J. B. S. 1936 *Ann. Eugen.* **7**, 28–57.

Haldane, J. B. S. 1937*a* *J. Hered.* **28**, 58–60.

Haldane, J. B. S. 1937*b* *Amer. Nat.* **71**, 337–348.

Haldane, J. B. S. 1938 *Ann. Eugen.* **8**, 255–262.

Haldane, J. B. S. 1941*a* *J. Genet.* **41**, 141–144.

Haldane, J. B. S. 1941*b* *New paths in genetics.* London: Allen and Unwin.

Haldane, J. B. S. 1946 *Ann. Eugen.* **13**, 122–134.

Haldane, J. B. S. 1947 *Ann. Eugen.* **13**, 262–271.

Haldane, J. B. S. 1948 Unpublished.

Haldane, J. B. S. & Smith, C. A. B. 1947 *Ann. Eugen.* **14**, 10–31.

Holford, F. F. 1938 *J. Infect. Dis.* **63**, 287–297.

Hirszfeld L. & Kostuch Z. 1938 *Schweiz. Z. Path. u. Bakt.* **1**, 23.

Hoogvliet, B. 1942 *Genetica*, **23**, 94.

Hyman, H. S. 1935 *J. Immunol.* **29**, no. 3.

Kemp, T. 1944 *Acta Path. microbiol. Scand.* suppl. LIV.

Kloepfer, H. W. 1946 *Ann. Eugen.* **13**, 35–71.

Landsteiner, K. & Levine, P. 1928 *J. Exp. Med.* **47**, 757–775.

Landsteiner, K. & Wienin, A. S. 1941 *J. Exp. Med.* **74**, 309–320.

Lattes & Garrasi 1932 *Atti IV Congr. Naz. Microbiol.* p. 146.

Lewis, T. & Embleton 1908 *Biometrika*, **6**, 26.

Mather, K. & Philip, U. 1940 *Ann. Eugen.* **10**, 403–416.

Matta, D. 1937 *Faculty Med. Publ. Egypt. Univ. Cairo*, no. 11.

Metz, C. W. 1938 Cooperation in research, *Carn. Inst. Wash. Pub.* **501**, 275–294.

Morch, T. 1941 *Chondrodystrophic dwarfs in Denmark.* Copenhagen: Ejnar Munksgaard.

Moureau, P. 1935 *Rev. Belg. Sci. Med.* **7**, 541–588.

Patau, K. & Nachtsheim, H. 1946 *Z. Naturforsch.* **1**, 345.

Pearson, K., Nettleship & Usher 1913 *Drap. Co. Res. Mem. Biom.*, Series IX.

Penrose, L. S. 1935 *Ann. Eugen.* **6**, 133–138.

Penrose, L. S. 1946*a* *Ann. Eugen.* **13**, 25.

Penrose, L. S. 1946*b* *J. Hered.* **37**, 285.

Philip, U. & Mather, K. 1940 *Ann. Eugen.* **10**, 403–416.

Pipkin, A. C. & Pipkin, S. 1945 *J. Hered.* **36**, 313.

Richsbieth, H. 1912 *Treas. Hum. Inher.* **1**, 355–553.

Rife, D. C. 1941 *Science*, **94**, 187.

Schiff, F. 1933 *Dtsch. Z. ges. gerichtl. Med.* **21**, 404–434.

Sjögren, T. 1931 *Hereditas*, **14**, 197–425.

Snyder, L. H. & Palmer, D. M. 1943 *J. Hered.* **34**, 207–212.

Taylor, G. L. & Prior, A. M. 1939*a* *Ann. Eugen.* **9**, 18–44.

Taylor, G. L. & Prior, A. M. 1939*b* *Ann. Eugen.* **9**, 97–108.

Weinberg, W. 1927 *Z. indukt. Abstamm.- u. VererbLehre*, **48**, 179–228.

White, M. 1940 *J. Genet.* **40**, 403–438.

Wiener, A. S. 1943 *Blood groups and transfusion.* Springfield: Charles C. Thomas.

Wiener, A. S. & Sonn, E. B. 1943 *Genetics*, **28**, 157–161.

Wiener, A. S. & Vaisberg, M. 1931 *J. Immunol.* **20**, 371–388.

Zieve, M. A., Wiener, A. S. & Fries, J. 1936 *Ann. Eugen.* **3**, 163–178.

J. B. S. HALDANE

Disease and evolution

Estratto dal volume:
SYMPOSIUM SUI FATTORI ECOLOGICI E GENETICI DELLA SPECIAZIONE NEGLI ANIMALI

Supplemento a « LA RICERCA SCIENTIFICA »
ANNO 19° - 1949

RIASSUNTO. – Negli esempi addotti dai biologi per mostrare come la selezione naturale agisce, la struttura o la funzione presa in esame è per lo più collegata con la protezione contro forze naturali avverse, contro predatori, oppure con la conquista di alimento o dell'altro sesso. L'A. mostra che la lotta contro le malattie, e in particolare contro le malattie infettive, ha rappresentato un fattore evolutivo molto importante e che alcuni dei suoi risultati sono diversi da quelli raggiunti attraverso le forme consuete della lotta per l'esistenza.

RÉSUMÈ. – Les exemples portés par les biologistes pour montrer comment la sélection naturelle opère tiennent compte d'ordinaire de structures ou de fonctions liées à la protection contre des forces naturelles hostiles, contre des prédateurs, ou bien liées à la conquête de la nourriture ou du sexe opposé. L'A. montre que la lutte contre les maladies, et en particulier contre les maladies infectieuses, a représenté un facteur évolutif très important et que qualques-uns parmi ses résultats diffèrent bien de ceux qui ont été atteints par les formes ordinaires de la lutte pour la vie.

SUMMARY. – Examples quoted by biologists, in order to show how natural selection is working, almost present structures or functions concerned either with protection against natural forces or against predators, or with purchase of food or mates. The Author suggests that the struggle against diseases, and especially infectious diseases, has been a very important evolutionary agent and that some of its results have been rather unlike those of the struggle for life in its common meaning.

It is generally believed by biologists that natural selection has played an important part in evolution. When however an attempt is made to show how natural selection acts, the structure or function considered is almost always one concerned either with protection against natural «forces» such as cold or against predators, or one which helps the organism to obtain food or mates. I want to suggest that the struggle against disease, and particularly infectious disease, has been a very important evolutionary agent, and that some of its results have been rather unlike those of the struggle against natural forces, hunger, and predators, or with members of the same species.

Under the heading infectious disease I shall include, when considering animals, all attacks by smaller organisms, including bacteria, viruses, fungi, protozoa, and metazoan parasites. In the case of plants it is not so clear whether we should regard aphids or caterpillars as a disease. Similarly there is every gradation between diseases due to a deficiency of some particular food constituent and general starvation.

The first question which we should ask is this. How important is disease as a killing agent in nature? On the one hand what fraction of members of a species die of disease before reaching maturity? On the other, how far does disease reduce the fertility of those members which reach maturity? Clearly the answer will be very different in different cases. A marine species producing millions of small eggs with planktonic larvae will mainly be eaten by predators. One which is protected against predators will lose a larger proportion from disease.

There is however a general fact which shows how important infectious disease must be. In every species at least one of the factors wich kills it or lowers its fertility must increase in efficiency as the species becomes denser. Otherwise the species, if it increased at all, would increase without limit. A predator cannot in general be such a factor, since predators are usually larger than their prey, and breed more slowly. Thus if the numbers of mice increase, those of their large enemies, such as owls, will increase more slowly. Of course the density-dependent check may be lack of food or space. Lack of space is certainly effective on dominant species such as forest trees or animals like *Mytilus*. Competition for food by the same species is a limiting factor in a few phytophagous animals such as defoliating caterpillars, and in very stenophagous animals such as many parasitoids. I believe however that the density-dependent limiting factor is more often a parasite whose incidence is disproportionately raised by overcrowding.

As an example of the kind of analysis which we need, I take Varley's (1947) remarkable study on *Urophora jaceana*, which forms galls on the composite *Centaurea nigra*. In the year considered 0.5 % of the eggs survived to produce a mature female. How were the numbers reduced to $\frac{1}{200}$ of the initial value?

If we put $200 = e^k$, we can compare the different killing powers of various environmental agents, writing $K = k_1 + k_2 + k_3 + \dots$, where k_r is a measure of the killing power of each of them. The result is given in Table 1. Surprisingly, the main killers appear to be mice and voles (*Mus*, *Microtus*, etc.) which eat the fallen galls and account for at least 22 %, and perhaps 43 % of k. Parasitoids account for 31 % of the total kill, and the effect of *Eurytoma curta* was shown to be strongly dependent on host density, and probably to be the main factor in controlling the numbers of the species, since the food plants were never fully occupied.

When we have similar tables for a dozen species we shall know something about the intensity of possible selective agencies. Of course in the case of *Urophora jaceana* analysis is greatly simplified by the fact that the imaginal period is about 2 % of the whole life cycle, so that mortality during it is unimportant.

A disease may be an advantage or a disadvantage to a species in competition with others. It is obvious that it can be a disadvantage. Let us consider an ecological niche which has recently been opened, that of laboratories where the genetics of small insects are studied. A number of species of *Drosophila* are well adapted for this situation. Stalker attempted to breed the related genus *Scaptomyza* under similar conditions, and found that his cultures died of bacterial disease. Clearly the immunity of *Drosophila* to such diseases must be of value to it in nature also.

Now let us take an example where disease is an advantage. Most, if not all, of the South African artiodactyls are infested by trypanosomes such as *T. rhodesiense* which are transmitted by species of *Glossina* to other mammals and, sometimes at least, to men. It is impossible to introduce a species such as *Bos taurus* into an area where this infection is prevalent. Clearly these ungulates have a very powerful defence against invaders. The latter may ultimately acquire immunity by natural selection, but this is a very slow process, as is shown by the fact that the races of cattle belonging to the native African peoples have not yet acquired it after some centuries of sporadic exposure to the infection. Probably some of the wild ungulates die of, or have their health lowered by the trypanosomes, but this is a small price to pay for protection from other species.

A non-specific parasite to which partial immunity has been acquired, is a powerful competitive weapon. Europeans have used their genetic resistance to such viruses as that of measles (rubeola) as a weapon against primitive peoples as effective as fire-arms. The latter have responded with a variety of diseases to which they are resistant. It is entirely possible that great and, if I may say so, tragic episodes in evolutionary history such as the extinction of the Noto-ungulata and Litopterna may have been due to infectious diseases carried by invaders such as the ungulates, rather than to superior skeletal or visceral developments of the latter.

A suitable helminth parasite may also prove a more efficient protection against predators than horns or cryptic coloration, though until much more is known as to the power of helminths in killing vertebrates or reducing their fertility, this must remain speculative.

However it may be said that the capacity for harbouring a non-specific parasite without grave disadvantage will often aid a species in the struggle for existence. An ungulate species which is not completely immune to *Trypanosoma rhodesiense* has probably (or had until men discovered the life history of this parasite) a greater chance of survival than one which does not harbour it, even though it causes some mortality directly or indirectly.

TABLE 1.

Month	Density per square metre	Cause of death	k.
July	203,0	—	—
»	184,7	Infertile eggs.	0,095
»	147,6	Failure to form gall.	0,224
»	144,6	? Disease.	0,021
»	78,8	*Eurytoma curta*	0.607
Aug., Sept.		Other parasitoids.	0,222
»	50,2	Caterpillars.	0,234
Winter	19,2	Disappearance, probably mice.	0 957
»	7,0	Mice.	1,009
»	5.2	Unknown	0.297
May-June		Birds.	0,090
»	3,6	Parasitoids	0.270
July	2.03	Floods.	0.581
			4,606

Mortality of *Urophora jaceana* in 1935-1946, after Varley.

The winter disappearance was probably due to galls carried off by mice. The mortality attributed to mice is based on counts of galls bitten open. The k due to *Eurytoma curta* in the preceding year was. 0.069, in the subsequent year 0,137. This cause of death depends very strongly on host and parasitoid densities. The caterpillars killed the larvae by eating the galls.

I now pass to the probably much larger group of cases where the presence of a disease is disadvantageous to the host. And here a very elementary fact must be stressed. In all species investigated the genetical diversity as regards resistance to disease is vastly greater than that as regards resistance to predators.

Within a species of plant we can generally find individuals resistant to any particular race of rust (Uredineae) or any particular bacterial disease. Quite often this resistance is determined by a single pair, or a very few pairs, of genes. In the same way there are large differences between different breeds of mice and poultry in resistance to a variety of bacterial and virus diseases. To put the matter rather figuratively, it is much easier for a mouse to get a set of genes which enable it to resist *Bacillus typhi murium* than a set which enable it to resist cats. The genes commonly segregating in plants have much more effect on their resistance to small animals which may be regarded as parasites, than to larger ones. Thus a semiglabrous mutant of *Primula sinensis* was constantly infested by aphids, which however are never found on the normal plant. I suppose thornless mutants of *Rubus* are less resistant to browsing mammals than the normal type, but such variations are rarer.

Anyone with any experience of plant diseases will of course point out that the resistance of which I have spoken is rarely very general. When a variety of wheat has been selected which is immune to all the strains of *Puccinia graminis* in its neighbourhood, a new strain to which it is susceptible usually appears within a few years, whether by mutation. gene recombination, or migration. Doubtless the same is true for bacterial and virus diseases. The microscopic and sub-microscopic parasites can evolve so much more rapidly than their hosts that the latter have little chance of evolving complete immunity to them. It is very remarkable that *Drosophila* is as generally immune as it is. I venture to fear that some bacillus or virus may yet find a suitable niche in the highly overcrowded *Drosophila* populations of our laboratories, and that if so this genus will lose its proud position as a laboratory animal. The most that the average species can achieve is to dodge its minute enemies by constantly producing new genotypes, as the agronomists are constantly producing new rust-resistant wheat varieties.

Probably a very small biochemical change will give a host species a substantial degree of resistance to a highly adapted microorganism. This has an important evolutionary effect. It means that it is an advantage to the individual to possess a rare biochemical phenotype. For just because of its rarity it will be resistant to diseases which attack the majority of its fellows. And it means that it is an advantage to a species to be biochemically diverse, and even to be mutable as regards genes concerned in disease resistance. For the biochemically diverse species will contain at least some members capable of resisting any particular pestilence. And the biochemically mutable species will not remain in a condition where it is resistant to all the diseases so far encountered, but an easy prey to the next one. A beautiful example of the danger of homogeneity is the case of the cultivated banana clone « Gros Michel » which is well adapted for export and has been widely planted in the West Indies. However it is susceptible to a root infection by the fungus *Fusarium cubense* to which many varieties are immune. and its exclusive cultivation in many areas has therefore had serious economic effects.

Now every species of mammal and bird so far investigated has shown a quite surprising biochemical diversity revealed by serological tests. The antigens concerned seem to be proteins to which polysaccharide groups are attached. We do not know their functions in the organism, though some of them seem to be part of the structure of cell membranes. I wish to suggest that they may play a part in disease resistance, a particular race of bacteria or virus being adapted to individuals of a certain range of biochemical constitution, while those of other constitutions are relatively resistant. I am quite aware that attempts to show that persons of a particular blood group are specially susceptible to a particular disease have so far failed. This is perhaps to be expected, as a disease such as diphtheria or tuberculosis is caused by a number of biochemically different races of pathogens. The kind of investigation needed is this. In a particular epidemic, say of diphtheria, are those who are infected (or perhaps those who are worst affected) predominantly drawn from one serological type (for example *AB*, *MM*, or *BMM*)? In a different epidemic a different type would be affected.

In addition, if my hypothesis is correct, it would be advantageous for a species if the genes for such biochemical diversity were particularly mutable, provided that this could be achieved without increasing the mutability of other genes whose mutation would give lethal or sublethal genotypes. Dr. P. A. Gorer informs me that there is reason to think that genes of this type are particularly mutable in mice. Many pure lines of mice have split up into sublines which differ in their resistance to tumour implantation. This can only be due to mutation. The number of loci concerned is comparable, it would seem, with the number concerned with coat colour. But if so their mutation frequency must be markedly greater.

We have here, then, a mechanism which favours polymorphism, because it gives a selective value to a genotype so long as it is rare. Such mechanisms are not very common. Among others which do so are a system of self-sterility genes of the *Nicotiana* type. Here a new and rare gene will always be favoured because pollen tubes carrying it will be able to grow in the styles of all plants in which it is absent, while common genes will more frequently meet their like. However this selection will only act on genes at one locus, or more rarely at two or three. A more generally important mechanism is that where a heterozygote is fitter than either homozygote, as in *Paratettix texanus* (Fisher 1939) and *Drosophila pseudoobscura* (Dobzhansky 1947). This does not, however, give an advantage to rarity as such. It need hardly be pointed out that, in the majority of cases where it has been studied, natural selection reduces variance.

I wish to suggest that the selection of rare biochemical genotypes has been an important agent not only in keeping species variable, but also in speciation. We know, from the example of the *Rh* locus in man, that biochemical differentiation of this type may lower the effective fertility of matings between different genotypes in mammals. Wherever a father can induce immunity reactions in a mother the same is likely to be the case. If I am right, under the pressure of disease, every species will pursue a more or less random path of biochemical evolution. Antigens originally universal will disappear because a pathogen had become adapted to hosts carrying them, and be replaced by a new set, not intrinsically more valuable, but favouring resistance to that particular pathogen. Once a pair of races is geographically separated they will be exposed to different pathogens. Such races will tend to diverge antigenically, and some of this divergence may lower the fertility of crosses. It is very striking that Irwin (1947) finds that related, and still crossable, species of *Columba*, *Streptopelia*, and allied genera differ in respect of large numbers of antigens. I am quite aware that random mutation would ultimately have the same effect. But once we have a mechanism which gives a mutant gene as such an advantage, even if it be only an advantage of one per thousand, the process will be enormously accelerated, particularly in large populations.

There is still another way in which parasitism may favour speciation. Consider an insect in which a parasitoid, say an ichneumon fly, lays its eggs. And let us suppose both host and parasite to have an annual cycle, the parasite being specific to that particular host. To simplify matters still further, we shall suppose that the parasite is the only density-dependent factor limiting the growth of the host population, whilst the density-dependent factor limiting the growth of the parasite population is the difficulty of finding hosts. It is further assumed that the parasitoid only lays one egg in each host, or that only one develops if several are laid. Varley showed that all these assumptions are roughly true for *Urophora jaceana* and *Eurytoma curta*.

Let e^k be the effective fertility of the host, that is to say let k be the mean value of the natural logarithm of the number of female-producing eggs laid per female. Let k_1 be the killing power of agents killing during the part of the life cycle before the host is not infested. Let k_2 be the killing power of agents other than the parasite killing during that part of the life cycle when it is infested, and therefore killing the same fraction $1-e^{-k_2}$ of parasites as of hosts. Let k_3 be the killing power of agents killing after the parasites have emerged as imagines.

Let x be the equilibrium density of adult hosts, y that of parasitoids, and a the mean area of search of the parasitoid.

Then the fraction of hosts which are not parasitized must be e^{-k_4}, where $k_1 + k_2 + k_3 + k_4 = K$. Nicholson and Bailey (1933) showed that $k_4 = ay$. But the host density available for parasitism is e^{K-k_1}. Of these $(1-e^{-k_4})\, e^{K-k_1}$ are parasitized. And $e^{K-k_1-k_2}(1-e^{-k_4})$ of the parasites live to emerge. This is diminished by a factor e^{-k_1}. The equilibrium densities are given by

$$x = \frac{e^{k_1-k_3}\, y}{e^{K-k_1-k_2-k_3} - 1},$$

$$y = \frac{K^{k_1-k_2-k_3}}{a},$$

though there is perpetual oscillation round this equilibrium. Now consider the effect of changes in these parameters. Any gene in the host which increases $K - k_1 - k_2 - k_3$ will give its carriers a selective advantage over their fellows, and will therefore spread through the population. This will cause an increase in the density of parasitoids. If it acts before or during parasitisation, thus diminishing k_1 or k_2, it will diminish the equilibrium value of x. If it acts after parasitisation is over, thus diminishing k_3, it will increase the equilibrium value of x, though not very much. But since we have supposed that the parasitoids only emerge shortly before the end of the hosts life cycle, every increase in its adaptation to environmental factors other than the specific parasite will diminish the numbers of adult hosts, though it may increase the number of their larvae at an early stage. This is a striking example of the way in which the survival of the fittest can make a species less fit.

A concrete case would be a gene which, by improving cryptic or aposematic coloration of the larvae, enabled more of them to escape predators, and therefore more parasites to do so. Since the host population is denser they will parasitise a larger fraction of the hosts and thus reduce their number. Since a larger fraction of parasites escape, equilibrium will be reached with a lower host density. Fewer of the caterpillars « nati a far l'angelica farfalla » will achieve this end. More of them will give rise to ichneumons or chalcids.

Natural selection will also favour genes which enable the host to resist the parasitoid, but the latter will also increase its efficiency by natural selection. As Nicholson and Bailey showed, every increase in the area searched by it will diminish the density of both hosts and parasites.

The best that can be said for this tendency, from the host's point of view, is that it makes it less likely to become extinct as the result of other agencies. For the parasitoid being dependent on the density of the host population, will allow its numbers to increase rapidly after any temporary fall.

The host can hardly hope to throw off the parasite permanently by changing its life cycle, developing immunity (if this is possible) or otherwise. But it can reduce its numbers by speciating. For suppose that the pair of species is replaced by two host-parasitoid pairs, the population will be doubled, in so far as the parasitoid is the regulator. It is unlikely that a species can divide sympatrically, but the reduction in numbers caused by parasitoidism will leave food available for other immigrant species of similar habits, even if they are equally parasitised.

Thus certain types of parasitism will tend to encourage speciation, as others encourage polymorphism. This will specially be the case where the parasite is very highly adapted to its host, the most striking cases of adaptation being probably those of the parasitoid insects.

We see then that in certain circumstances, parasitism will be a factor promoting polymorphism and the formation of new species. And this evolution will in a sense be random. Thus any sufficiently large difference in the times of emergence or oviposition of two similar insect species will make it very difficult for the same parasitoid to attack both of them efficiently. So will any sufficiently large difference in their odours. We may have here a cause for some of the apparently unadaptive differences between related species.

Besides these random effects, disease will of course have others. It is clear that natural selection will favour the development of all kinds of mechanisms of resistance, including tough cuticles, phagocytes, the production of immune bodies, and so on. It will have other less obvious effects. It will be on the whole an antisocial agency. Disease will be less of a menace to animals living singly or in family groups than to those which live in large communities. Thus it is doubtful if all birds could survive amid the faecal contamination which characterises the colonies of many sea birds. A factor favouring dispersion will favour the development of methods of sexual recognition at great distances such as are found in some Lepidoptera.

Again, disease will set a premium on the finding of radically new habitats. When our ancestors left the water, they must have left many of their parasites behind them. A predator which ceases to feed on a particular prey, either through migration or changed habits, may shake off a cestode which depends on this feeding habit. When cerebral development has gone far enough to make this possible, it will favour a negative reaction to faecal odours and an objection to cannibalism, and will so far be of social value. A vast variety of apparently irrelevant habits and instincts may prove to have selective value as a means of avoiding disease.

A few words may be said on non-infectious diseases. These include congenital diseases due to lethal and sub-lethal genes. Since mutation seems to be non-specific as between harmful and neutral or beneficial genes, and mutation rate is to some extent inherited, it follows that natural selection will tend to lower the mutation rate, and this tendency may perhaps go so far as to slow down evolution. It will also tend to select other genes which neutralise the effect of mutants, and thus to make them recessive or even ineffective, as Fisher has pointed out. Whether the advantage thus given to polyploids is ever important, we do not know. But the evolution of dominance must tend to make the normal genes act more intensely and thus probably earlier in ontogeny, so that a character originally appearing late in the life cycle will tend to develop earlier as time goes on.

Deaths from old age are due to the breakdown of one organ or another, in fact to disease, and the study of the mouse has shown that senile diseases such as cancer and nephrosis are often congenital. In animals with a limited reproductive period senile disease does not lower the fitness of the individual, and increases that of the species. A small human community where every woman died of cancer at 55, would be more prosperous and fertile than one where this did not occur. Senile disease may be an advantage wherever the reproductive period is limited; and even where it is not, a genotype which lead to disease in the 10 % or so of individuals which live longest may be selected if it confers vigour on the majority. As Simpson (1944) has emphasized, some of the alleged cases of hypertely can be explained in this way.

Deficiency diseases are due to the lack of a particular food constituent which an organism or its symbionts cannot synthesize or make from larger molecules. They must act as a selective agent against the loss of synthetic capacity which is a very common type of mutation in simple organisms at least, and in favour of genotypes with a varied symbiotic flora. They might thus have speeded up the evolution of the ruminants, whose symbionts probably make vitamins as well as simple nutrients like acetic acid. To be precise it might be an advantage to have a small rumen where symbionts made B vitamins before it got large enough to add appreciably to the available calories.

On the other hand Rudkin and Schulz (1948) have shown that deficiency diseases can select mutants which utilize the nutrilite in question less than does the normal type. In particular the vermilion mutant of *Drosophila melanogaster* does not form the brown eye pigment ommatin from tryptophane. It is more viable than the wild type on a diet seriously deficient in tryptophane. Thus deficiency diseases may cause a regressive type of evolution characterized by the loss of capacity to utilise rare nutrilites for synthesis.

In this brief communication I have no more than attempted to suggest some lines of thought. Many or all of them may prove to be sterile. Few of them can be followed profitably except on the basis of much field work.

REFERENCES

DOBZHANSKY, T. 1947. Genetics of natural populations XIV. A response of certain gene arrangements in the third chromosome of *Drosophila subobscura* to natural selection. *Genetics*, 32: 142.

FISHER, R. A. 1939. Selective forces in wild populations of *Paratettix texanus*. *Ann. Eugen.*, 9: 109.

IRWIN, M. R. 1949. Immunogenetics. *Advances in Genetics*, 1: 133.

NICHOLSON, I. J. and BAILEY, V. A. 1935. The balance of animal populations Pt. I. *Proc. Zool. Soc. London*: 551-598.

RUDKIN, G. T. and SCHULZ, J. 1948. A comparison of the Tryptophane requirements of mutant and wild type *Drosophila melanogaster*. *Proc. Int. Cong. Genetics, Stockholm*. July 1948.

SIMPSON, G. G. 1944. *Tempo and mode in Evolution*. New York.

VARLEY, G. C. 1947. Natural control of population balance in the knapweed gallfly (*Urophora jaceana*). *Journ. Anim. Ecol.*, 16: 139.

DISCUSSION

MONTALENTI. Sottolinea l'importanza delle vedute espresse dal Prof. Haldane. Ricorda il caso della microcitemia o talassemia, studiato da Silvestroni, Bianco e Montalenti. Qui un gene, letale allo stato omozigote (morbo di Cooley) si trova, allo stato eterozigote, con tale frequenza in alcune popolazioni (più del 10 %) che bisogna ammettere che esso rappresenti in questa condizione un vantaggio per gli individui che lo portano. Poichè da alcune ricerche, tutt'altro che complete, sembra che il gene sia più frequente in zone malariche, il Prof. Haldane ha suggerito in comunicazione verbale che gli individui microcitemici, i quali fra l'altro hanno resistenza globulare aumentata, possano essere più resistenti all'infezione malarica. Comunque è questo un caso interessante di eterosi, che si ricollega a quanto ha illustrato il Prof. Haldane.

JUCCI. La relazione del Prof. Haldane ha sviluppato magistralmente, in modo quanto mai suggestivo, un argomento del più alto interesse. Desidero fare qualche commento su qualcuno dei tanti aspetti del problema. Non conoscevo le ricerche di

Varley su *Urophora*. Certo gli insetti gallicoli offrono un materiale particolarmente adatto. Anni fa cominciai a raccogliere dati analoghi sul cecidomide *Mikiola fagi*. Ma la mia attenzione fu particolarmente assorbita dal fatto che nella zona da me esplorata – ogni singolo faggio lungo la strada che sale al Terminillo, nel tratto da 1000 a 1200 metri di altezza – si presentava una varietà di comportamento spiccatissima. Accanto a un faggio carico di galle spesso un altro ne era del tutto sprovvisto, come per una variabilità genetica di comportamento della pianta ospite. Le ricerche verranno riprese ed approfondite ora che stiamo per organizzare una Stazione montana di Genetica sul Terminillo, all'altezza di 1700 m. Suggestive le considerazioni del Prof. Haldane sul pericolo che per la specie presenta una eccessiva omogeneità e sul vantaggio di una capacità a presentare mutazioni biochimiche in rapporto alla possibilità di esprimere dalla costituzione genetica razze resistenti a parassiti Io ho avuto occasione di studiare a lungo le diverse recettività di due bombici serigeni, *Phylosamia ricini* e *Ph. cynthia*, al virus del giallume. La *ricini*, forma domestica, è resistente: portatore sano; la *cynthia*, selvatica sull'ailanto,recettiva come il *Bombyx*. Forse è per questa ragione che in Italia la *cynthia* è diffusa largamente, ma ovunque poco abbondante. Una o poche mutazioni (nella F2 dell'incrocio si ha la disgiunzione dei fattori con ritorno a forme resistenti e recettive, come le parentali) possono aver determinato nella *ricini* la capacità ad essere allevate in massa. A proposito della tendenza antisociale che il periodo delle malattie infettive può imprimere a molte specie di organismi, noterò che per l'evoluzione degli insetti sociali deve certo avere avuto larga importanza l'acquisizione di forte resistenza alle infezioni. Sarebbe interessante paragonare a questo riguardo la recettività della forma domestica (*Apis mellifica*) e di forme affini selvatiche alla peste delle api e simili forme epidemiche. Una delle vie per le quali il fattore malattia da infestione o infezione deve avere profondamente influenzato il processo evolutivo è stata certo quella della simbiosi, che va considerata come uno stato di alleanza subentrato a un periodo più o meno lungo di guerra fra due organismi. Caratteristico il caso dei batteri simbionti nel tessuto adiposo di Blattidi e di Termiti. La simbiosi risale ai Protoblattoidi del Carbonifero, come lo dimostra l'identità dei processi di trasmissione dei batteri da una generazione all'altra nei Blattidi e nel *Mastotermes*. Gli Isotteri hanno lasciato cadere lungo la via filogenetica la simbiosi con i batteri forse perché hanno trovato assai più vantaggiosa la simbiosi con i flagellati dell'intestino che hanno loro permesso la conquista del mondo della cellulosa. Interessantissimo l'accenno del Prof. Haldane alle malattie di carenza: mutazioni in questo senso possono aver sollecitato lo stabilirsi di simbiosi nelle quali l'associato veniva ad offrire il fattore accessorio che l'ospite non era più capace di produrre e che non poteva trovare nell'ambiente.

HADORN. Bei Bakterien gibt es zahlreiche Beispiele, die zeigen dass biochemische Mutationen die zu synthetischen Defekten führen, gleichzeitig eine Resistenz gegen Infektionen (Phagen) bedingen. Vielleicht könnte dies als Modell dienen für den positiven Selektionswert im Falle von Thalassemia.

Wie kann man erklären, dass die Negerbevölkerung von Zentralafrika gegenüber der tropischen Schlafkrankheit weniger resistent ist als die eingewanderten Europäer ? Es wäre vielmehr zu erwarten dass die Selektion bei der schwarzen Bevölkerung eine erhöhte Immunität begünstigt hätte.

HALDANE. 1. I agree with Dr. Montalenti's project. Another possibility is that (by analogy with the advantage possessed by vermilion *Drosophila* on media deficient in tryptophan) microcythemic heterozygotes may be at an advantage on diets deficient in iron or other substances, thus leading to anaemia.

2. Perhaps the theory that most diseases evolve into symbioses is somewhat panglossist. I doubt if it occurs as a general rule, though it may do so. The position for the original host is however best.

THE ASSOCIATION OF CHARACTERS AS A RESULT OF INBREEDING AND LINKAGE

By J. B. S. HALDANE

Department of Biometry, University College, London

The effect of inbreeding in increasing the frequency of homozygosis, and therefore of recessive phenotypes, is well known, and its theory in a population was firmly established by Wright (1922). In the present paper a step is taken to extend it to pairs of linked or unlinked genes. The effects of linkage in human genetics are by no means fully worked out. It is frequently found that two abnormal characters are associated, that is to say, that zygotes possessing one of them are more likely than the average of the population to possess the other also. This phenomenon is sometimes attributed to linkage between the genes responsible for these two characters. In most cases this explanation is incorrect. The association is often due to pleiotropism of a single gene, which may, but does not always, manifest itself by producing two different characters, the manifestation in one or both cases depending on other genes or environmental factors. As a reaction against this view it is sometimes stated that linkage between two genes does not give rise to any association between the phenotypes determined by them in a population. This is true only in a random mating population. It will be shown that if there is partial inbreeding even unlinked recessive characters show a certain amount of association, while linked ones may show it to a much greater degree. As a preliminary I shall summarize Malécot's (1948) proof of Wright's theory as applied to a single locus, and show how association arises in the absence of linkage.

Coefficients of relationship and inbreeding

Consider an ideal population in which, at a certain locus, every chromosome in the gametes forming it carried a different allelomorph. That is to say, the different zygotes are $\mathbf{a}^1\mathbf{a}^2$, $\mathbf{a}^3\mathbf{a}^4$, $\mathbf{a}^5\mathbf{a}^6$, and so on. If this population is allowed to breed for some generations, matings being between unrelated individuals except as specified, we ask the following question. What is the probability f_{XY} that, if the zygote X has produced a gamete carrying a particular allelomorph **a**, a gamete produced by the zygote Y will carry the same allelomorph? f_{XY} is called the coefficient of relationship of X and Y. If these gametes unite to form a zygote Z, $f_Z = f_{XY}$ is the probability that Z will be a homozygote **aa**, and is called the coefficient of inbreeding of Z. We say that X and Y are related by a chain of relationship of m links if they have a common ancestor P, and m is the sum of the numbers of generations separating P from X and Y. X and Y are often related by several chains. For example, an uncle and niece are related by two chains of three links. Clearly each link in a single chain halves the value of f. Wright showed that $f_{XX} = \frac{1}{2}(1+f_X)$, and that if X and Y are related by a number of chains of which the rth consists of m_r links, while the common ancestor P_r had a coefficient of inbreeding f_r, then

$$f_{XY} = \Sigma\,[2^{-m_r-1}(1+f_r)]. \tag{1}$$

If **a** mutates to other allelomorphs with frequency μ per generation, then

$$f_{XY} = \Sigma\left[\left(\frac{1-\mu}{2}\right)^{-m_r-1}(1+f_r)\right],$$

so that f_{XY} is not unity or near it in a population derived from a few ancestors in the very remote past. Selection in favour of heterozygotes has a similar, and sometimes larger, effect.

If we now pass to the more concrete case where the gene **a** has a frequency p, its allelomorphs, collectively described as **A**, a frequency $p' = 1-p$, we see that if X produces a gamete **a**, in a fraction f of all cases it will meet a gamete of Y derived from a common ancestral gamete and carrying **a**. In $1-f$ of all cases it will meet a gamete not so derived, and with a probability p of carrying **a**. Thus the probability that it will unite with a gamete carrying **a** is $f+(1-f)p$, or $p+fp'$; and since the probability that any particular gamete of X carries **a** is p, the probability that Z is **aa** is $p^2+fp'p$. Thus the frequency distribution of genotypes in a group of Z zygotes with the same coefficient of inbreeding f is

$$(p'^2+fp'p)\,\mathbf{AA}+2(1-f)\,p'p\mathbf{Aa}+(p^2+fp'p)\,\mathbf{aa}.$$

The values of f for different relationships are known. The mean value $\bar{f}$ in a population is Bernstein's (1930) coefficient of inbreeding α. This is not known at all exactly for any human population, the values given by Haldane & Moshinsky (1939) being minimum values. f is $\frac{1}{16}$ for first-cousin marriages, and $\bar{f}$ is at least 0·001 in several large European populations, and at least 0·01 in some small and isolated ones.

The association of phenotypes due to unlinked genes

Let **a** and **b** be two genes in different chromosomes, their frequencies being p and q, where $p+p' = q+q' = 1$. Then in a series of zygotes with the same coefficient of inbreeding the frequencies of **aa**, **bb** and **aabb** are $p^2+fp'p$, $q^2+fq'q$, and $(p^2+fp'p)\,(q^2+fq'q)$. There is no association. But in the whole population the frequency of **aa** is $p^2+\bar{f}p'p$, that of **bb** is $q^2+\bar{f}q'q$, and that of **aabb** is

$$p^2q^2+\bar{f}(p^2q'q+p'pq^2)+\overline{f^2}p'pq'q,$$

or

$$(p^2+\bar{f}p'p)\,(q^2+\bar{f}q'q)+V_fp'pq'q, \qquad (2)$$

where $V_f = \overline{f^2}-(\bar{f})^2$ is the variance of f in the population. Thus unless the coefficient of inbreeding is the same in all members of the population, there is an excess of double homozygotes over the product of the frequencies of single homozygotes. The excess frequency is clearly the same for **AABB**, **AAbb**, **aaBB** and **aabb**. On drawing up a 3×3 table we see that the frequency of each class of single heterozygotes is reduced by $2V_fp'pq'q$; for example, the frequency of **AaBB** is

$$2(1-\bar{f})\,p'p(q^2+\bar{f}q'q)-2V_fp'pq'q.$$

The frequency of double heterozygotes **AaBb** is

$$4[(1-\bar{f})^2+V_f]\,p'pq'q.$$

Thus, to take an example, the frequency of albinism must be greater among infantile amaurotic idiots than in the rest of the population, even if the genes responsible are on different chromosomes.

If we could divide up our population into groups, each of which had exactly the same coefficient of inbreeding, this association would vanish within each such group. But we cannot do so. Thus the progeny of supposedly unrelated parents includes some members whose parents were distantly related; the progeny of first-cousin marriages includes many cases drawn from rural populations in which there is a further inbreeding. A correlation of this type is sometimes, but in my opinion with doubtful propriety, described as spurious.

A numerical example may make the situation clearer. Suppose $p = 0{\cdot}01$, $q = 0{\cdot}003$, then in outbred individuals the frequencies of **aa**, **bb** and **aabb** would be 10^{-4}, 9×10^{-6}, and 9×10^{-10}. Among the progeny of unions of first cousins the corresponding frequencies would be $7{\cdot}2 \times 10^{-4}$, $195{\cdot}9 \times 10^{-6}$, and $1408{\cdot}3 \times 10^{-10}$. Thus the frequency of **aa** would be increased 7·2 times, of **bb** 21·8 times, and of **aabb** 156·5 times. Now if 1 % of all marriages were between first cousins, while 99 % of married couples were unrelated, the overall frequencies of **aa**, **bb** and **aabb** in the population would be $1{\cdot}062 \times 10^{-4}$, $1{\cdot}087 \times 10^{-5}$ and $2{\cdot}299 \times 10^{-9}$, as compared with an expected value of $1{\cdot}154 \times 10^{-9}$ in the absence of association. Moreover, 61·2 % of all **aabb** individuals would be the progeny of the 1 % of cousin marriages. This example, however, shows that an effect of this kind could rarely be detected even in a survey of a whole nation, since when p and q are larger the association is less marked.

If the genes **a** and **b** are fully recessive, and their effects additive, the product-moment correlation of the characters determined by them in the whole population is

$$\rho = V_f\left[\frac{p'pq'q}{(p+\bar{f}p')(1+p-\bar{f}p)(q+\bar{f}q')(1+q-\bar{f}q)}\right]^{\frac{1}{2}}, \tag{3}$$

which approximates to $\frac{V_f\sqrt{(pq)}}{\bar{f}}$ when p and q are small, and has a maximum near $\frac{V_f}{\sqrt{2\bar{f}}}$ when $p = q = \left[\sqrt{\left(\frac{2}{\bar{f}}-1\right)}+1\right]^{-1}$. However, for small values of p and q Yule's coefficient of association is much larger. This is

$$Q = \frac{V_f}{2(p+\bar{f}p')(q+\bar{f}q')(1+p-\bar{f}p)(1+q-\bar{f}q)+(1-2p^2-2\bar{f}p'p)(1-2q^2-2\bar{f}q'q)V_f+2p'pq'qV_f^2},$$

which can be nearly 1 when p and q are small and f very variable. It may be remarked that ρ is zero if either gene is completely without dominance, the heterozygote being intermediate.

A MEASURE OF THE EFFECT OF LINKAGE

First consider a hypothetical population in which all genes at the **a** and **b** loci are different. Let c be the frequency of recombination between these loci, and $c' = 1-c$. If X has produced an **ab** gamete we ask what is the probability F_{XY} that Y will also do so. First consider the case where X and Y are identical and outbred. In $1-c$ of all cases X is $\frac{++}{\mathbf{ab}}$, and the probability is $\frac{1}{2}(1-c)$. In c of all cases X is $\frac{\mathbf{a}+}{+\mathbf{b}}$, and the probability is $\frac{1}{2}c$. Thus

$$F_{XX} = \tfrac{1}{2}(c'^2+c^2) = \tfrac{1}{2}-c'^2.$$

If **a** and **b** have entered a zygote in the same gamete the probability that a gamete from this zygote will contain both is $\frac{1}{2}c'$; and the probability that, if a zygote has produced an **ab** gamete, a specified parent of it produced an **ab** gamete which went to form it is the same. Thus with each link in a chain of relationship the value of F must be multiplied by $\frac{1}{2}c'$. It follows that if X and Y are related by a single chain of m links through a single outbred common ancestor P (who may be identical with X, Y, or both),

$$F_{XY} = (\tfrac{1}{2}c')^m(\tfrac{1}{2}-c'c). \tag{4}$$

We see that if $c = 0$ (complete linkage), $F = f$, while if $c = \frac{1}{2}$ (independence), $F = f^2$. In general $f \geqslant F \geqslant f^2$. The same is clearly true for any type of relationship whatever. To take a concrete example, if X and Y are half first cousins, $f_{XY} = \frac{1}{32}$, and $F_{XY} = (\frac{1}{2}c')^4 (\frac{1}{2} - c'c)$.

In human pedigrees relatives are usually related by a pair of equal chains passing to a married pair of ancestors. We first determine F_{XY} when X and Y are sibs with outbred and unrelated parents. Suppose X produced an **ab** gamete. In c' of all cases X is $\frac{++}{\mathbf{ab}}$. In c' of these **a** and **b** came from a $\frac{++}{\mathbf{ab}}$ parent, so the probability that Y is $\frac{++}{\mathbf{ab}}$ is $\frac{1}{2}c'$; the further probability that a given gamete from Y is **ab** being also $\frac{1}{2}c'$. In c cases **a** and **b** came from an $\frac{\mathbf{a}+}{+\mathbf{b}}$ parent, so the probability that Y is $\frac{++}{\mathbf{ab}}$ is $\frac{1}{2}c$; and the further probability that a given gamete from Y is **ab** is $\frac{1}{2}c'$. Thus the total probability so far is $\frac{1}{2}c'^2 (\frac{1}{2}c'^2 + \frac{1}{2}c^2)$.

In c of all cases X is $\frac{\mathbf{a}+}{+\mathbf{b}}$. One parent was $\frac{++}{\mathbf{a}+}$, the other $\frac{++}{+\mathbf{b}}$. So the probability that Y is $\frac{\mathbf{a}+}{+\mathbf{b}}$ is $\frac{1}{4}$. If so the probability that a given gamete from Y is **ab** is $\frac{1}{2}c$. The total probability of this set of events is $\frac{1}{8}c^2$. Hence

$$F_{XY} = \tfrac{1}{8}(2c'^4 + 2c'^2c^2 + c^2).$$

And since with every further link in the chains F_{XY} must be multiplied by $\frac{1}{2}c'$, the value of the coefficient when X and Y are related by two equal chains of relationship of m links going back to a pair of mated outbred ancestors is

$$F_{XY} = (\tfrac{1}{2}c')^{m-2}\tfrac{1}{8}(2c'^4 + 2c'^2c^2 + c^2). \tag{5}$$

Each type of multiple relationship between X and Y involves a separate polynomial in c' and c. Thus if X and Y are double half first cousins, that is to say, if their parents were half-sibs who had married another pair of half-sibs,

$$F_{XY} = 2^{-7}(8c'^6 + 8c'^4c^2 + c^2).$$

There are similar complications if one or more of the common ancestors of X and Y are inbred. I have been unable to devise a general formula comparable with Wright's which will give F in all cases, though I deal with some more cases later in this paper. Until this is done the theory will be very incomplete, even though it is not very hard to work out the formula in any particular pedigree.

Next suppose the frequencies of **a** and **b** to be p and q, with $p' + p = q' + q = 1$. Suppose also that the population has reached equilibrium, so that the frequencies of the four gametic types are given by

$$p'q'\mathbf{AB} + p'q\mathbf{Ab} + pq'\mathbf{aB} + pq\mathbf{ab}.$$

This is a stable equilibrium, and unless c is very small or inbreeding very intense the stability is high. For in an outbred population if $pq + x_n$ be the frequency of **ab** in the nth generation, $x_n \propto c'^n$.

X produces an **ab** gamete with frequency pq. Y may produce an **ab** gamete for four reasons:

(1) **a** and **b** are derived from one or two common ancestors. This event has a probability F_{XY}.

(2) **a** is derived from a common ancestor and **b** from another source. **a** is so derived in f_{XY} of all cases. In $f_{XY} - F_{XY}$ **a** but not **b** is derived from a common ancestor. In $q(f_{XY} - F_{XY})$ it is associated with **b** from another source. Thus the probability is $q(f_{XY} - F_{XY})$.

(3) **b** is derived from a common ancestor, **a** from another source. The probability is $p(f_{XY} - F_{XY})$.

(4) Both **a** and **b** are derived from another source. In $1 - 2f_{XY} + F_{XY}$ cases neither **a** nor **b** is derived from a common ancestor. Hence the probability of this event is $pq(1 - 2f_{XY} + F_{XY})$.

The total probability that Z, a child of X and Y, should be **aabb** is therefore, if we put $f_Z = f_{XY}$,

$$\begin{aligned} &pq[F_Z + (p+q)(f_Z - F_Z) + pq(1 - 2f_Z + F_Z)] \\ &\qquad = pq(F_Z p'q' + f_Z p'q + f_Z pq' + pq) \\ &\qquad = pq(f_Z p' + p)(f_Z q' + q) + \phi_Z p'pq'q, \qquad (6) \end{aligned}$$

where $\phi_Z = F_Z - f_Z^2$. $\phi_{XY} = \phi_Z$ may be called the coefficient of relationship or inbreeding for a linked gene pair. Table 1 gives the values of ϕ for a number of relationships. $c' - c$ or $1 - 2c$ is always a factor of ϕ. So $\phi = f(1-f)$ when $c = 0$, and vanishes when $c = \frac{1}{2}$. It is also clear that the frequencies of all the four doubly homozygous genotypes are increased by the same amount, as the result of linkage, namely, $\phi_Z p'pq'q$, just as, in the case of a single gene, the frequencies of the two homozygous genotypes **aa** and **AA** are increased by $f_Z p'p$. As before, the frequencies of single homozygous genotypes are each diminished by $2\phi_Z p'pq'q$, those of each of the two doubly heterozygous genotypes $\frac{\mathbf{+\,+}}{\mathbf{ab}}$ and $\frac{\mathbf{a\,+}}{\mathbf{+\,b}}$ being increased by $2\phi_Z p'pq'q$. These frequencies are set out in Table 2. Linkage leads to an association between the homozygous types within a group with the same type of inbreeding, for example, the progeny of unions between first cousins. In this case

$$\phi = 2^{-8}[8c'^2(2c'^4 + 2c'^2c^2 + c^2) - 1],$$

Table 1. *Values of* ϕ_{XY}

Relation of X to Y	ϕ_{XY}	f_{XY}
Identical	$\frac{1}{4}(c'-c)^2$	$\frac{1}{2}$
Parent-offspring	$\frac{1}{16}(c'-c)(3c'^2+c^2)$	$\frac{1}{4}$
Whole sibs	$\frac{1}{16}(4c'^4+4c'^2c^2+2c^2-1)$	$\frac{1}{4}$
Half sibs	$\frac{1}{64}(8c'^4+8c'^2c^2-1)$	$\frac{1}{8}$
Uncle-niece, aunt-nephew	$\frac{1}{64}(8c'^5+8c'^3c^2+4c'c^2-1)$	$\frac{1}{8}$
Double first cousins	$2^{-6}(8c'^6+8c'^4c^2+4c'^2c^2+2c^2-1)$	$\frac{1}{8}$
First cousins	$2^{-8}[8c'^2(2c'^4+2c'^2c^2+c^2)-1]$	$\frac{1}{16}$
Half first cousins	$2^{-10}[32c'^4(c'^2+c^2)-1]$	$\frac{1}{32}$
Second cousins	$2^{-12}[32c'^2(2c'^4+2c'^2c^2+c^2)-1]$	$\frac{1}{64}$

These formulae can of course be written in terms of c or c' alone, or in a homogeneous form. They all contain $c' - c$ or $1 - 2c$, as a factor. Thus the formula for first cousins can be written

$$\begin{aligned} \phi_{XY} &= 2^{-8}(c'-c)(15c'^5 + 9c'^4c + 18c'^3c^2 + 14c'^2c^3 + 14c'c^4 + c^5) \\ &= 2^{-8}(1-2c)(15 - 66c + 132c^2 - 136c^3 + 72c^4 - 16c^5) \\ &= 2^{-8}(2c'-1)[1 + 2c'\{1 + 2c'(2c'-1)(2c'^2+1)\}]; \end{aligned}$$

but the forms given in the table seem to be the simplest.

Table 2. *Frequencies with which the four classes of gametes from X unite with members of the four classes from Y if f and* ϕ *are their coefficients of relationship*

	AB	**Ab**	**aB**	**ab**
AB	$(p'^2+fp'p)(q'^2+fq'q)+\lambda$	$(1-f)(p'^2+fp'p)q'q-\lambda$	$(1-f)p'p(q'^2+fq'q)-\lambda$	$(1-f)^2p'pq'q+\lambda$
Ab	$(1-f)(p'^2+fp'p)q'q-\lambda$	$(p'^2+fp'p)(q^2+fq'q)+\lambda$	$(1-f)^2p'pq'q+\lambda$	$(1-f)p'p(q^2+fq'q)-\lambda$
aB	$(1-f)p'p(q'^2+fq'q)-\lambda$	$(1-f)^2p'pq'q+\lambda$	$(p^2+fp'p)(q'^2+fq'q)+\lambda$	$(1-f)(p^2+fp'p)q'q-\lambda$
ab	$(1-f)^2p'pq'q+\lambda$	$(1-f)p'p(q^2+fq'q)-\lambda$	$(1-f)(p^2+fp'p)q'q-\lambda$	$(p^2+fp'p)(q^2+fq'q)\pm\lambda$

$$\lambda = \phi p'pq'q.$$

which is tabulated in Table 3, ranges from $\frac{15}{256}$ to 0 as c rises from 0 to $\frac{1}{2}$, and is 0·02997 when $c = 0{\cdot}10$. The correlation of phenotypes is

$$\rho = \phi\left[\frac{p'pq'q}{(p+fp')(1+p-fp)(q+fq')(1+q-fq)}\right]^{\frac{1}{2}}$$

$$= \phi\left[\frac{1}{p'p} - (1-f)\left(\frac{1}{p} - \frac{1}{p'}\right) - (1-f)^2\right]^{-\frac{1}{2}}\left[\frac{1}{q'q} - (1-f)\left(\frac{1}{q} - \frac{1}{q'}\right) - (1-f)^2\right]^{-\frac{1}{2}}.$$

In the case of first-cousin marriage

$$\rho = 256\phi\left[\frac{256}{p'p} - 240\left(\frac{1}{p} - \frac{1}{p'}\right) - 225\right]^{-\frac{1}{2}}\left[\frac{256}{q'q} - 240\left(\frac{1}{q} - \frac{1}{q'}\right) - 225\right]^{-\frac{1}{2}}.$$

Table 3

c	0	0·05	0·1	0·2	0·3	0·4	0·5
ϕ (first cousins)	0·05859	0·04211	0·02997	0·01430	0·006176	0·0002106	0
ϕ (second cousins)	0·01538	0·01014	0·006616	0·002669	0·0009909	0·00004651	0

Thus ρ would be $\frac{256\phi}{799}$ when $p = q = \frac{1}{2}$, or 0·0135 if $c = 0{\cdot}10$. To detect this we should need a sample of about 1400 progeny of cousins, and many more would be needed were either gene rare. For example, if $p = q = 0{\cdot}01$, we should expect the frequency of **aa** and **bb** among the progeny of first-cousin marriages to be $7{\cdot}2 \times 10^{-4}$, as compared with 10^{-4} in that of unrelated parents. In the absence of linkage $7{\cdot}2 \times 10^{-4}$ of either of these classes should be **aabb**. With 10 % recombination the fraction would rise to $47{\cdot}2 \times 10^{-4}$. In order to detect it, we should need a sample of the order of 400 recessives known to be the progeny of first cousins. Such samples do not exist at present. However, if among fifty or so single recessives from parents known to be related, a single double recessive were found, this would create a suspicion of linkage, which would become strong if two or more double recessives were found. We should not expect anything like so many among the progeny of unrelated parents. But the presence of one or two would not disprove the hypothesis of linkage, since the group in which consanguinity is not reported must include some cases where it exists but has not been recorded.

It seems that a systematic search of the existing literature might reveal cases suggesting linkage in this manner.

If we consider the whole population, the frequency of **aa** is $p(\bar{f}p' + p)$, that of **aabb** is

$$pq[(\bar{f}p' + p)(\bar{f}q' + q) + (\bar{\phi} + V_f)\, p'q'],$$

and we can substitute $(\bar{\phi} + V_f)\, p'pq'q$ for λ throughout Table 2.

Thus the overall association of **aa** and **bb** is due both to the variance of f and to the existence of linkage. The fraction of **aa** which are also **bb** is $q(\bar{f}q' + q) + \frac{(\bar{\phi} + V_f)\, p'q'}{p(\bar{f}p' + p)}$.

It should be possible to determine V_f in the future, as it is a fairly important constant of any population, and is probably a little below 10^{-4} for many European peoples. $\bar{\phi}$ must certainly exceed V_f when linkage is strong. It may therefore be possible to use data on whole populations to detect linkage, but it would seem more hopeful to deal separately with consanguineous unions.

If, for example, we take the values $p = 0{\cdot}01$, $q = 0{\cdot}003$ of the former numerical example, and suppose that there is 5 % recombination between the loci of **a** and **b**, then the frequency of **aabb** among outbred individuals will be $1{\cdot}154 \times 10^{-9}$ as before, or about two in the whole human race. The frequency among the progeny of unions of first cousins will be $1{\cdot}388 \times 10^{-6}$, or 1200 times greater. This is an effect of inbreeding which we should only get with a single gene of frequency 5×10^{-6}, which is probably too small to allow of genetical investigation. It must, however, be emphasized that the calculated effects are at most on a small scale, and the object of this paper has been to place the theory on a firm basis rather than to suggest concrete research. There is only one human situation where double recessives for rare gene pairs are likely to be relatively very common. This is when there is assortative mating over several generations on the basis of somatic resemblance. This certainly occurs in the case of recessive deaf-mutism, and may do so in the case of other defects.

The calculation of ϕ_{XY} in more complex pedigrees

First let us find the value of ϕ_{XX} when ϕ_X and f_X are known. This enables us to calculate ϕ_{XY} in any pedigree where X and Y are related through a single common ancestor who was inbred. To do so we go back to the original hypothetical population, which is essentially the limiting case of an actual population when the gene frequencies p and q tend to zero. We see at once that if X is inbred, the frequencies of the four genotypes which can produce **ab** gametes are as

$$2[(1-f)^2+\phi]\,\frac{\mathbf{+\,+}}{\mathbf{ab}} : 2[(1-f)^2+\phi]\,\frac{\mathbf{a\,+}}{\mathbf{+\,b}} : 2(f-f^2-\phi)\,\frac{\mathbf{a\,+}}{\mathbf{ab}} : 2(f-f^2-\phi)\,\frac{\mathbf{+\,b}}{\mathbf{ab}} : (f^2+\phi)\,\frac{\mathbf{ab}}{\mathbf{ab}},$$

where $f = f_X$, $\phi = \phi_X$.

Now $\frac{1}{2}c'$ of the gametes from $\frac{\mathbf{+\,+}}{\mathbf{ab}}$ are **ab**, as are $\frac{1}{2}c$ of those from $\frac{\mathbf{a\,+}}{\mathbf{+\,b}}$, $\frac{1}{2}$ of those from $\frac{\mathbf{a\,+}}{\mathbf{ab}}$, and so on. Hence

$$\left.\begin{aligned} F_{XX} &= \tfrac{1}{4}c'^2 . 2[(1-f)^2+\phi] + \tfrac{1}{4}c^2 . 2[(1-f)^2+\phi] + \tfrac{1}{4} . 4(f-f^2-\phi) + f^2 + \phi \\ &= f + \tfrac{1}{2}(c'^2+c^2)\,[(1-f)^2+\phi], \\ \phi_{XX} &= \tfrac{1}{4}(1-f_X)^2\,(c'-c)^2 + \tfrac{1}{2}\phi_X(c'^2+c^2) \\ &= (\tfrac{1}{2}-c'c)\,(1-f_X)^2 + (\tfrac{1}{4}-c'c)\,\phi_X, \end{aligned}\right\} \quad (7)$$

while $f_{XX} = \frac{1}{2}(1+f_X)$. This formula enables us to deal with cases where one common ancestor P is inbred, provided we can calculate ϕ_P. We can similarly deal with the case where each of the two common ancestors P and Q are inbred, provided $f_{PQ} = 0$, that is to say they are unrelated. However, I have not found a formula covering the case when P and Q are related. It is possible that f_{PQ} and ϕ_{PQ} do not give all the needful information. There is no particular difficulty in cases where X and Y are more than doubly related, provided that ancestors are not inbred or related. I give the formula when X and Y are double first cousins in Table 1.

Evolutionary consequences

In a population all of whose members are not equally inbred it is clear that the lethal or sublethal character of some homozygotes will lessen the viability of homozygotes at other loci. For example, if the frequency of the genes for the various group A agglutinogens is 0·30, the frequency of **AA** zygotes will be 9 % when the parents are unrelated, 10·31 % if they are first cousins. There is reason to think that, on the whole, the progeny of first cousins are slightly less viable and fertile than that of unrelated parents. If so **AA** zygotes will, for this reason, be a little less fit than AO and AB. If any sublethal genes are in the same chromosome with the blood-group genes, this will have a further effect in the same direction. It is true that in the case of incompatibility between mother and foetus, heterozygotes are less fit than homozygotes. However, it is unlikely that this influence is enough to counteract the general disadvantage of homozygosis.

I naturally thought that this selective 'force' would tend to encourage heterozygosis at all loci. But like so many verbal arguments concerning evolution, this is fallacious. Consider the pairs of genes **Aa** and **Bb**, linked or otherwise, as before, and let **bb** have a fitness $(1-K)$ of those of **AA** and **Aa**, while **BB**, **Bb** and **bb** have the same fitness of unity. Of the $q(\bar{f}q'+q)$ **bb** zygotes,

$$p(\bar{f}p'+p)(\bar{f}q'q+q^2)+(\phi+V_f)\,p'pq'q \quad \text{are } \mathbf{aa},$$

$$2(1-\bar{f})\,p'p(\bar{f}q'q+q^2)-2(\phi+V_f)\,p'pq'q \quad \text{are } \mathbf{Aa},$$

$$p'(p'+\bar{f}p)(\bar{f}q\,q+q^2)+(\phi+V_f)\,p'pq'q \quad \text{are } \mathbf{AA}.$$

Thus from an original population of

$$(p'^2+\bar{f}p'p)\,\mathbf{AA}+2(1-\bar{f})\,p'p\mathbf{Aa}+(p^2+\bar{f}p'p)\,\mathbf{aa},$$

the survivors will be in the frequencies

$$(p'^2+\bar{f}p'p-kp'p)\,\mathbf{AA}+2(p'p-\bar{f}p'p+kp'p)\,\mathbf{Aa}+(p^2+\bar{f}p'p-kp'p)\,\mathbf{aa},$$

where $k=\dfrac{K(\phi+V_f)\,q'q}{1-K(\bar{f}q'q+q^2)}$. Thus k is independent of p. Hence in the next generation p becomes

$$(1-f)\,p'p+kp'p+p^2+fp'p-kp'p,$$

that is to say, p is not altered. Hence, although selection against homozygotes at some loci reduces the frequency of homozygosis at other loci, it does so in such a way as to leave gene frequencies unaltered, and thus has no evolutionary consequences.

Discussion

It should be emphasized that the formulae here given are subject to two suppositions, both rather unrealistic. First, it is assumed that we are dealing with the whole population. For example, of the group of single recessives, **aa**, a fraction of at least $2p(p'+\bar{f}p)$ would have one or both parents **aa**. In any collection of pedigrees these would be separately classified. Secondly, it is assumed that the viability of the recessives is normal, while in fact they are often lethal or sub-lethal. These considerations invalidate the well-known formulae such as $\frac{1}{16}p(1+15p)$. In fact, if we ask what is the frequency of recessive zygotes from the mating $X\times Y$, when X and Y are first cousins, but it is also known that neither X, Y, nor any of their parents or grandparents, are homozygous recessives, we raise a rather complicated problem, whose solution is not without interest.

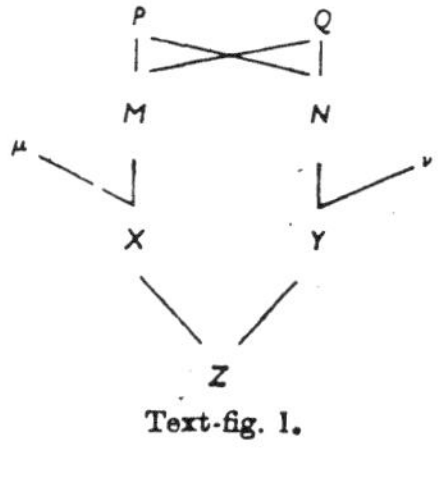

Text-fig. 1.

Consider the pedigree of Fig. 1, where P, Q, μ, ν are supposed to be outbred individuals, and P, Q, M, N, μ, ν, X and Y are all known to be **AA** or **Aa**. Since outbred individuals occur in the frequencies p'^2**AA** $+ 2p'p$**Aa** $+ p^2$**aa**, the probability that an outbred dominant is **Aa** is $\frac{2p}{1+p}$, which will be written as x. We require the probability that Z shall be **aa**. This can occur in seven cases:

(1) P or Q is **Aa** (probability $2x$).
(2) P and Q are **Aa** (probability x^2).
(3) μ and ν are **Aa** (probability x^2).
(4) P and μ, P and ν, Q and μ, or Q and ν are **Aa** (probability $4x^2$).
(5) P, Q and μ, or P, Q and ν are **Aa** (probability $2x^3$).
(6) P, μ, and ν, or Q, μ, and ν are **Aa** (probability $2x^3$).
(7) P, Q, μ, and ν are all **Aa** (probability x^4).

Now the probability that M or N shall be **Aa** is $\frac{1}{2}$ whether one or both of P and Q are **Aa**. Thus cases (1) and (2) give the same fraction of homozygous Z. Cases (4) and (5) are equivalent, as are cases (6) and (7). In case (1) 2^{-6} of Z are **aa**. In case (3) 2^{-4} of Z are **aa**. In case (4) suppose P and μ are **Aa**. The genotype of M is irrelevant, for whatever it may be the chance that X is **Aa** is $\frac{1}{2}$. Hence 2^{-5} of Z are **aa**. Similarly, cases (6) and (7) are equivalent to case (3). Hence the probability that Z shall be **aa** is

$$\begin{aligned} 2^{-6}(2x+x^2) + 2^{-4}(x^2+2x^3+x^4) + 2^{-5}(4x^2+2x^3) &= 2^{-6}x(2+13x+12x^2+4x^3) \\ &= \frac{p(1+16p+53p^2+54p^3)}{16(1+p)^4} \\ &= \tfrac{1}{16}p(1+12p-p^2-18p^3+\ldots). \end{aligned} \tag{8}$$

Similar expressions could be found in other cases, notably that where M and N had several normal sibs, but it is clear that they would often be very complicated. The first term in each polynomial, which is multiplied by a coefficient of inbreeding, is always unaltered. But the effect of omitting pedigrees where homozygous recessives occur among the parents and other relatives will be a slight decrease in the various frequencies calculated for inbred progeny.

Summary

Partial inbreeding, such as occurs in human communities, leads to a slight tendency for recessive characters due to unlinked genes to be associated. This is because as a result of consanguineous unions the frequency of double recessives is more augmented than that of single recessives. Linkage between recessive genes leads to a further association of recessive characters, but it is still so slight as to be of doubtful value for the detection of linkage. Finally, an expression is found for the frequency of recessives in the progeny of cousin marriages where a number of ancestors are known to have been normal.

REFERENCES

Bernstein, F. (1930). Fortgesetzte Untersuchungen aus der Theorie der Blutgruppen. *Z. indukt. Abstamm.- u. VererbLehre*, **56**, 223.

Haldane, J. B. S. & Moshinsky, P. (1939). Inbreeding in Mendelian populations with special reference to human cousin marriages. *Ann. Eugen., Lond.*, **9**, 321.

Malécot, S. (1948). *Les mathématiques de l'Hérédité.* Paris: Masson et Cie.

Wright, S. (1922). Coefficients of inbreeding and relationship. *Amer. Nat.* **56**, 330.

REPRINTED FROM *ANNALS OF EUGENICS*, Vol. 14, Part 4, pp. 288–292, 1949
 PRINTED IN GREAT BRITAIN

PARENTAL AND FRATERNAL CORRELATIONS FOR FITNESS

By J. B. S. HALDANE, *Department of Biometry, University College, London*

The fitness of a genotype in the Darwinian sense is measured by the mean numbers of its progeny, different generations being counted at the same stage of the life cycle. Fisher's (1930) Malthusian parameter is the natural logarithm of the fitness, and his more detailed definition may be accepted. The Malthusian parameter has the advantage that when it varies with time we can use its arithmetic mean. However, the fitness has the important property that, over a sufficiently long time, the arithmetic mean of the fitnesses of all individuals must be very near unity. More accurately the geometric mean of the arithmetic means in each generation must approximate to unity. For if it were 1·01 over only 10,000 generations (which is a short time geologically) the population would increase by a factor of 10^{43}, which is impossible even for bacteria. If we are concerned with changes in the composition of a population, we need only consider the relative fitness of different genotypes. It is hardly necessary to emphasize that fitness throughout will be taken to mean fitness in this strictly Darwinian sense, and not fitness for football, industry, music, self-government, or any other activity.

In the absence of mutation natural selection acts so as to maximize the mean fitness of the population, some genotypes being eliminated, others being present in the proportions which are optimal under the given mating system, though in general a higher fitness could be achieved under a different mating system. Mutation in general lowers the fitness below what would otherwise be its value. Fitness can only be maximized so as long as all possible genes or chromosomal arrangements making for maximal fitness are present in the population. But of course any mutation producing a gene or chromosomal pattern which can further increase fitness will ultimately shift the equilibrium. Since the mean fitness must always be very close to unity over long periods it is a little paradoxical to speak of maximizing it. However, a move towards the equilibrium will increase the fitness possible at the particular population density in question, though it may cause an increase in density which again lowers the fitness to unity.

If a gene has a marked effect on fitness, natural selection must affect its frequency considerably, and it must approach its stable equilibrium rapidly. Hence such genes must generally be near their equilibrium frequencies, unless there has been a recent change in the environment, altering the relative fitnesses of genotypes, a change in the mating system, or one in the mutation rate. It is therefore interesting to consider the correlations between relatives to be expected in a population in equilibrium. It will be seen that these are sometimes very different from those found by Fisher (1918) for genes which affect a metrical character, but whose effect on fitness was not explicitly considered.

If we are dealing with a pair of autosomal allelomorphs **A** and **a**, whose effects on fitness are additive with those of other genes, there are three possible conditions for equilibrium, apart from the complete disappearance of one of them:

(1) **Aa** is fitter than **AA** or **Aa** (heterosis).

(2) **Aa** is less fit than **aa**, but **A** is constantly arising by mutation. If the difference of fitnesses is many times the mutation rate, **AA** is so rare that its fitness is irrelevant.

(3) **AA** and **Aa** are equally fit, but **aa** is less fit than either, while **a** is constantly arising by mutation.

A combination of (1) and (3) is also possible, i.e. the fitnesses may be in the order **Aa**, **AA**, **aa**, with **A** and **a** arising by mutation, but usually (1) or (3) will be nearly a correct description of the situation. Other causes of equilibrium are negligible if differences of fitness greatly exceed mutation rates. Where genes interact on fitness, numerous stable equilibria may be possible, as Wright (1935) has pointed out. However, the above conditions will hold near any one of them. Thus if **AABB** is substantially fitter than **AaBB** or **AABb**, there will be a stable equilibrium with the population composed mainly of **AABB**, even though **aabb** is fitter than **AABB**.

EQUILIBRIUM UNDER HETEROSIS AND RANDOM MATING

Suppose the fitnesses of **AA**, **Aa**, and **aa** to be in the ratios $1-K:1:1-k$. Then there is a stable equilibrium when the gene frequencies of **A** and **a**, both at birth and after selection has operated, are $\frac{k}{K+k}$ and $\frac{K}{K+k}$ respectively. The population at birth is thus

$$\frac{k^2}{(K+k)^2}\,\mathbf{AA}+\frac{2Kk}{(K+k)^2}\,\mathbf{Aa}+\frac{K^2}{(K+k)^2}\,\mathbf{aa}.$$

Its mean fitness is $1-\frac{Kk}{K+k}$ and its variance in fitness $\left(\frac{Kk}{K+k}\right)^2$. Let us suppose selection to act by differential mortality before maturity, rather than by differences in fertility or in mortality during the fertile period. This simplifies calculation without essentially altering the situation. The effective breeders are thus

$$\frac{k^2(1-K)}{(K+k)(K+k-Kk)}\,\mathbf{AA}+\frac{2Kk}{(K+k)(K+k-Kk)}\,\mathbf{Aa}+\frac{K^2(1-k)}{(K+k)(K+k-Kk)}\,\mathbf{aa}.$$

The progeny of different matings are therefore as shown in Table 1. It is a well-known and easily calculable result that the progeny of **AA** parents are k**AA** : K**Aa**, those of **Aa** parents k**AA** : $(K+k)$ **Aa** : K**aa**, and those of **aa** parents k**Aa** : K**aa**. All these progenies have the same fitness. Thus as regards fitness the correlation between parent and offspring is zero.

Table 1

Mating	Frequency $\times (K+k)^2(K+k-Kk)^2$	Progeny	Mean fitness of progeny	Variance of progeny's fitness
AA × **aa**	$2K^2k^2(1-K)(1-k)$	**Aa**	1	0
Aa × **AA**	$4Kk^3(1-K)$	½**AA**, ½**Aa**	$1-\frac{1}{2}K$	$\frac{1}{4}K^2$
Aa × **aa**	$4K^3k(1-k)$	½**Aa**, ½**aa**	$1-\frac{1}{2}k$	$\frac{1}{4}k^2$
Aa × **Aa**	$4K^2k^2$	¼**AA**, ½**Aa**, ¼**aa**	$1-\frac{1}{2}(K+k)$	$\frac{1}{16}(3K^2-2Kk+3k^2)$
AA × **AA**	$k^4(1-K)^2$	**AA**	$1-K$	0
aa × **aa**	$K^4(1-k)^2$	**aa**	$1-k$	0

But it must be emphasized that if the gene affects any measurable character this character will in general show a high parent-offspring correlation. Thus **AA** babies might, on an average, weigh 500 g. more than **Aa** at birth, **aa** 1000 g. less. As babies of unusually high or low birth weights are in general more likely to die than those near the average, the heterozygotes could be fitter than the homozygotes. There would then be a high parent-offspring correlation for birth weight, but none for fitness.

On the other hand, the fitnesses of sibs are positively correlated. The variance of the total progeny at birth is $\sigma^2 = \left(\frac{Kk}{K+k}\right)^2$. The mean variance within a sibship is

$$(K+k)^{-2}(K+k-Kk)^{-2}[(1-K)K^3k^3+(1-k)K^3k^3+\tfrac{1}{4}(3K^2-2Kk+3k^2)K^2k^2],$$

or $\frac{\sigma^2(3-4\sigma)}{4(1-\sigma)^2}$. Hence the fraternal correlation is $\frac{1-2\sigma}{2-2\sigma}$. This varies between $\frac{1}{2}$ when K or k, and therefore σ, is small, and nearly zero when K and k are both near unity. If a number of gene pairs are acting in this way with additive effects on fitness, each with a small value of σ, the fraternal correlation due to all of them will be just below $\frac{1}{2}$.

The above calculations will not be much affected if inbreeding occurs with the moderate intensity usual in man. For if we consider a group of children of first cousins, the frequency of **AA** and **aa** will each be increased by $\frac{Kk}{16(K+k)^2}$ and the mean fitness therefore only diminished from $1-\frac{Kk}{K+k}$ to $1-\frac{17Kk}{16(K+k)}$. However, assortative mating on the basis, not of fitness, but of some other character determined by **A** and **a**, might lead to a substantial parent-offspring correlation, besides diminishing the fitness of the population appreciably. The work of Pearson & Lee (1900, p. 150) suggests that this may be true for some of the genes responsible for human iris colour.

EQUILIBRIUM BETWEEN MUTATION AND ELIMINATION OF A DOMINANT

Suppose that **a** mutates to **A** with frequency μ per generation, and that the fitness of **Aa** is $1-k$. Then a stable equilibrium is reached when the population at birth consists of $\frac{2\mu}{k}$ **Aa** + $\left(1-\frac{2\mu}{k}\right)$ **aa** provided $\frac{\mu}{k}$ is so small that its square can be neglected, i.e. that **AA** zygotes do not occur with appreciable frequency (Haldane, 1927). This also implies that inbreeding is irrelevant. If $1-x$ be the fitness at birth, it can be seen that $\bar{x} = 2\mu$, $\overline{x^2} = 2\mu k$. Supposing selection to act before maturity, the breeders are

$$\frac{2\mu(1-k)}{k}\,\mathbf{Aa} + \left[1-\frac{2\mu(1-k)}{k}\right]\mathbf{aa}.$$

So if $1-y$ be the fitness of a parent,

$$\bar{y} = 2\mu(1-k), \quad \overline{y^2} = 2\mu k(1-k).$$

The variances are clearly almost equal to the mean squares. It is assumed that almost all mutations occur late in the formation of gametes, so that we very rarely find two sibs due to the same mutation which has affected a number of gametes from the same zygote.

We see that $\overline{xy} = \frac{4\mu(1-k)}{k}\,\frac{1}{4}k^2 = \mu k(1-k)$. So the parent-offspring correlation is

$$\frac{\mu k(1-k)}{\sqrt{[2\mu k \,.\, 2\mu k(1-k)]}} = \tfrac{1}{2}\sqrt{(1-k)}.$$

The fraternal correlation table is:

	Aa	**aa**
Aa	$\mu k^{-1}(1-k)$	$\mu k^{-1}(1+k)$
aa	$\mu k^{-1}(1+k)$	$1-\mu k^{-1}(3+k)$

neglecting terms of the order of μ^2, so the fraternal correlation is $\frac{1}{2}(1-k)$. Both are very nearly $\frac{1}{2}$ if k is small. They are clearly equal to the correlations for metrical characters. Only if **Aa** is sublethal will they be substantially less than $\frac{1}{2}$.

Equilibrium between mutation and elimination of a recessive

Here if **A** mutates to **a** with frequency μ, and the fitness of **aa** is $1-k$, the frequency of **aa** at equilibrium is μ/k under any mating system, provided this is a small quantity, though the equilibrium is approached very slowly (Haldane, 1939). Since almost all **aa** progeny are derived from **Aa** × **Aa** unions, the parent-offspring correlation for fitness is very small, and the fraternal correlation about $\frac{1}{4}$. The same values are found for metrical characters if Aa is indistinguishable from **AA**.

Discussion

We see that the correlation in fitness between parent and offspring is practically zero except where unfavourable dominants are arising by mutation, whereas the fraternal correlations range between 0·5 and 0·25, except in the case of nearly lethal dominants. This is, however, only true for populations in equilibrium. If the effects of a number of genes on fitness have recently altered through changed environmental conditions, there may be an appreciable parental correlation in the fitness due to heterotic genes. But even so we should expect fraternal correlations to be a good deal higher than parental.

A number of characters, notable longevity (Beeton & Pearson, 1901) and fertility (Pearson, Lee & Bramley-Moore, 1899) have been measured, and fairly high parental correlations found. While there may well be a substantial non-genetical element in these, due to family tradition as regards over-eating, birth control, and so on, it is hard to believe that much of the correlation is not of genetical origin. Unfortunately, however, I know of no work where fitness has been directly estimated in men. It is entirely possible that were this done, the parental correlations would be much attenuated. Thus it is possible that, in so far as length of life is inherited, it may be negatively correlated with fertility. This would not mean that it was so in general. Pearson, Lee & Moore were essentially of this opinion when they stressed the antagonistic effects of natural selection (i.e. selection for longevity) and reproductive selection (i.e. selection for fertility).

However the statistics, so far as they go, are suggestive. Thus Beeton & Pearson pointed out that the causes of death in infancy and later life are very different, and dealt particularly with durations of life of children who died at 21 or later, and who were therefore potential or actual parents. The four parent-offspring correlations range from 0·1301 to 0·1493, with mean 0·1365. The three sib-sib correlations range from 0·2139 to 0·3322 with mean 0·2611, brother-sister correlation being given double weight. The remarkable difference certainly bears out the theory here developed.

It is not easy to see how the inheritance of human fitness could be quantitatively investigated. Probably the best method would be to correlate the mean numbers of children born to a group of persons who had died before the age of 60 or had reached that age, with the corresponding numbers for their parents and sibs. It would be essential to follow up entire families. Records may possibly be available for certain groups such as the peerage and the Society of Friends

The parents would be a highly selected group, those with many children being more represented than those with few. If the thesis of this paper be correct, the parental correlations should be quite small, the sib correlations large.

If this were so we could say that unfavourable dominants balanced by mutation did not play an important part in determining human fitness. We should not be able to distinguish between recessive genes and those acting through heterosis. But an investigation of the fitness of the children of first cousins would enable us to obtain some estimate of the importance of recessives. For inbreeding would have a much larger effect with rare recessive genes than with those responsible for heterosis.

Finally it is worth emphasizing what I have not said. If there is a very small correlation between the fitness of a group of children and that of their parents, this does not imply that fitness is not inherited, in one sense of this vague word. It can be genetically determined, but not inherited in the ordinary sense. I have not discussed the problem of selection against heterozygotes such as occurs in connexion with neonatal jaundice. Either human populations are very far from equilibrium with regard to genes having an effect of this kind, or it is balanced by some other effect of which we know nothing at present. But it is clear that the *prima facie* effect will be to add a factor to the sib-sib correlation for fitness, without increasing that between parents and offspring.

Summary

In so far as fitness in the Darwinian sense is a measurable character, it should be substantially correlated in sibs, and not at all in parent and offspring, in the case of genes where the heterozygote is fitter than either or both homozygotes. Only in the case where the heterozygote is less fit, that is to say of dominant genes lowering fitness, is a parental correlation to be expected.

References

M. Beeton & K. Pearson (1901). On the inheritance of the duration of life, and on the intensity of natural selection in man. *Biometrika*, **1**, 50–89.

R. A. Fisher (1918). The correlation between relatives on the supposition of Mendelian inheritance. *Proc. Roy. Soc. Edinb.* **52**, 399–433.

R. A. Fisher (1930). *The Genetical Theory of Natural Selection*. Oxford.

J. B. S. Haldane (1927). A mathematical theory of natural and artificial selection. Part V. *Proc. Camb. Phil. Soc.* **23**, 363–72.

J. B. S. Haldane (1939). The spread of harmful autosomal recessive genes in human populations. *Ann. Eugen., Lond.*, **9**, 232–7.

K. Pearson, A. Lee & L. Bramley-Moore (1899). Mathematical contributions to the theory of evolution. VI. *Philos. Trans.* A, **192**, 257–330.

K. Pearson & A. Lee (1900). Mathematical contributions to the theory of evolution. VIII. *Philos. Trans.* A, **195**, 79–150.

S. Wright (1935). Evolution in populations in approximate equilibrium. *J. Genet.* **30**, 257–66.

AN ENUMERATION OF SOME HUMAN RELATIONSHIPS

By J. B. S. HALDANE AND S. D. JAYAKAR

Genetics & Biometry Research Unit, C.S.I.R.

Introduction

In view of the importance attached to relationship in most human cultures, religions, and legal codes, it might be thought that at least the simpler ones, for example those not more distant than that of uncle, would have been enumerated, and a terminology adopted for them, either in colloquial or legal language, or in that of anthropologists. This is not the case. For example if we say that *B* is *A*'s first cousin we shall show that this may mean any of 48 relationships if the sexes of *A* and *B* are not specified, and 192 if they are specified. Only a few of these are given special names in any language known to us. All but 6 of the 48 involve at least one multiple marriage, or its biological equivalent, among the grandparents of *A* and *B*. However even when simultaneous polygamy and divorce are both illegal, remarriage after the death of a spouse is permitted and may be enjoined, and its frequency is shown by the existence of such words as "stepmother" and "half-sister". With increasing study of the extent and effects of human inbreeding an exact terminology is desirable, though we do not suppose that our own cannot be improved. We venture to hope that our enumeration may be of value to anthropologists.

(*a*) As we are concerned with biological relationships, it is irrelevant whether the parents of any member of the pedigree were married when he or she was born. Nevertheless we shall frequently use the word "marriage" to mean "marriage or its biological equivalent".

(*b*) We confine ourselves to cognate or "blood" relationships, that is to say relationships between two persons who have at least one known latest common ancestor in common, or of whom one is the ancestor of the other. By "latest common ancestor" is meant the last-born common ancestor. Thus two sons of the same man by different women have two grandparents in common, but their father is their latest common ancestor.

(*c*) We also confine ourselves to relationships of *B* to *A* where no latest common ancestor is more remote than a grandparent of *A* or *B*.

(*d*) We further neglect the possibility of any inbreeding in the ancestry of *A* or *B* (though of course their offspring, if any, are inbred). For it can be seen that by condition (*c*) this would imply a fertile sexual union between parent and offspring or between whole or half brother and sister. A union between grandparent and grandchild, uncle and niece, or aunt and nephew would violate condition (*c*). Thus if *A* is the child of a man and his niece, this means that the same person is *A*'s grandparent and great-grandparent. Incestuous unions between parent and offspring, or between sibs, rarely occur, and are still more rarely discovered with certainty. We are aware that in Bali (*fide* Karve, 1953) twins of opposite sex were compelled to marry. A consideration of such possibilities would greatly extend our analysis. We do however consider unions, such as that of a man with a woman and her daughter by another man, which are forbidden in many cultures. Such unions do not involve inbreeding.

(*e*) Finally we adopt the convention that the sexes of the relatives *A* and *B* are irrelevant to the relationship. This convention reduces the number of relationships listed to one quarter of the possible number, and greatly simplifies the symbolism. However it involves some complication in the consideration of sex-linked genes. The structure of most languages is illogical. Thus a man or a woman usually uses the same word for his or her brother, and another for his or her sister, though in India different words of older and younger brothers, and for older and younger sisters, are usual. However a man and a woman almost always use the same words. Thus the description of the relationship of *B* to *A* depends on the sex of *B* and not that of *A*. But according to Karve (1953) the Nambudri Brahmins of Kerala are more logical. A woman calls her elder brother "*oppa*", a man "*jyesthan*". A woman calls her elder sister "*cheltati*" or "*jyesthati*", a man calls her "*oppol*". The terms for younger sibs do not appear to depend on *A*'s sex.

Ignoring the sexes of *A* and *B* we have to enumerate 129 distinct relationships, or 516 if the sexes of *A* and *B* are considered. This large number is mainly due to the possibilities of polygamy, remarriage, and their biological equivalents. If no member of the pedigree has a child by more than one spouse or sexual partner, these numbers are reduced to 17 and 68.

Monozygotic twinning leads to a slight complication. Monozygotic twins have the same genotype apart from mutation, and their children presumably resemble one another as closely as those of the same individual. The effect of such twinning is considered in a special section.

The classification adopted in Roman law (see Morton, 1961 for diagrams) is excellent so far as it goes, and will be adopted here. The degree of consanguinity is the number of "steps" between two relatives, the parent-child relationship being regarded as a step. Thus parents are relatives of degree 1, sibs of degree 2. This system does not take cognizance of half-relationships, and even with the restrictions which we have adopted, *B* can be simultaneously related to *A* in two different degrees.

A geneticist asks three main types of question about a given relationship:

(1) What correlations may be expected between the phenotypic characters of *A* and *B* as the result of their relationship ?

(2) If *A* and *B* are of different sexes, and have children, how may these children be expected to differ from the general population ?

(3) What are the frequencies in a population studied, of marriages, or their biological equivalent, between relatives of various different kinds, and of progeny of such marriages ? These two frequencies are not quite the same if inbreeding affects the net fertility of a marriage, or the viability of its children.

The first two questions can be answered with the aid of coefficients of relationship which are here calculated. It must however be stated that these coefficients may be misleading for at least five reasons. The population studied may be divided into more or less endogamous groups, based either on geographical isolation, or on religious, occupational, or caste differences. In some societies spouses are positively correlated for certain phenotypic characters, presumably as a result of choice. Selective deaths may alter correlations; thus maternal-foetal incompatibility must raise the correlation between mothers and surviving children with respect to some antigens. There is presumably a tendency for relationships to accumulate. Thus those who are first cousins are probably more often also second or third cousins than are persons unrelated in the fourth degree. Finally the environments of relatives are correlated. All these causes must tend to increase correlations.

All the relationships which we shall consider are irreflexive in the terminology of logic. If *B* is *A*'s paternal half-brother, he cannot be identical with *A*. So we must be careful not to define *A*'s paternal half-brother as *A*'s father's son, and if we are using symbolic logic, to add the non-identity symbol *J* where it is needed to ensure irreflexivity (see Carnap, 1958, pp. 117, 223). None of the relations in our list is transitive, like "ancestor" and "descendant". Some are intransitive, others non-transitive, for example the relation "whole sib". The symmetry or otherwise of relationships is more important. It is clear that some relationships are symmetric, for example if *B* is *A*'s mother's whole sister's child, *A* is *B*'s mother's whole sister's child. Others are asymmetric. Thus if *B* is *A*'s mother's whole brother's child, *A* is *B*'s father's whole sister's child. Such asymmetric relations evidently occur in pairs, each member of a pair being the converse of the other. A third class of relations, the non-symmetric, also exists. If *B* has a relation *R* of this class to *A*, then *A* may or may not have it to *B*. Thus if *B* is *A*'s sister, *A* may be *B*'s sister or her brother. None of the relations in our classification fall into this class, as they would do if *B*'s sex were specified while *A*'s was not. We avoid this class either by specifying the sex of neither *A* nor *B*, or by specifying the sex of both. We can thus classify all our 129 relationships as symmetrical or fully asymmetrical. In fact 37 are symmetrical, and the other 92 occur in converse pairs.

COEFFICIENTS OF RELATIONSHIP

The terminology of coefficients of relationship is unfortunately imprecise. Wright (1922) used the lower case letter f for his coefficient, which is much the most important of the group. Recent authors have however used F. Haldane and Moshinsky (1939) used f' for sex-linked loci. This had however been used by Wright for f_{n-1} when f denoted f_n. We suggest that the Greek letter ϕ be used. f and ϕ enable us to make statements about the gametes of *B*, given information about a gamete of *A*. But we also require information about the diploid genotype of *B*, given that of *A*. This information may be given by two more coefficients, F for autosomal loci, and Φ for sex-linked loci in members of the homogametic sex. A similar coefficient for *Y*-linked genes would be unity for males with a latest common male ancestor connected to each by a series of males, (e.g. if *B* is *A*'s father's paternal half-brother) and otherwise zero.

The logical products of all these four symbols are null for the human species. Thus $M.P$ would mean that x was both mother and father of y, which is only possible in self-fertilized organisms. However their relative products are meaningful. Thus $M|M$ means maternal grandmother, and $M|P$ paternal grandmother (mother of father). Cognate relationships involving a common ancestor are symbolized by a series of one or more inverse signs followed by one or more direct signs. The first direct sign must be the converse of the last converse sign. Thus $M|P$ is null. It means that x's mother is y's father. $M|M$ means that x and y have the same mother. To ensure that x is not identical with y we must use the non-identity sign J. Thus $\breve{M}|M.\ J$ means that x has the same mother as y but is not identical. x and y often have several latest common ancestors. Thus $M|M.\ \breve{P}|P.\ J$ means that x has the same mother as y, and also the same father, and is not identical; hence x is y's whole sister or brother. This is however a somewhat cumbrous expression, which we replace by a single letter. However we are aware that logicians may prefer a symbolism which fits into the corpus of symbolic logic. And it may also readily be translated into the symbols of binary arithmetic. Thus if x is the child of y's mother's father and of y's father's whole sister, a relation which we symbolize by $\left.\begin{matrix} wH \\ hMw \end{matrix}\right\}$, the relationship in the terminology of this section is $(\breve{P}|P.J)\ |M.\breve{M}|\ (\breve{M}|M.\ \breve{P}|P.J)\ |P$. If we write *0* for $\breve{M}$ and M and 1 for $\breve{P}$ and P, using a decimal point for the latest common ancestor, with the convention that children of the same parent are not identical, this becomes $1\cdot10\frown00\cdot01\frown01\cdot11$, using Russell's sign for logical product. It is instructive to note why we could not use symbols for "Son of" and "Daughter of" as our primitive signs.

Symbolism

In the interests of brevity we use the following symbolism. Each letter stands for a human being. w means a wife, woman, Weib, etc. h means a man (husband, homme, Herr, homo, etc.). The symbols m (which may mean male, man, maschio, mother, Mutter, mā (Hindi) etc.) and f (which may mean father, female, femme, etc.) are liable to be misleading. Any set of letters (not more than three in this paper) symbolises a relationship of B to A through a common ancestor, beginning with A's parent. The common ancestor is written with a capital letter, and letters subsequent to it represent descendants of the common ancestor, and ancestors of B. Thus wH means that A's mother w was a daughter of H, the father of B. Thus B is A's maternal half-uncle. Similarly hWh means that B is the child of A's maternal half-brother. If there are several common ancestors we use a bracket. Thus $\left.\begin{matrix} hH \\ wWw \end{matrix}\right\}$ means that A's paternal grandfather H had a child B by the maternal half sister of A's mother. That is to say H married his son's wife's maternal half-sister. Thus both H and W must have married twice (or had children by two sexual partners). Where a pair of common ancestors are married, we use the symbol M. Thus hM replaces $\left.\begin{matrix} hW \\ hH \end{matrix}\right\}$ and means that B is a whole sib of A's father h, that is to say a paternal aunt or uncle of A.

We are aware that we have no symbols for the relationships in a direct ancestral line, namely parent and child, and the symbols are ambiguous for grandparent, and grandchild, which come within our scope. But here unambiguous words or phrases are available in most languages. The Indian languages are richer than the European in terms for relationships. Thus in Hindi "brother" is "*bhai*" and "sister" "*bahin*" or "*bahan*". The four types of male first cousin, namely the sons of *A*'s mother's sister, mother's brother, father's sister, and father's brother (in our symbolism *w.Mw*, *w.Mh*, *h.Mw*, and *h.Mh*) are called *mausera-bhai*, *mamera-bhai*, *phuphera-bhai*, and *chachera-bhai*, respectively, their sisters being called *mauseri-bahan*, etc. These are derived from the names of the four types of aunt and uncle. But although remarriage of widowers is normal in northern India, and polygyny was not rare, there are no special words for *wHw*, etc. There is therefore a need for a symbolism.

In translating our symbolism into that of symbolic logic, the order should be reversed. *w* before the capital becomes $\breve{M}$, after it M. *h* before the capital becomes $\breve{P}$, after it P. W becomes $\breve{M}|M.\ J$; H becomes $\breve{P}|P.\ J$, and M becomes $(\breve{M}|M.\ \breve{P}|P.\ J)$. Inclusion in a bracket is replaced by the full stop or other sign for a logical product or intersection class.

THE ENUMERATION

Table 1 gives our enumeration. The third column gives the converse of each relationship. *S* denotes that a relationship is symmetrical, and is therefore its own converse. There are only 17 relationships which do not involve at least one remarriage. They are the six relations between ancestor and descendant which head our list, and the following:—

M, wM, Mw, hM, Mh, $w.Mw$, $w.Mh$, $h.Mw$, $h.Mh$, $\left.\begin{matrix} w.Mw \\ h.Mh \end{matrix}\right\}$, and $\left.\begin{matrix} w.Mh \\ h.Mw \end{matrix}\right\}$. In Indian communities where widows do not remarry, relationships containing the letter *W* do not occur, or are not recognized.

Some of the multiple relationships involving remarriage or polygamy are no doubt bizarre, and several of them can only occur after marriages to agnates (spouse's blood-relatives) which are forbidden in some cultures. However they are often encouraged in others. Thus where a man marries two full sisters, simultaneously or successively, their children will be in the relation $\left.\begin{matrix} H \\ w.Mw \end{matrix}\right\}$ (paternal half sib and full cousin) to one another. Again in some polygamous cultures, and particularly in ruling families, a man might inherit his father's wives and concubines, and have access to all of them but his own mother. The child of a woman by her first husband and by his son by another wife are in the relationship $\left.\begin{matrix} W \\ Hh \end{matrix}\right\}$, that is to say *B* is *A*'s maternal half-brother and paternal nephew. Mythology furnishes examples of still stranger relationships. Thus in the Mahabharata the children of the brothers Yudhiṣṭhira and Arjuna by their co-wife Draupadi were legally $\left.\begin{matrix} W \\ h.Mh \end{matrix}\right\}$; but since according to the epic Yudhiṣṭhira

6

Table 1. *Relationships and coefficients of relationship*

	Relation	Symbol	Converse	f	F	ϕ_{11}	ϕ_{12}	ϕ_{21}	ϕ_{22}	Φ
	Degree 1									
1, 2	Parent	—	Child	1/4	0	0	1/2	1/2	1/4	0
	Degree 2									
1, 2	Mother's Parent	—	Daughter's child	1/8	0	1/4	1/4	1/4	1/8	0
3, 4	Father's Parent	—	Son's child	,,	,,	0	0	0	1/4	0
5	Maternal half sib	W	S	1/8	0	1/2	1/4	1/4	1/8	0
6	Paternal half sib	H	S	,,	,,	0	0	0	1/4	0
7	Full sib	M	S	1/4	1/4	1/2	1/4	1/4	1/8	1/2
	Degree 3									
1, 2	Half aunt or uncle	wW	Ww	1/16	0	1/4	1/8	1/8	1/16	0
3, 4	,, ,, ,,	wH	Hw	,,	,,	0	1/4	0	1/8	,,
5, 6	,, ,, ,,	hW	Wh	,,	,,	0	0	1/4	1/8	,,
7, 8	,, ,, ,,	hH	Hh	,,	,,	0	0	0	0	,,
9, 10	Aunt or uncle	wM	Mw	1/8	0	1/4	1/8	1/8	1/16	0
11, 12	,, ,, ,,	hM	Mh	,,	,,	0	0	1/4	1/8	0
13, 14	Double half aunt or uncle (Fig. 1)	wW } hH }	Ww } Hh }	1/8	1/16	1/4	1/8	1/8	1/16	0
15, 16	,, ,, ,,	wH } hW }	Hw } Wh }	,,	,,	0	1/4	1/4	1/4	1/4
17, 18	Half aunt or uncle and half niece or nephew (Fig. 2)	wW } Hh }	Ww } hH }	1/8	1/16	1/4	1/8	1/8	1/16	0
19	,, ,, ,, ,, ,, ,,	wH } Hw }	S	,,	,,	0	1/4	1/4	1/4	1/4
20	,, ,, ,, ,, ,, ,,	hW } Wh }	S	,,	,,	0	1/4	1/4	1/4	1/4
	Degree 4									
I	One common grandparent									
1	Half first cousin Fig. 3	wWw	S	1/32	0	1/8	1/16	1/16	1/32	0
2	,, ,, ,,	wHw	S	,,	,,	1/4	1/8	1/8	1/16	,,
3, 4	,, ,, ,,	wWh	hWw	,,	,,	0	1/8	0	1/16	,,
5, 6	,, ,, ,,	wHh	hHw	,,	,,	0	0	0	0	,,
7	,, ,, ,,	hWh	S	,,	,,	0	0	0	1/8	,,
8	,, ,, ,,	hHh	S	,,	,,	0	0	0	0	,,
II	Two common grandparents									
A	No remarriage									
9	Full first cousin (Fig. 4)	wMw	S	1/16	0	3/8	3/16	1/16	3/32	0
10, 11	,, ,, ,,	wMh	hMw	,,	,,	0	1/8	0	1/16	,,
12	,, ,, ,,	hMh	S	,,	,,	0	0	0	1/8	,,
B	Two remarriages									
13	Double half first cousin (Fig. 5)	wWw } hWh }	S	1/16	1/64	1/8	1/16	1/16	5/32	1/16
14	,, ,, ,, ,,	wWw } hHh }	S	,,	,,	1/8	1/16	1/16	1/32	0
15	,, ,, ,, ,,	wHw } hWh }	S	,,	,,	1/4	1/8	1/8	3/16	1/8

Table 1. *Relationships and coefficients of relationship*—(Contd.)

	Relation	Symbol	Converse	f	F	ϕ_{11}	ϕ_{12}	ϕ_{21}	ϕ_{22}	Φ
B	Two remarriages									
16	Double half first cousin	*wHw* *hHh*	*S*	$\frac{1}{16}$	$\frac{1}{64}$	$\frac{1}{4}$	$\frac{1}{8}$	$\frac{1}{8}$	$\frac{1}{16}$	0
17	„ „ „ „	*wWh* *hWw*	*S*	„	„	0	$\frac{1}{8}$	$\frac{1}{8}$	$\frac{1}{8}$	$\frac{3}{16}$
18	„ „ „ „	*wHh* *hHw*	*S*	„	„	0	0	0	0	0
19, 20	„ „ „ „	*wWh* *hHw*	*wHh* *hWw*	„	„	0	$\frac{1}{8}$	0	$\frac{1}{16}$	0
C	Double remarriage									
21, 22	Double half first cousin (Fig. 6)	*wWw* *wHh*	*wWw* *hHw*	$\frac{1}{16}$	0	$\frac{1}{8}$	$\frac{1}{16}$	$\frac{1}{16}$	$\frac{3}{32}$	0
23, 24	„ „ „ „	*wWh* *wHw*	*wHw* *hWw*	„	„	$\frac{1}{4}$	$\frac{1}{4}$	$\frac{1}{8}$	$\frac{1}{8}$	0
25, 26	„ „ „ „	*wWh* *hHh*	*hWw* *hHh*	„	„	0	$\frac{1}{8}$	0	$\frac{3}{16}$	0
27, 28	„ „ „ „	*wHh* *hWh*	*hHw* *hWh*	„	„	0	0	0	$\frac{1}{8}$	0
III	Three common grand-parents									
A	One remarriage									
29	Full and half first cousin (Fig. 7)	*wMw* *hWh*	*S*	$\frac{3}{32}$	$\frac{1}{32}$	$\frac{3}{8}$	$\frac{3}{16}$	$\frac{3}{16}$	$\frac{5}{32}$	$\frac{3}{16}$
30	„ „ „ „	*wMw* *hHh*	*S*	„	„	$\frac{3}{8}$	$\frac{3}{16}$	$\frac{1}{16}$	$\frac{3}{32}$	0
31, 32	„ „ „ „	*wMh* *hWw*	*hMw* *wWh*	„	„	0	$\frac{1}{8}$	$\frac{1}{8}$	$\frac{1}{16}$	0
33, 34	„ „ „ „	*wMh* *hHw*	*hMw* *wHh*	„	„	0	$\frac{1}{8}$	0	$\frac{1}{16}$	0
35	„ „ „ „	*hMh* *wWw*	*S*	„	„	$\frac{1}{8}$	$\frac{1}{16}$	$\frac{3}{16}$	$\frac{5}{32}$	$\frac{3}{16}$
36	„ „ „ „	*hMh* *wHw*	*S*	„	„	$\frac{1}{4}$	$\frac{1}{8}$	$\frac{1}{8}$	$\frac{1}{16}$	$\frac{1}{8}$
B	Triple remarriage									
37	Triple half first cousin (Fig. 8)	*wWh* *hWw* *wHw*	*S*	$\frac{3}{32}$	$\frac{1}{64}$	$\frac{1}{4}$	$\frac{1}{4}$	$\frac{1}{4}$	$\frac{9}{16}$	$\frac{1}{16}$
38, 39	„ „ „	*wWw* *wHh* *hWh*	*wWw* *hHw* *hWh*	„	„	$\frac{1}{8}$	$\frac{1}{16}$	$\frac{1}{16}$	$\frac{5}{32}$	$\frac{1}{16}$
40	„ „ „	*wWw* *wHh* *hHw*	*S*	„	„	$\frac{1}{8}$	$\frac{1}{16}$	$\frac{1}{16}$	$\frac{3}{32}$	0
41	„ „ „	*wWh* *hHh* *hWw*	*S*	„	„	0	$\frac{1}{8}$	$\frac{1}{8}$	$\frac{1}{8}$	$\frac{1}{16}$
42, 43	„ „ „	*wHw* *wWh* *hHh*	*wHw* *hWw* *hHh*	„	„	$\frac{1}{4}$	$\frac{1}{4}$	$\frac{1}{8}$	$\frac{1}{8}$	0
44	„ „ „	*wHh* *hHw* *hWh*	*S*	„	„	0	0	0	$\frac{1}{8}$	0

Table 1. *Relationships and coefficients of relationship*—(Contd.)

	Relation	Symbol	Converse	f	F	ϕ_{11}	ϕ_{12}	ϕ_{21}	ϕ_{22}	Φ
IV	Four common grandparents									
A	Two marriages									
45	Double first cousin (Fig. 9)	*wMw* *hMh*	*S*	$\frac{1}{8}$	$\frac{1}{16}$	$\frac{3}{8}$	$\frac{1}{16}$	$\frac{1}{16}$	$\frac{7}{32}$	$\frac{1}{16}$
46	,, ,, ,,	*wMh* *hMw*	*S*	,,	,,	0	$\frac{1}{8}$	$\frac{1}{8}$	$\frac{1}{8}$	$\frac{1}{16}$
B	Cyclical remarriage									
47	Quadruple half first cousin (Fig. 10)	*wWw* *wHh* *hWh* *hHw*	*S*	,,	$\frac{1}{32}$	$\frac{1}{8}$	$\frac{1}{16}$	$\frac{1}{16}$	$\frac{5}{32}$	$\frac{1}{16}$
48	,, ,, ,,	*wWh* *wHw* *hWw* *hHh*	*S*	,,	,,	$\frac{1}{4}$	$\frac{1}{4}$	$\frac{1}{4}$	$\frac{3}{16}$	$\frac{1}{16}$
	Degrees 2 and 3									
1, 2	Half sib and half aunt or uncle (Fig. 11)	*W* *hH*	*W* *Hh*	$\frac{3}{16}$	$\frac{1}{8}$	$\frac{1}{2}$	$\frac{1}{4}$	$\frac{1}{4}$	$\frac{1}{8}$	0
3, 4	,, ,, ,,	*H* *wW*	*H* *Ww*	,,	,,	$\frac{1}{4}$	$\frac{1}{8}$	$\frac{1}{8}$	$\frac{5}{16}$	$\frac{1}{4}$
	Degrees 2 and 4									
I	Two remarriages									
1	Half sib and half first cousin (Fig. 12)	*W* *hWh*	*S*	$\frac{5}{32}$	$\frac{1}{16}$	$\frac{1}{2}$	$\frac{1}{4}$	$\frac{1}{4}$	$\frac{1}{4}$	$\frac{1}{4}$
2	,, ,, ,,	*W* *hHh*	*S*	,,	,,	$\frac{1}{2}$	$\frac{1}{4}$	$\frac{1}{4}$	$\frac{1}{8}$	0
3	,, ,, ,,	*H* *wWw*	*S*	,,	,,	$\frac{1}{8}$	$\frac{1}{16}$	$\frac{1}{16}$	$\frac{9}{32}$	$\frac{1}{8}$
4	,, ,, ,,	*H* *wHw*	*S*	,,	,,	$\frac{1}{4}$	$\frac{1}{8}$	$\frac{1}{8}$	$\frac{5}{16}$	$\frac{1}{4}$
II	One remarriage									
5	Half sib and full cousin (Fig. 13)	*W* *hMh*	*S*	$\frac{3}{16}$	$\frac{1}{8}$	$\frac{1}{2}$	$\frac{1}{4}$	$\frac{1}{4}$	$\frac{1}{4}$	$\frac{1}{4}$
6	,, ,, ,,	*H* *wMw*	*S*	,,	,,	$\frac{3}{8}$	$\frac{3}{16}$	$\frac{3}{16}$	$\frac{11}{32}$	$\frac{3}{8}$
	Degrees 3 and 4									
I A	One remarriage									
1, 2	Half aunt or uncle and half cousin (Fig. 14)	*wW* *wHh*	*Ww* *hHw*	$\frac{3}{32}$	0	$\frac{1}{4}$	$\frac{1}{8}$	$\frac{1}{8}$	$\frac{1}{16}$	0
3, 4	,, ,, ,,	*wH* *wWw*	*Hw* *wWw*	,,	,,	$\frac{1}{8}$	$\frac{5}{16}$	$\frac{1}{16}$	$\frac{5}{32}$	0
5, 6	,, ,, ,,	*hW* *hHh*	*Wh* *hHh*	,,	,,	0	0	$\frac{1}{4}$	$\frac{1}{8}$	0
7, 8	,, ,, ,,	*hH* *hWw*	*Hh* *wWh*	,,	,,	0	0	$\frac{1}{8}$	$\frac{1}{16}$	0

Table 1. *Relationships and coefficients of relationship*—(Contd.)

	Relation	Symbol	Converse	f	F	ϕ_{11}	ϕ_{12}	ϕ_{21}	ϕ_{22}	Φ
B	Two remarriages									
9, 10	Half aunt or uncle and half cousin (Fig. 15)	*wW* *hWh*	*Ww* *hWh*	1/32	1/32	1/4	1/8	1/8	1/16	1/8
11, 12	,, ,, ,,	*wW* *hHh*	*Ww* *hHh*	,,	,,	1/4	1/8	1/8	1/16	0
13, 14	,, ,, ,,	*wH* *hWw*	*Hw* *wWh*	,,	,,	0	1/4	1/8	1/16	1/8
15, 16	,, ,, ,,	*wH* *hWw*	*Hw* *wHh*	,,	,,	0	1/4	0	1/8	0
17, 18	,, ,, ,,	*hW* *wWh*	*Wh* *hWw*	,,	,,	0	1/8	1/4	1/16	1/8
19, 20	,, ,, ,,	*hW* *wHh*	*Wh* *hHw*	,,	,,	0	1/8	1/4	1/8	0
21, 22	,, ,, ,,	*hH* *wWw*	*Hh* *wWw*	,,	,,	1/8	1/16	1/16	1/32	0
23, 24	,, ,, ,,	*hH* *wHw*	*Hh* *wHw*	,,	,,	1/4	1/8	1/8	1/16	0
II A	Double remarriage									
25, 26	Half aunt or uncle and double half cousin (Fig. 16)	*wW* *wHh* *hWh*	*Ww* *hHw* *hWh*	1/8	1/32	1/4	1/8	1/8	1/16	1/8
27, 28	,, ,, ,,	*wH* *wWw* *hHw*	*Hw* *wWw* *wHh*	,,	,,	1/8	1/16	1/16	3/32	0
29, 30	,, ,, ,,	*hW* *hHh* *wWh*	*Wh* *hHh* *hWw*	,,	,,	0	1/4	1/8	1/16	1/8
31, 32	,, ,, ,,	*hH* *hWw* *wHw*	*Hh* *wWh* *wHw*	,,	,,	1/4	1/8	1/4	1/8	0
II B	One remarriage									
33, 34	Half aunt or uncle and cousin (Fig. 17)	*wW* *hMh*	*Ww* *hMh*	1/8	1/16	1/4	1/8	1/8	1/16	1/8
35, 36	,, ,, ,,	*wH* *hMw*	*Hw* *wMh*	,,	,,	0	1/4	1/8	1/16	1/8
37, 38	,, ,, ,,	*hW* *wMh*	*Wh* *hMw*	,,	,,	0	1/8	1/4	1/16	1/8
39, 40	,, ,, ,,	*hH* *wMw*	*Hh* *wMw*	,,	,,	3/8	1/16	3/16	3/32	0
III	Two remarriages									
41	Half aunt or uncle, half nephew or niece, and half cousin (Fig. 18)	*wH* *Hw* *wWw*	*S*	5/32	1/16	1/8	3/16	3/16	9/32	1/4
42	,, ,, ,,	*hW* *Wh* *hHh*	*S*	,,	,,	0	1/4	1/4	1/4	1/4

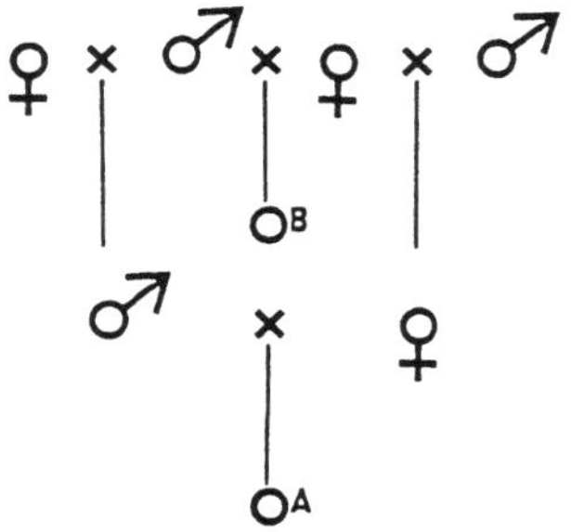

Fig. 1 The relationship symbolised by $\left\{\begin{matrix} \text{wW} \\ \text{h H} \end{matrix}\right.$

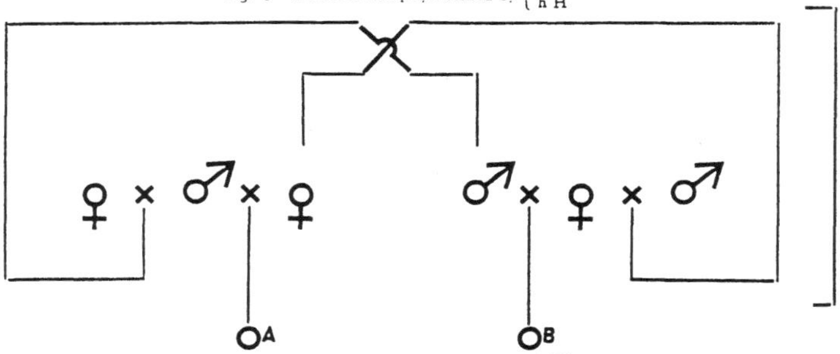

Fig. 2 The relationship symbolised by $\left\{\begin{matrix} \text{wW} \\ \text{H h} \end{matrix}\right.$

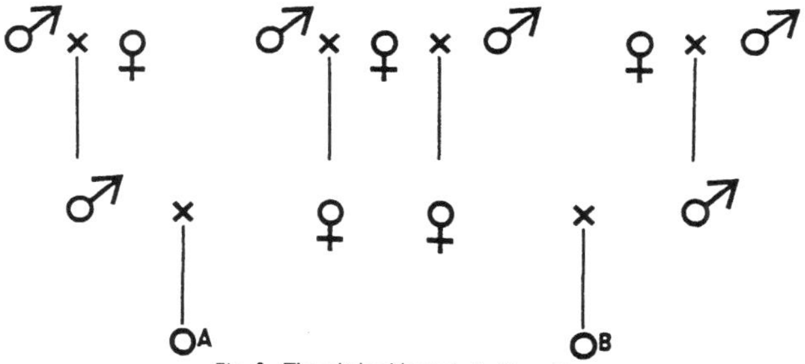

Fig. 3 The relationship symbolised by wWw

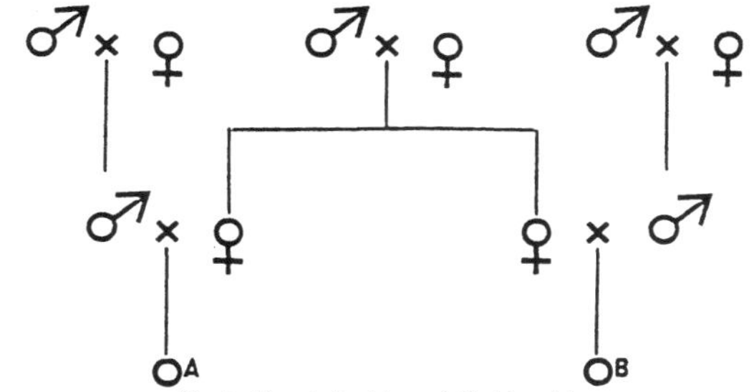

Fig. 4 The relationship symbolised by wMw

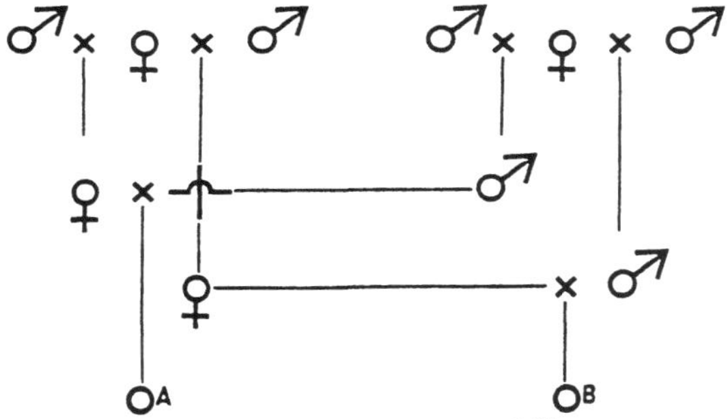

Fig. 5 The relationship symbolised by $\left\{\begin{matrix} wWw \\ hWh \end{matrix}\right.$

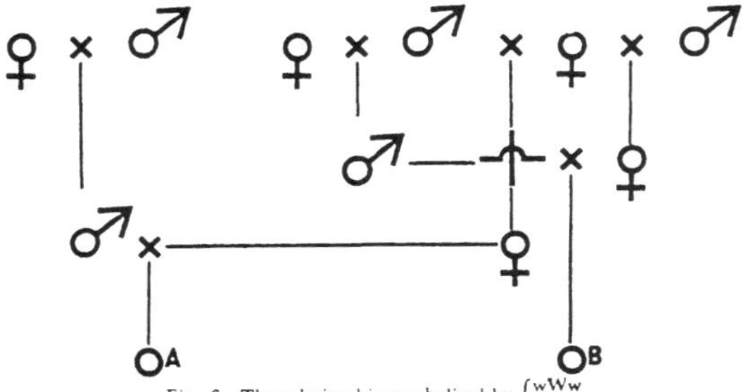

Fig. 6 The relationship symbolised by $\left\{\begin{matrix} wWw \\ wHh \end{matrix}\right.$

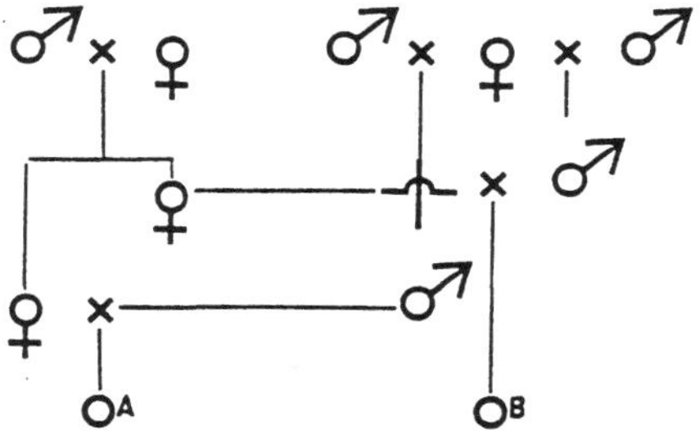

Fig. 7 The relationship symbolised by $\left\{\begin{matrix} wMw \\ hWh \end{matrix}\right.$

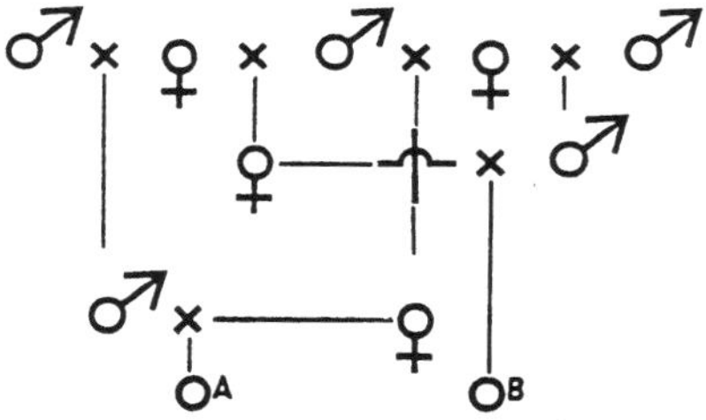

Fig. 8 The relationship symbolised by $\left\{\begin{matrix} wWw \\ hWh \\ wHw \end{matrix}\right.$

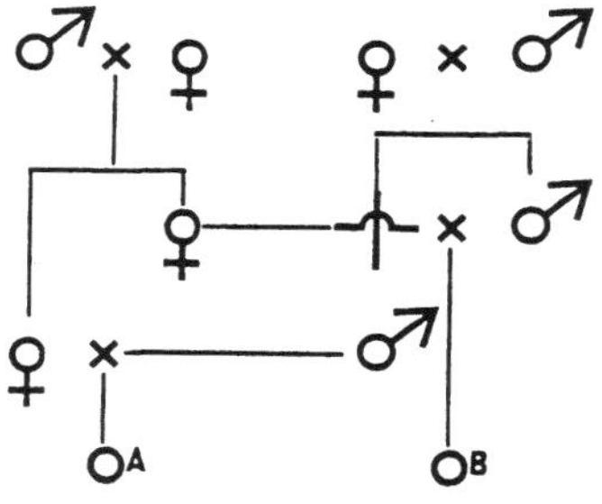

Fig. 9 The relationship symbolised by $\left\{\begin{matrix} wMw \\ hMh \end{matrix}\right.$

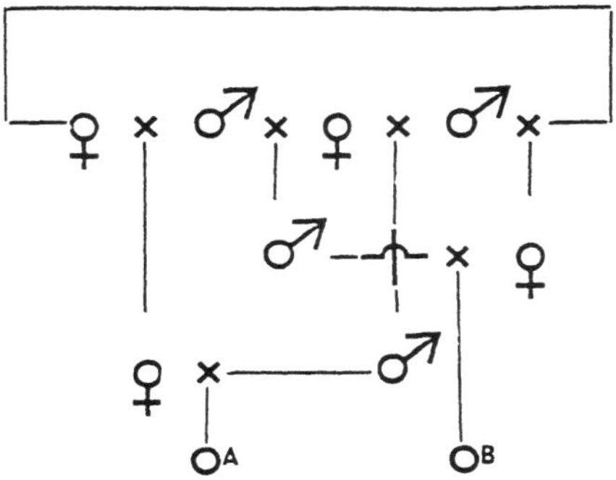

Fig. 10 The relationship symbolised by $\begin{cases} wWw \\ wHh \\ hWh \\ hHw \end{cases}$

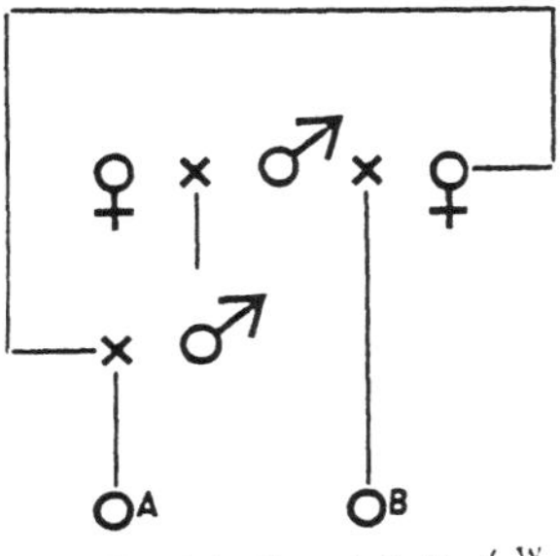

Fig. 11 The relationship symbolised by $\begin{cases} W \\ hH \end{cases}$

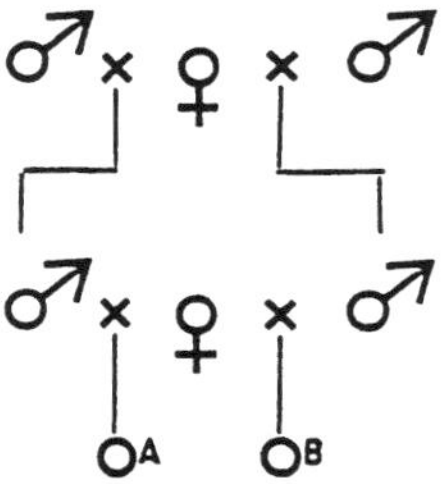

Fig. 12 The relationship symbolised by $\left\{\begin{matrix} W \\ hWh \end{matrix}\right.$

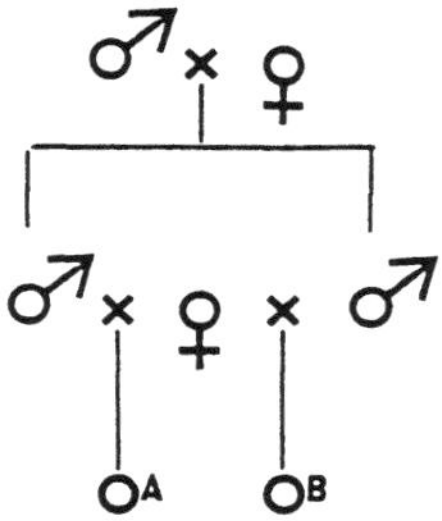

Fig. 13 The relationship symbolised by $\left\{\begin{matrix} W \\ hMh \end{matrix}\right.$

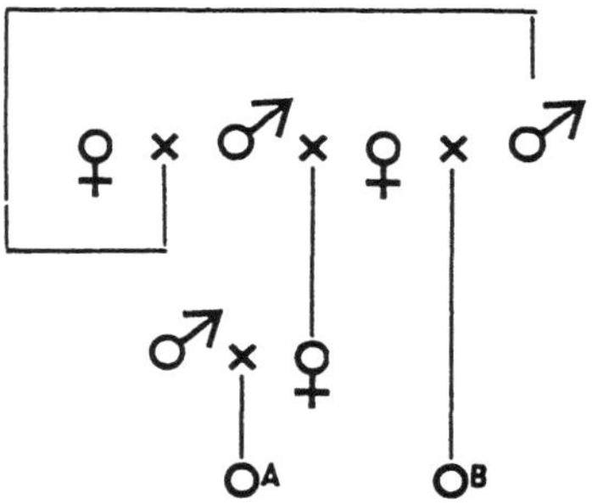

Fig. 14 The relationship symbolised by $\left\{\begin{matrix} wW \\ wHh \end{matrix}\right.$

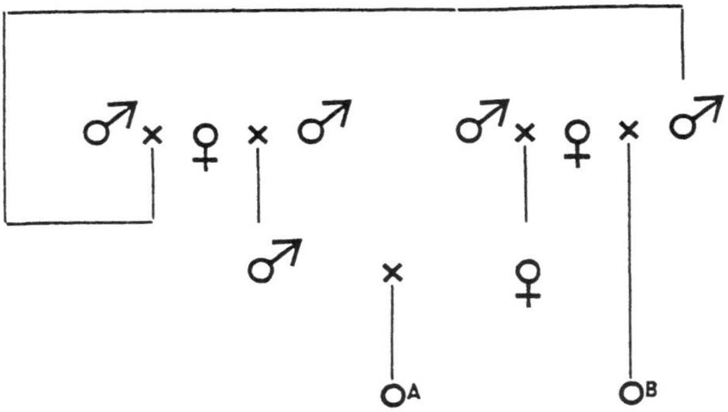

Fig. 15 The relationship symbolised by $\left\{\begin{array}{l} wW \\ hWh \end{array}\right.$

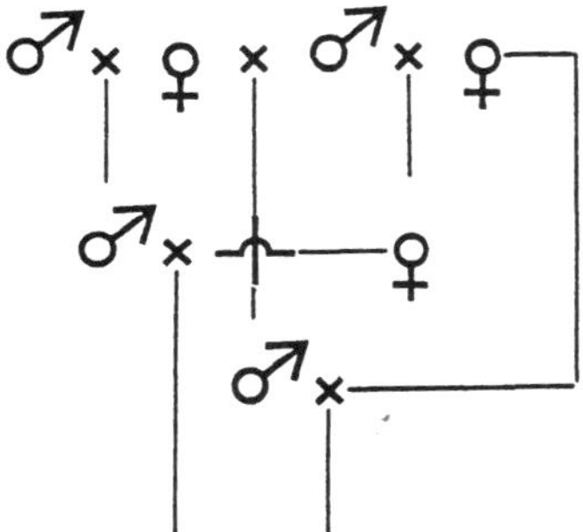

Fig. 16 The relationship symbolised by $\left\{\begin{array}{l} wW \\ wHh \\ hWh \end{array}\right.$

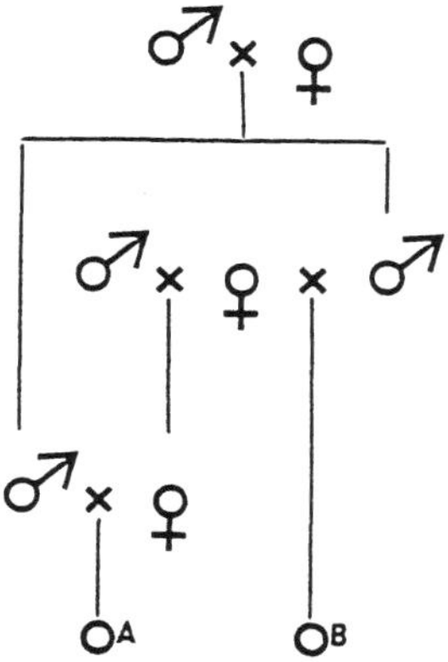

Fig. 17 The relationship symbolised by $\begin{cases} \text{wW} \\ \text{hMh} \end{cases}$

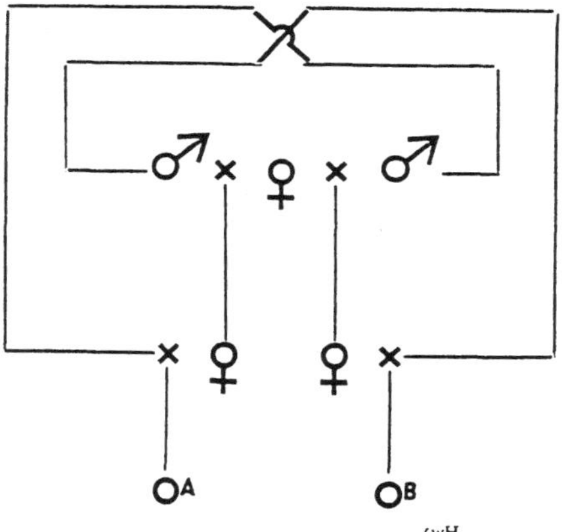

Fig. 18 The relationship symbolised by $\begin{cases} \text{wH} \\ \text{Hw} \\ \text{wWw} \end{cases}$

and Arjuna, though legally sons of Pandu, were in fact children of their mother Kunti by different males, their relationship was $\left.\begin{matrix} W \\ hWh \end{matrix}\right\}$. To take a still more startling relationship, according to some Greek mythologists, after Odysseus' death his son Telemachus by Penelope married Circe, his son Telegonos by Circe married Penelope. The children of these second marriages were in the relation $\left.\begin{matrix} Wh \\ hW \\ hHh \end{matrix}\right\}$. Each, if a male, was half-uncle, half-nephew, and half-first cousin of the other. It is perhaps unlikely that this relationship, which closes our list, has occurred outside mythology.

While relationships whose symbol contains a single H or a single W are not rare, those with several such are much rarer, and those involving a triple remarriage of five persons must be very rare, even though such a chain of marriages could occur without divorce. On the other hand a cyclical remarriage (Fig. 10) must be rare, though it occurs in communities where divorce is easy and spouses exchanged. But the sequel of two marriages between the unrelated progeny of the cyclical remarriage must be very rare indeed, whereas a marriage between two brothers and two sisters, which yields similar coefficients of relationship, is not unusual.

The relationships fall into 24 groups, in each of which the structure, as shown by the pedigree, is the same, apart from differences of sex. Hence in each group the values of f and F, which refer to autosomal genes, and are thus not affected by sex, are constant. The groups are separated in Table 1. The values of f and F may of course be the same in two groups of different structure, for example the grandparent and grandchild group and the half sib group. There is no difficulty in being sure that one has enumerated all the possible relationships in such a group. One has merely to permute the sexes of all relevant ancestors of A and B in every way consistent with the condition that the parents of any individual are of different sexes. The number of relationships in a group then ranges from 1 to 16 (subject to multiplication by 4 if the sexes of A and B are taken into account). It is a little harder to lay down rules to ensure that the enumeration of the isomorphic groups is exhaustive.

The following argument shows that there are 48 and only 48 types of first cousin relationship. A has four grandparents, his mother's mother C_2, his father's mother C_1, his mother's father γ_2, his father's father γ_1. Similarly B's four grandparents may be labelled C_2', C_1', γ_2', γ_1'. A and B may have 1, 2, 3, or 4 grandparents in common.

First consider in how many ways they may have one in common. We can choose any of A's four grandparents, say C_1. This grandparent must be a female grandparent of B, and can be assigned to B in two ways, either as C_1' or C_2'. Thus there are 8 different relationships. We can choose two like-sexed grandparents of A in 2 ways, and assign them to B in 2 ways. So they can have two like-sexed grandparents in 4 ways. We can choose two unlike-sexed grandparents of A in 4 ways, and assign them in 4 ways. So A and B can have 2 unlike-sexed grandparents in 16 ways, and 2 grandparents in 20 ways. We can choose 3 grandparents of A in 4 ways, and assign them to B in 4 ways, making 16 possibilities. Finally if they have all 4 grandparents in common the grandmothers may be assigned to B in 2 ways, and the grandfathers in 2 ways, making 4 in all. This agrees with the figures 8, 20, 16, and 4, given in Table 1.

However we actually used a method which can be illustrated from the relations between first cousins. We write down the 8 single path relationships:—

wWw, *wWh*, *hWw*, *hWh*, *wHw*, *wHh*, *hHw*, and *hHh*.

Any one of these is compatible with any other differing from it by two or more steps. A capital letter represents two steps. Thus *wWw* is compatible with all the others except *wWh* and *hWw*. Thus 8 of the 28 possible pairs of paths are excluded because they involve incest, e.g. $\left.\begin{matrix} wWw \\ wWh \end{matrix}\right\}$. This leaves 20 admissible relationships with 2 grandparents in common. A third path may be added to each pair provided it is not incompatible with either of the first two. The triad of paths must include two with the same common capital letter. There are only 4 such pairs, and each such pair can be associated with any path with the other capital letter. For example $\left.\begin{matrix} wWh \\ hWw \end{matrix}\right\}$ can be associated with any path including H. Thus there are 16 relationships involving 3 grandparents. Similarly each of the two compatible pairs including W can be associated with either of the two including H, giving 4 quadruple relationships. In fact we represented each single path by a point, joined the compatible points by 20 lines, and then picked out triangles and quadrilaterals with both diagonals. Two paths differing only in their capital letters are condensed, e.g. $\left.\begin{matrix} wWw \\ wHw \end{matrix}\right\}$ to *wMw*. The same principles can be applied to the relationships of mixed degree, though here some multiple relationships are excluded because they involve more than 3 generations.

The calculation of coefficients of relationship is not difficult. B may be related to A by at most 4 single paths; and since a gene found in A and B can only be inherited from one of their common ancestors, the contributions of these paths to f and ϕ are additive. The single paths are symbolized by W, H, numbers 1 to 8 of degree 3, and numbers 1 to 8 of degree 4. Thus having calculated the values of f and ϕ for these paths we can obtain them for all the rest by addition. Thus the values for $\left.\begin{matrix} wMw \\ hWh \end{matrix}\right\}$ are obtained by adding those for *wWw*, *wHw*, and *hWh*. The values of F and Φ are sums of two products of f and ϕ values which may be looked up in the earlier parts of Table 1, and of the values when $A \equiv B$, which are given in the first line of Table 2.

The most important of the coefficients is Wright's f, which among other things, determines the biological dangers of inbreeding, and its biological advantage in reducing the risk of maternal-foetal incompatibility. As the latter, though it has probably been detected by Goldschmidt (1961), has not been calculated, we discuss it in the next section. The prohibitions against marriage with cognate relatives, if, as has been suggested, they are based on the observation that inbreeding produces more defective children than outbreeding, are not very logical, as has often been pointed out. Marriage between half brother and half sister is generally prohibited, and a union between them is criminal in many legal codes. However, by the standard of f, they are no more closely related than niece and uncle or aunt and nephew, whose union is legal in some codes, and criminal in few or none, double first cousins (who may marry where uncle and niece may not, as in Britain) and several complex relations. In British law a man may not marry his half-niece, who is less closely related ($f=\frac{1}{16}$) than his double first cousin.

THE EFFECT OF INBREEDING ON DISEASE AND DEATH DUE TO MATERNAL-FOETAL INCOMPATIBILITY

Consider an autosomal locus where a gene **A** determines the production of an antigen such that an **Aa** child may immunize an **aa** mother, and cause its own death, or more usually that of a subsequent **Aa** child. The symbol **A** is used both for genes such a $\mathbf{A}_1$ which appear often to immunize a mother to her first **Aa** child, and those such as **D** which rarely immunize the mother during the first pregnancy.

If p is the frequency of **A**, q that of **a**, i.e. of all alleles not producing the antigen in question, the frequency of mothers lacking the antigen is q^2. In a random mating population a fraction p of their children, or pq^2 of all children, is liable to be immunized. Of these p^2q^2 are in families consisting of **Aa** children only, pq^3 in families consisting of **Aa** and **aa.** In the case of genes such as **D** the former are at a considerably greater risk. If the father is a relative of the mother with given values of f and F, the frequency of **Aa** among the children of **aa** mothers is reduced from p to $(1-2f)p$. The fraction belonging to all-**Aa** families is reduced from p^2 to $(1-4f-F)p^2$, while that belonging to mixed families is changed from pq to $p[q+2f(p-q)-Fp]$, which may be an increase or decrease according to the value of p. If K of the **Aa** children of homozygous, and k of the children of heterozygous fathers are killed by incompatibility, the death-rate from this cause is $pq^2\ (Kp+kq)$ when parents are unrelated, and

$$pq^2[Kp+kq-f\ (2Kp-kp+kq)+F(K-k)p]$$

when they are related. Thus inbreeding saves the lives of a fraction

$$f+\frac{(f-F)\ (K-k)\ p}{Kp+kq}$$

of the babies which would otherwise die from the effect of incompatibility. $f>F$ and $K>k$, so the fraction exceeds f, but cannot exceed $2f-F$. This however is the fraction saved at any one locus. If the number of independent loci concerned is large enough, it is conceivable that the death-rate may be reduced quite considerably by cousin marriage.

Sex-linked genes responsible for human antigens are not yet known.* Still less is there any evidence that such genes are ever responsible for incompatibility between mother and foetus. However it is interesting to calculate what effect they have if they exist. Let **S** and **s** be a pair of sex-linked allelomorphs, or groups of allelomorphs, such that **S** determines the production of an antigen capable of immunizing **ss** mothers, while **s** does not. A **ss** mother cannot bear **S** sons, but may bear **Ss** daughters, who may be eliminated. Let p and q be the frequencies of **S** and **s,** and k the fraction of **Ss** daughters of **ss** mothers eliminated. The fraction of daughters eliminated if parents

* We learn that one has at last been discovered.

are unrelated is clearly kpq^2, and it can be seen that there is unstable equilibrium when $p = q = \frac{1}{2}$, as in the autosomal case. The frequency of males among the surviving offspring would thus be $\frac{1}{2 - kpq^2}$ if no other causes were disturbing the sex ratio.

If the parents are related, the frequency of **Ss** among the daughters of **ss** mothers is reduced from p to $(1 - \phi)p$ where ϕ is the coefficient of relationship of the parents. Thus the frequency of males would be reduced from $(2 - kpq^2)^{-1}$ to $[2 - k(1 - \phi)pq^2]^{-1}$. Goldschmidt however found more males when the parents were related. So incompatibility, if it accounts for a lower abortion rate, cannot account for a higher frequency of males when parents are related. If $p = \frac{1}{3}$, which gives the maximal elimination, and $k = 0{\cdot}1$, which is very high, the frequency of males would only be 50·373%, and if the coefficient of sex-linked relationship of parents were 1/8, it would only be reduced to 50·326%, which could hardly be verified on a sample less than a million. There might be several such loci on the X chromosome, but a high mortality rate and a high frequency of the rarer allele could seldom coexist. Even if, between them, they accounted for the whole excess of males observed, inbreeding would rarely reduce the ratio by even one eighth of the way towards equality. We conclude that such effects, if they occur, are unimportant.

The effect of inbreeding in raising the male frequency, if it is confirmed, is perhaps more likely to be due to the same group of causes which eliminate male mammals, and in general members of the heterogametic sex, in interspecific hybrids (Haldane, 1922).

The Effect of Monozygotic Twinning

If B is A's monozygotic twin, the effect on the coefficients of relationship is as shown in the first line of Table 2. If a pair of like-sexed sibs are monozygotic twins they are believed to be genetically identical. If any pair of "paths" connecting B to A passes through a pair of whole brothers or sisters, these may be monozygotic twins. In double first cousinship of the first type, either the sisters, the brothers, or both, may be monozygotic twins. The relationships which can be transformed by monozygotic twinning are listed in Table 2. The first one can of course only be transformed if A and B are of like sex, the second if B is a woman, the third if A is a woman, the fourth if B is a man and the fifth if A is a man. Altogether 18 relationships can be so transformed. The second column gives the original value of f, the fourth and later those of the transformed relationship. The value of f is always increased, but never more than doubled. That of F can be increased up to four times. The marriage of two pairs of monozygotic twins may not be as rare as might be thought. A biometric study of the resemblance between the children of monozygotic twins would be well worth carrying out.

Relationships when Relatives are Inbred

We shall not consider these in any detail, but it may be instructive to work out the number of first cousinships possible if A, B, or both are inbred. A may have only 3

Table 2. *Enhancement of relationship by monozygotic twinning*

Original relationship	f	Enhanced relationship	f	F	ϕ_{11}	ϕ_{12}	ϕ_{21}	ϕ_{22}	Φ
M	$\frac{1}{2}$	Identity	$\frac{1}{2}$	1	1	..	..	$\frac{1}{2}$	1
w.M	$\frac{1}{4}$	Mother	$\frac{1}{4}$	0	..	$\frac{1}{2}$	..	$\frac{1}{4}$	0
Mw	,,	Woman's child	,,	,,	..	..	$\frac{1}{2}$	$\frac{1}{4}$	0
h.M	,,	Father	,,	,,	0	..	$\frac{1}{2}$	..	..
Mh	,,	Man's child	,,	,,	0	$\frac{1}{2}$	..	..	..
w.Mw	$\frac{1}{16}$	*W*	$\frac{1}{8}$	0	$\frac{1}{2}$	$\frac{1}{4}$	$\frac{1}{4}$	$\frac{1}{8}$	0
h.Mh	,,	*H*	,,	,,	0	0	0	$\frac{1}{4}$	0
w.Mw } *hWh* }	$\frac{7}{32}$	*W* } *hWh* }	$\frac{5}{32}$	$\frac{1}{16}$	$\frac{1}{2}$	$\frac{1}{4}$	$\frac{1}{4}$	$\frac{1}{4}$	$\frac{1}{4}$
w.Mw } *hHh* }	,,	*W* } *hHh* }	,,	,,	$\frac{1}{2}$	$\frac{1}{4}$	$\frac{1}{4}$	$\frac{1}{8}$	0
h.Mh } *wWw* }	,,	*H* } *wWw* }	,,	,,	$\frac{1}{8}$	$\frac{1}{16}$	$\frac{1}{16}$	$\frac{9}{32}$	$\frac{1}{8}$
h.Mh } *wHw* }	,,	*H* } *wHw* }	,,	,,	$\frac{1}{4}$	$\frac{1}{8}$	$\frac{1}{8}$	$\frac{5}{16}$	$\frac{1}{4}$
w.Mw } *h.Mh* }	$\frac{1}{8}$	*W* } *h.Mh* }	$\frac{1}{16}$	$\frac{1}{8}$	$\frac{1}{2}$	$\frac{1}{4}$	$\frac{1}{4}$	$\frac{1}{4}$	$\frac{1}{4}$
,,	,,	*H* } *w.Mw* }	,,	,,	$\frac{3}{8}$	$\frac{3}{16}$	$\frac{3}{16}$	$\frac{11}{32}$	$\frac{3}{8}$
,,	,,	*M*	$\frac{1}{4}$	$\frac{1}{4}$	$\frac{1}{2}$	$\frac{1}{4}$	$\frac{1}{4}$	$\frac{3}{8}$	$\frac{1}{2}$
W } *hMh* }	$\frac{3}{16}$	*M*	,,	,,	,,	,,	,,	,,	,,
H } *wMw* }	,,	*M*	,,	,,	,,	,,	,,	,,	,,
wW } *hMh* }	$\frac{1}{8}$	*H* } *wW* }	$\frac{3}{16}$	$\frac{1}{8}$	$\frac{1}{4}$	$\frac{1}{8}$	$\frac{1}{8}$	$\frac{5}{16}$	$\frac{1}{4}$
Ww } *hMh* }	,,	*H* } *Ww* }	,,	,,	$\frac{1}{4}$	$\frac{1}{8}$	$\frac{1}{8}$	$\frac{5}{16}$	$\frac{1}{4}$
hH } *wMw* }	,,	*W* } *hH* }	,,	,,	$\frac{1}{2}$	$\frac{1}{4}$	$\frac{1}{4}$	$\frac{1}{8}$	0
Hh } *wMw* }	,,	*W* } *Hh* }	,,	,,	$\frac{1}{2}$	$\frac{1}{4}$	$\frac{1}{4}$	$\frac{1}{8}$	0

grandparents in two ways. His double grandfather had a son and daughter by different women, and *A* is the offspring of their union. Or he may have only one grandmother as a result of a union between her offspring by two men. In either case the three grandparents can be specified uniquely. *A* can have only two grandparents in three ways. His grandfather may have united with a daughter, and is therefore *A*'s father and grandfather. Or his grandmother may have united with a son. We do not consider these possibilities further, as they give rise to mixed relationships of degree 3 and 4. Finally *A* may be the offspring of the union of a whole brother and sister.

7

This possibility will be considered. All these possibilities are of course realised in animal breeding.

Table 3. *Summary of Tables* 1 *and* 2

Degree of relationship	Symmetrical relationships	Pairs of converse relationships	Number enhanced by monozygosity
1	0	1	0
2	3	2	1
3	2	9	4
4	24	12	7
2+3	0	2	0
2+4	6	0	2
3+4	2	20	4
	37	46	18

It is convenient to denote the relationships where *A* has *m* grandparents and *B* has *n* by (m, n). We have shown that there are 48 relationships of class (4, 4). Let us now find the number in class (3, 4). First consider the relationships with 1 grandparent in common. If *A* has only one grandfather he can be assigned to *B* in 2 ways. But *A*'s grandmother can be chosen in 2 ways and assigned in 2. So they may have one grandparent in common in 6 ways, with 6 more when *A* has only one grandmother, making 12. Again if *A* has only one grandfather we can choose two grandmothers in one way and assign them to *B* in 2 ways; we can choose a grandfather and grandmother in 2 ways and assign them in 4. Similarly if *A* has only one grandmother. Thus *A* and *B* can have 2 common grandparents in 20 ways. Similarly *A*'s 3 grandparents may be assigned in 4 ways if he has one grandmother, or 8 in all. The total number of cousinships of class (3, 4) is thus 12+20+8, or 40.

Similar calculations may be made for other classes, and we find the following numbers

(4, 4)	48
(3, 4) and (4, 3)	80
(2, 4) and (4, 2)	16
(3, 3)	40
(2, 3) and (3, 2)	20
(2, 2)	3
	207

Thus the number of possible first cousin-ships has been increased from 48 to 207, or 828 if the sexes of *A* and *B* are considered. The grand total of all relationships would be considerably increased, since new relationships of mixed degree are possible, for example A may be B's parent and grandparent, parent and half-sib, and so on. Our h, w symbolism is not adapted to describe relationships involving inbreeding of either relative, that is to say relation through a line of intermediaries which forks.

RELATIONSHIPS OF HIGHER DEGREE

It is quite possible to enumerate relationships of higher degree, and to calculate their coefficients. We have not attempted this task for two reasons. The first is its gigantic character. As will be seen, a list of relationships between second cousins on the lines of Table 1 would occupy several volumes. The second is that as soon as we reach asymmetrical relations of degree 4 such as that of great-uncle, or relations of higher degree such as first cousin once removed, it becomes possible for A or B to be inbred, and related through chains of relatives which split. We shall merely calculate the number of distinct relationships between second cousins which do not involve inbreeding, so that both A and B have 8 distinct grandparents. Clearly they are all built up of 32 constituents such as *whWhh*, though at most 8 of these can be combined, since there are at most 8 common grandparents. Let the great-grandmothers of A be C_1, C_2, C_3, C_4, the great-grandfathers γ_1, γ_2, γ_3, γ_4, each defined by her or his relation to A. Thus C_2 might be A's mother's father's mother. Let C'_1, C'_2, C'_3, C'_4, γ'_1, γ'_2, γ'_3, γ'_4 be the great grandparents of B, similarly defined. From 1 to 8 of these may be common great grandparents of both. Consider the grandmothers. If a single one is common to A and B this can occur in 4^2 or 16 ways, for that of A can be any of C_1, C_2, C_3, and C_4, and that of B can be any one of C'_1, C'_2, C'_3 and C'_4. Thus the same woman could be A's mother's father's mother and B's father's father's mother. Similarly a second identical pair can be chosen in $3^2 = 9$ ways, but since the order of the pairs is irrelevant we have $16 \times 9 \div 2$ or 72 possibilities. Similarly 3 identities can be chosen in $4^2.3^2.2^2 \div 3!$, or 96 ways, and four identities in $4^2.3^2.2^2.1^2 \div 4!$, or 24 ways. In fact the identity of i great grandmothers allows of $\frac{(4!)^2}{[(4-i)!]^2 i!}$ possibilities. The same is clearly true for the great grandfathers. Now suppose A and B have 5 great-grandparents in common, 4 may be great grandmothers and 1 great-grandfather, or 1 great-grandmother and 4 great-grandfathers, each giving 24×16, or 384 possibilities. Or they may have 3 great-grandmothers and 2 great-grandfathers, or 2 and 3, in common, each giving 72×96, or 6912 possibilities. We thus have the possibilities given in Table 4.

There are thus 43,680 or $2^5.3.5.7.13$ distinct relationships when neither A nor B is inbred. But A's or B's parents may, without incest, be any one of the 48 types of first cousin, descended from only 7 to 4 great-grandparents. When allowance is made for this there may be about 9 million types of second cousin.

DISCUSSION

Our main results are summarized in Table 3. Perhaps the most unexpected is the large number of possible relationships of mixed degrees 3 and 4. Some of these may

Table 4. *Possible relations of outbred second cousins*

Number of common greatgrandparents	Partitions	Possible relationships	Total
1	0+1	2×16	32
2	0+2, 1+1	$2\times 72+16^2$	400
3	0+3, 1+2	$2\times 96+2\times 16\times 72$	2,496
4	0+4, 1+3, 2+2	$2\times 24+2\times 16\times 96+72^2$	8,304
5	1+4, 2+3	$2\times 16\times 24+2\times 72\times 96$	14,592
6	2+4, 3+3	$2\times 72\times 24+96^2$	12,672
7	3+4	$2\times 96\times 24$	4,608
8	4+4	24^2	576
			43,680

not be very rare. Where it is permitted, there is nothing surprising in a widower marrying a woman, and his son by another marriage marrying her younger sister. The children of these marriages are in the relationship symbolized by $\left.\begin{matrix}Hh\\ wMw\end{matrix}\right\}$.

We are aware that we may have made errors both by omitting relationships permitted by our hypothesis, by miscalculation, or by the overlooking of misprints. We shall be thankful to receive corrections, and to publish them if they are accepted. Our symbolism may be found unacceptable. We have given reasons for preferring it to a bulkier if more logical symbolism, and for using *w* and *h* rather than *f* and *m*, *m* and *f*, or *m* and *p*. It has the grave demerits of not covering ancestral relationships or their converses, relations beyond the fourth degree, or relationships involving incest. It has however the merit that it can readily be extended to cover the distinction between older and younger brothers or sisters where this is sociologically important. If by putting a sign above or below that of the common ancestor or ancestors we denote younger and elder sibs, while an asterisk denotes twins, this need can be met. Thus $\overline{W}$ would denote a younger maternal half sib, $\underline{Mw}$ the child of an elder full sister, wM^* a twin of *A*'s mother, and so on.

There is a very serious gap between genetics and anthropology, and anything which can help to bridge that gap is worth attempting.

Summary

The logical structure of human relationships is discussed. When the relatives are not inbred their genetical implications can be summarized by four coefficients of relationship, namely Wright's coefficient of single autosomal relationship, a coefficient of double autosomal relationship, a coefficient of single sex-linked relationship, and one of double sex-linked relationship between women only. A simple symbolism for human relationships is developed. There are 516 possible relationships between *A* and *B*, not involving an ancestor of either more remote than a grandparent, and not involving incest. Table 1 gives the coefficients of relationship for all of them. 192 are relationships between first cousins. In 66 cases the coefficients may be raised by monozygotic twinning. The effect of relationship on incompatibility between mother and foetus is described. There is a brief discussion of relationships involving incest, and those between second cousins.

REFERENCES

CARNAP, R. (1958). *Introduction to symbolic logic and its applications.* Dover, New York.

FISHER, R. A. (1918). The correlation between relatives on the supposition of Mendelian inheritance. *Trans. Roy. Soc. Ed.*, **52**, II, no. 15.

GOLDSCHMIDT, E. (1961). Viability studies in Jews from Kurdistan. Conference on Human Population Genetics in Israel. Abstracts of Communications.

HALDANE, J. B. S. (1922). Sex ratio and unisexual sterility in hybrid animals. *J. Genet.*, **12**, 101-109.

HALDANE, J. B. S. AND MOSHINSKY, P. (1939). Inbreeding in Mendelian populations with special reference to human cousin marriage. *Ann. Eug.*, **9**, 321-340.

KARVE, I. (1953). Kinship organisation in India. *Deccan College Monograph Series*, 11.

KEMPTHORNE, O. (1957). *Introduction to Genetic Statistics.* John Wiley & Sons, Inc., New York.

LERNER, I. M. (1950). *Population Genetics and Animal Improvement.* Cambridge University Press.

MALÉCOT, G. (1948). *Les mathématiques de l'Hérédité.* Masson, Paris.

MORTON, N. E. (1961). Morbidity of children from consanguineous marriages. *Progress in medical genetics.* Vol. **1**, 261-291. Grune and Stratton, New York.

RUSSELL, B. (1903). *The principles of mathematics.* Cambridge.

WRIGHT, S. (1922). Coefficients of inbreeding and relationship. *Amer. Nat.*, **56**, 330-339.

Linkage

Haldane's first study in genetics involved the discovery of linkage in mice, the first known case in vertebrates when he first reported it in a seminar of E.S. Goodrich at Oxford in 1911. However, R.C. Punnett advised him to obtain confirmatory evidence by conducting his own experiments. The paper was published in 1915 with his sister N.M. Haldane (now Lady Naomi Mitchison) and A.D. Sprunt, who died later in World War I. (See "An Autobiography in Brief," p. 19).

A number of papers dealt with the estimation of linkage in special situations. The first of these provided the first mapping function relating crossover values with map distances (1919). The same paper contains the suggestion that map distances can be conveniently measured in units of "centimorgans" (cM), which is now universally used in gene mapping. Another paper (with C.H. Waddington) dealt with an analysis of the effects of inbreeding on linked factors, especially in complex situations that Jennings found so frustrating to deal with.[1] The final paper of the section is especially concerned with the analysis of linkage in the tetraploid *Primula sinensis*, the first such study ever undertaken in plants.

1. Jennings, H.S., The numerical results of diverse systems of breeding with respect to two characters, etc. *Genetics*, 2: 97–154, 1917.

REDUPLICATION IN MICE.

(Preliminary Communication.)

By J. B. S. HALDANE, B.A.,
Lieut. 3rd Black Watch, New College, Oxford;

A. D. SPRUNT, B.A.,
Late 2nd Lieut. 4th Bedfordshire Regt., New College, Oxford;

and N. M. HALDANE,
Home Student, Oxford.

(From the Laboratory of the Department of Comparative Anatomy, Oxford.)

Darbishire's (1) experiments indicated the existence of Reduplication in Mice, and this work was undertaken to verify and extend his results. Owing to the war it has been necessary to publish prematurely, as unfortunately one of us (A. D. S.) has already been killed in France. He was a man of considerable promise, and his death is a real loss to Zoology.

The reduplication occurs between the factors named by Miss Durham (2) **C** and **E**, the absence of **C** producing albinism, that of **E** (when **C** is present) pink eyes and a coloured but pale coat. It is thus not possible to distinguish **ce** (albino) and **Cee** (pink eyed pigmented) mice on birth: hence mice with pink eyes dying before the hair is grown cannot be distinguished, whereas **CE** (dark eyed) mice are at once identifiable.

8 **cc** and 8 **Cee** mice were mated. All the **cc**'s were of composition **ccEE**, two of the **Cee**'s were **Ccee**, the rest **CCee**.

The F_1 generation consisted of 96 **CE** and 6 **cc**, the **CE**'s being therefore of composition **Ce . cE**.

They were mated together and produced 111 **CE**, 116 **Cee** or **cc**. Of these latter 74 survived to grow hair and 33 were **Cee**, 41 **cc**. If the rate of mortality is equal for **Cee** and **cc**, as Darbishire's figures suggest, the original numbers were approximately 111 **CE**, 51·7 **Cee**, 64·3 **cc**.

If the gametic series of F_1 was 1 **CE** : 1 **Ce** : 1 **cE** : 1 **ce**, the expectation would be 9 : 3 : 4, or 127·7 **CE**, 42·6 **Cee**, 56·7 **cc**. If it was 1 **CE** : 3 **Ce** : 3 **cE** : 1 **ce**, the expectation would be 33 : 15 : 16, or 117 **CE**, 53·2 **Cee**, 56·7 **cc**, a much closer fit.

Darbishire mated his F_1 to albinos, obtaining 378 **CE**, 368 **cc**, or nearly equality. We mated F_1 to **CCee** mice, obtaining 18 **CE**, 23 pink eyed, of which the 16 survivors were all **Cee**. This ratio suggests equality.

We next mated the F_2 mice of composition **cc** (albinos) to those of composition **ee** (pink eyed pigmented). We thus discovered which albinos were **ccEE**, **ccEe**, and **ccee**, the former giving no **Cee** offspring, the latter no **CE**, and similarly the **Cee**'s were separated into **CCee** and **Ccee**. Of the albinos 11 were **ccEE**, 9 **ccEe**, 6 either **ccEE** or **ccEe**, 1 **ccEe** or **ccee**. Of the **Cee**'s 7 were **CCee**, 11 **Ccee**, 4 doubtful.

Having thus produced a number of **Ccee** mice (either F_2 or offspring of **ccEe** × **CCee**), they were mated together, and all their albino offspring were therefore **ccee**. These were mated back to the F_1. The result was 3 **CE**, 24 **Cee** or **cc**, of which 7 survivors were **cc**.

Supposing the gametic series to have been 1 **CE**, x **Ce**, y **cE**, z **ce**, we have from the above matings:—

$1 + x = y + z$, and probably $1 + y = x + z$, also $x + y + z = \frac{24}{3}$. Hence $y = x$, $z = 1$, and $2x + 1 = 8$, $\therefore x = 3\frac{1}{2}$. Assuming however that $x = 3$, the expectation from the mating $F_1 \times$ **ccee** is 1 : 7 or $3\frac{3}{8}$ **CE**, $23\frac{5}{8}$ **Cee** and **cc**, a close enough agreement, while without reduplication we should expect $6\frac{3}{4}$, $20\frac{1}{4}$.

The experiments are being continued and extended to rats.

Part of our expenses were met by a grant from the Royal Society.

CONCLUSION.

Reduplication of the "repulsion" type, probably on the basis 1 : 3 : 3 : 1, occurs between the colour factors in mice named by Miss Durham (2) **C** and **E**, by Hagedoorn (3) **A** and **E**.

REFERENCES.

1. DARBISHIRE. *Biometrika*, Vol. III. p. 1, 1904.
2. DURHAM. *Reports to Evolution Committee of the Royal Society*, IV. 1908.
   —— *Journal of Genetics*, Vol. I. No. 2, 1911.
3. HAGEDOORN. *Zeitschrift für induktive Abstammungs- und Vererbungslehre*, Vol. VI. No. 3, 1911.

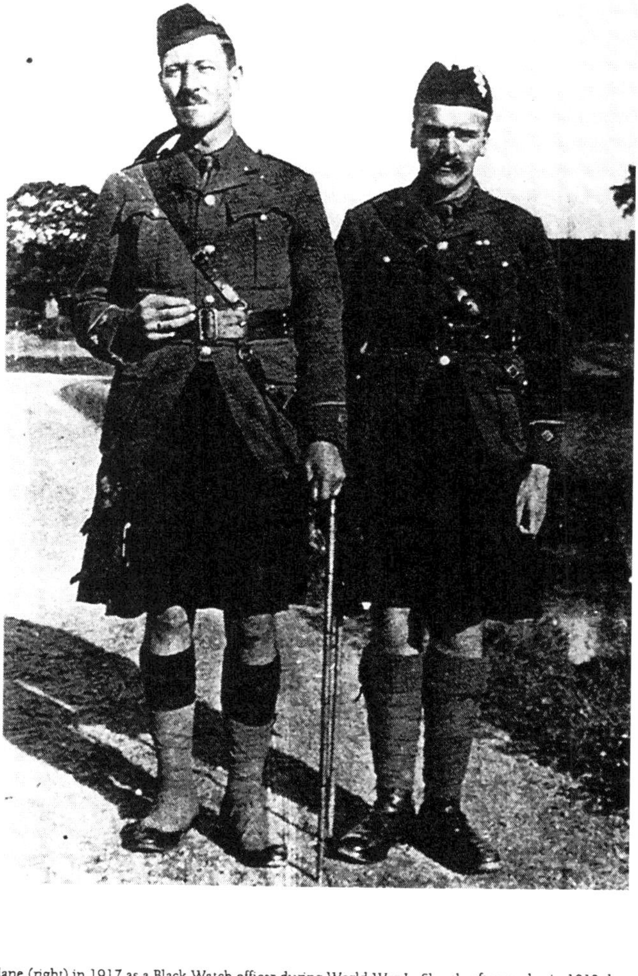

Haldane (right) in 1917 as a Black Watch officer during World War I. Shortly afterwards, in 1919, he wrote a paper on the estimation of linkage, inventing the first mapping function and the unit 'centimorgan' (cM) for measuring map distances.

THE COMBINATION OF LINKAGE VALUES, AND THE CALCULATION OF DISTANCES BETWEEN THE LOCI OF LINKED FACTORS.

BY J. B. S. HALDANE, M.A.,
Fellow of New College, Oxford.

(With One Text-figure.)

ON the theory that the degree of linkage between two factors depends on the distance apart of their loci in a chromosome, Morgan and his fellow-workers have taken the distance between two loci as proportional to the cross-over value[1] of the factors located in them. This theory gives consistent results when the cross-over values are small, but, as recognised by Sturtevant, and by Morgan and Bridges(1), is not accurate for larger values. On the reduplication theory Trow(2) has given a formula for the combination of linkage values which is shown below to be inaccurate when the linkage is not close. In the present paper a more accurate theory of the relations *inter se* of the cross-over values, and of their connexion with the distances apart of the loci of factors in a chromosome, is developed. Some such theory is especially necessary when dealing with a group of factors containing few members not very closely linked.

Suppose A, B, C to be three factors whose loci lie in that order in the same chromosome. Let m be the cross-over value for A and B, n that for A and C. If the chromosomes were perfectly flexible, so that the fact of their having crossed between A and B did not diminish the probability of their crossing again between B and C, we should expect a triply heterozygous organism to produce gametes in the fol-

[1] If zygotes of composition $AB \,.\, ab$ and $Ab \,.\, aB$ give gametic series

$$(1-m)\,AB : m\,Ab : m\,aB : (1-m)\,ab \quad \text{and} \quad m\,AB : (1-m)\,Ab : (1-m)\,aB : m\,ab$$

respectively, then m is said to be the cross-over value for the factors A and B.

lowing proportions if it were of composition $ABC.abc$, and similarly for other compositions: .

No cross-over	(ABC and abc).	$(1-m)(1-n)$.
Cross-over between loci of A and B only	(aBC and Abc).	$m(1-n)$.
,, ,, ,, B and C only	(ABc and abC).	$(1-m)n$.
,, ,, ,, A and B and of B and C	(AbC and aBc).	mn.

Actually the last class has been shown to be in defect in many cases. This has been thought to be due to the loops formed by the chromosomes during synapsis having a modal length(3). If this were so, we should expect to find an excessive number of double cross-overs when the distance between the loci of A and C was equal to twice the modal distance between points of crossing over. This phenomenon has however not been recorded. The shortage of double cross-overs can equally well be explained by the mere rigidity of the chromosomes, which makes sharp bending difficult. In the sex chromosome of Drosophila the ratio[1] of observed to calculated numbers of double cross-overs is ·58 : 1 for eosin (white), vermilion, and sable (4) (where $m + n = \cdot 406$), and ·21 : 1 for vermilion, sable, and bar (3) (where $m + n = \cdot 239$).

If the calculated number mn of double cross-overs occurred, the cross-over value for A and C would be equal to the total number of single cross-overs, *i.e.* to $m(1-n) + (1-m)n$, or $m + n - 2mn$.

If double cross-overs were impossible, but the full numbers of single cross-overs occurred, as would happen if the chromosomes were straight rigid rods, the cross-over value for A and C would obviously be $m + n$ (Morgan and Bridges' formula).

Finally if double cross-overs were impossible, and in every case where one should have occurred according to the calculation above, a single cross-over took its place, the cross-over value for A and C would be $m + n - 2mn + mn$, or $m + n - mn$. This case might be approximately realised if the chromosome could not form loops shorter than some definite length.

Hence the cross-over values for A and C should be approximately $m + n$ when m and n are small, $m + n - 2mn$ when their sum is large, and $m + n - mn$ for intermediate values.

Table I contains the observed values(5) for all triads of factors in the sex chromosome of Drosophila for which each of the cross-over values exceeds ·1 (10 °/₀). The first column gives the three factors concerned in each case; the second and third columns give the cross-

[1] Called by Muller the "coincidence."

over values for the first and second, and second and third factors respectively, *i.e.* m and n. The fourth, fifth, and sixth columns give the results of the three provisional summation formulae obtained above; the seventh gives the observed cross-over value for the first

TABLE I.

1 Factors	2 m	3 n	4 $m+n$	5 $m+n-mn$	6 $m+n-2mn$	7 Observed	8 Class
White sable lethal *sc*	·412	·236	·648	·531	·454	·460	γ
Yellow vermilion rudimentary .	·345	·241	·586	·503	·420	·429	γ
,, ,, bar	·345	·239	·584	·502	·419	·479	γ
White depressed bar	·203	·380	·583	·506	·429	·436	γ ?
,, sable forked	·412	·160	·572	·506	·440	·457	γ
Yellow sable rudimentary ...	·429	·143	·572	·511	·449	·429	δ
,, bar	·429	·138	·567	·508	·449	·479	γ
White vermilion fused	·305	·258	·563	·484	·406	·433	γ
Bifid vermilion forked	·311	·245	·556	·480	·404	·425	γ ?
White sable rudimentary ...	·412	·143	·555	·496	·437	·424	δ
Bifid vermilion rudimentary ...	·311	·241	·552	·477	·402	·427	γ
White vermilion forked ...	·305	·245	·550	·475	·401	·457	γ
,, sable bar	·412	·138	·550	·493	·436	·436	γδ
Yellow miniature bar	·343	·205	·548	·478	·407	·479	β
White vermilion rudimentary ...	·305	·241	·546	·472	·399	·424	γ
,, ,, bar	·305	·239	·544	·471	·398	·436	γ
,, miniature bar	·332	·205	·537	·469	·401	·436	γ
Yellow miniature rudimentary...	·343	·179	·522	·471	·419	·429	γ
White miniature rudimentary .	·332	·179	·511	·452	·392	·424	γ
,, reduplicated bar ...	·289	·206	·495	·435	·375	·436	β
,, furrowed forked	·303	·191	·494	·436	·378	·457	β?
Bifid miniature rudimentary ...	·306	·179	·485	·430	·375	·427	γ?
White furrowed bar	·303	·179	·482	·428	·374	·436	β?
Yellow vermilion sable	·345	·101	·446	·411	·376	·429	β
Facet vermilion sable	·326	·101	·427	·394	·361	·430	α?
Depressed vermilion bar ...	·170	·239	·409	·368	·328	·380	β?
White vermilion sable	·305	·101	·406	·375	·344	·412	α
Shifted vermilion bar... ...	·155	·239	·394	·357	·320	·314	δ?
White depressed vermilion ...	·203	·170	·373	·338	·304	·305	γ?
Yellow club vermilion	·177	·188	·365	·332	·298	·345	β
White lethal *sb* miniature ...	·156	·199	·355	·325	·295	·332	β
White club vermilion	·143	·188	·331	·304	·2	·305	β
,, lemon vermilion ...	·145	·120	·265	·248	·230	·305	α?
Vermilion sable forked ...	·101	·160	·261	·245	·229	·245	βγ
,, ,, rudimentary ...	·101	·143	·244	·230	·215	·241	β
,, ,, bar	·101	·138	·239	·225	·211	·239	αβ

and third factors. In the eighth column these observed values are classified as follows:

Greater than $m + n$	α
Between $m + n$ and $m + n - mn$ . . .	β
,, $m + n - mn$ and $m + n - 2mn$ . .	γ
Less than $m + n - 2mn$	δ.

Those exactly equal to $m + n$ are classified as αβ, and so on. The data are placed in the order of the magnitudes of $m + n$. Where any of the three observed values is based on a count of less than 500 individuals (in which case the probable error of the cross-over value may exceed 1·5 °/₀, as pointed out by the author(6) elsewhere) a query is placed in the last column.

It will be seen that the observed values, when $m+n$ exceeds ·5, lie almost wholly between $m+n-mn$ and $m+n-2mn$, as demanded by the theory above. The three discordant values out of 19 are no more than would be expected in view of the probable errors of the observations due both to small numbers and differential mortality. When $m+n$ is less than ·5 the results are somewhat more irregular, as the calculated values from the three formulae are not very different, but the majority of observations lie between $m+n$ and $m+n-mn$, as demanded by the theory.

This table also enables us to test the formulae given by Trow(2), based on the reduplication theory. If reduplication takes place so that A and B when coupled give the gametic series

$$qAB:1Ab:1aB:qab\left(\text{cross-over value } m=\frac{1}{q+1}\right),$$

whilst B and C give the series

$$rBC:1Bc:1bC:rbc\left(\text{cross-over value } n=\frac{1}{r+1}\right),$$

then A and C should give the series

$$(qr+1)\,BC:(q+r)\,Bc:(q+r)\,bC:(qr+1)\,bc$$

$$\left(\text{cross-over value}=\frac{q+r}{qr+q+r+1}\right).$$

This latter value $=\dfrac{1}{q+1}+\dfrac{1}{r+1}-\dfrac{2}{(q+1)(r+1)}=m+n-2mn$. Hence on this hypothesis the observed cross-over values for A and C should cluster round $m+n-2mn$, and approximately equal numbers should be greater or less than it. In other words, as many values should fall in class δ as in classes α, β, and γ together.

The expectation is therefore 18 (δ), 18 (α, β, and γ); the actual numbers are 3·5 (δ), 32·5 (α, β, and γ), reckoning the single value $\gamma\delta$ as half in each class. Hence the above form of Trow's theory is untenable.

On a more complicated form of the same theory, which Sturtevant(7) has shown to be impossible on other grounds, A and C when coupled alone give a primary series $sAC:1Ac:1aC:sac$, and in zygotes of composition $ABC.abc$, a series

$$(qrs+s)\,AC:(q+r)\,Ac:(q+r)\,aC:(qrs+s)\,ac$$

$$\left(\text{cross-over value} = \frac{q+r}{qrs+q+r+s}\right).$$

As this value is less than that of $m+n-2mn$, it is still more clearly impossible.

The supporters of the reduplication theory must therefore explain the deficiency of the double cross-over classes of gamete (which from a zygote of composition $ABC.abc$ are AbC and aBc). On the chromosome theory this is due to the rigidity of the chromosomes, and until an equally plausible explanation on the reduplication theory is given, the chromosome theory must be considered the more probable of the two, so far as the class of evidence dealt with in this paper is concerned.

It has been shown above that if A, B and C are three factors whose loci lie in that order in the same chromosome, and if m and n are the cross-over values for A, B, and B, C respectively, then the value for A and C is $m+n-pmn$, where p is a number between 0 and 2, increasing on the whole with $m+n$, and having the value 1 when $m+n=$ about ·5. The distances between loci may now be calculated as follows:

Let x be the distance between the loci of two factors, y their cross-over value, and let the unit of distance be chosen so that when y is sufficiently small x becomes equal to y. This assumption is legitimate if we suppose that crossing over is as likely to occur (other things being equal) at one point in the chromosome as another, *i.e.* that the chromosome is equally flexible and breakable at all points. The unit of distance is thus 100 times Morgan's unit.

If now we write $y=f(x)$, the form of this function being indeterminate,

$$\therefore\ f(x+h)=f(x)+f(h)-pf(x)f(h), \text{ where } h \text{ is any increment of } x.$$

$$\therefore\ \frac{f(x+h)-f(x)}{h}=\frac{f(h)-pf(x)f(h)}{h}.$$

Now as h is decreased towards 0, $\frac{f(h)}{h}$ tends to the limit 1.

$$\therefore\ \frac{dy}{dx}=\operatorname*{Lt}_{h\to 0}\frac{f(x+h)-f(x)}{h}$$

$$=\operatorname*{Lt}_{h\to 0}\frac{f(h)-pf(x)f(h)}{h}$$

$=1-pf(x)$, where p has the value assumed when $m=y$, $n=0$,

$=1-py$.

Therefore

$$x = \int_0^y \frac{dt}{1-pt},$$ since x and y vanish together, and $py < 1$.

Hence if p were constant we should have

$$x = \frac{-1}{p}\log_e(1-py), \text{ or } y = \frac{1-e^{-px}}{p} \quad\ldots\ldots\ldots\ldots\ldots(1).$$

Since however p varies between 0 and 2, the values of x must lie between y and $\frac{-1}{2}\log_e(1-2y)$, those of y between x and $\frac{1-e^{-2x}}{2}$; the equation

$$y = x \quad\ldots\ldots\ldots\ldots\ldots\ldots\ldots\ldots\ldots\ldots\ldots(2)$$

being nearly accurate for small values of x and y, the equation

$$y = \frac{1-e^{-2x}}{2}, \text{ or } x = \frac{-1}{2}\log_e(1-2y) \quad\ldots\ldots\ldots\ldots\ldots(3)$$

for large values of x and y, as is obvious, since for large values of x, y approaches the value ·5 asymptotically. The equation (2) corresponds to Morgan's summation formula $m+n$, the equation (3) to Trow's formula $m+n-2mn$.

The equation (3) may be deduced more directly as follows for a perfectly flexible chromosome:

Let a length x of the chromosome be considered as divided into a very large number N of small equal portions. Then the chance of a cross-over in each of these is approximately $\frac{x}{N}$. Hence the chance of a cross-over in t of these segments and no more is

$$\frac{N!}{t!\,(N-t)!}\left(\frac{x}{N}\right)^t\left(1-\frac{x}{N}\right)^{N-t}.$$

When N becomes infinite the limiting value of this expression, *i.e.* the probability of exactly t and no more cross-overs in a length x, is

$$c_t = \frac{x^t e^{-x}}{t!} \quad\ldots\ldots\ldots\ldots\ldots\ldots\ldots\ldots\ldots\ldots(4).$$

Hence the value of y for a given value of x is the sum of the probabilities of all odd numbers of cross-overs.

$$\begin{aligned}\therefore\ y &= c_1 + c_3 + c_5 + c_7 + \ldots\ldots \\ &= e^{-x}\left(\frac{x}{1!} + \frac{x^3}{3!} + \frac{x^5}{5!} + \frac{x^7}{7!} + \ldots\ldots\right) \\ &= e^{-x}\sinh x \\ &= \frac{1-e^{-2x}}{2} \quad\ldots\ldots\ldots\ldots\ldots\ldots\ldots\ldots\ldots\ldots\ldots\ldots(3).\end{aligned}$$

In practice, however, owing to the rigidity of the chromosome, the value of c_1 thus calculated is too small, and those of c_0, c_2, etc. too large. They are however more accurate for great lengths, where the rigidity of the chromosomes affects the results to a less extent.

It is suggested that the unit of distance in a chromosome as defined above be termed a "morgan," on the analogy of the ohm, volt, etc. Morgan's unit of distance is therefore a centimorgan.

To obtain a more accurate relation between x and y we may plot the curves representing equations (2) and (3), and then obtain empirically a curve lying between the two which fits the observed results as closely as possible. This has been done in the figure, where line (a) represents equation (2), curve (b) equation (3), and curve (c)

$$x = \cdot 7y - \frac{\cdot 3}{2} \log_e (1 - 2y) \quad \ldots\ldots\ldots\ldots\ldots\ldots\ldots (5).$$

Equation (5) is merely chosen to give as good a fit as possible and has probably no theoretical significance. The points representing observations are plotted as follows:

The values of y in columns 2 and 3 of Table I are taken, and the corresponding distances in morgans (values of x) read off from curve (c) or Table II. which is calculated from equation (5). These latter are added together, and a point plotted with their sum as abscissa and the observed cross-over value from column 7 of Table I as ordinate. For example the first row of Table I gives the following result:

The cross-over values ·412 and ·236 correspond, according to the curve (c), or better, by interpolation from Table II, to distances of ·549 and ·261 morgans respectively. The sum of these distances is ·810, and the observed cross-over value from column 7 is ·460. The point farthest to the right is accordingly plotted with abscissa ·810 and ordinate ·460. Curve (c) gives the value ·479 for y, and the error of y is accordingly ·019, or 1·9 °/$_\circ$.

It will be seen that 18 of the observations lie above the curve (c), 18 below, and that in only 4 cases, 3 of which are among the results queried in Table I, does the error of y exceed ·04 or 4 °/$_\circ$. The probable error of the cross-over values, as calculated from the curve, is 1·8 °/$_\circ$, or, omitting the queried results, 1·6 °/$_\circ$. This result is not large considering the probable errors of the values of y for the points plotted, which range from 3·1 °/$_\circ$ downwards.

The curve gives satisfactory results for smaller cross-over values, but these are not plotted, as they do not allow of much discrimination between the three equations. If the points had been plotted from either line (*a*) or curve (*b*), $3\frac{1}{2}$ would have lain on one side, $32\frac{1}{2}$ on the other, as may be seen from Table I.

Hence the curve (*c*) may be taken as a fairly accurate guide to the combination of linkage values, and this remains equally true whether the chromosome theory is adopted or not. For this reason a series of values of $100x$ and $100y$ (*i.e.* distances in centimorgans and cross-over values as percentages) calculated from equation (5) are given in Table II. As more results accumulate it should be possible to correct these values, which are rather uncertain for large values of x and y.

TABLE II.

$100y$ (Cross-over value as percentage)					0·0	5·0	8·0	10·0	11·0	12·0	13·0
$100x$ (Distance in centimorgans)				...	0·0	5·1	8·2	10·3	11·4	12·5	13·6
$100y$ ...	14·0	15·0	16·0	17·0	18·0	19·0	20·0	21·0	22·0	23·0	24·0
$100x$ ...	14·7	15·9	17·0	18·1	19·3	20·5	21·7	22·9	24·1	25·3	26·6
$100y$ ...	25·0	26·0	27·0	28·0	29·0	30·0	31·0	32·0	33·0	34·0	35·0
$100x$ ...	27·9	29·2	30·5	31·9	33·3	34·7	36·2	37·7	39·3	40·9	42·6
$100y$ ...	36·0	37·0	38·0	39·0	40·0	41·0	42·0	43·0	44·0	45·0	46·0
$100x$ ...	44·3	46·1	48·0	50·0	52·2	54·4	56·9	59·6	62·6	66·0	70·1
$100y$ ...	47·0	48·0	49·0	49·5	49·7	49·8	49·9	50·0			
$100x$ ...	75·1	81·9	93·0	99·2	109·4	117·7	128·1	∞			

As an example of the use of this table the following problem may be taken:

"The factors A and B give a cross-over value of 38·5 °/₀, the factors B and C a value of 22·7 °/₀. What is the value for A and C?"

From the table we find by interpolation that the distance AB is 49·0 centimorgans, the distance BC 24·9. Hence the distance

$$AC = AB \pm BC = 73{\cdot}9 \text{ or } 24{\cdot}1 \text{ centimorgans.}$$

The cross-over value is therefore 46·8 °/₀ or 22·0 °/₀, according as C lies outside AB or between A and B. Morgan's formula would have given 61·2 °/₀ (an impossible value), or 15·8 °/₀; Trow's formula 43·7 °/₀, or 28·9 °/₀ (by solving the equation $m + {\cdot}227 - 2m \times {\cdot}227 = {\cdot}385$). On the reduplication theory the result from $AB + BC$ corresponds to the view that the reduplication between A and C is "secondary" to those between A, B and B, C; the result from $AB - BC$ to the view that the reduplication between A and B is secondary to those between A, C and C, B.

It should be remarked that the existence of a quantity x which has the property demonstrated above is not a conclusive proof of the chromosome theory, and indeed such a quantity may occur in certain forms (*e.g.* Trow's) of the reduplication theory. However the fact that the values of x correspond to those demanded for the distance on the hypothesis that the factors are located in a semi-rigid chromosome is a strong point in favour of that hypothesis.

We have now the data for a fairly accurate estimate of the total length of the known portion of a chromosome, *e.g.* the sex chromosome in Drosophila. Taking some of the best authenticated measurements we have:

Factors			$100y$ (Cross-over value in per cent.)	$100x$ (from Table II)
Yellow-White	...	...	1·1	1·1
White-Vermilion	...	...	30·5	35·4
Vermilion-Bar	...	...	23·9	26·5
Bar-Lethal *sc*	...	...	8·3	8·5
Totals	...	...	63·8	71·5

This gives a total length of 71·5 centimorgans against Morgan and Bridges' estimate(8) of 66·2. The discrepancy is due to the fact that in some comparatively long segments of the chromosome (*e.g.* between the loci of Sable and Rudimentary, a distance of about 15 centimorgans) no factors have been located, and such distances tend to be underestimated. It may also be due in part to the large probable error involved in using a large number of small distances.

From equation (4) we may calculate the proportion of chromosomes giving t cross-overs in the known region. These values are incorrect, owing to the rigidity of the chromosome, c_1 being too low, the remainder too high. The theoretical values are:

No cross-over in	$c_0 = e^{-\cdot 715}$,	or 49·1 %	of the chromosomes
One " in	$c_1 = \cdot 715 e^{-\cdot 715}$,	or 34·4 %	" "
Two cross-overs in	$c_2 = \dfrac{\cdot 715^2 e^{-\cdot 715}}{2}$,	or 12·6 %	" "
Three " in	$c_3 = \dfrac{\cdot 715^3 e^{-\cdot 715}}{6}$,	or 3·0 %	" "
Four " in	$c_4 = \dfrac{\cdot 715^4 e^{-\cdot 715}}{24}$,	or ·36 %	" "

and so on.

The value of c_1 is too low, the others too high. The real value of $c_1 + c_3 + c_5 + \ldots$ is the cross-over value of 46·3 %, and Morgan(8) gives $c_2 + c_4 + c_6 + \ldots$, the number of double cross-overs (including quadruples, etc.), as about 10 %, so that c_0 should be about 43 %. When the relation between x and y is accurately known it will be possible to calculate the values of c_t with accuracy by integration.

It is believed that the above method of estimating distances will prove of considerable value when applied to comparatively long chromosomes in which factors are sparsely located, such as the second and third in Drosophila, since there is no reason to suppose that the relation arrived at between distance and cross-over value is peculiar to the sex chromosome in Drosophila. The results of investigations on these chromosomes should go far to confirm or refute the theory.

Outside Drosophila the best series of results on which to test it are those of Altenburg(9) with the three factors *M*, *S*, and *G* in Primula sinensis, quoted by Punnett(10) in a recent paper. Here the cross-over value for *M* and *S* is 11·6 %, for *M* and *G* 34·0 %, for *S* and *G* 40·6 %, each result being based on 3684 individuals. By Table II the distance *SM* is 12·1 centimorgans, *MG* 40·9, and hence *SG* is 55·0 centimorgans (assuming the loci to lie in the order *SMG*). Hence the cross-over value for *S* and *G* should be 40·4 %, the observed value being 40·6 %, a very nearly perfect fit. The addition formula gives 45·6 %, Trow's formula 37·7 %. The probable error of the calculated result is ·64 %, of the observed ·55 %. Hence the probable value of their difference is ·84 %, and though the close agreement is accidental, both the alternative formulae are impossible.

In the case of Punnett's(10) results for sweet peas the agreement is also good, but owing to the closeness of the linkage, the three formulae give nearly equal values. There is, however, no reason to suppose that Table II does not represent with fair accuracy the relation between distance and cross-over value in all organisms, though the absolute value in $\mu\mu$ of the unit of distance, or morgan, is presumably different in different cases.

Summary.

By a consideration of the observed gametic ratios of the sex-linked factors in Drosophila, the following results, among others, are arrived at:

1. If *A*, *B*, and *C* are three factors lying in a chromosome in that order, and if m is the cross-over value for *A* and *B*, n that for *B* and *C*, then the value for *A* and *C* lies between $m+n$ and $m+n-2mn$, being nearer to the former when $m+n$ is small, to the latter when it is large.

2. A relation is arrived at, on the hypothesis that the chromosomes are partially rigid, between cross-over value and distance, which permits of the calculation of one of the cross-over values for three factors from the other two, with a probable error of less than 2 %.

3. This relation may also be used to calculate the total length of a chromosome, and the number of double and triple cross-overs to be expected in a large distance.

4. The results from Drosophila are incompatible with Trow's form of the reduplication theory, but perhaps not with other possible forms of it.

5. The theory developed above fits all the observed data in plants.

REFERENCES.

1. MORGAN and BRIDGES. "Sex-linked inheritance in Drosophila." *Carnegie Institution of Washington*, 1916, p. 21.
2. TROW. "Primary and Secondary Reduplication." *Journal of Genetics*, Vol. II. p. 22, 1913.
3. MORGAN and BRIDGES. *Loc. cit.* p. 43.
4. —— —— *Loc. cit.* p. 37.
5. —— —— *Loc. cit.* p. 84.
6. HALDANE. "The Probable Errors of Observed Linkage Values." *Journal of Genetics*, Vol. VIII. p. 291, 1919.
7. STURTEVANT. "The Reduplication hypothesis applied to Drosophila." *American Naturalist*, Vol. XLVIII. p. 535, 1914.
8. MORGAN and BRIDGES. *Loc. cit.* p. 8.
9. ALTENBURG. *Genetics*, Vol. I. p. 354, 1916.
10. PUNNETT. "Reduplication series in Sweet Peas." *Journal of Genetics*, Vol. VI. No. 3, 1917.

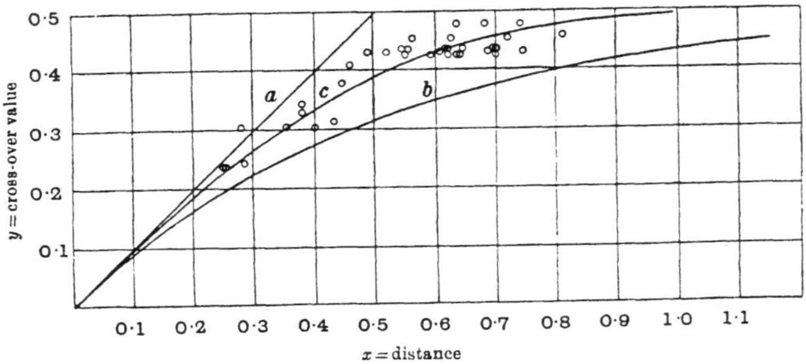

INBREEDING AND LINKAGE*

J. B. S. HALDANE AND C. H. WADDINGTON
John Innes Horticultural Institution, London, England

Received August 9, 1930

TABLE OF CONTENTS

When a heterozygous population is self-fertilized or inbred the ultimate result (apart from effects of mutation) is complete homozygosis. The final proportions of the various genotypes are usually independent of the system of inbreeding adopted, although, as JENNINGS (1916) and others have shown, the speed at which equilibrium is approached is greater in the case of self-fertilization than of brother-sister mating, and so on.

If however the population be heterozygous for linked genes, the final proportions depend on the system of mating, for crossing over can only occur in double heterozygotes, and the proportion of double heterozygotes falls off at a different rate in different mating systems. JENNINGS (1917) stated that he "would find it a relief if someone else would deal thoroughly with the laborious problem of the effects of inbreeding on two pairs of linked factors." This is the object of the present paper. ROBBINS (1918) solved the problem in the case of self-fertilization.

In what follows we employ a direct method to obtain the final proportions of the population. The rate of approach can be calculated, but this is a very laborious process, and always involves the irrational roots of quadratic, sometimes those of quartic or higher equations. In each case we shall suppose that the number of dominant and recessive genes of each type in the population is equal throughout the progress of the inbreeding. This enormously simplifies the mathematics. Thus a system of 55 equa-

* Part of the cost of the mathematical composition in this article is paid by the GALTON AND MENDEL MEMORIAL FUND.

GENETICS 16: 357 Jl 1931

tions described by JENNINGS (1917) is at once reduced to 22. This restriction is later removed.

SELF-FERTILIZATION

This problem has been solved by ROBBINS, but the shorter solution here given serves to illustrate our method. Consider the results of crossing *AABB* and *aabb*, where *A* and *B* are linked. The crossover values on the two sides of a hermaphrodite are taken as 100β percent and 100δ percent, so that the two gametic series given by *AB.ab* are:

$$(1-\beta)AB:\beta Ab:\beta aB:(1-\beta)ab.$$

$$(1-\delta)AB:\delta Ab:\delta aB:(1-\delta)ab.$$

For the sake of symmetry we suppose the original population to be entirely *AB.ab*. Then in the nth generation which is self-fertilized, let the 10 zygotic types occur in the proportions:

C_n *AABB* and *aabb*.
D_n *AAbb* and *aaBB*.
E_n *AABb*, *AaBB*, *Aabb*, and *aaBb*.
F_n *AB.ab*.
G_n *Ab.aB*.

We assume $2C_n+2D_n+4E_n+F_n+G_n=2$, so that $C_1=D_1=E_1=G_1=0$, and $F_1=2$. Clearly $E_\infty=F_\infty=G_\infty=0$, and D_∞ is the final proportion of crossover zygotes. Then considering the results of selfing each generation, we have:

$$\begin{aligned}
C_{n+1} &= C_n+\tfrac{1}{2}E_n+\tfrac{1}{4}(1-\beta-\delta+\beta\delta)F_n+\tfrac{1}{4}\beta\delta G_n \\
D_{n+1} &= D_n+\tfrac{1}{2}E_n+\tfrac{1}{4}\beta\delta F_n+\tfrac{1}{4}(1-\beta-\delta+\beta\delta)G_n \\
E_{n+1} &= \tfrac{1}{2}E_n+\tfrac{1}{4}(\beta+\delta-2\beta\delta)(F_n+G_n) \\
F_{n+1} &= \tfrac{1}{2}(1-\beta-\delta+\beta\delta)F_n+\tfrac{1}{2}\beta\delta G_n \\
G_{n+1} &= \tfrac{1}{2}\beta\delta F_n+\tfrac{1}{2}(1-\beta-\delta+\beta\delta)G_n
\end{aligned} \qquad (1.1)$$

These equations are derived as follows. The homozygous types when selfed reproduce themselves only, so C_n and D_n contribute only to C_{n+1} and D_{n+1}. *AABb* selfed gives $\tfrac{1}{4}$*AABB*, $\tfrac{1}{4}$*AAbb*, $\tfrac{1}{2}$*AABb*. Hence the contribution of E_n to E_{n+1} is $\tfrac{1}{2}E_n$. Since there are twice as many classes in the proportion E_n as C_{n+1}, the coefficient of its contribution to C_{n+1} must be doubled, and similarly for its contribution to D_{n+1}. The contributions of F_n and G_n are similarly calculated.

Now put $C_n-D_n=c_n$, $F_n-G_n=d_n$, and the average crossover value,

$\frac{1}{2}(\beta+\delta)=x$. Then subtracting the equations for C_{n+1}, D_{n+1}, and F_{n+1}, G_{n+1}, we have:

$$\left.\begin{aligned} c_{n+1} &= c_n + \tfrac{1}{4}(1-2x)d_n \\ d_{n+1} &= \tfrac{1}{2}(1-2x)d_n \end{aligned}\right\} \qquad (1.2)$$

Now choose λ so that $c_{n+1}+\lambda d_{n+1}\equiv c_n+\lambda d_n$ for all values of n.

Then $c_n+\lambda d_n \equiv c_n + \frac{1}{4}(1-2x)d_n + \frac{1}{2}\lambda(1-2x)d_n$

$$\therefore\ \lambda = \frac{1-2x}{2+4x}\cdot$$

Then since $d_\infty = 0$, and $c_1 = 0$, $d_1 = 2$,

$$c_\infty = c_\infty + \lambda d_\infty = c_1 + \lambda d_1 = \frac{1-2x}{1+2x}\cdot$$

Put $y = D_\infty$ (the final proportion of crossover zygotes)

$$\therefore\ C_\infty + D_\infty = 1,\ C_\infty - D_\infty = c_\infty\ \therefore\ y = \tfrac{1}{2}(1-c_\infty).$$

$$\therefore\ y = \frac{2x}{1+2x}\cdot \qquad (1.3)$$

Hence the proportion of crossover zygotes is approximately equal to twice the mean gametic crossover value when the latter is small, rising to 50 percent with 50 percent crossing over (see figure 1). The actual proportions of the different zygotic types in each generation can be calculated from equations (1.1). Equations (1.2) are not sufficient. The method of solution is given by ROBBINS, and the principal result in our terminology, putting $p=\beta\delta$, the product of the crossover values, is:

$$\left.\begin{aligned} C_n &= \frac{1-(\frac{1}{2}-x)^n}{1+2x} + \tfrac{1}{2}(\tfrac{1}{2}-x+p)^{n-1} - (\tfrac{1}{2})^{n-1} \\ D_n &= \frac{2x+(\frac{1}{2}-x)^n}{1+2x} + \tfrac{1}{2}(\tfrac{1}{2}-x+p)^{n-1} - (\tfrac{1}{2})^{n-1}. \end{aligned}\right\} \qquad (1.4)$$

Thus the final proportion of crossover zygotes, D_∞, depends on x only; the rate of approach to this value depends on p. Indeed if crossing over were restricted to one side of a hermaphrodite, as it is to one sex in the higher insects, we should have $p=0$, and no crossover zygotes would appear before F_3. D_n is 0 in F_1, $\frac{1}{2}p$ in F_2, rising sharply to $\frac{1}{2}(x+p-2px+p^2)$ in F_3, and over half way to its final value in F_4. Except in F_2 the figures depend almost entirely on the mean crossover value. Thus with a mean value of 10 percent we have in successive generations the percentages of crossover homozygotes given in table 1.

TABLE 1

CROSSOVER VALUES PERCENT	F_2	F_3	F_4	F_5	F_6	F_∞
10, 10	0.50	5.405	9.746	12.683	14.462	$16.\dot{6}$
20, 0	0	5.0	9.5	12.55	14.395	$16.\dot{6}$

Hence in a plant propagated by self-fertilization, where new combinations are required after a cross, there is a very great advantage in growing on a large progeny as far as F_3, and rather little advantage in growing it beyond F_4. As will appear later, this is also true when double crossing over is taken into account.

BROTHER-SISTER MATING. SEX-LINKED GENES

Two sex-linked genes provide four types of zygotes in the heterogametic sex, and ten in the homogametic. There are thus forty different types of mating. If we consider the results of an original mating $AABB \times ab$, or $aabb \times AB$, the numbers of A and a genes are unequal, and there is a lack of symmetry in the equations, just as there would be in the case last considered if we did not begin with equal numbers of the allelomorphs. We therefore suppose that at the beginning both reciprocal crosses were made in equal numbers. The crossover percentage is taken as 100β, and $\alpha = 1 - \beta$. The fourteen variables of equations (2.1) refer to the proportions of matings of each type. Under the circumstances considered all matings fall into one of fourteen classes having the same frequency in each generation, which is calculable when we know the frequencies in the preceding generation.

MATINGS	PROPORTION
$AABB \times AB$ $aabb \times ab$	$C_{n+1} = C_n + \frac{1}{2}I_n + \frac{\alpha^2}{4}M_n + \frac{\beta^2}{4}Q_n$
$AAbb \times Ab$ $aaBB \times aB$	$D_{n+1} = D_n + \frac{1}{2}J_n + \frac{\alpha^2}{4}P_n + \frac{\beta^2}{4}R_n$
$AABB \times Ab$ $AABB \times aB$ $aabb \times aB$ $aabb \times Ab$	$E_{n+1} = \frac{1}{4}I_n + \frac{\alpha\beta}{4}(M_n + Q_n)$

Matings	
AAbb × *AB* *AAbb* × *ab* *aaBB* × *AB* *aaBB* × *ab*	$F_{n+1} = \frac{1}{4}J_n + \frac{\alpha\beta}{4}(P_n + R_n)$
AABB × *ab* *aabb* × *AB*	$G_{n+1} = \frac{\alpha^2}{4}M_n + \frac{\beta^2}{4}Q_n$
AAbb × *aB* *aaBB* × *Ab*	$H_{n+1} = \frac{\alpha^2}{4}P_n + \frac{\beta^2}{4}R_n$
AaBB × *AB* *AABb* × *AB* *Aabb* × *ab* *aaBb* × *ab*	$I_{n+1} = E_n + \frac{1}{4}(I_n + J_n + K_n) + \frac{\alpha\beta}{4}(M_n + Q_n) + \frac{\beta^2}{4}P_n + \frac{\alpha^2}{4}R_n$
AaBB × *aB* *AABb* × *Ab* *Aabb* × *Ab* *aaBb* × *aB*	$J_{n+1} = F_n + \frac{1}{4}(I_n + J_n + L_n) + \frac{\alpha\beta}{4}(P_n + R_n) + \frac{\beta^2}{4}M_n + \frac{\alpha^2}{4}Q_n$
AaBB × *Ab* *AABb* × *aB* *Aabb* × *aB* *aaBb* × *Ab*	$K_{n+1} = \frac{1}{4}K_n + \frac{\alpha\beta}{4}(P_n + R_n) + \frac{\beta^2}{4}M_n + \frac{\alpha^2}{4}Q_n$
AaBB × *ab* *AABb* × *ab* *Aabb* × *AB* *aaBb* × *AB*	$L_{n+1} = \frac{1}{4}L_n + \frac{\alpha\beta}{4}(M_n + Q_n) + \frac{\beta^2}{4}P_n + \frac{\alpha^2}{4}R_n$
AB·ab × *AB* *AB·ab* × *ab*	$M_{n+1} = G_n + \frac{1}{2}L_n + \frac{\alpha^2}{2}M_n + \frac{\beta^2}{2}Q_n$
Ab·aB × *Ab* *Ab·aB* × *aB*	$P_{n+1} = H_n + \frac{1}{2}K_n + \frac{\alpha^2}{2}P_n + \frac{\beta^2}{2}R_n$
Ab·aB × *AB* *Ab·aB* × *ab*	$Q_{n+1} = K_n + \frac{\alpha\beta}{2}(P_n + R_n)$
AB·ab × *Ab* *AB·ab* × *aB*	$R_{n+1} = L_n + \frac{\alpha\beta}{2}(M_n + Q_n)$.

(These equations are referred to as 2.1.)

As an illustration of how these equations are derived we may take the distribution of K_n in the following generation. The mating *AaBB*×*Ab* gives *AABb*, *Ab.aB*, *AB*, and *aB* offspring in equal numbers. Hence in the next generation the matings *AABb*×*AB*, *AABb*×*aB*, *Ab.aB*×*AB*, and *Ab.aB*×*aB* occur in equal numbers among its progeny. Hence K_n contributes to I_{n+1}, K_{n+1}, Q_{n+1}, P_{n+1} as shown. To reduce the equations (2.1) we put:

$c_n = C_n - D_n$, $d_n = E_n - F_n$, $e_n = G_n - H_n$, $f_n = I_n - J_n$, $g_n = K_n - L_n$, $h_n = M_n - P_n$, $i_n = Q_n - R_n$.

$$\left.\begin{aligned}
\therefore\ c_{n+1} &= c_n + \tfrac{1}{2}f_n + \frac{\alpha^2}{4}h_n + \frac{\beta^2}{4}i_n \\
d_{n+1} &= \tfrac{1}{4}f_n + \frac{\alpha\beta}{4}(h_n + i_n) \\
e_{n+1} &= \frac{\alpha^2}{4}h_n + \frac{\beta^2}{4}i_n \\
f_{n+1} &= d_n + \tfrac{1}{4}g_n + \frac{\alpha\beta - \beta^2}{4}h_n - \frac{\alpha^2 - \alpha\beta}{4}i_n \\
g_{n+1} &= \tfrac{1}{4}g_n - \frac{\alpha\beta - \beta^2}{4}h_n + \frac{\alpha^2 - \alpha\beta}{4}i_n \\
h_{n+1} &= e_n - \tfrac{1}{2}g_n + \frac{\alpha^2}{2}h_n + \frac{\beta^2}{2}i_n \\
i_{n+1} &= \tfrac{1}{2}g_n - \frac{\alpha\beta}{2}(h_n + i_n)
\end{aligned}\right\} \qquad (2.2)$$

When $n = 0$, G_n and therefore $e_n = 1$, the other variables are zero. When $n = \infty$, all but C_n, D_n, and consequently c_n vanish. It is required to find the value of c_∞. To do so we have to find values of ϵ, ζ, η, θ, ϕ, ψ, such that

$$c_{n+1} + \epsilon d_{n+1} + \zeta e_{n+1} + \eta f_{n+1} + \theta g_{n+1} + \phi h_{n+1} + \psi i_{n+1}$$
$$\equiv c_n + \epsilon d_n + \zeta e_n + \eta f_n + \theta g_n + \phi h_n + \psi i_n.$$

Substituting in the above identity the values of c_{n+1}, etc. and equating coefficients of d_n, etc. we have:

$$\left.\begin{aligned}
\epsilon &= \eta \\
\zeta &= \phi \\
\eta &= \tfrac{1}{2} + \tfrac{1}{4}\epsilon \\
\theta &= \tfrac{1}{4}(\eta + \theta - 2\phi + 2\psi) \\
\phi &= \frac{\alpha^2}{4}(1 + \zeta + 2\phi) + \frac{\alpha\beta}{4}(\epsilon - 2\psi) + \frac{\alpha\beta - \beta^2}{4}(\eta - \theta) \\
\psi &= \frac{\beta^2}{4}(1 + \zeta + 2\phi) + \frac{\alpha\beta}{4}(\epsilon - 2\psi) + \frac{\alpha\beta - \alpha^2}{4}(\eta - \theta)
\end{aligned}\right\} \qquad (2.3)$$

Eliminating $\epsilon = \eta = \frac{2}{3}$, and $\phi = \zeta$, we have

$$9\theta = 2 - 6\zeta + 6\psi$$

$$12(\zeta - \psi) = (\alpha - \beta)(5 + 9\zeta - 3\theta).$$

$$12(\zeta + \psi) = 1 + 3(\alpha^2 + \beta^2)(3\zeta + \theta) - 6\alpha 3\psi.$$

Hence, putting $\beta = x$,

$$\epsilon = \zeta = \tfrac{2}{3}, \zeta = \phi = \frac{3 - 4x}{3(1 + 4x)}, \quad \theta = 2\psi = \frac{2(4x - 1)}{3(1 + 4\beta)}.$$

Hence, for all values of n,

$$c_\infty = c_n + \tfrac{2}{3}(d_n + f_n) + \frac{(3 - 4x)(e_n + h_n)}{3(1 + 4x)} + \frac{(4x - 1)(2g_n + i_n)}{3(1 + 4x)} \quad (2.4)$$

and since $C_n + D_n = 1$, $C_n - D_n = c$

$$\therefore\ y = D_n = \tfrac{1}{2}(1 - c_n).$$

In the case here considered $e_0 = 1$

$$\therefore\ c_\infty = \frac{3 - 4x}{3(1 + 4x)}$$

$$\therefore\ y = \frac{8x}{3(1 + 4x)}. \quad (2.5)$$

This is plotted in figure 1. It will be seen that if two sex-linked genes give 50 percent crossing over in the homogametic sex, the final proportion of crossover zygotes will be 4/9. In order to study the rate at which the final values are approached it is necessary to solve the equations (2.2), and also a corresponding set of seven equations for $C_n + D_n$, etc. This is quite possible. Thus it can easily be shown that

$$(h_{n+2} - i_{n+2}) - \alpha(h_{n+1} - i_{n+1}) - (\alpha - \beta)(h_n - i_n) = 0$$

$$\therefore\ h_n - i_n = \frac{1}{\sqrt{5\alpha^2 - 4\beta^2}}\left[\left(\frac{\alpha + \sqrt{5\alpha^2 - 4\beta^2}}{2}\right)^n - \left(\frac{\alpha - \sqrt{5\alpha^2 - 4\beta^2}}{2}\right)^n\right].$$

As, however, any variable, such as C_n, may be the sum of a large number of terms from geometrical series, numerical calculation is easier than algebraic. The expressions given by JENNINGS and ROBBINS for the proportion of heterozygotes in the nth generation are wholly independent of linkage. Hence it is clear that by about F_{10} the population contains only 10 percent of *Aa* and as many *Bb* in the homogametic sex, so that equilibrium is nearly reached.

BROTHER-SISTER MATING. AUTOSOMAL GENES

We consider the results of an initial mating $AABB \times aabb$ or reciprocally. The gametic series from an $AB.ab$ ♀ is assumed to be $\alpha AB : \beta Ab : \beta aB : \alpha ab$, from $AB.ab$ ♂, $\gamma AB : \delta Ab : \delta aB : \gamma ab$, so that 100β and 100δ are the crossover values. In general these are different, but in mammals β and δ are nearly equal; in the higher insects one of them is zero. There are 100 different types of mating, and owing to the different crossover values in the two sexes, reciprocal crosses do not always yield the same progeny, and therefore the same numbers of matings in the next generation. However, reciprocal crosses occur in the same numbers, and can be grouped together. In the following scheme only one example is given of each type of mating. The total number of types is given in column 2. Thus the following 7 types of mating occur in equal numbers with $AABB \times AAbb$:

$$AAbb \times AABB,\ aaBB \times AABB,\ AABB \times aaBB,\ aabb \times aaBB,$$
$$aaBB \times aabb,\ aabb \times AAbb,\ AAbb \times aabb.$$

In the third column the numbers of each kind of mating in the (n+1)th generation are given in terms of similar numbers in the nth. To save space the suffixes of the latter are omitted, for example, H is written for H_n. The method of calculation is similar to that in the sex-linked case. We thus have equations (3.1):

Typical mating	*Number of types*	
$AABB \times AABB$	2	$C_{n+1} = C_n + H + \frac{1}{4}(\alpha^2+\gamma^2)L + \frac{1}{4}(\beta^2+\delta^2)N + \frac{1}{4}Q + \frac{1}{4}R + \frac{1}{8}(\alpha^2+\gamma^2)U + \frac{1}{8}(\beta^2+\delta^2)V + \frac{1}{16}\alpha^2\gamma^2W + \frac{1}{16}(\alpha^2\delta^2+\beta^2\gamma^2)X + \frac{1}{16}\beta^2\delta^2Y.$
$AAbb \times AAbb$	2	$D_{n+1} = D + I + \frac{1}{4}(\alpha^2+\gamma^2)M + \frac{1}{4}(\beta^2+\delta^2)P + \frac{1}{4}Q + \frac{1}{4}S + \frac{1}{8}(\beta^2+\delta^2)U + \frac{1}{8}(\alpha^2+\gamma^2)V + \frac{1}{16}\beta^2\delta^2W + \frac{1}{16}(\alpha^2\delta^2+\beta^2\gamma^2)X + \frac{1}{16}\alpha^2\gamma^2Y.$
$AABB \times aabb$	2	$E_{n+1} = \frac{1}{16}\alpha^2\gamma^2W + \frac{1}{16}(\alpha^2\delta^2+\beta^2\gamma^2)X + \frac{1}{16}\beta^2\delta^2Y.$
$AAbb \times aaBB$	2	$F_{n+1} = \frac{1}{16}\beta^2\delta^2W + \frac{1}{16}(\alpha^2\delta^2+\beta^2\gamma^2)X + \frac{1}{16}\alpha^2\gamma^2Y.$
$AABB \times AAbb$	8	$G_{n+1} = \frac{1}{16}(\alpha\beta+\gamma\delta)(U+V) + \frac{1}{16}\alpha\beta\gamma\delta(W+2X+Y).$
$AABB \times AABb$	8	$H_{n+1} = \frac{1}{2}H + \frac{1}{4}(\alpha\beta+\gamma\delta)(L+N) + \frac{1}{4}R + \frac{1}{16}(\alpha^2+2\alpha\beta+\gamma^2+2\gamma\delta)U + \frac{1}{16}(2\alpha\beta+\beta^2+2\gamma\delta+\delta^2)V + \frac{1}{16}\alpha\gamma(\alpha\delta+\beta\gamma)W + \frac{1}{16}(\alpha\gamma+\beta\delta)(\alpha\delta+\beta\gamma)X + \frac{1}{16}\beta\delta(\alpha\delta+\beta\gamma)Y.$
$AAbb \times AABb$	8	$I_{n+1} = \frac{1}{2}I + \frac{1}{4}(\alpha\beta+\gamma\delta)(M+P) + \frac{1}{4}S + \frac{1}{16}(2\alpha\beta+\beta^2+2\gamma\delta+\delta^2)U + \frac{1}{16}(\alpha^2+2\alpha\beta+\gamma^2+2\gamma\delta)V + \frac{1}{16}\beta\delta(\alpha\delta+\beta\gamma)W + \frac{1}{16}(\alpha\gamma+\beta\delta)(\alpha\delta+\beta\gamma)X + \frac{1}{16}\alpha\gamma(\alpha\delta+\beta\gamma)Y.$
$AABB \times Aabb$	8	$J_{n+1} = \frac{1}{16}(\alpha^2+\gamma^2)U + \frac{1}{16}(\beta^2+\delta^2)V + \frac{1}{16}\alpha\gamma(\alpha\delta+\beta\gamma)W + \frac{1}{16}(\alpha\gamma+\beta\delta)(\alpha\delta+\beta\gamma)X + \frac{1}{16}\beta\delta(\alpha\delta+\beta\gamma)Y.$
$AAbb \times AaBB$	8	$K_{n+1} = \frac{1}{16}(\beta^2+\delta^2)U + \frac{1}{16}(\alpha^2+\gamma^2)V + \frac{1}{16}\beta\delta(\alpha\delta+\beta\gamma)W + \frac{1}{16}(\alpha\gamma+\beta\delta)(\alpha\delta+\beta\gamma)X + \frac{1}{16}\alpha\gamma(\alpha\delta+\beta\gamma)Y.$
$AABB \times AB.ab$	4	$L_{n+1} = \frac{1}{4}(\alpha^2+\gamma^2)L + \frac{1}{4}(\beta^2+\delta^2)N + \frac{1}{8}(\alpha^2+\gamma^2)U + \frac{1}{8}(\beta^2+\delta^2)V + \frac{1}{8}\alpha^2\gamma^2W + \frac{1}{8}(\alpha^2\delta^2+\beta^2\gamma^2)X + \frac{1}{8}\beta^2\delta^2Y.$
$AAbb \times Ab.aB$	4	$M_{n+1} = \frac{1}{4}(\alpha^2+\gamma^2)M + \frac{1}{4}(\alpha^2+\delta^2)P + \frac{1}{8}(\beta^2+\delta^2)U + \frac{1}{8}(\alpha^2+\gamma^2)V + \frac{1}{8}\beta^2\delta^2W + \frac{1}{8}(\alpha^2\delta^2+\beta^2\gamma^2)X + \frac{1}{8}\alpha^2\gamma^2Y.$

Typical mating	Number of types	
$AABB \times Ab.aB$	4	$N_{n+1} = \frac{1}{8}R + \frac{1}{8}(\alpha\beta+\gamma\delta)(U+V) + \frac{1}{8}\alpha\beta\gamma\delta(W+2X+Y).$
$AAbb \times AB.ab$	4	$P_{n+1} = \frac{1}{8}S + \frac{1}{8}(\alpha\beta+\gamma\delta)(U+V) + \frac{1}{8}\alpha\beta\gamma\delta(W+2X+Y).$
$AABb \times AABb$	4	$Q_{n+1} = 2G + \frac{1}{2}(H+I+J+K) + \frac{1}{4}(\alpha^2+\gamma^2)(L+M) + \frac{1}{4}(\beta^2+\delta^2)(N+P) + \frac{1}{4}Q + \frac{1}{8}(R+S+T) + \frac{1}{8}(\alpha^2+\alpha\beta+\beta^2+\gamma^2+\gamma\delta+\delta^2)(U+V) + \frac{1}{16}(\alpha\delta+\beta\gamma)^2(W+Y) + \frac{1}{8}(\alpha\gamma+\beta\delta)^2X.$
$AABb \times AaBB$	4	$R_{n+1} = \frac{1}{4}(\beta^2+\delta^2)L + \frac{1}{4}(\alpha^2+\gamma^2)N + \frac{1}{8}R + \frac{1}{8}(\beta+\delta)U + \frac{1}{8}(\alpha+\gamma)V + \frac{1}{16}(\alpha\delta+\beta\gamma)^2(W+Y) + \frac{1}{8}(\alpha\gamma+\beta\delta)^2X.$
$AABb \times Aabb$	4	$S_{n+1} = \frac{1}{4}(\beta^2+\delta^2)M + \frac{1}{4}(\alpha^2+\gamma^2)P + \frac{1}{8}S + \frac{1}{8}(\alpha+\gamma)U + \frac{1}{8}(\beta+\delta)V + \frac{1}{16}(\alpha\delta+\beta\gamma)^2(W+Y) + \frac{1}{8}(\alpha\gamma+\beta\delta)^2X.$
$AABb \times aaBb$	4	$T_{n+1} = \frac{1}{8}(\alpha\beta+\gamma\delta)(U+V) + \frac{1}{16}(\alpha\delta+\beta\gamma)^2(W+Y) + \frac{1}{8}(\alpha\gamma+\beta\delta)^2X.$
$AABb \times AB.ab$	8	$U_{n+1} = \frac{1}{2}J + \frac{1}{4}(\alpha\beta+\gamma\delta)(L+N) + \frac{1}{8}(S+T) + \frac{1}{8}(\alpha+\gamma)U + \frac{1}{8}(\beta+\delta)V + \frac{1}{8}\alpha\gamma(\beta\gamma+\alpha\delta)W + \frac{1}{8}(\alpha\gamma+\beta\delta)(\alpha\delta+\beta\gamma)X + \frac{1}{8}\beta\delta(\beta\gamma+\alpha\delta)Y.$
$AABb \times Ab.aB$	8	$V_{n+1} = \frac{1}{2}K + \frac{1}{4}(\alpha\beta+\gamma\delta)(M+P) + \frac{1}{8}(R+T) + \frac{1}{8}(\beta+\delta)U + \frac{1}{8}(\alpha+\gamma)V + \frac{1}{8}\beta\delta(\beta\gamma+\alpha\delta)W + \frac{1}{8}(\alpha\gamma+\beta\delta)(\alpha\delta+\beta\gamma)X + \frac{1}{8}\alpha\gamma(\beta\gamma+\alpha\delta)Y.$
$AB.ab \times AB.ab$	1	$W_{n+1} = 2(E+J) + \frac{1}{2}(\alpha^2+\gamma^2)L + \frac{1}{2}(\beta^2+\delta^2)N + \frac{1}{4}(S+T) + \frac{1}{4}(\alpha^2+\gamma^2)U + \frac{1}{4}(\beta^2+\delta^2)V + \frac{1}{4}\alpha^2\gamma^2W + \frac{1}{4}(\alpha^2\delta^2+\beta^2\gamma^2)X + \frac{1}{4}\beta^2\delta^2Y.$
$AB.ab \times Ab.aB$	2	$X_{n+1} = \frac{1}{2}T + \frac{1}{2}(\alpha\beta+\gamma\delta)(U+V) + \frac{1}{2}\alpha\beta\gamma\delta(W+2X+Y).$
$Ab.aB \times Ab.aB$	1	$Y_{n+1} = 2(F+K) + \frac{1}{2}(\alpha^2+\gamma^2)M + \frac{1}{2}(\beta^2+\delta^2)P + \frac{1}{4}(R+T) + \frac{1}{4}(\beta^2+\delta^2)U + \frac{1}{4}(\alpha^2+\gamma^2)V + \frac{1}{4}\beta^2\delta^2W + \frac{1}{4}(\alpha^2\delta^2+\beta^2\gamma^2)X + \frac{1}{4}\alpha^2\gamma^2Y.$

Now let $c_n = C_n - D_n$, $d_n = E_n - F_n$, $e_n = H_n - I_n$, $f_n = J_n - K_n$, $g_n = L_n - M_n$, $h_n = N_n - P_n$, $i_n = R_n - S_n$, $j_n = U_n - V_n$, $k_n = W_n - Y_n$.

Hence we have the equations (3.2):

$$c_{n+1} = c_n + e_n + \tfrac{1}{4}(\alpha^2+\gamma^2)g_n + \tfrac{1}{4}(\beta^2+\delta^2)h_n + \tfrac{1}{8}i_n + \tfrac{1}{8}(\alpha-\beta+\gamma-\delta)j_n + \tfrac{1}{16}(\alpha^2\gamma^2-\beta^2\delta^2)k_n.$$

$$d_{n+1} = \tfrac{1}{16}(\alpha^2\gamma^2-\beta^2\delta^2)k_n.$$

$$e_{n+1} = \tfrac{1}{2}e_n + \tfrac{1}{4}(\alpha\beta+\gamma\delta)(g_n+h_n) + \tfrac{1}{8}i_n + \tfrac{1}{16}(\alpha-\beta+\gamma-\delta)j_n + \tfrac{1}{16}(\alpha\gamma-\beta\delta)(\alpha\delta+\beta\gamma)k_n.$$

$$f_{n+1} = \tfrac{1}{16}(\alpha-\beta+\gamma-\delta)j_n + \tfrac{1}{16}(\alpha\gamma-\beta\delta)(\alpha\delta+\beta\gamma)k_n.$$

$$g_{n+1} = \tfrac{1}{4}(\alpha^2+\gamma^2)g_n + \tfrac{1}{4}(\beta^2+\delta^2)h_n + \tfrac{1}{8}(\alpha-\beta+\gamma-\delta)j_n + \tfrac{1}{8}(\alpha^2\gamma^2-\beta^2\delta^2)k_n.$$

$$h_{n+1} = \tfrac{1}{8}i_n.$$

$$i_{n+1} = \tfrac{1}{4}(\beta^2+\delta^2)g_n + \tfrac{1}{4}(\alpha^2+\gamma^2)h_n + \tfrac{1}{8}i_n - \tfrac{1}{8}(\alpha-\beta+\gamma-\delta)j_n.$$

$$j_{n+1} = \tfrac{1}{2}f_n + \tfrac{1}{4}(\alpha\beta+\gamma\delta)(g_n+h_n) - \tfrac{1}{8}i_n + \tfrac{1}{8}(\alpha-\beta+\gamma-\delta)j_n + \tfrac{1}{8}(\alpha\gamma-\beta\delta)(\alpha\delta+\beta\gamma)k_n.$$

$$k_{n+1} = 2(d_n+f_n) + \tfrac{1}{2}(\alpha^2+\gamma^2)g_n + \tfrac{1}{2}(\beta^2+\delta^2)g_n - \tfrac{1}{4}i_n + \tfrac{1}{4}(\alpha-\beta+\gamma-\delta)j_n + \tfrac{1}{4}(\alpha^2\gamma^2-\beta^2\delta^2)k_n.$$

When $n=0$, $E_0=1 \therefore d_0=1$, the other terms being zero.

When $n=\infty$, $C_\infty+D_\infty=1$, and c_∞ is finite, the other terms being zero.

We now have to find $\xi, \eta, \theta, \kappa, \lambda, \mu, \nu, \phi$ so that:

$$c_{n+1} + \zeta d_{n-1} + \eta e_{n-1} + \theta f_{n-1} + \kappa g_{n-1} + \lambda h_{n-1} + \mu i_{n-1} + \nu j_{n-1} + \phi k_{n+1}$$
$$\equiv c_n + \zeta d_n + \eta e_n + \theta f_n + \kappa g_n + \lambda h_n + \mu i_n + \nu j_n + \phi k_n.$$

The conditions for this to be the case are equations (3.3)

$$\zeta = 2\phi$$
$$\eta = 1 + \tfrac{1}{2}\eta$$
$$\theta = \tfrac{1}{2}\nu + 2\phi$$
$$\kappa = \tfrac{1}{4}(\alpha^2 + \gamma^2)(1 + \kappa + 2\phi) + \tfrac{1}{4}(\beta^2 + \delta^2)\mu + \tfrac{1}{4}(\alpha\beta + \gamma\delta)(\eta + \nu).$$
$$\lambda = \tfrac{1}{4}(\beta^2 + \delta^2)(1 + \kappa + 2\phi) + \tfrac{1}{4}(\alpha^2 + \gamma^2)\mu + \tfrac{1}{4}(\alpha\beta + \gamma\delta)(\eta + \nu).$$
$$\mu = \tfrac{1}{8}(1 + \eta + \lambda + \mu - \nu - 2\phi).$$
$$\nu = \tfrac{1}{16}(\alpha - \beta + \gamma - \delta)(2 + \eta + \theta + 2x - 2\mu + 2\nu + 4\phi).$$
$$\phi = \tfrac{1}{16}(\alpha^2\gamma^2 - \beta^2\delta^2)(1 + \zeta + 2\kappa + 4\phi) + \tfrac{1}{16}(\alpha\gamma - \beta\delta)(\alpha\delta + \beta\gamma)(\eta + \theta + 2\nu).$$

We eliminate $\eta = 2$, and $\phi = \tfrac{1}{2}\zeta$. We also subtract and add together the fourth and fifth of these equations. We put $x = \tfrac{1}{2}(\beta + \delta)$, the average cross-over value, and also $y = \tfrac{1}{2}(\alpha\beta + \gamma\delta)$, $z = \alpha\gamma + \beta\delta$, $q = \tfrac{1}{2} - x$. Hence:

$$2\theta = \nu + 2\zeta.$$
$$\kappa - \lambda = q(1 + \zeta + \kappa - \mu).$$
$$2\kappa + 2\lambda = 1 + y + (1 - y)(\zeta + \kappa) + y\nu.$$
$$7\mu = 3 - \zeta + \lambda - \nu.$$
$$8\nu = q(3 + 2\zeta + \theta + 2\kappa - 2\mu + 2\nu).$$
$$4\zeta = q(3 + \theta + 2\nu) - qz(2 + 3\zeta - \theta + 2\kappa - 2\nu).$$

Omitting some rather tedious algebra, the solution of these equations is:

$$\zeta = \frac{q}{2 - 3q}, \quad \theta = \frac{2q}{2 - 3q}, \quad \kappa = \frac{1}{2 - 3q},$$
$$\lambda = \frac{1 - 2q}{2 - 3q}, \quad \mu = \frac{1 - 2q}{2 - 3q}, \quad \nu = \frac{2q}{2 - 3q}$$

as may easily be verified.

$$\therefore\ c_\infty = c_n + 2e_n + \frac{1}{1 + 6x}\big[(1 - 2x)(d_n + 2f_n + 2j_n + \tfrac{1}{2}k_n) + 2g_n + 4x(h_n + i_n)\big] \tag{3.4}$$

and $y = \tfrac{1}{2}(1 - c_\infty)$.

In the case considered, $d_0 = 1$, $\therefore c_\infty = \zeta d_0 = 1 - 2x/1 + 6x$. Hence the proportion of crossover zygotes, $y = 4x/1 + 6x$ (3.5).

This is plotted in figure 1. If there is 50 percent crossing over in both sexes, $x = \frac{1}{2}$, $y = \frac{1}{2}$. If there is 50 percent in one sex, and none in the other, $x = \frac{1}{4}$, $y = 5/12$, that is 5/12 only of the zygotes are crossovers.

To solve the equations (3.1) completely, we require, besides the equations (3.2), a group of 13 equations for $C_n + D_n$, etc. and also for the symmetrical terms G_n, Q_n, T_n, and X_n. The full expression for D_n is the sum of a constant term with the nth terms of 19 geometrical series. Their ratios are $\frac{1}{2}$ and the irrational roots of two algebraic equations of the 7th and 11th degrees. These equations can, in part at least, be reduced to quartics, but at least one quartic is irreducible. Hence only numerical calculation is practicable.

PARENTS AND OFFSPRING MATING. SEX-LINKED GENES

In this system of mating a father is mated to his own daughter, a son of this union to his mother and subsequently to his daughter, and so on indefinitely. JENNINGS (1917) has dealt with it in the case of unlinked genes. We consider the results of inbreeding where the matings $AABB \times ab$ and $aabb \times AB$ are made in equal numbers and the daughters (assuming the female sex to be homogametic) backcrossed to the fathers. If the sons were backcrossed to their mothers they would of course give 100 percent non-crossover homozygotes at once. The result of the cross considered, between fathers and F_1 daughters, is the same as if the F_1 were crossed with one another, and their children (F_2) backcrossed to parents. It will be shown later that this latter procedure gives the maximum of crossing over of autosomal genes. The case is fairly simple, since many types of mating are impossible after the first generation. For example *aabb* mothers have only *ab* sons. β is the crossover proportion, and $\alpha = 1 - \beta$.

Typical mating	*Number of types*	
$AABB \times AB$	2	$C_{n+1} = C_n + \frac{1}{2}E_n + \frac{1}{4}\alpha G_n + \frac{1}{4}\beta J_n$.
$AAbb \times Ab$	2	$D_{n+1} = D_n + \frac{1}{2}F_n + \frac{1}{4}\alpha H_n + \frac{1}{4}\beta I_n$.
$AABb \times AB$	4	$E_{n+1} = \frac{1}{2}E_n + \frac{1}{4}F_n + \frac{1}{4}\beta G_n + \frac{1}{4}\alpha J_n$.
$AABb \times Ab$	4	$F_{n+1} = \frac{1}{4}E_n + \frac{1}{2}F_n + \frac{1}{4}\beta H_n + \frac{1}{4}\alpha I_n$. (4.1)
$AB.ab \times AB$	2	$G_{n+1} = \frac{3}{4}\alpha G_n + \frac{1}{2}\alpha I_n + \frac{1}{4}\beta J_n$.
$Ab.aB \times Ab$	2	$H_{n+1} = \frac{3}{4}\alpha H_n + \frac{1}{4}\beta I_n + \frac{1}{2}\beta J_n$.
$AB.ab \times Ab$	2	$I_{n+1} = \frac{1}{2}\beta(G_n + I_n)$.
$Ab.aB \times AB$	2	$J_{n+1} = \frac{1}{2}\beta(H_n + J_n)$.

Putting $c_n = C_n - D_n$, $d_n = E_n - F_n$, $e_n = G_n - H_n$, $f_n = I_n - J_n$

$$\begin{aligned} \therefore\ c_{n+1} &= c_n + \tfrac{1}{2}d_n + \tfrac{1}{4}\alpha e_n - \tfrac{1}{4}\beta f_n \\ d_{n+1} &= \tfrac{1}{4}d_n + \tfrac{1}{4}\beta e_n - \tfrac{1}{4}\alpha f_n \\ e_{n+1} &= \tfrac{3}{4}\alpha e_n + \tfrac{3}{4}(2\alpha - \beta)f_n \\ f_{n+1} &= \tfrac{1}{2}\beta(e_n + f_n) \end{aligned} \qquad (4.2)$$

Put $c_{n+1}+\zeta d_{n+1}+\eta e_{n+1}+\theta f_{n+1} \equiv c_n+\zeta d_n+\eta e_n+\theta f_n$.

$$\left.\begin{aligned} \therefore\ \zeta &= \tfrac{1}{2} + \tfrac{1}{4}\zeta \\ \eta &= \tfrac{1}{4}\alpha + \tfrac{1}{4}\beta\zeta + \tfrac{3}{4}\alpha\eta + \tfrac{1}{2}\beta\theta \\ \theta &= -\tfrac{1}{4}\beta - \tfrac{1}{4}\alpha\zeta + \tfrac{1}{4}(2\alpha-\beta)\eta + \tfrac{1}{2}\beta\theta \end{aligned}\right\} \tag{4.3}$$

Putting $\beta = x$,

$$\left.\begin{aligned} \zeta = \tfrac{2}{3},\quad \eta = \frac{6-7x}{3(2+3x)},\quad \theta = \frac{2-9x}{3(2+3x)} \\ \therefore\ c_\infty = c_n + \tfrac{2}{3}d_n + \frac{(6-7x)e_n + (2-9x)f_n}{3(2+3x)}. \end{aligned}\right\} \tag{4.4}$$

In the case considered $e_1 = G_1 = 1$

$$\therefore\ c_\infty = \frac{6-7x}{6+9x}$$

$$\therefore\ y = \frac{8x}{6+9x}. \tag{4.5}$$

Hence with 50 percent crossing over in the homogametic sex the final proportion of crossover zygotes is 8/21. If both sexes of F_1 are crossed back to the parents,

$$y = \frac{4x}{6+9x}.$$

In this case it is quite possible to solve the equations (4.1) completely. C_n differs from C_∞ by the sum of six terms of geometric series, whose ratios are

$$\frac{1}{4},\ \frac{3}{4},\ \frac{2x \pm \sqrt{9-26x+19x^2}}{4}.\ \frac{2x \pm \sqrt{9-26x+23x^2}}{4}$$

Even here however the expression is rather complicated.

PARENT AND OFFSPRING MATING. AUTOSOMAL GENES

The mating system is the same as in the last case, except that both sons and daughters in F_1 are crossed back to the parents. This case has been considered, for unlinked genes, by both JENNINGS (1917) and WRIGHT (1921b). If 100β and 100δ are the crossover percentages, and $\alpha+\beta=\gamma+\delta=1$, we arrive at equations (5.1).

Typical mating	Number of types	
$AABB \times AABB$	2	$C_{n+1}=C+F+\frac{1}{4}(\alpha+\gamma)J+\frac{1}{4}(\beta+\delta)L.$
$AAbb \times AAbb$	2	$D_{n+1}=D+G+\frac{1}{4}(\alpha+\gamma)K+\frac{1}{4}(\beta+\delta)M.$
$AABb \times AABb$	4	$E_{n+1}=\frac{1}{2}(E+F+G)+\frac{1}{4}(H+I+N+P).$
$AABB \times AABb$	8	$F_{n+1}=\frac{1}{8}E+\frac{1}{2}F+\frac{1}{8}H+\frac{1}{8}(\beta+\delta)J+\frac{1}{8}(\alpha+\gamma)L+\frac{1}{16}(\alpha+\gamma)N+\frac{1}{16}(\beta+\delta)P.$
$AAbb \times AABb$	8	$G_{n+1}=\frac{1}{8}E+\frac{1}{2}G+\frac{1}{8}I+\frac{1}{8}(\beta+\delta)K+\frac{1}{8}(\alpha+\gamma)M+\frac{1}{16}(\beta+\delta)N+\frac{1}{16}(\alpha+\gamma)P.$
$AABb \times AaBB$	4	$H_{n+1}=\frac{1}{4}H+\frac{1}{8}(\beta+\delta)N+\frac{1}{8}(\alpha+\gamma)P.$
$AABb \times Aabb$	4	$I_{n+1}=\frac{1}{4}I+\frac{1}{8}(\alpha+\gamma)N+\frac{1}{8}(\beta+\delta)P.$
$AABB \times AB.ab$	4	$J_{n+1}=\frac{1}{4}(\alpha+\gamma)J+\frac{1}{8}(\beta+\delta)L+\frac{1}{8}(\alpha+\gamma)N+\frac{1}{8}\alpha\gamma Q+\frac{1}{16}(\alpha\delta+\beta\gamma)R.$
$AAbb \times Ab.aB$	4	$K_{n+1}=\frac{1}{4}(\alpha+\gamma)K+\frac{1}{8}(\beta+\delta)M+\frac{1}{8}(\alpha+\gamma)P+\frac{1}{8}\alpha\gamma S+\frac{1}{16}(\alpha\delta+\beta\gamma)R.$
$AABB \times Ab.aB$	4	$L_{n+1}=\frac{1}{8}(\beta+\delta)(L+P)+\frac{1}{16}(\alpha\delta+\beta\gamma)R+\frac{1}{8}\beta\delta S.$
$AAbb \times AB.ab$	4	$M_{n+1}=\frac{1}{8}(\beta+\delta)(M+N)+\frac{1}{16}(\alpha\delta+\beta\gamma)R+\frac{1}{8}\beta\delta Q.$
$AABb \times AB.ab$	8	$N_{n+1}=\frac{1}{8}I+\frac{1}{8}(\beta+\delta)J+\frac{1}{8}(\alpha+\gamma)M+\frac{1}{16}(4+\alpha+\gamma)N+\frac{1}{16}(\beta+\delta)P+\frac{1}{8}(\alpha\delta+\beta\gamma)Q+\frac{1}{16}(\alpha\gamma+\beta\delta)R.$
$AABb \times Ab.aB$	8	$P_{n+1}=\frac{1}{8}H+\frac{1}{8}(\beta+\delta)K+\frac{1}{8}(\alpha+\gamma)L+\frac{1}{16}(4+\alpha+\gamma)P+\frac{1}{16}(\beta+\delta)N+\frac{1}{8}(\alpha\delta+\beta\gamma)S+\frac{1}{16}(\alpha\gamma+\beta\delta)R.$
$AB.ab \times AB.ab$	1	$Q_{n+1}=\frac{1}{2}(\alpha+\gamma)(J+N)+\frac{1}{2}\alpha\gamma Q+\frac{1}{4}(\alpha\delta+\beta\gamma)R.$
$AB.ab \times Ab.aB$	2	$R_{n+1}=\frac{1}{4}(\beta+\delta)(L+M+N+P)+\frac{1}{4}\beta\delta(Q+S)+\frac{1}{4}(\alpha\delta+\beta\gamma)R.$
$Ab.aB \times Ab.aB$	1	$S_{n+1}=\frac{1}{2}(\alpha+\gamma)(K+P)+\frac{1}{2}\alpha\gamma S+\frac{1}{4}(\alpha\delta+\beta\gamma)R.$

Let $c_n=C_n-D_n$, $d_n=F_n-G_n$, $e_n=H_n-I_n$, $f_n=J_n-K_n$, $g_n=L_n-M_n$, $h_n=N_n-P_n$, $i_n=Q_n-S_n$. Let $\beta+\delta=2x$, $\beta\delta=p$.

$$\left.\begin{aligned}
\therefore\ c_{n+1} &= c_n + d_n + \tfrac{1}{2}(1-x)f_n + \tfrac{1}{2}xg_n.\\
d_{n+1} &= \tfrac{1}{2}d_n + \tfrac{1}{8}e_n + \tfrac{1}{4}xf_n + \tfrac{1}{4}(1-x)g_n + \tfrac{1}{8}(1-2x)h_n.\\
e_{n+1} &= \tfrac{1}{4}e_n - \tfrac{1}{4}(1-2x)h_n.\\
f_{n+1} &= \tfrac{1}{2}(1-x)f_n + \tfrac{1}{4}xg_n + \tfrac{1}{4}(1-x)h_n + \tfrac{1}{8}(1-2x+p)i_n.\\
g_{n+1} &= \tfrac{1}{4}x(g_n-h_n) - \tfrac{1}{8}pi_n.\\
h_{n+1} &= -\tfrac{1}{8}e_n + \tfrac{1}{4}xf_n - \tfrac{1}{4}(1-x)g_n + \tfrac{1}{8}(3-2x)h_n + \tfrac{1}{4}(x-p)i_n.\\
i_{n+1} &= (1-x)(f_n+h_n) + \tfrac{1}{2}(1-2x+p)i_n.
\end{aligned}\right\}\quad(5.2)$$

In order to have $c_n+\zeta d_n+\eta e_n+\theta f_n+\kappa g_n+\lambda h_n+\mu i_n$ independent of n, it is necessary that:

$$\left.\begin{aligned}
\zeta &= 1+\tfrac{1}{2}\zeta.\\
\eta &= \tfrac{1}{8}\zeta+\tfrac{1}{4}\eta-\tfrac{1}{8}\lambda.\\
\theta &= \tfrac{1}{2}(1-x)+\tfrac{1}{4}x\zeta+\tfrac{1}{2}(1-x)\theta+\tfrac{1}{4}x\lambda+(1-x)\mu.\\
\kappa &= \tfrac{1}{2}x+\tfrac{1}{4}(1-x)\zeta+\tfrac{1}{4}x(\theta+\kappa)-\tfrac{1}{4}(1-x)\lambda.\\
\lambda &= \tfrac{1}{8}(1-2x)\zeta-\tfrac{1}{4}(1-2x)\eta+\tfrac{1}{4}(1-x)\theta-\tfrac{1}{4}x\kappa+\tfrac{1}{8}(3-2x)\lambda+(1-x)\mu.\\
\mu &= \tfrac{1}{8}(1-2x+p)\theta-\tfrac{1}{8}p\kappa+\tfrac{1}{4}(x-p)\lambda+\tfrac{1}{2}(1-2x+p)\mu.
\end{aligned}\right\}\quad(5.3)$$

Hence $\zeta = 2,\ \eta = \dfrac{2x}{1+4x},\ \theta = \dfrac{2}{1+4x},\ \kappa = \dfrac{4x}{1+4x},\ \lambda = \dfrac{2(1-2x)}{1+4x},$

$$\mu = \frac{1-2x}{1+4x},$$

as may readily be verified.

$$\therefore\ c_\infty = c_n + 2d_n + \frac{1}{1+4x}[2f_n + 2x(e_n + 2g_n) + (1-2x)(2h_n + i_n)] \quad (5.4)$$

In the case considered $J_0 = f_0 = \frac{1}{2}\ \therefore c_\infty = 1/1+4x$

$$\therefore\ y = \frac{2x}{1+4x}. \quad (5.5)$$

Hence with 50 percent crossing over in both sexes, $y = \frac{1}{3}$, with 50 percent crossing over in one only, $y = \frac{1}{4}$. In order to obtain the maximum proportion of crossovers, we should mate F_1 *inter se*, and then mate F_2 back to F_1 of the opposite sex. In this case

$$Q_1 = i_1 = 2,\ \text{so}\ c_\infty = \frac{1-2x}{1+4x},\ \text{and}\ y = \frac{3x}{1+4x}.$$

Hence when $x = \frac{1}{2}$, $y = \frac{1}{2}$, and with 50 percent crossing over in one sex only, $y = \frac{3}{8}$. The approach to equilibrium involves the solution of equations (5.2) and a set of nine similar equations for $C_n + D_n$, etc. along with E_n and R_n. C_n differs from C_∞ by the sum of terms from 14 geometric series.

INBREEDING WITH ANY INITIAL POPULATION

The five systems of equations (1.1), (2.1), (3.1), (4.1) and (5.1) are true whatever be the initial composition of the population, provided that it contains the genes *A*, *a*, *B*, and *b* in equal numbers. This is not in general so. But we can render any population symmetrical by adding to it three other suitably chosen populations, these latter being added after one generation of inbreeding, so as not to mate with the group first considered. This addition does not affect the proportion of crossover zygotes, and the proportion of the genes is of course unaltered by inbreeding.

An example will make the method clear. We desire to know the final fate of a population consisting of zygotes in the proportion 1*AABB*:4*aaBb*, when mating is at random for one generation, and afterwards brothers and sisters only are mated. After one generation we add to it equal numbers of the children of three populations consisting of (1*AABB*:4*Aabb*), (1*aabb*:

4*AABb*) and (1*aabb*:4*AaBB*). Hence, out of 100 typical matings of the mixed F_1, 2 are *AABB*×*AABB*, 2 *aabb*×*aabb*, 4 of each of the 8 types exemplified by *AABB*×*aaBb*, 16 of each of the 4 types exemplified by *AABb* ×*AABb*. Dividing by 50, to give a total of 2:

$$c_1 = C_1 = \frac{1}{25};\ f_1 = J_1 = \frac{2}{25};\ Q_1 = \frac{8}{25}.$$

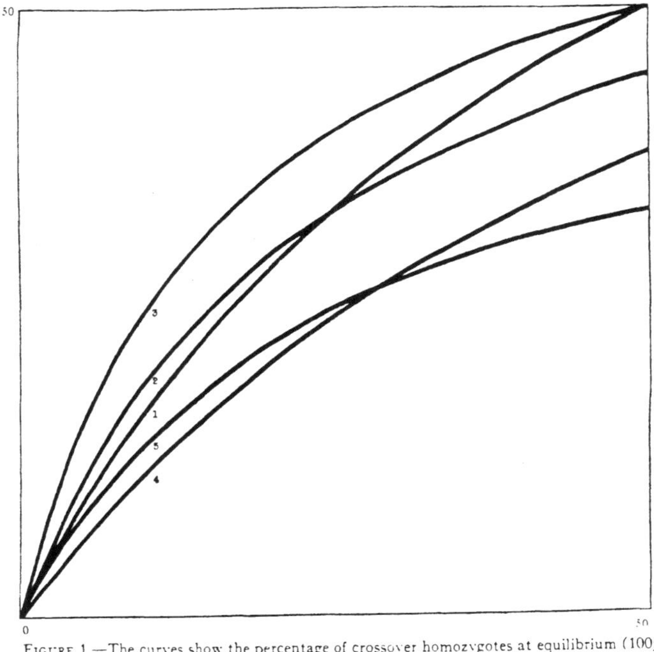

FIGURE 1.—The curves show the percentage of crossover homozygotes at equilibrium (100y), plotted as ordinates against the average crossover value (100x) as abscissa, for the following five systems of mating:

1. Self-fertilization.
2. Brother-sister mating. Sex-linked genes.
3. Brother-sister mating. Autosomal genes.
4. Parent-offspring mating, F_1 daughters backcrossed to father, sex-linked genes.
5. Parent-offspring mating, both F_1 sons and daughters backcrossed to parents, autosomal genes.

Hence by equation (3.4), $c_x = 1/25 + 2/25 \cdot 2(1-2x)/(1+6x)$.

$$\therefore\ y = \frac{10 + 76x}{25(1 + 6x)}.$$

This is the proportion of crossover zygotes. In the population first considered the ratio $A:a$ is 1:4, that of $B:b$ is 3:2. Hence if $[AABB]$ is the proportion of that type in the final population,

$$[AABB] + [AAbb] = \frac{1}{5},\ [AABB] + [aaBB] = \frac{3}{5},\ [AAbb] + [aaBB] = y$$

$$\therefore\ [AABB] = \frac{5 + 22x}{25(1 + 6x)}, \quad [AAbb] = \frac{8x}{25(1 + 6x)}.$$

$$[aaBB] = \frac{10 + 68x}{25(1 + 6x)}, \quad [aabb] = \frac{10 + 52x}{25(1 + 6x)}.$$

Similarly the final composition of any other population may be found. It is often more convenient to split it up into groups, and consider each separately. Thus in the above case 1/25 of the final population is derived from $AABB \times AABB$, that is, is all $AABB$; 16/25 is derived from the mating $aaBb \times aaBb$, that is, consists of equal numbers of $aaBB$ and $aabb$; 8/25 is derived from $AABb \times aaBb$, and the reciprocal cross. This gives all four zygotic types in proportions depending on the value of x. It is quite possible to form equations for the results of breeding from a population containing arbitrary numbers of each of the 20 zygotic types, but the expressions obtained are neither short nor elegant.

DOUBLE CROSSING OVER

Consider the inbreeding of zygotes ABC/abc, where the 3 genes A, B, C are linked and in that order. Let p be the proportion of crossing over between AB (that is, 100p the crossover value), and let q, r be the same proportions for BC, AC. Then the proportion of double crossovers is obviously $\frac{1}{2}(p+q-r)$. Similarly if, after inbreeding, the proportions of crossover zygotes are f(p), f(q), f(r), the proportion of double crossover zygotes, that is, $aaBBcc$ and $AAbbCC$, is $\frac{1}{2}[f(p)+f(q)-f(r)]$. Now f(p) is always of the form kp/(1+lp). Hence we have, for the proportion Z of double crossovers,

$$2Z = \frac{kp}{1 + lp} + \frac{kq}{1 + lq} + \frac{kr}{1 + lr}$$

$$\therefore\ Z = \frac{k(p + q - r + 2lpq + l^2pqr)}{2(1 + lp)(1 + lq)(1 + lr)}.$$

Now $\frac{1}{2}(p+q-r)$ is the proportion of gametic double crossovers, and therefore smaller than pq, owing to interference, unless p and q are quite large. Hence since $l>1$ the last two terms in the nominator are the most important. When p and q are small, r is practically equal to their sum, and $Z = klpq$, approximately.

That is to say whereas the proportion of single gametic crossovers is k times the corresponding gametic value when the latter is small, the proportion of zygotic double crossovers is kl times the proportion of gametic double crossovers calculated if there were no interference, and many more times the real value. The values of k and kl, collected from equations (1.3), (2.5), (3.5), (4.5), (5.5) and their modifications, are given in table 2.

TABLE 2

TYPE OF INBREEDING	TYPE OF LINKAGE	k	kl
Self-fertilization	Autosomal	2	4
Brother-sister mating	Autosomal	4	24
Brother-sister mating	Sex-linked	8/3	32/3
Parent-offspring mating	Autosomal	2	8
Parent-offspring mating after F_1	Autosomal	3	12
Parent-offspring mating both ways	Sex-linked	2/3	1
Parent-offspring mating father-daughter, or after F_1	Sex-linked	4/3	2

DISCUSSION

The method of calculation here employed cannot be applied to most other types of inbreeding. It is wholly inapplicable to the important case where a male is bred to a large group of his half-sisters in each generation. The case of double first cousin matings with autosomal linkage involves the consideration of 10,000 different pairs of mating types, and other systems are still more complex. It may prove possible to solve such problems by an extension of WRIGHT'S (1921a) correlation method, but we have been unable to do so.

Inbreeding may be undertaken for several purposes. It may be desired to obtain and fix as many types as possible after crossing two different varieties, to obtain a pure line of a desired type, or merely a pure line of any sort. In each case it is desirable to encourage crossing over. If the genetics of the organism concerned are known already, this can doubtless be done by *ad hoc* matings. In general this is not possible. The reason why crossing over, that is, recombination, is desirable in all types of inbreeding is as follows. Hybrid vigor may be due partly to heterozygosis as such, but it is probably also in part due to the presence in the hybrid of dominant genes contributed by the two parents. If so the vigor of an extracted pure line will depend on the numbers of such dominants which are combined in it. In so far as they are linked, the probability of such a combination will depend on the type of mating practised.

It is clear from table 2 that the differences are very considerable. For example a recombination involving three fairly closely linked genes is about 3 times as likely with brother-sister mating as with parent-offspring mating, and six times as likely as with self-fertilization. In the case of sex-linked genes the probability is over 10 times as great with brother-sister mating as with parent-offspring mating. However the disadvantages of the latter are considerably diminished if instead of beginning it by crossing the F_1 to the parents, the first parent-offspring mating is between F_1 and F_2. If the ideal genotype requires the occurrence of a number of crossings over the differences between different mating systems are greatly increased.

For example if two pure lines of Drosophila whose males are of composition $Ab(CdE/CdE)(FgH/FgH)$, and $aB(cDe/cDe)(fGh/fGh)$, respectively, are crossed, the proportion of pure lines finally containing all the dominants is 0.98 percent with brother-sister mating, 0.0372 percent with unrestricted parent-offspring mating, even when all crossover values are 50 percent.

It is clear then that the proportion of homozygosis reached is not the sole possible criterion of intensity of inbreeding. But the difference between different systems due to the considerations here outlined will be far more intense in an organism with high linkage, such as Apotettix, Lebistes, Drosophila, or Funaria, than in one with little linkage, such as a mammal or *Triticum vulgare*.

SUMMARY

Formulae are given for the amount of crossing over which is found in the final population when organisms heterozygous for linked genes are inbred according to various systems.

LITERATURE CITED

JENNINGS, H. S., 1916 The numerical results of diverse systems of breeding. Genetics 1: 53.

JENNINGS, H. S., 1917 The numerical results of diverse systems of breeding with respect to two characters, etc. Genetics 2: 97–154.

ROBBINS, R. B., 1918 Some applications of mathematics to breeding problems. III. Genetics 3: 375–379.

WRIGHT, S., 1921a Systems of mating. I. Genetics 6: 111–123.

1921b Systems of mating. II. Genetics 6: 124–143.

[FROM JOURNAL OF GENETICS, VOL. XXIV. No. 1,
pp. 121–144, FEBRUARY, 1931.]

LINKAGE IN THE TETRAPLOID *PRIMULA SINENSIS.*

BY D. DE WINTON AND J. B. S. HALDANE.
(*John Innes Horticultural Institution, Merton.*)

CONTENTS.

INTRODUCTION.

LINKAGE has so far been almost exclusively studied in diploids and allopolyploids such as wheat. In the latter the phenomenon is not essentially different from that in diploids, as each chromosome, save for rare exceptions, has a definite mate. The only case of true polyploid linkage so far studied is that in the triplo-**X** *Drosophila melanogaster* of Bridges and Anderson (1925). No linked factors were known in autotetraploid plants other than *Primula sinensis* until 1930, but our colleague Dr Sansome is now studying linkage in tetraploid tomatoes.

The present work was begun in 1909 by the late R. P. Gregory. Sverdrup Sömme (1930) has analysed the data up to 1927. We incorporate counts of 2867 more plants, but reject some of her data on various grounds.

The factors here considered are **S**, **B** and **G**. **S** converts a pin plant, with long style and short stamens, into a thrum with short style and long stamens. **B** converts red flower pigment into magenta, **G** inhibits the formation of anthocyanin pigment in the centre of the flower, producing a green stigma and ovary in place of a red. In the diploid they are completely dominant. In the tetraploid **S** is completely so, but **Bbbb** and **Gggg**, though generally easily distinguished from **bbbb** and **gggg**, are on the whole not so different from them as are **BBBB** and **GGGG**. There is no possibility of a mistake in scoring **S**. In some families **Bbbb** and **bbbb** may have been confused. It is possible, though not very likely, that errors may have been made regarding **G**. No attempt has been made to separate different grades of dominant, *e.g.* **BBbb** and **Bbbb**, though in some cases this was partly possible.

The linkage values of these factors in the diploid are based on a mass of material, partly given by Gregory, de Winton and Bateson (1923). Table I is based entirely on back-cross data as regards the diploid; the F_2 data are concordant, but do not enable a distinction to be made between the male and female sides of the plant. The data on which the tetraploid figures are based will be given later.

TABLE I.

Cross-over values per cent., with standard errors.

Factors	Diploid ♀	Diploid ♂	Tetraploid ♀	Tetraploid ♂
SB	7·35 ± 0·40	12·91 ± 0·50	8·01 ± 0·69	8·41 ± 0·99
SG	33·29 ± 0·74	40·47 ± 0·78	37·58 ± 1·92	38·91 ± 2·23
BG	31·15 ± 0·53	36·24 ± 0·68	35·18 ± 1·85	34·38 ± 2·17

In order to understand the linkage data we must first consider the genetical behaviour of the factors one at a time. Apart from aneuploids, *e.g.* plants with $4n + 1$ (49) chromosomes, the following types of zygote are to be expected with regard to a single pair of allelomorphs **X** and **x**: **XXXX**, quadruplex; **XXXx**, triplex; **XXxx**, duplex; **Xxxx**, simplex; **xxxx**, nulliplex.

Quadruplex and triplex plants give no recessive offspring, duplex by nulliplex give 5 dominant : 1 recessive, simplex by nulliplex 1 dominant : 1 recessive. In Table II actual figures are given for the factors concerned. These figures do not represent all the material available, but only those in which the composition of the dominant parent was known from its ancestry. All the duplex plants included in them were from the cross **XXXX** × **xxxx** or reciprocal. The only element of doubt here is the possibility of an alleged **XXXX** grand-parent having been **XXXx**, such triplex plants being indistinguishable from quadruplex by a single generation of breeding, and being eliminated rather slowly on self-fertilisation. Plants known by their genetic behaviour, but not their ancestry, to have been **XXxx** are excluded. Such plants occurred, for example, among the progeny when **XXxx** was selfed.

Similarly the only **Xxxx** plants whose progeny is included are those from **Xxxx** × **xxxx** or the reciprocal cross, the constitution of the simplex grand-parent being assumed, if necessary, from its genetical behaviour. Dominant progeny of 73 crosses of simplex × nulliplex have been tested, and all have proved simplex. On the hypothesis of random assortment of chromatids (Haldane, 1930) one in thirteen would have been duplex.

TABLE II.

Single factor ratios.

Parents	No. of families	Dominant	Recessive	D	$D \div \sigma$
$\mathbf{Ss_3} \times \mathbf{Ss_3}$	40	1282	395	−24·25	1·20
$\mathbf{Bb_3} \times \mathbf{Bb_3}$	17	358	124	+ 3·5	0·37
$\mathbf{Gg_3} \times \mathbf{Gg_3}$	10	265	91	+ 2	0·24
$\mathbf{Ss_3} \times \mathbf{s_4}$	75	1001	1009	− 4	0·18
$\mathbf{Bb_3} \times \mathbf{b_4}$	38	559	542	− 8·5	0·51
$\mathbf{Gg_3} \times \mathbf{g_4}$	25	368	371	+ 1·5	0·11
$\mathbf{s_4} \times \mathbf{Ss_3}$	45	456	534	−39	2·48
$\mathbf{b_4} \times \mathbf{Bb_3}$	28	291	380	−44·5	3·43
$\mathbf{g_4} \times \mathbf{Gg_3}$	24	293	315	+11	0·89
$\mathbf{S_2s_2} \times \mathbf{S_2s_2}$	1	44	2	+ 0·7	0·65
$\mathbf{G_2g_2} \times \mathbf{G_2g_2}$	23	1204	44	+10	1·74
$\mathbf{G_2g_2} \times \mathbf{g_4}$	34	643	125	− 3	0·29
$\mathbf{g_4} \times \mathbf{G_2g_2}$	9	87	22	+ 3·8	0·98

Table II shows the genetical behaviour of simplex and duplex plants. The results are not independent, owing to linkage. It will be seen that the only really serious deviations from expectation occur in the cross of $\mathbf{x_4} \times \mathbf{Xx_3}$, the heterozygotes giving an excess of recessive gametes on the male side. The fact that the same families are included in the **B** and **S** totals accounts for the similar discrepancy in both cases, since **B** and **S** were coupled in many of the plants. Five $\mathbf{Bb_3}$ plants as males gave 66 **B**, 106 **b**, which accounts for nearly half the discrepancy. Used as females they gave 90 **B**, 85 **b**. We have clearly to deal with a case of anisogeny, the **B** pollen grains being handicapped while the **B** ovules are not. A possible explanation is that these plants were **Bbbbb**, *i.e.* 49 chromosome plants, and that as in *Datura* $2n + 1$ ovules are functional, $2n + 1$ pollen not so in competition with $2n$ pollen. In this case the ovules would give a ratio of 1 **B** : 1 **b**, the pollen grains 2 **B** : 3 **b**, which agrees with observation. If the divergence from expectation were due to random pairing of chromatids we should expect similar gametic ratios on both sides, for the equality of linkage values suggests that meiosis is similar on the two sides of the plant. If non-disjunction of the **SBG** chromosome is at all common we should expect to find **Bbbbb** plants among the parents of Table II: on the other hand **Bbbb** bbbb or the reciprocal cross could not give **BBbbb** apart from double reduction.

Exceptions due to double reduction may occur, but they are too rare to be considered in an admittedly preliminary theory of linkage.

Hence in what follows we assume that two chromatids from the same chromosome always go into different gametes. This is borne out by the behaviour of linked factors. The further question whether two chromatids which have paired and exchanged factors by crossing-over may enter the same gamete is considered later. Both these anomalies would involve non-disjunction.

THEORY OF LINKAGE IN TETRAPLOIDS.

In a diploid organism heterozygous for two factors we can only study two types of gametic series, those characteristic of coupling and repulsion, which are closely related, and their relation could be deduced on many different theories of segregation. For example, it was consistent with the reduplication theory, or with several different theories as to the relation between factors and chromosomes.

In the tetraploid, however, there should be seven distinct types of gametic series: (1) single coupling, (2) single repulsion, (3) asymmetrical coupling, (4) asymmetrical repulsion, (5) double coupling, (6) double repulsion, (7) coupling *and* repulsion. It will be difficult to construct zygotes giving combined coupling and repulsion, or to identify them with certainty if they have been constructed.

We consider only the ratios to be expected in the case of completely dominant factors. In order to obtain visible segregation the number of these factors in a zygote must be one or two. Suppose two factors **X** and **Y** to be linked, crossing-over occurring in the formation of a proportion p of the gametes; and a plant known from its genetical performance to be of the composition

XY
xy
xy
xy

Then if, after crossing-over has occurred, two chromosomes can enter the same gamete, some of its **XY** offspring when it is crossed with (**xy**)[4] will exhibit repulsion of **X** and **Y**. As will be seen later, such an event is rare, if it occurs at all. In what follows we will assume that it does not occur, *i.e.* that after two chromosomes have paired, they must proceed to different poles. The absence of such a conversion of coupling into repulsion also renders pairing of three chromosomes leading to "progressive" crossing-over unlikely, and further reasons are given later to show that it is a rare or non-existent phenomenon.

Case 1. Single coupling.

$$\begin{array}{c}\mathbf{XY}\\ \mathbf{xy}\\ \mathbf{xy}\\ \mathbf{xy}\end{array}$$

The chromosome containing **X** and **Y** must pair with one of the others. Crossing-over occurs in p of the total cases, the gametic series is therefore:

$$(1-p)\genfrac{}{}{0pt}{}{\mathbf{XY}}{\mathbf{xy}} : p\genfrac{}{}{0pt}{}{\mathbf{Xy}}{\mathbf{xy}} : p\genfrac{}{}{0pt}{}{\mathbf{xY}}{\mathbf{xy}} : (1-p)\genfrac{}{}{0pt}{}{\mathbf{xy}}{\mathbf{xy}}$$

a series similar to that of the diploid.

Case 2. Single repulsion.

$$\begin{array}{c}\mathbf{Xy}\\ \mathbf{xY}\\ \mathbf{xy}\\ \mathbf{xy}\end{array}$$

Calling the four chromosomes A, B, C and D, in two-thirds of all cases A does not pair with B, so the gametes are:

$$1\genfrac{}{}{0pt}{}{\mathbf{Xy}}{\mathbf{xY}} : 1\genfrac{}{}{0pt}{}{\mathbf{Xy}}{\mathbf{xy}} : 1\genfrac{}{}{0pt}{}{\mathbf{xY}}{\mathbf{xy}} : 1\genfrac{}{}{0pt}{}{\mathbf{xy}}{\mathbf{xy}}$$

In the remaining one-third A and B pair, so there is a chance of crossing-over, the gametes being:

$$p\genfrac{}{}{0pt}{}{\mathbf{XY}}{\mathbf{xy}} : (1-p)\genfrac{}{}{0pt}{}{\mathbf{Xy}}{\mathbf{xy}} : (1-p)\genfrac{}{}{0pt}{}{\mathbf{xY}}{\mathbf{xy}} : p\genfrac{}{}{0pt}{}{\mathbf{xy}}{\mathbf{xy}}$$

Hence the total gametic series is:

$$1\genfrac{}{}{0pt}{}{\mathbf{Xy}}{\mathbf{xY}} : p\genfrac{}{}{0pt}{}{\mathbf{XY}}{\mathbf{xy}} : (2-p)\genfrac{}{}{0pt}{}{\mathbf{Xy}}{\mathbf{xy}} : (2-p)\genfrac{}{}{0pt}{}{\mathbf{xY}}{\mathbf{xy}} : (1+p)\genfrac{}{}{0pt}{}{\mathbf{xy}}{\mathbf{xy}}$$

Case 3. Asymmetrical coupling.

$$\begin{array}{c}\mathbf{XY}\\ \mathbf{Xy}\\ \mathbf{xy}\\ \mathbf{xy}\end{array}$$

Here in one-third of all cases AB, CD pair and the gametes are:

$$1\genfrac{}{}{0pt}{}{\mathbf{XY}}{\mathbf{xy}} : 1\genfrac{}{}{0pt}{}{\mathbf{Xy}}{\mathbf{xy}}$$

In the other cases crossing-over may occur between A and C or D, and the resulting chromosome has an equal chance of entering an **Xy** or an **xy** gamete. The total gametic series is therefore:

$$(1-p)\genfrac{}{}{0pt}{}{\mathbf{XY}}{\mathbf{Xy}} : (2-p)\genfrac{}{}{0pt}{}{\mathbf{XY}}{\mathbf{xy}} : p\genfrac{}{}{0pt}{}{\mathbf{Xy}}{\mathbf{xY}} : p\genfrac{}{}{0pt}{}{\mathbf{Xy}}{\mathbf{Xy}} : 2\genfrac{}{}{0pt}{}{\mathbf{Xy}}{\mathbf{xy}} : p\genfrac{}{}{0pt}{}{\mathbf{xY}}{\mathbf{xy}} : (1-p)\genfrac{}{}{0pt}{}{\mathbf{xy}}{\mathbf{xy}}$$

Case 4. Asymmetrical repulsion.

$$\begin{matrix}\mathbf{Xy}\\ \mathbf{Xy}\\ \mathbf{xY}\\ \mathbf{xy}\end{matrix}$$

In one-third of all cases *AB*, *CD* pair and the gametes are:

$$1\ \genfrac{}{}{0pt}{}{\mathbf{Xy}}{\mathbf{xY}} : 1\ \genfrac{}{}{0pt}{}{\mathbf{Xy}}{\mathbf{xy}}$$

In the other two-thirds pairing of *C* with *A* or *B* renders crossing-over possible, the resulting chromosomes as above entering a gamete with **Xy** or **xy** in equal numbers. The total gametic series is thus:

$$p\ \genfrac{}{}{0pt}{}{\mathbf{XY}}{\mathbf{Xy}} : p\ \genfrac{}{}{0pt}{}{\mathbf{XY}}{\mathbf{xy}} : (2-p)\ \genfrac{}{}{0pt}{}{\mathbf{Xy}}{\mathbf{xY}} : (1-p)\ \genfrac{}{}{0pt}{}{\mathbf{Xy}}{\mathbf{Xy}} : 2\ \genfrac{}{}{0pt}{}{\mathbf{Xy}}{\mathbf{xy}} : (1-p)\ \genfrac{}{}{0pt}{}{\mathbf{xY}}{\mathbf{xy}} : p\ \genfrac{}{}{0pt}{}{\mathbf{xy}}{\mathbf{xy}}$$

Case 5. Double coupling.

$$\begin{matrix}\mathbf{XY}\\ \mathbf{XY}\\ \mathbf{xy}\\ \mathbf{xy}\end{matrix}$$

In one-third of all cases *AB*, *CD* pair and the gametes are $\genfrac{}{}{0pt}{}{\mathbf{XY}}{\mathbf{xy}}$. In two-thirds of the cases crossing-over may occur. The following question now arises. Does the fact that crossing-over has occurred between chromosomes *A* and *C* alter the probability of crossing-over between *B* and *D*? This probability would be increased if certain variable conditions in the nucleus as a whole favoured crossing-over in both cases. It would be diminished if, for example, only a finite amount of energy was available for twisting or breaking the chromosomes, and this might be concentrated on one pair or the other. In what follows we shall assume that the probabilities are independent, an hypothesis which agrees fairly well with experience. The gametic output where crossing-over is possible is therefore symbolised by

$$[(1-p)\,\mathbf{XY} : p\,\mathbf{Xy} : p\,\mathbf{xY} : (1-p)\,\mathbf{xy}]^2$$

and the total gametic series is:

$$(1-2p+p^2)\ \genfrac{}{}{0pt}{}{\mathbf{XY}}{\mathbf{XY}} : (2p-2p^2)\ \genfrac{}{}{0pt}{}{\mathbf{XY}}{\mathbf{Xy}} : (2p-2p^2)\ \genfrac{}{}{0pt}{}{\mathbf{XY}}{\mathbf{xY}} :$$

$$2\,(2-2p-p^2)\ \genfrac{}{}{0pt}{}{\mathbf{XY}}{\mathbf{xy}} : 2p^2\ \genfrac{}{}{0pt}{}{\mathbf{Xy}}{\mathbf{xY}} : p^2\ \genfrac{}{}{0pt}{}{\mathbf{Xy}}{\mathbf{Xy}} : (2p-2p^2)\ \genfrac{}{}{0pt}{}{\mathbf{Xy}}{\mathbf{xy}} :$$

$$p^2\ \genfrac{}{}{0pt}{}{\mathbf{xY}}{\mathbf{xY}} : (2p-p^2)\ \genfrac{}{}{0pt}{}{\mathbf{xY}}{\mathbf{xy}} : (1-p)^2\ \genfrac{}{}{0pt}{}{\mathbf{xy}}{\mathbf{xy}}$$

In the event of a positive or negative correlation between the two cross-overs the terms whose coefficients are divisible by p would be increased or diminished respectively.

Case 6. Double repulsion.

$$\begin{matrix}\mathbf{Xy}\\ \mathbf{Xy}\\ \mathbf{xY}\\ \mathbf{xY}\end{matrix}$$

In one-third of all cases AB, CD pair and the gametes are all $\begin{matrix}\mathbf{Xy}\\ \mathbf{xY}\end{matrix}$. In the remaining two-thirds crossing-over may occur. If it is independent the output is symbolised by

$$[p\ \mathbf{XY} : (1-p)\ \mathbf{Xy} : (1-p)\ \mathbf{xY} : p\ \mathbf{xy}]^2$$

and the total gametic series is:

$$p^2 \begin{matrix}\mathbf{XY}\\ \mathbf{XY}\end{matrix} : (2p-2p^2) \begin{matrix}\mathbf{XY}\\ \mathbf{Xy}\end{matrix} : (2p-2p^2) \begin{matrix}\mathbf{XY}\\ \mathbf{xY}\end{matrix} : 2p^2 \begin{matrix}\mathbf{XY}\\ \mathbf{xy}\end{matrix} : (4-4p+2p^2) \begin{matrix}\mathbf{Xy}\\ \mathbf{xY}\end{matrix} :$$

$$(1-p)^2 \begin{matrix}\mathbf{Xy}\\ \mathbf{Xy}\end{matrix} : (2p-2p^2) \begin{matrix}\mathbf{Xy}\\ \mathbf{xy}\end{matrix} : (1-p)^2 \begin{matrix}\mathbf{xY}\\ \mathbf{xY}\end{matrix} : (2p-2p^2) \begin{matrix}\mathbf{xY}\\ \mathbf{xy}\end{matrix} : p^2 \begin{matrix}\mathbf{xy}\\ \mathbf{xy}\end{matrix}$$

subject to the above reservation.

Case 7. Coupling and repulsion.

$$\begin{matrix}\mathbf{XY}\\ \mathbf{Xy}\\ \mathbf{xY}\\ \mathbf{xy}\end{matrix}$$

In one-third of all cases AB, CD pair and the gametes are:

$$1 \begin{matrix}\mathbf{XY}\\ \mathbf{xY}\end{matrix} : 1 \begin{matrix}\mathbf{XY}\\ \mathbf{xy}\end{matrix} : 1 \begin{matrix}\mathbf{Xy}\\ \mathbf{xY}\end{matrix} : 1 \begin{matrix}\mathbf{Xy}\\ \mathbf{xy}\end{matrix}$$

In one-third of all cases AC, BD pair and the gametes are:

$$1 \begin{matrix}\mathbf{XY}\\ \mathbf{Xy}\end{matrix} : 1 \begin{matrix}\mathbf{XY}\\ \mathbf{xy}\end{matrix} : 1 \begin{matrix}\mathbf{Xy}\\ \mathbf{xY}\end{matrix} : 1 \begin{matrix}\mathbf{xY}\\ \mathbf{xy}\end{matrix}$$

In one-third of all cases AD. CB pair and in the absence of correlation the gametic series is represented by

$$[p\ \mathbf{XY} : (1-p)\ \mathbf{Xy} : (1-p)\ \mathbf{xY} : p\ \mathbf{xy}]$$
$$[(1-p)\ \mathbf{XY} : p\ \mathbf{Xy} : p\ \mathbf{xY} : (1-p)\ \mathbf{xy}]$$

Hence the total gametic series is:

$$(p-p^2)\,\frac{\mathbf{XY}}{\mathbf{XY}} : (2-2p+2p^2)\,\frac{\mathbf{XY}}{\mathbf{Xy}} : (2-2p+2p^2)\,\frac{\mathbf{XY}}{\mathbf{xY}} :$$

$$(2+2p-2p^2)\,\frac{\mathbf{XY}}{\mathbf{xy}} : (2+2p-2p^2)\,\frac{\mathbf{Xy}}{\mathbf{xY}} : (p-p^2)\,\frac{\mathbf{Xy}}{\mathbf{Xy}} :$$

$$(2-2p+2p^2)\,\frac{\mathbf{Xy}}{\mathbf{xy}} : (p-p^2)\,\frac{\mathbf{xY}}{\mathbf{xY}} : (2-2p+2p^2)\,\frac{\mathbf{xY}}{\mathbf{xy}} : (p-p^2)\,\frac{\mathbf{xy}}{\mathbf{xy}}$$

provided that, in the third case, crossing-over is not correlated.

Since in the case of complete dominance, the various classes of gamete containing at least one **X** and **Y** produce indistinguishable zygotes, the above results may be summarised in Table III. p and q are the cross-over ratios on the two sexual sides of the plant.

TABLE III.

Type of zygote	Types of gametes	Gametes in general	Gametes, $p=0$	Gametes, $p=\frac{1}{2}$	Gametes in absence of linkage	Zygotic ratio on selfing
1. **XY.(xy)$_3$**	**XY**	$1-p$	1	1	1	$2+(1-p)(1-q)$
	Xy	p	0	1	1	$1-(1-p)(1-q)$
	xY	p	0	1	1	$1-(1-p)(1-q)$
	xy	$1-p$	1	1	1	$(1-p)(1-q)$
2. **Xy.xY.(xy)$_2$**	**XY**	$1+p$	1	1	1	$18+(1+p)(1+q)$
	Xy	$2-p$	2	1	1	$9-(1+p)(1+q)$
	xY	$2-p$	2	1	1	$9-(1+p)(1+q)$
	xy	$1+p$	1	1	1	$(1+p)(1+q)$
3. **XY.Xy.(xy)$_2$**	**XY**	$3-p$	3	5	5	$26+(1-p)(1-q)$
	Xy	$2+p$	2	5	5	$9-(1-p)(1-q)$
	xY	p	0	1	1	$1-(1-p)(1-q)$
	xy	$1-p$	1	1	1	$(1-p)(1-q)$
4. **(Xy)$_2$.xY.xy**	**XY**	$2+p$	2	5	5	$26-pq$
	Xy	$3-p$	3	5	5	$9-pq$
	xY	$1-p$	1	1	1	$1-pq$
	xy	p	0	1	1	pq
5. **(XY)$_2$.(xy)$_2$**	**XY**	$5-2p-p^2$	5	17	25	$34-(1-p)^2(1-q)^2$
	Xy	$2p-p^2$	0	3	5	$1-(1-p)^2(1-q)^2$
	xY	$2p-p^2$	0	3	5	$1-(1-p)^2(1-q)^2$
	xy	$1-2p+p^2$	1	1	1	$(1-p)^2(1-q)^2$
6. **(Xy)$_2$.(xY)$_2$**	**XY**	$4-p^2$	4	17	25	$34-p^2q^2$
	Xy	$1-p^2$	1	3	5	$1-p^2q^2$
	xY	$1-p^2$	1	3	5	$1-p^2q^2$
	xy	p^2	0	1	1	p^2q^2
7. **XY.Xy.xY.xy**	**XY**	$8+p-p^2$	4	33	25	$136-pq(1-p)(1-q)$
	Xy	$2-p+p^4$	1	7	5	$4-pq(1-p)(1-q)$
	xY	$2-p-p^2$	1	7	5	$4-pq(1-p)(1-q)$
	xy	$p-p^2$	0	1	1	$pq(1-p)(1-q)$

For purposes of calculation it is convenient to put $1-p=P$, $1-q=Q$.

The gametic series in double coupling may then be written $4-P^2 : 1-P^2 : 1-P^2 : P^2$, and the expressions for the following zygotic series may be simplified:

Single coupling, $2-PQ : 1-PQ : 1-PQ : PQ$.
Asymmetrical coupling, $26-PQ : 9-PQ : 1-PQ : PQ$.
Double coupling, $34-P^2Q^2 : 1-P^2Q^2 : 1-P^2Q^2 : P^2Q^2$.
Coupling and repulsion, $136-pqPQ : 4-pqPQ : 4-pqPQ : pqPQ$.

The second column gives the gametic series in general, the third the expected ratios when linkage is so strong that crossing-over may be neglected, the fourth when linkage is so weak that crossing-over amounts to 50 per cent. In the fifth column the ratios are given which are found when the factors are in different chromosomes. In the last column are given the zygotic ratios to be expected on selfing. In the case of single coupling the ratios are the same as in a diploid. But in the case of single repulsion this is not so, since two factors in different chromosomes can still enter the same gamete. The asymmetrical cases call for no special comment.

Whereas in the first four cases no difference is to be expected when the factors, though in the same chromosome, are far apart, from the ratios obtained when they are in different chromosomes, this is not so in the last three. If the factors are in different chromosomes each tetrad of homologous chromosomes can pair in three ways giving two pairs each, so the total number of distinct cases to be considered is 36. But if the factors are far apart in the same chromosome each of the six possible pairs of chromosomes can produce one, two or four different types of gametes; the total number of cases is therefore 24 or 48. It is thus theoretically possible, in a tetraploid plant, to distinguish between 50 per cent. crossing-over and the absence of linkage.

Similar calculations have been made to meet the possibility that, after pairing, the chromosomes can enter gametes at random, so that in one-third of all cases, two chromosomes which have paired so as to permit of crossing-over may enter the same gamete. The expected ratios are somewhat different. As, however, it will be shown that this event occurs rarely if ever in *Primula sinensis*, the possibility need not be further considered here. It is however possible that it may occur in other tetraploid organisms, or that a state of affairs may be found in them intermediate between the above condition and that here described. If after pairing, chromosomes always went to the same pole, only **XY** and **xy** gametes would be found in the case of single or double coupling. This, of course, is not the case.

When three factors are concerned, matters are much more complicated: 44 possible zygotic types must be considered. Moreover two different types of double crossing-over are theoretically possible. Consider four homologous chromosomes *A*, *B*, *C*, *D*, in a zygote

XYZ
xyz
xyz
xyz

Chromosome *A* may pair with *B*, crossing-over twice, and giving **XyZ** and **xYz** gametes. Or it may pair with both *B* and *C*, giving **Xyz**, **xYz** and **xyZ**. Both these types of crossing-over were found by Bridges and Anderson (1925) in the triploid *Drosophila melanogaster*, the first being termed recurrent, the second progressive. In the case of progressive crossing-over in a tetraploid we should expect that, as the result of a situation such as that shown in Fig. 1, the two gametes formed would be

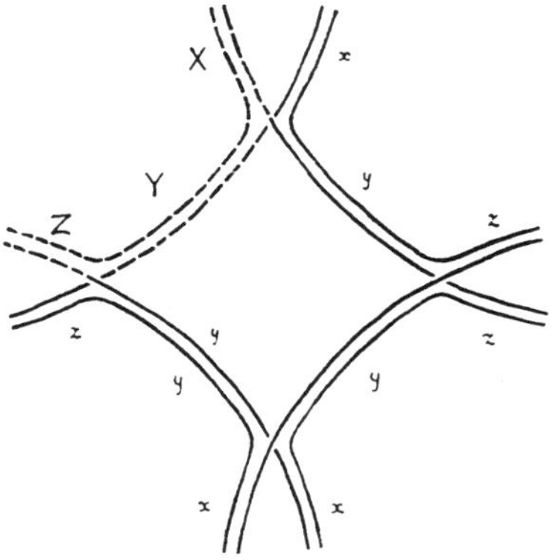

Fig. 1. Configuration in the diplotene stage which might yield **Xyz**/**xyZ** gametes. The chromosome containing the three dominants is dotted.

xYz/xyz and **Xyz**/xyZ. The fact that in such a case **X** and **Z** would exhibit repulsion in the progeny shows that such cases, if they occur, are rare. If they are at all frequent, however, **XyZ** and **xYz** gametes should be more commonly produced by the zygote

XYZ
xyz
xyz
xyz

than by **XYZ**/**xyz**, provided that the cross-over values are the same in both. Double cross-overs are not more common in the tetraploid, not at least to any significant extent. Hence it is considered that, for the present, a theory based on crossing-over involving two chromosomes only, which is not presented as final, will cover all the facts found, to a first approximation.

In view of the somewhat complicated nature of the theory, it is perhaps worth pointing out simpler, if less rigorous, methods of calculating some of the above gametic and zygotic series. Consider the case of double repulsion. The **yy** gametes form one-sixth of the whole, from the single factor theory. But in order that a **yy** gamete should also be **xx**, crossing-over must have occurred twice. The chance of this is p^2: hence the ratio of **Xyy** to **xxyy** gametes is $1 - p^2 : p^2$. The relative proportion of **xxY** gametes is also $1 - p^2$. But since the total proportion of **X** gametes is five for every one **xx**, there must be $4 + p^2$ **XY** gametes. Similarly the proportion of **xxyy** gametes in double coupling is P^2, this being the chance that no crossing-over has occurred on two distinct occasions.

In the corresponding zygotic series the proportions of bottom recessives are $\frac{p^2q^2}{36}$ and $\frac{P^2Q^2}{36}$. In the first case crossing-over must have occurred twice on the male and twice on the female side (a most improbable occurrence), in the second it must have failed to occur on four independent occasions. So that even in a doubly coupled zygote, double recessives rarely occur as a result of selfing. Thus if the cross-over value in each sex is $33\frac{1}{3}$ per cent., $p = \frac{1}{3}$, $P = \frac{2}{3}$, therefore the proportion of double recessives is $\frac{1}{36}\left(\frac{2}{3}\right)^4$, or 4 in 729. This is greater than the proportion of 1 in 1296 expected in the absence of linkage, but is still small.

EXPERIMENTAL RESULTS.

In the interpretation of the experimental results there is a certain danger of circularity in the argument. Thus a number of plants, from their genetical behaviour, agree with the expectation on the assumption that they are of the composition

SBG
sbg
sbg
sbg

Some of these plants are derived from a cross between a triple recessive plant and a triple dominant of uncertain composition. Others arise from selfing, and so on. Only their genetical behaviour makes their composition more or less certain. On the other hand, many such plants are derived from the cross of a plant known from its ancestry, genetical behaviour, or both, to be of the above composition, crossed with a triple

9-2

recessive. On the theory here developed, all plants in such families, provided that they carry the three dominants, should be of the above composition, unless some exceptional event such as progressive crossing-over has occurred. Such plants, and no others, may legitimately be used to test the theory.

We may however legitimately include with them other plants of similar genetical behaviour, provided their offspring occur in the theoretical proportions, and use the total of such families for the purpose of calculating linkage intensities. In the tables three distinct classes of parents are considered.

(*a*) Parents whose genetic composition can be predicted from those of their ancestors on the assumption that neither double reduction, non-disjunction, nor progressive crossing-over has occurred.

(*b*) Parents in which the ancestry does not suffice to determine the number of factors, but where the linkages are certain once the numbers of factors are known. Now the number of factors (*i.e.* whether the plant is simplex or duplex) can be determined from the ratios in which the single factors segregate in their progeny. In families of ten or more plants there is very little chance of confusing a 1 : 1 with a 5 : 1 ratio, and little chance of confusing a 3 : 1 with a 35 : 1. Hence the progeny of such plants furnish reliable data on linkage. For example 161[1]/24 was derived from a cross between **SSSsBBbb** and **ssssbbbb**, and being a thrum magenta, was either duplex or simplex in **S** and **B**. Crossed with an **ssssbbbb** plant it gave 18 **S**, 2 **s** and 7 **B**, 13 **b**. Hence its composition was **SSssBbbb**. But since one of the gametes which formed it was **ssbb**, its own composition was necessarily

SB
Sb
sb
sb

Most of our data on asymmetrical linkage are derived from such plants, though it would be theoretically possible to make them from a cross between **SSSSBbbb** (derived from a cross of **SSSSBbbb** and **SSSSbbbb**) and **ssssbbbb**. Such a parent would be of class (*a*).

(*c*) Parents whose composition is only deducible from their offspring. As an example

SBG
sbg
sbg
sbg

selfed has given several plants which behaved as

SBG
SBG
sbg
sbg

But even after the single-factor ratios were determined they might as well have been of composition

SBG	or of	**SBg**
SBg		**SBg**
sbG		**sbG**
sbg		**sbG**

to name only two possibilities.

We are quite aware that the inclusion of class (*b*) leads to a certain distortion of the single factor ratios, and class (*c*) may also distort the linkage ratios, owing to the omission, in each case, of parents of uncertain composition. Nevertheless we think their inclusion justifiable, with the above caution. It will be seen that even if attention is confined to the class (*a*) plants, the general features of the linkage are quite clear. We have allowed ourselves the inclusion of a few families of 1930 which are not quite complete, certain plants not yet having flowered. These are not included in the totals of Table II, but we consider that on the whole more is gained than lost by including them in Tables IV–XI.

Origin of the plants considered.

Tetraploids of the following origins have been used:

(*a*) Gregory's (1914) **GX** race which originated in a plant from Messrs Sutton in 1909. This plant lacked **S** and was at least duplex for **B**, **G**, **D** (white), and **Y** (palmate as opposed to fern leaf).

(*b*) Gregory's (1914) **GT** race which originated in 1911 from a cross made by him between two diploids. It was at least duplex for **S**, **B** and **G**, and also carried **D**.

(*c*) Sutton's "Symmetry," introduced into the experiments in 1920, and Sutton's "Mosscurl" in 1922. Both lacked **S** and **B** and were at least triplex for **G**. Most of our numbers for **S**. **G** asymmetrical repulsion come from these races crossed to others lacking **G** and simplex for **S**.

Linkage between two factors.

The single coupling figures (Table IV) require little comment. Only two of the families considered are in any way abnormal. Among the class (*a*) families from **SB** . $(\mathbf{sb})_3$ × $(\mathbf{sb})_4$ occurs one (149, 22) consisting of

19 **SB**, 20 **Sb**, 11 **sB**, 19 **sb**. It seems probable that its parent $43^1/21$ was of the composition mentioned, and it behaved more normally in another similar cross, giving 5 **SB**, 1 **Sb**, 1 **sB**, 2 **sb**. It is clear, however, that

TABLE IV.

Single coupling $\mathbf{\frac{XY}{xy\ xy\ xy}}$

Parents*		No. of families	SB	Sb	sB	sb
$\mathbf{SB.(sb)_3 \times (sb)_4}$	(*a*)	35	475	59	45	453
,, ,,	(*b*)	19	191	21	12	148
,, ,,	(*c*)	2	101	6	11	83
,, ,,	(Total)	56	767	86	68	684
,, ,,	(Calc.)	—	738·2	64·3	64·3	738·2
$\mathbf{(sb)_4 \times SB.(sb)_3}$	(*a*)	24	229	25	23	303
,, ,,	(*b*)	15	88	9	8	72
,, ,,	(*c*)	2	13	1	0	14
,, ,,	(Total)	41	330	35	31	389
,, ,,	(Calc.)	—	359·5	33	33	359·5
$\mathbf{SB.(sb)_3 \times SB.(sb)_3}$	(*a*)	14	304	18	17	96
,, ,,	(*b*)	8	145	7	8	53
,, ,,	(*c*)	7	137	4	9	40
,, ,,	(Total)	29	586	29	34	189
,, ,,	(Calc.)	—	595·5	33·0	33·0	176·5
			SG	**Sg**	**sG**	**sg**
$\mathbf{SG.(sg)_3 \times (sg)_4}$	(*a*)	15	178	114	101	169
,, ,,	(*b*)	2	26	12	12	24
,, ,,	(Total)	17	204	126	113	193
,, ,,	(Calc.)	—	198·5	119·5	119·5	198·5
$\mathbf{(sg)_4 \times SG.(sg)_3}$	(*a*)	16	124	80	95	155
,, ,,	(*b*)	4	8	9	2	5
,, ,,	(Total)	20	132	89	97	160
,, ,,	(Calc.)	—	146	93	93	146
$\mathbf{SG.(sg)_3 \times SG.(sg)_3}$	(*a*)	7	179	47	40	27
,, ,,	(Calc.)	—	174·4	45·3	45·3	27·9
			BG	**Bg**	**bG**	**bg**
$\mathbf{BG.(bg)_3 \times (bg)_1}$	(*a*)	16	190	105	93	180
,, ,,	(*b*)	4	33	16	21	30
,, ,,	(Total)	20	223	121	114	210
,, ,,	(Calc.)	—	216·5	117·5	117·5	216·5
$\mathbf{(bg)_1 \times BG.(bg)_3}$	(*a*)	16	135	69	84	165
,, ,,	(*b*)	4	8	9	2	5
,, ,,	(Total)	20	143	78	86	170
,, ,,	(Calc.)	—	156·5	82	82	156·5
$\mathbf{BG.(bg)_3 \times BG.(bg)_3}$	(*a*)	7	177	48	42	26
,, ,,	(*b*)	2	14	1	4	2
,, ,,	(Total)	9	191	49	46	28
,, ,,	(Calc.)	—	190·4	45·1	45·1	33·4

* Throughout these tables the parent used as a female is put first. The groups in which the parents are of the same composition almost all arise from self-fertilisation.

some anomaly is occurring here (possibly a mistake was made in crossing). The chance of obtaining such a family by random sampling is much less than one in a billion. It has therefore been omitted from the total figures used in calculating the **SB** cross-over value of 8·01 per cent. Its in-

TABLE V.

Single repulsion **Xy**
xY
xy
xy

Parents		No. of families	**SB**	**Sb**	**sB**	**sb**
Sb.sB.(sb)$_2$ × (sb)$_4$	(*a*)	3	36	43	39	28
,, ,,	(*c*)	1	8	12	6	6
,, ,,	(Total)	4	44	55	45	34
,, ,,	(Calc.)	—	32	57	57	32
(sb)$_4$ × Sb.sB.(sb)$_2$	(*a*)	3	11	25	15	15
,, ,,	(Calc.)	—	11·9	21·1	21·1	11·9
Sb.sB.(sb)$_2$ × Sb.sB.(sb)$_2$	(*b*)	2	40	17	11	0
,, ,,	(Calc.)	—	36·2	14·8	14·8	2·2
			SG	**Sg**	**sG**	**sg**
Sg.sG.(sg)$_2$ × (sg)$_4$	(*a*)	11	72	76	77	61
,, ,,	(*b*)	12	54	60	69	41
,, ,,	(Total)	23	126	136	146	102
,, ,,	(Calc.)	—	116·9	138·1	138·1	116·9
(sg)$_4$ × Sg.sG.(sg)$_2$	(*a*)	9	31	43	46	40
,, ,,	(*b*)	5	7	14	14	12
,, ,,	(Total)	14	38	57	60	52
,, ,,	(Calc.)	—	47·9	55·6	55·6	47·9
			BG	**Bg**	**bG**	**bg**
Bg.bG.(bg)$_2$ × (bg)$_4$	(*a*)	7	32	32	38	31
,, ,,	(*b*)	10	47	48	62	37
,, ,,	(Total)	17	79	80	100	68
,, ,,	(Calc.)	—	73·7	89·8	89·8	73·7
(bg)$_4$ × Bg.bG.(bg)$_2$	(*a*)	4	10	22	30	24
,, ,,	(*b*)	5	6	14	15	12
,, ,,	(Total)	9	16	36	45	36
,, ,,	(Calc.)	—	29·8	36·7	36·7	29·8
Bg.bG.(bg)$_2$ × Bg.bG.(bg)$_2$	(*c*)	1	8	5	4	1
,, ,,	(Calc.)	—	9·9	3·6	3·6	0·9

clusion would bring this value up to 9·53 per cent. Another plant 180^3/28, believed from its ancestry to be **SBG**.(**sbg**)$_3$, when used as a female with (**sbg**)$_4$ gave normal coupling of **S** and **B**, but 7 **SG**, 10 **Sg**, 9 **sG**, 6 **sg** and 6 **BG**, 10 **Bg**, 10 **bG**, 6 **bg**, as if **G** were being repelled from **S** and **B**. As male and when selfed the numbers were too small to be decisive. However, three **SBG** plants from the anomalous family 70–73/29 whose numbers are given above were selfed, and all behaved as if **SBG** were coupled, the totals being 29 **SG**, 10 **Sg**, 17 **sG**, 7 **sg**. The family 70–73/29 is therefore included, although the proportion of cross-overs between **B** and **G** deviates by more than six times the standard error of sampling. It must be realised, however, that cross-over values probably do vary in reality, and not only as a result of sampling.

The calculated figures are obtained directly from the back-cross data, so that the agreement in the case of back-crosses is no proof of the correctness of the theory. The agreement is, however, quite satisfactory in the case of the families due to selfing. The inclusion of class (*c*) plants only alters the **SB** cross-over values from 7·93 to 8·01, and from 8·59 to 8·41 per cent.

The data for single repulsion are given in Table V. The figures are decidedly irregular, but this is mainly due to the single factor ratios. If there is any systematic difference between observed and calculated linkage, it should show up in a difference between observed and calculated numbers of **XY** + **xy** zygotes (*i.e.* **SB** + **sb**, etc.) in the crosses giving 1 : 1 single factor ratios. The observed numbers are 621 (**XY** + **xy**), 800 (**Xy** + **xY**), the calculated 624·4 and 796·6. The agreement is thus very good, and the theory as a whole is confirmed. It is at once clear that the phenomenon is quite different from repulsion in a diploid.

In the case of asymmetrical coupling and repulsion a number of families have not been included which illustrate linkage of **G** with **S** and **B**. These are class (*c*) families. That is to say, the type of linkage is deduced from the family concerned, and is not certain from the ancestry. In the case of linkage between **S** and **B**, however, such families are included. The linkage being strong, there is little chance of mistaking coupling for repulsion, especially when the plant whose composition is doubtful has been both crossed and selfed. Except in the case of the asymmetrical repulsion of **S** and **G**, which arose from frequent crosses between horticultural varieties homozygous for **S** and **G**, and $\mathbf{Ss_3g_4}$ plants, the data are scrappy, and it is difficult to be sure how far the disagreements of theory and observation are fortuitous.

Summing the asymmetrical coupling figures from

$$\mathbf{XY}\ .\ \mathbf{Xy}\ .\ (\mathbf{xy})_2\ .\ (\mathbf{xy})_4$$

and the reciprocal we have:

	XY	Xy	xY	xy
Found	558	431	33	158
Calculated	544·5	455·5	35·9	144·1

TABLE VI.

Asymmetrical coupling **XY**
Xy
xy
xy

Parents		No. of families	SB	Sb	sB	sb
$SB.Sb.(sb)_2 \times (sb)_4$	(*b*)	1	6	12	1	1
,, ,,	(*c*)	7	49	32	0	11
,, ,,	(Total)	8	55	44	1	12
,, ,,	(Calc.)	—	54·5	38·8	1·5	17·2
$SB.sB.(sb)_2 \times (sb)_4$	(*b*)	8	100	1	51	18
,, ,,	(*c*)	1	18	0	13	11
,, ,,	(Total)	9	118	1	64	29
,, ,,	(Calc.)	—	103·2	2·8	73·5	32·5
$(sb)_4 \times SB.Sb.(sb)_2$	(*c*)	6	22	11	0	6
,, ,,	(Calc.)	—	18·9	13·6	0·55	5·9
$(sb)_4 \times SB.sB.(sb)_2$	(*c*)	1	2	0	2	0
,, ,,	(Calc.)	—	2·1	0·05	1·4	0·6
$SB.Sb.(sb)_2 \times SB.Sb.(sb)_2$	(*b*)	3	33	14	1	1
,, ,,	(*c*)	1	2	1	0	0
,, ,,	(Total)	4	35	15	1	1
,, ,,	(Calc.)	—	38·8	11·8	0·2	1·2
$SB.sB.(sb)_2 \times SB.sB.(sb)_2$	(*b*)	5	71	1	32	0
,, ,,	(Calc.)	—	77·5	0·5	23·6	2·4
			SG	**Sg**	**sG**	**sg**
$SG.Sg.(sg)_2 \times (sg)_4$	(*b*)	3	26	15	3	5
,, ,,	(Calc.)	—	21·4	19·4	3·1	5·1
$SG.sG.(sg)_2 \times (sg)_4$	(*a*)	1	3	0	4	2
,, ,,	(*b*)	13	153	9	104	33
,, ,,	(Total)	14	156	9	108	35
,, ,,	(Calc.)	—	134·7	19·3	122	32
$(sg)_4 \times SG.sG.(sg)_2$	(*a*)	1	12	5	20	7
,, ,,	(*b*)	4	36	2	30	6
,, ,,	(Total)	5	48	7	50	13
,, ,,	(Calc.)	—	51·4	7·7	47	12
$SG.sG.(sg)_2 \times SG.sG.(sg)_2$	(*a*)	3	101	1	30	2
,, ,,	(*b*)	7	272	6	88	8
,, ,,	(Total)	10	373	7	118	10
,, ,,	(Calc.)	—	371·2	9·8	121·6	5·4
			BG	**Bg**	**bG**	**bg**
$BG.bG.(bg)_2 \times (bg)_4$	(*b*)	10	122	7	88	23
,, ,,	(Calc.)	—	105·9	14·1	94·1	25·9
$(bg)_4 \times BG.bG.(bg)_2$	(*a*)	1	12	3	20	9
,, ,,	(*b*)	4	37	2	29	6
,, ,,	(Total)	5	49	5	49	15
,, ,,	(Calc.)	—	52·2	6·8	46·1	12·9
$BG.bG.(bg)_2 \times BG.bG.(bg)_2$	(*b*)	8	175	5	70	4
,, ,,	(Calc.)	—	186·4	4·1	69·5	3

The disagreement in the case of the small cross-over class **xY** is serious. But it is partly due to the very bad single factor ratio for **X**, the number of recessives being only 171 instead of 200. Making allowance for this the number of **xY** would be increased to 39·3. The divergence is now only just over twice the standard error, and not certainly significant. Only further work can decide whether the theory holds in this case. On the other hand in the case of selfed plants we have:

	XY	Xy	xY	xy
Found	654	235	14	15
Calculated	675·9	218·6	13·5	12·0

The agreement is much better, and the cross-overs are in excess of expectation, which suggests that the disagreement in the former case is due to bad luck.

In the case of asymmetrical repulsion, theory agrees very well with observation. The figures could be used to calculate linkage intensity. Thus if, the expectation being $3 - p : 2 + p : 1 - p : p$, the numbers found are a, b, c and d, the method of maximum likelihood (cf. Fisher and Balmukand (1928)) shows that p is a root of

$$\frac{a}{p-3} + \frac{b}{p+2} + \frac{c}{p-1} + \frac{d}{p} = 0,$$

or

$$(a + b + c + d)\,p^3 - (-a + 4b + c + 2d)\,p^2 - (2a - 3b + 6c + 5d)\,p + 6d = 0.$$

Applying this equation to the data of **Sg**.(**sG**)$_2$.**sg** × (**sg**)$_4$, where $a = 439$, $b = 422$, $c = 98$, $d = 70$, we have:

$$1029p^3 - 1487p^2 - 550p + 420 = 0,$$

whence $p = 12{\cdot}2$ per cent. as compared with 37·[illegible] per cent. from the single coupling data. We have not however used such figures to correct the linkage values used, since the agreement of observation and calculation is more logically demonstrated when the latter is based on single coupling only.

The majority of figures for double coupling of **S** and **B** come from a few plants which are placed in class (*c*) but whose composition is not really in the least doubt. They were derived from the self-fertilisation of known **SB**.(**sb**)$_3$ plants, and have given large families which make it clear that they are of the composition (**SB**)$_2$.(**sb**)$_2$. Actually of the $\mathbf{S_2s_2B_2b_2}$ plants from such ancestry [illegible] per cent. should be of the above composition, and the remainder should give many more **Sb** and **sB** than **sb** plants when crossed to a recessive. The progeny of two of these plants is also included in the tables for double coupling of **G** with **S** and **B**, but the

TABLE VII.

Asymmetrical repulsion **Xy**
Xy
xY
xy

Parents		No. of families	SG	Sg	sG	sg
Sg.(**sG**)$_2$.**sg** × (**sg**)$_4$	(*a*)	25	260	64	297	45
,, ,,	(*b*)	19	162	34	142	25
,, ,,	(Total)	44	422	98	439	70
,, ,,	(Calc.)	—	407·5	107	450	64·5
(**sg**)$_4$ × **Sg**.(**sG**)$_2$.**sg**	(*a*)	8	24	6	31	4
,, ,,	(*b*)	2	9	1	7	0
,, ,,	(Total)	10	33	7	38	4
,, ,,	(Calc.)	—	32·7	8·3	35·7	5·3
Sg.(**sG**)$_2$.**sg** × **Sg**.(**sG**)$_2$.**sg**	(*a*)	12	520	25	152	5
,, ,,	(*b*)	13	327	6	115	2
,, ,,	(Total)	25	847	31	267	7
,, ,,	(Calc.)	—	836·8	27·2	283·2	4·8
			BG	**Bg**	**bG**	**bg**
Bg.(**bG**)$_2$.**bg** × (**bg**)$_4$	(*b*)	3	39	8	39	10
,, ,,	(Calc.)	—	37·5	10·4	42·5	5·6
(**bg**)$_4$ × **Bg**.(**bG**)$_2$.**bg**	(*b*)	4	13	2	8	0
,, ,,	(Calc.)	—	9	2·5	10·2	1·3
(**Bg**)$_2$.**bG**.**bg** × (**Bg**)$_2$.**bG**.**bg**	(*b*)	2	69	32	3	1
,, ,,	(Calc.)	—	76·6	25·9	2·1	0·35
Bg.(**bG**)$_2$.**bg** × **Bg**.(**bG**)$_2$.**bg**	(*a*)	1	15	3	9	1
,, ,,	(*b*)	3	24	1	9	0
,, ,,	(Total)	4	39	4	18	1
,, ,,	(Calc.)	—	45	1·5	15·3	0·21

propriety of this step is less certain. The total number of cross-overs, 118, is less than the expectation, 134·2, but not sufficiently so to warrant the deduction that crossing-over between one pair of chromosomes hinders simultaneous crossing-over between the other pair. Certainly, however, there is no suggestion of a positive correlation between the two processes.

The double repulsion figures are less satisfactory. Nevertheless the class (*b*) families demonstrate the existence of the phenomenon in the case of **B** and **G**. Some of the class (*c*) families here included may really be examples of the seventh type of linkage, viz. coupling with repulsion. However, in each case considerations favour the assignment here given. There is possibly, as in the last case, a deficiency of the zygotic type (here the double recessive) which is due to simultaneous crossing-over. Besides the families of Tables VIII and IX a large number of other families are on record which are derived from parents duplex for two factors. But the evidence regarding their linkage is quite inconclusive. They may in most cases be examples either of double coupling, of double repulsion or of coupling and repulsion. Unfortunately we have as yet no clear case of the latter type of linkage.

We are aware that the data on double coupling and repulsion are unsatisfactory. In order to remedy this defect it is proposed to establish pure (*i.e.* quadruplex) lines of dominants. Since, however, two generations are required to test the homozygosity of such lines, satisfactory data will not be available for some years, and it has been thought best to publish the present evidence, which clearly demonstrates the existence of double coupling and repulsion, although the precise laws which they obey are still in some doubt.

TABLE VIII.

Double coupling **XY XY xy xy**

Parents		No. of families	SB	Sb	sB	sb
$(SB)_2.(sb)_2 \times (sb)_4$	(*b*)	1	14	1	0	0
,, ,,	(*c*)	7	274	7	4	54
,, ,,	(Total)	8	288	8	4	54
,, ,,	(Calc.)	—	285·9	9·1	9·1	49·9
$(sb)_4 \times (SB)_2.(sb)_2$	(*c*)	2	84	5	3	16
,, ,,	(Calc.)	—	87·1	2·9	2·9	15·1
$(SB)_2.(sb)_2 \times (SB)_2.(sb)_2$	(*c*)	5	146	1	0	3
,, ,,	(Calc.)	—	144·6	1·2	1·2	3·0
			SG	**Sg**	**sG**	**sg**
$(SG)_2.(sg)_2 \times (sg)_4$	(*b*)	3	16	0	3	1
,, ,,	(*c*)	3	130	18	10	17
,, ,,	(Total)	[illegible]	[illegible]	18	13	18
,, ,,	(Calc.)	—	[illegible]	19·8	19·8	12·7
$(sg)_4 \times (SG)_2.(sg)_2$	[illegible]	1	45	6	3	11
,, ,,	[illegible]	1	36	7	6	6
,, ,,	(Total)	2	81	13	9	17
,, ,,	(Calc.)	—	87·5	12·5	12·5	7·5
$(SG)_2.(sg)_2 \times (SG)_2.(sg)_2$	(*b*)	3	80	2	2	2
,, ,,	(*c*)	1	24	1	2	0
,, ,,	(Total)	4	104	3	4	2
,, ,,	(Calc.)	—	107·2	2·7	2·7	0·45
			BG	**Bg**	**bG**	**bg**
$(BG)_2.(bg)_2 \times (bg)_4$	[illegible]	1	101	13	0	13
,, ,,	(Calc.)	—	100·2	13·1	13·1	9·5
$(bg)_4 \times (BG)_2.(bg)_2$	[illegible]		[illegible]	7	3	6
,, ,,	(Calc.)	—	[illegible]	5·2	5·2	3·9
$(BG)_2.(bg)_2 \times (BG)_2.(bg)_2$	[illegible]	1	24	0	2	1
,, ,,	(Calc.)	—	25·6	0·61	0·61	0·14

TABLE IX.

Double repulsion **Xy** **Xy** **xY** **xY**

Parents		No. of families	SG	Sg	sG	sg
$(\mathbf{Sg})_2.(\mathbf{sG})_2 \times (\mathbf{sg})_4$	(*c*)	12	124	21	19	0
,, ,,	(Calc.)	—	113·3	23·4	23·4	3·9
$(\mathbf{sg})_4 \times (\mathbf{Sg})_2.(\mathbf{sG})_2$	(*c*)	2	11	0	1	0
,, ,,	(Calc.)	—	8·3	1·7	1·7	0·30
			BG	**Bg**	**bG**	**bg**
$(\mathbf{Bg})_2.(\mathbf{bG})_2 \times (\mathbf{bg})_4$	(*b*)	5	110	24	14	2
,, ,,	(*c*)	3	40	14	8	0
,, ,,	(Total)	8	150	38	22	2
,, ,,	(Calc.)	—	145·7	31·0	31·0	4·4
$(\mathbf{bg})_4 \times (\mathbf{Bg})_2.(\mathbf{bG})_2$	(*b*)	1	4	0	0	0
,, ,,	(Calc.)	—	2·7	0·54	0·54	0·08
$(\mathbf{Bg})_2.(\mathbf{bG})_2 \times (\mathbf{Bg})_2.(\mathbf{bG})_2$	(*b*)	5	102	1	1	0
,, ,,	(Calc.)	—	98·2	2·8	2·8	0·04

Linkages between three factors.

The totals of 30 families, all of class (*a*), in which all three factors were singly coupled, are collected in Table X. In 15 the cross was

$$\mathbf{SBG}.(\mathbf{sbg})_3 \times (\mathbf{sbg})_4,$$

in the other 15 $$(\mathbf{sbg})_4 \times \mathbf{SBG}.(\mathbf{sbg})_3.$$

The ratios expected are the same as in diploid linkage. The expectations given in the table are calculated from the linkage values found for the factors two at a time. The agreement found merely shows that the families considered are a fair sample.

The interest centres on the double cross-overs, which are fewer than expected. If there were no interference, *i.e.* if crossing-over between **S** and **B** did not diminish the probability of crossing-over between **B** and **G**, the expected values in these families would be $\frac{41 \times 183}{543}$, or 13·8 on the female side, and $\frac{29 \times 147}{420}$, or 10·15 on the male side. The average coincidence is thus 67 per cent., most marked on the male side. On the basis of the cross-over values of Table I the coincidence is 99 per cent. on the female side, and 69 per cent. on the male side. But these estimates are less reliable because the figures used are not all drawn from the same families. In the diploid the data of Gregory, de Winton and Bateson give a coincidence of 89 per cent. on the female side and 83 per cent. on the male side. The concordance is quite satisfactory in view of the small numbers. There is no suggestion that double crossing-over is easier in the tetraploid owing to exchanges involving three chromosomes.

TABLE X.

Progeny of **SBG**.**(sbg)**$_3$ × **(sbg)**$_4$ *and reciprocally.*

	Ex Het. ♀		Ex Het. ♂	
SBG	173	330 (323·7)	112	249 (248·6)
sbg	157		137	
Sbg	15	30 (28·3)	11	24 (27·0)
sBG	15		13	
SBg	92	172 (175·8)	66	142 (136·0)
sbG	80		76	
SbG	5	11 (15·2)	2	5 (8·4)
sBg	6		3	

TABLE XI.

SBG.**(sbg)**$_3$ *selfed. Six families.*

	SBG	**SBg**	**SbG**	**Sbg**	**sBG**	**sBg**	**sbG**	**sbg**
Found	169	45	10	2	8	3	32	24
Calculated	169·2	39	5·2	6·3	8·4	3·1	36·9	24·8

TABLE XII.

Sbg.**sBG**.**(sbg)**$_2$ × **(sbg)**$_4$ *and reciprocally.*

SBG	14	25 (23·5 = $1 - r - y - z$)
sbg	11	
SBg	10	20 (12·2 = $y - 2z$)
sbG	10	
SbG	10	24 (22·1 = $2y + z$)
sBg	14	
Sbg	18	30 (41·2 = $2 - r - 2y - 2z$)
sBG	12	

In a diploid, satisfactory data regarding the linkage of three factors can be obtained even when one is repelled from the other two. This is not so in a tetraploid. Four class (*a*) families are derived from the mating **Sbg**.**sBG**.**(sbg)**$_2$ × **(sbg)**$_4$, and from the reciprocal cross. They are summarised in Table XII. The expectation is calculated on the basis that x is the expected proportion of cross-overs between the loci of **S** and **B**, y between those of **B** and **G**, and z the proportion of double cross-overs. The values taken, weighted to allow for the fact that reciprocal crosses are added together, are $x = 0{\cdot}0582$, $y = 0{\cdot}3220$, $z = 0{\cdot}0243$. It will be seen that the agreement of theory and expectation is poor. But it is also clear that such data would be useless for calculating z. Other families exist in which **S**, **B** and **G** were all in different chromosomes. But they are mostly in class (*b*), and cannot be expected to agree very well with theory; nor do they throw any light on double crossing-over.

In Table XI are collected six families, all of class (a), from the selfing of **SBG**.(**sbg**)$_3$ plants. The agreement with theory is on the whole good. The only class which is necessarily due to double crossing-over of one chromosome is **sBg**. **SbG** can of course be formed by one cross-over on the female side and another on the male side.

DISCUSSION.

It is at once clear that the various results obtained agree fairly well with expectation on the chromosome theory. In fact the agreement is rather surprising in view of the numerous irregularities in meiosis which Darlington (1930) has described in this plant. We should have expected to find single factor ratios nearer to those deduced from a basis of random segregation between chromatids, and also evidence of crossing-over involving three chromosomes, double reduction, and other anomalies. The regularity observed may be due to several causes. The chromosome considered may have little tendency to form quadrivalents at meiosis. This is rather unlikely, as it contains 6 of the 27 known factors, and is therefore probably fairly long.

A somewhat more likely view, suggested to me by Dr Darlington, is that the three factors in question are located rather near the attachment constriction of the chromosome in which they are situated. In this case segregation would be little affected by the fact that pairing is between chromatids, and not whole chromosomes. The only common type of non-disjunction to be expected in such a case would be that leading to $2n + 1$ or $2n - 1$ gametes, which are doubtless largely eliminated, though as pointed out earlier in the paper, it is probable that some of our parent plants possessed an extra chromosome in the set carrying the factors discussed.

Table I gives a comparison of linkage values. It is obvious that the difference in linkage intensity which exists in the diploid between the male and the female sides of the plant is here absent or very slight. In each case the tetraploid values found are intermediate between those found on the two sides of the diploid. The differences, however, are not always large compared with their standard errors; but that between the cross-over values for **S** and **B** on the male side is 4·50 per cent., with a standard error of only 1·11 per cent.; the difference being four times its standard error, the odds in favour of its significance are nearly 10,000 to 1, assuming the errors to be due to sampling only. Even though, as pointed out above, a few families are aberrant, so that errors are not solely due to sampling, the difference is probably real.

The work is being continued. Recent observations, both on the diploid and tetraploid, have made it probable that the factor **V**, in whose absence the stem is green, is linked with **S**, **B** and **G**. We hope to compare this linkage in the diploid and tetraploid. The linked factors **F** (for flat as opposed to crimped leaves) and **Ch** (for *sinensis* as opposed to *stellata* type) are also available in the tetraploid. But the dominance of both is so incomplete as to render them unsuitable for accurate work. Before the theory here given can be regarded as generally applicable to autotetraploids it is desirable that it should be tested on other plants. Dr Sansome is at present engaged in a study of linkage in the tetraploid tomato at this Institution.

SUMMARY.

1. An account is given of six types of linkage observed between three pairs of factors in the tetraploid *Primula sinensis*, and of a seventh theoretically possible type.

2. The intensity of linkage is nearly, but not quite, the same in the tetraploid as in the diploid. It is the same on the two sides in the tetraploid.

3. As regards the factors considered, there is no evidence of crossing-over involving more than two chromosomes at a time, or of two chromosomes going to the same pole after crossing-over.

4. The six readily available gametic series contain only one adjustable constant p, and since the experimental results in other cases agree reasonably well with prediction when p has been calculated from the results of single coupling, this affords substantial support of the chromosome theory of inheritance.

REFERENCES.

BRIDGES, C. B. and ANDERSON, E. G. (1925). "Crossing-over in the X chromosomes of triploid females of *Drosophila melanogaster*." *Genetics*, X, 418.

DARLINGTON, C. D. (1931). "Meiosis in Diploid and Tetraploid *Primula sinensis*." *Journ. Gen.* XXIV, 65.

FISHER, R. A. and BALMUKAND, B. (1928). "The estimation of linkage from the offspring of selfed heterozygotes." *Ibid.* XX, 79.

GREGORY, R. P., DE WINTON, D. and BATESON, W. (1923). "Genetics of *Primula sinensis*." *Ibid.* XIII, 219.

GREGORY, R. P. (1914). "On the genetics of tetraploid plants in *Primula sinensis*." *Proc. Roy. Soc.* B, LXXXVII, 484.

HALDANE, J. B. S. (1930). "Theoretical genetics of Autopolyploids." *Journ. Gen.* XXII, 359.

SVERDRUP SOMME, A. (1930). "Genetics and Cytology of the Tetraploid Form of *Primula sinensis*." *Ibid.* XXIII, 447.

Biochemical Genetics and Immunogenetics

Starting in the 1920s, Haldane wrote a great deal about the biochemical basis of gene action. Although Sir Archibald E. Garrod pioneered this field in the early 1900s through his study of human metabolic errors, his work was largely ignored. It was Haldane, through his direction of research on plant pigments at the John Innes Institution (1925–35) and through his numerous publications, who continued to influence the biochemical viewpoint of gene action. By the time Beadle and collaborators published their experimental findings, first with *Drosophila* (1936) and later with *Neurospora* (1941), Haldane had already prepared the ground for the establishment of biochemical genetics. Indeed, the work of George W. Beadle was deeply influenced by the early publications of and personal contacts with Haldane (see Kay[1]).

The first of these papers appeared in a journal that is not readily accessible. Among its speculative ideas are the nucleoprotein nature of the gene and the gene-enzyme concept. The second paper refers to the "one gene–one antigen" theory, which Haldane pioneered.

1. Kay, L.E., Selling pure science in wartime: The Biochemical Genetics of G.W. Beadle. *Jour. Hist. Biol.*, 22: 73–101, 1989.

3

SOME RECENT WORK ON HEREDITY.

By J. B. S. HALDANE, M.A. (New College).

ONE of the most striking features in the physics of this century has been the extension of the atomic theory to two quantities which were formerly supposed to vary continuously, namely, electric charge and moment of momentum. In biology a similar development is occurring, and has already proved as fruitful as either of the physical theories mentioned, although from the nature of the material under investigation progress must be slow, especially in the study of comparatively large animals and plants. I refer to the discovery that inheritance, to a large extent at least, obeys the laws discovered by Mendel in 1855, and since applied to hundreds of different plants and animals, and greatly broadened in their scope. I will give brief examples illustrating the two ordinary types of Mendelian heredity before I turn to the work which, as I believe, has discovered their physical basis.

If we mate pure-bred coloured and white mice the first generation are all coloured. On mating these to white we get half white and half coloured. The latter behave like their coloured parents. Coloured mice which if mated to white give 50 per cent. whites, when mated together produce 25 per cent. of coloured mice which give no whites on mating to whites, 50 per cent. of coloured mice which give equal numbers of coloured and white on mating to whites, and 25 per cent. of whites. These results, and those of all possible matings of such mice can be explained if, and only if, we adopt the following hypothesis. A factor *C* is necessary for the presence of colour; the absence of *C* is denoted by *c**. A mouse can get this from either or both parents. *CC* mice are coloured and all their eggs and spermatozoa carry *C*. *Cc*

*I do not necessarily mean that there is a hole where *C* should be. *C* might conceivably be replaced by something larger but less active, as an *OH* group is replaced by an OC_2H_5 group.

mice are coloured and half their eggs and spermatozoa (we may use the term gametes to denote either) carry *C*, half *c*. *cc* mice are white, and all their gametes carry *c*. Finally fertilisation is at random; one sort of spermatozoon is no more likely to fuse with a given egg than another.

This type of inheritance was discovered by Mendel. In the second type, discovered by Horner, Doncaster and Durham, the sexes do not behave alike. One sex (the male in mammals, flies, and probably most other animals, the female in birds and lepidoptera) can only carry one factor instead of two. Thus vermilion eye colour is due to the absence of a factor *V* required for the normal eye colour in the fly *Drosophila ampelophila*. The wild male is *V*, the female *VV*, the vermilion male *v*, the female *vv*. The male produces two kinds of spermatozoa, one carrying *V* or *v*, one carrying neither, whilst the eggs all carry one or other. The first kind of spermatozoa on fusion with an egg produce females, so that the father can influence the eye colour of his daughters; the second produce males, whose eye colour does not depend on their father's.

Thus we have the following results :—

Parents	Normal ♀ VV	x	vermilion ♂ v	Vermilion ♀ vv	x	normal ♂ V
Gametes	Eggs V V		Spermatozoa v o	Eggs v v		Spermatozoa V o
Children	Normal* ♀ Vv		Normal ♂ V	Normal* ♀ Vv		Vermilion ♂ v

Parents	Normal ♂ V	x	Normal* ♀ Vv	x	Vermilion ♂ v
Gametes	Spermatozoa V o		Eggs V v		Spermatozoa v o
Children	Normal and vermilion ♂'s V, v. Normal ♀s VV, Vv.			Normal and vermilion ♂s V, v. Normal and vermilion ♀s Vv, vv.	

* These females, though normal in appearance, transmit vermilion to half their sons.

To these rules there are certain exceptions which, as we shall see, prove them. As they stand, however, they show clearly that there must be two classes of spermatozoa, male and female producing. This is also the case in man, where colour blindness is inherited in this way. Thus a colour blind man and a normal woman have normal children, but his daughters transmit colour blindness to about half their sons.

Now in many groups of animals the number of chromosomes* in the nucleus can be counted, and it is found that the female has an even number, often in pairs of similar appearance, half being derived from each parent, and the male has an odd number, or an unequal pair. The eggs contain half the parental number, and of the spermatozoa half get the same number as the eggs, while half get one less, or get that member of the unequal male pair which is only found in the male. The chromosome of this pair found in both sexes is generally denoted by X, that found in the male only, if at all, by Y. Thus in *Drosophila* the female has three pairs and a pair of X's, the male three pairs, an X and a Y. It is clear that the X-bearing spermatozoa produce males, the Y-bearing females, and it is an obvious conjecture that the factors like V are carried by the X chromosome.

This hypothesis was proved by Bridges to be correct. I can only give a very brief summary of what is perhaps the most important single piece of work on heredity since Mendel's paper. Certain vermilion females, when mated to normal males, gave about 4 per cent. of vermilion daughters, and as many normal sons, along with 96 per cent. of the expected classes as given above. Bridges came to the conclusion that these females, as the result of an exceptional cell division, such as has been observed in certain forms, must have come into the possession of a Y chromosome, as well as of the two X's. He tested this hypothesis by breeding

*A chromosome is a minute darkly staining body to be seen in the nucleus, or central portion of a cell when it is divided. The number is usually constant in a given species.

experiments involving some hundreds of thousands of flies, and many different factors, and by microscopical examination. Both confirmed his theory, and we are thus able at last to predict from an animal's hereditary behaviour the appearance of the nuclei in its cells, a step comparable to the observation during the last fifteen years of the actual behaviour of individual chemical atoms, though here, too, it was the exceptional radioactive atoms which finally proved the reality of Dalton's theory. The behaviour of the XXY female when mated to a normal male is as follows (X chromosomes carrying 'vermilion' are denoted X') :—

Parents	Vermilion female X′X′Y			Normal male XY
Gametes	Eggs 4% X′X′, 4% Y, 46% X′, 46% X′Y			Spermatozoa 50% X, 50% Y
Children	Duds 2% XX′X′	Normal ♂s 2% XY	Normal ♀s 23% XX′	Normal ♀s 23% XX′Y
	Vermilion ♀s 2% X′X′Y	Duds 2% YY	Vermilion ♂s 23% X′Y	Vermilion ♂s 23% X′YY

Those classes described as 'duds' do not develop. Half the regular and all the exceptional daughters have abnormal families, as do half the daughters of half the regular males. The reason that most eggs are X' and $X'Y$ is that, for certain reasons which cannot be dwelt upon in so short a paper, the two X chromosomes generally separate when the chromosome number is being reduced. The Y chromosome does not affect the sex of the animal, nor does it carry any hereditary factors. It is, in fact, a dummy, but males without it are sterile, so it must somehow balance the X in the formation of spermatozoa.

It is an obvious step to attempt to locate the other factors in the other chromosomes, and this has been done in *Drosophila ampelophila*. A male of this species, however many may be the differences in factors carried by the gametes which formed him, can only produce sixteen kinds of spermatozoa. We can divide the factors into four groups such that factors belonging to the same group, if they came in in the same gamete, go out in the same spermatozoön. One of these groups consists of the sex-linked factors, two others are large groups comprising scores of factors corresponding to two pairs of long chromosomes, the fourth corresponding to a very small pair of chromosomes, contains only three factors so far known.

But we can go further than this and say how the factors are packed in the chromosome. When two factors carried by the same chromosome come into the female from the same parent they have a tendency, but no more, to stick together. Thus if we mate a female with white eyes and miniature wings (*wm.wm*) to a normal male (*WM*) the daughters will be of normal appearance (*WM.wm*), but if we mate them to white-eyed miniatured-winged males (*wm*) we get four classes of children :—

White-eyed, miniature-winged wm and wm.wm 33·5 per cent.	Normal WM and WM.wm 33·5 per cent.	White-eyed, normal-winged wM and wM.wm 16·5 per cent.	Normal-eyed miniature-winged Wm and Wm.wm 16·5 per cent.

Thus in 33 per cent. of the eggs there has been a re-arrangement of the *X* chromosomes, so that the 'top' half of a paternal *X*, with *W*, has fused with the 'bottom' half of a maternal chromosome, with *m*. Now supposing another factor, *e.g.* the factor *T* in whose absence the body colour is tan, and the insects do not move towards a light, lies between the loci of *W* and *M*, then we find that if we bring this factor also into the experiment, it sometimes goes with the top, sometimes with the bottom part of the chromosome when the re-arrangement occurs, but only rarely is there a double break, so that a *WTM.wtm* female gives *WtM* or *wTm* eggs.

In this way we can make a map of the chromosomes, and calculate the distances of the loci of the factors with very fair accuracy. The longest chromosome in *Drosophila* is only 3 μ (·003 mm.), and the shortest calculated distance between the loci of factors is about 2 $\mu\mu$, about 100 times the diameter of a hydrogen molecule, and about the diameter of a very large protein molecule. The cell anatomists will have to be careful if they are not to be accused of poaching on the preserves of the organic chemist!

Partial linkage between factors, which on Morgan's theory given above means that they lie in the same chromosome, was discovered by Bateson and Punnett in the sweet pea, and exists in many other plants, and at least eight animals. For example, in the mouse, the first case found in vertebrates, linkage was discovered between the factors whose absences turn a normal mouse into a white and a pink-eyed grey respectively, by the late A. D. Sprunt (then President of this Club), my sister and myself. We have already the beginning of a comparative anatomy of the nucleus, but the task of bringing it even to the degree of perfection which the comparative anatomy of the body has already reached would probably occupy the entire surplus energies of the human race for as long as it is likely to continue.

Another interesting relation between factors is what is called 'multiple allelomorphism.' In the case of colour *versus* albinism in mice we have two factors, C and c, of which only one can get into a gamete. In the rabbit there are three factors, C, c^h, and c^a, which have this relation. Any rabbit with C in it is fully coloured, c^hc^h and c^hc^a are white with black feet and ears, whilst c^ac^a rabbits are pure white. Factors which have this relationship always affect the same character, and always give the same linkage values with other factors, thus proving that they lie at the same spot in the chromosome. They may thus be regarded as representing the same nuclear organ in different phases of activity, each phase being hereditary from one generation of cells to another.

It is only fair to say that I have so far been stating a case, and that some of the facts given above can be explained on a different hypothesis, whilst there are a few facts, mainly in plants, which have not yet been reconciled with the hypothesis here given. It is certainly speculative, but it has the great merit of enabling one to predict on so large a scale that if it is false it will certainly be disproved within the next ten years. And even a false theory is valuable to science if it suggests new problems to be attacked.

I will now mention a few of the more bizarre factors which have been discovered within the last few years. Factors may be necessary to the life of an organism. For example, yellow mice never breed true. If mated to normals they give 50 per cent. yellow, 50 per cent. normal, and are thus of composition *Yy*. If mated together they ought to give 25 per cent. *YY*, 50 per cent. *Yy*, and 25 per cent. *yy*. But the *YY* mice are never found. The reason for this is that the *YY* embryos begin to degenerate at a very early stage, and are eaten by phagocytes from the mother. There is reason to suspect that without a *y* they cannot oxidise fats. The converse case, where embryonic cells destroy the mother, occurs in man, and is known as chorion-epithelioma. It is conceivable that this may some day be explained on Mendelian lines.

Cancer in mice appears to be due to the absence of a factor found in the normal mouse. This is certainly so for a fatal tumour found in *Drosophila* which appears in half the male children of some mothers. We can easily map these lethals, because animals lacking the vital factor will also generally lack other factors which were absent from the same chromosome in the mother, and the nearer these factors lie to the deficient one, the fewer will appear in the offspring.

Other factors affect fertility. Thus a race of *Drosophila* lacking a factor *A* is fertile with itself or the normal form, and so is another race lacking the factor *B*, but crossed together they give no offspring, or only sterile females. The fact that mutually infertile races of the same animal can be obtained removes one of the classical objections to the Darwinian theory. Other factors govern the actual fertility of females. Two such factors are known in hens.

And from such fundamental factors as these we have every gradation down to factors which give a mouse a few white hairs on its nose, or which only come into play at all if other factors or external conditions are present. Many hundreds of such, with their effects, are described in *Mendel's Principles of Heredity*, or *Genetics and Eugenics*.

Very rarely—perhaps once in 10,000 individuals—a new factor appears or an old one ceases to function with visible effect. As to the cause of this we have no idea. The majority of variations are merely a re-shuffling of factors. How they got there we know no more than how the chemical elements did. We can occasionally observe one changing to another, but we cannot influence the rate of change in either case.

To sum up, we are left with the idea that the nucleus of every animal or plant cell consists very largely of some tens or hundreds of thousands of factors or 'genes,' each of which has a definite function and position. The chemist may regard them as large nucleoprotein molecules, but the biologist will perhaps remind him that they exhibit one of the most fundamental characteristics of a living organism: they reproduce themselves without any perceptible change in various different environments. The precise nature of their activity is uncertain, but in some cases we have very strong evidence that they produce definite quantities of enzymes, and that the members of a series of multiple allelomorphs produce the same enzyme in different quantities. They may for example produce the same change at varying rates, so that a caterpillar with one is black by its second moult, with another by its fourth, and so on. Similarly one combination will produce normal females, others will give females with imperfectly developed structures or instincts, or even with male structures and instincts.

In conclusion, I can only say that animal breeding requires no special technique in many cases, and that hundreds of problems in mammals and birds are still untouched. For example, I might suggest as a subject for research the question whether bulldogs, pugs, and Pekinese contain the same structural factor; whether it is related to any colour factors, and whether one can make a synthetic bulldog from, say, pugs and bull terriers. For the chemist the action of ferments in producing plant and animal pigments offers a fascinating field for investigation.

The Secretary has asked me to mention a few books on the subject of Genetics for the further information of anyone whom I may have interested in it. The best book for the beginner is :—

Mendelism. R. C. Punnett. (Macmillan, 1919.)

More advanced are :—

Mendel's Principles of Heredity. W. Bateson. (Cambridge University Press.)

This contains all the Mendelian results up to 1911.

Genetics and Eugenics. W. E. Castle.

This is more popular, less exhaustive, and more up to date, but contains a view which the author has since abandoned.

For the chromosome theory, of which I have mentioned some of the main features above :—

The Material Basis of Heredity. T. H. Morgan. (Lippincott.)

For practical applications of this work one may suggest :—

Genetics in Relation to Agriculture. Babcock and Claisen. (McGraw-Hill Co., N.Y.)

The Genetics of Cancer*

By PROF. J. B. S. HALDANE, F.R.S.

THE statement is occasionally made, and as frequently denied, that cancer is hereditary. It is, of course, clear that environmental influences can play a leading part in determining the production of cancer.

The question is whether nature, as well as nurture, is of importance. By far the most satisfactory evidence on this point comes from a study of genetically homogeneous populations of mice. By brother-sister mating for many generations (more than fifty in certain cases) pure lines can be built up in which the individuals are all homozygous for the same genes, apart from rare cases of mutation. By crossing two pure lines we obtain a population which is also genetically uniform, but not homozygous. Their progeny, however, is not genetically uniform.

In such a population, we can study three types of cancer :

(1) due to transplantation of a tumour from another animal.

(2) due to a carcinogenic agent. These include tar, the hydrocarbons shown to be carcinogenic by Kennaway and his colleagues, certain parasitic worms, and X-rays.

(3) spontaneous tumours ; that is, tumours arising for no, at present, assignable cause.

Now the order of ease of study is the above. An inoculated tumour can be judged as a 'take' or otherwise within a month. Tar painting may produce tumours within six months ; but spontaneous tumours in many lines do not reach their maximum incidence until an age of eighteen or more months. Hence our knowledge of tumour etiology is in the above order, though the order of practical importance for medicine is clearly the reverse.

It may be said at once that there are enormous differences between different lines as regards all three types of cancer. The genetics of reaction to transplantable tumours have been very fully worked out by Little and his colleagues. The laws disclosed are precisely similar to those which govern the transplantation of normal tissue or the transfusion of blood or of leukæmic corpuscles. A tumour arising spontaneously in one member of a pure line can be transplanted into all other members of it (actually more than 99 per cent of successful 'takes' can be achieved). Further, it can be transplanted into every F_1 mouse one of whose parents belonged to the pure line, but if these are mated together or outcrossed, only a minority of their offspring are susceptible. This at once suggests that susceptibility is due to the possession of certain dominant genes. This theory is fully confirmed by experiment. Supposing that a line X carries n pairs of genes $AABBCC$.... which are needed for tumour growth, and are not found in a line Y, then the F_1 will be $AaBbCc$...., and 100 per cent susceptible. Of the back-cross from mating of the F_1 with Y, only $(\frac{1}{2})^n$ will carry all n genes, and of the F_2, $(\frac{3}{4})^n$ will carry them, and thus be susceptible. In a number of cases, Cloudman[1] found that the two values of n so calculated were in agreement. The number of genes ranged from 2 to about 12.

Similarly, a tumour arising spontaneously in a F_1 individual, between two pure lines, in general requires in its host m genes contributed by one parent, and n contributed by the other. In such cases the tumour will grow in all the F_1, in $(\frac{1}{2})^m$ of one back-cross, $(\frac{1}{2})^n$ of the other, and $(\frac{3}{4})^{m+n}$ of the F_2. Thus Bittner[2] found in one case $m=4$, $n=1$, while the observed value of $m+n$ was 5.

Occasionally a tumour in the course of transplantation changes its character, so that it becomes transplantable into a larger proportion of a mixed population (F_2 or back-cross). It is then found that one or more genes less are required for susceptibility in the host.

These facts can be explained if the host only reacts to a transplanted tumour so as to destroy it as the result of foreign antigens in that tumour, just as a recipient agglutinates the corpuscles of a donor if they carry foreign isoagglutinogens. On this hypothesis each gene is responsible for the manufacture of a particular antigen, as in the case of the red corpuscles. However, the genetical facts are quite independent of this hypothesis.

A thorough study of these phenomena is under way in Little's laboratory. The genes required for susceptibility to different tumours are being compared. Thus it was found that a number of tumours arising in the same line required the same basic gene for susceptibility, but each demanded a different assortment of extra genes. Some of these genes have been located, by means of linkage studies, in the same chromosomes as genes responsible for colour differences.

The tendency to develop cancer as the result of tarring varies greatly in different lines. Thus Lynch[3] compared two lines A and B which differed in their spontaneous tumour rates, A having a higher incidence of spontaneous lung cancer than B. These tumours, however, never appeared before the age of 15 months. By tarring a large area of skin between the ages of 2 and 6 months, she induced lung tumours before the age of 13 months in 85 per cent of line A, and 22 per cent of line B. The difference was 6·3 times its standard error. On crossing A and B she found 79 per cent susceptibility. The back-cross to A gave 81 per cent susceptibility, while that to B gave 39 per cent. These figures suggest that susceptibility is

* Substance of lectures delivered at the Royal Institution on February 2 and 9, 1933.

determined, among other things, by a number of dominant genes. Other workers have obtained essentially similar results. Their importance for non-genetical workers on cancer is considerable. It is clear that in comparing the efficacy of two different carcinogenic agents, far fewer mice need be used in a pure line than in a mixed population, and it is worth noting that the variance in a mixed population is only about halved when litter mates instead of individuals taken at random are used as controls.

In the same way, Curtis, Dunning and Bullock[4] state that in the rat they have found that susceptibility to cancer, on infection with the cestode *Cysticercus*, is strongly inherited.

The problem of spontaneous cancer presents much greater difficulties. In no line can one obtain 100 per cent of deaths from cancer, because over the long period necessary, deaths from other causes cannot be prevented. But some idea of the conditions in a highly cancerous line can be obtained from the work of Murray[5]. In a particular inbred line, 1,938 females lived to be more than 7 months of age. Of these, 65 per cent died of mammary carcinoma, or were killed when severely affected with it. Above 80 per cent of deaths in females more than twelve months old were due to this cause. None survived for 23 months and probably none would have reached two years without cancer had all deaths from other causes been prevented.

In such a line we can observe the effects on spontaneous cancer of prophylactic measures. Thus of 198 females ovariotomised at 7 months, only 40 per cent died of mammary cancer, and one of these reached the age of 30 months. Still more striking is the fact that not a single operated female living beyond 22 months developed mammary cancer. It follows that in this stock the ovary plays an important part in the causation of mammary carcinoma. It is clear that a pure line (or the F_1 hybrids of two pure lines) furnish ideal material for the determination of factors in the environment favourable or otherwise to the development of cancer.

In contrast with such lines are others with an extremely low susceptibility to spontaneous tumours under ordinary laboratory conditions. A cross between such lines generally gives a hybrid generation with a cancer mortality nearly so high as that of the more susceptible line. Indications of linkage with colour genes have been obtained in one case.

It is important that the location of tumours is highly specific. One line has a high death-rate from mammary carcinoma in females only, and few tumours elsewhere. Another line has a heavy incidence of primary lung carcinomata in both sexes, and little mammary carcinoma. A third has few carcinomata of any kind, but sarcoma is not very rare. The genetics of spontaneous cancer will clearly be very complicated, and it is quite ludicrous to ascribe it to the activity of one gene, dominant or recessive.

Besides the work described above, a good deal has been done on stock which was not genetically homogeneous. From this work it is clear that, while a tendency to spontaneous cancer is hereditary, it is not due to a single gene, dominant or recessive, and also that a particular localisation of cancer may be hereditary. Thus Zavadskaia[6] found 13 out of 45 tumours in the occipital region in one particular line, and only 1 out of 212 in other lines. But all work with genetically heterogeneous material is unsatisfactory, because any individual may die before reaching the cancer age, and no other individual will be of just the same genetical make-up. Hence really exact work is impossible.

In the same way, human cancer tends to 'run in families' to some extent, but precise analysis is only possible where, as with retinoblastoma and some sarcomata, its victims are attacked early in life. Here there is reason to believe that a single dominant gene is mainly responsible for the cancerous diathesis, though environmental and possibly other genetic factors may be concerned as well.

A particularly clear case of the interaction of nature and nurture in cancer production is found in the case of human xeroderma pigmentosum, almost certainly a recessive character. Here the skin becomes inflamed, and ultimately cancerous, under the influence of light. We could speak with equal logical propriety of the recessive gene or the light as the 'cause' of the cancer, but as the former is rare, and the latter universal, it is more natural to regard the cancer as genetically determined.

Thus we have evidence of many different types of genetical predisposition to cancer, and although the data available on mice suggest that this predisposition is generally due to multiple dominant genes, it would certainly be incorrect to apply this theory to all human types of malignant disease.

The theory has been held by Boveri, Strong, and others, that the difference between a cancer and a normal cell is of the same character as that between the cells of two different varieties, that is to say, due to chromosomal aberration or gene mutation. This theory cannot of course be proved or disproved by genetical methods, as cancer cells do not reproduce sexually, and it is only by sexual reproduction that the geneticist can distinguish nuclear changes from plasmatic changes or virus infections.

The geneticist is concerned with the differences of 'nature' (in Galton's sense of the word) which play their part, along with environmental differences, in determining whether a given animal will or will not develop cancer. He is not particularly qualified to determine whether the difference between a normal cell and a cancer cell is analogous to that between sister gametes produced at meiosis, or to the difference which comes about at other cell divisions in the course of differentiation. The recognition of the importance of genetics for the study of cancer need not lead to any decision on this point.

To sum up, we can devise conditions under which either nature or nurture will play a predominant part in determining the incidence of cancer. Neither factor can possibly be neglected in a comprehensive survey. Except in a few cases, such as retinoblastoma, our knowledge is not sufficient to warrant interference with human breeding on eugenic grounds. Nevertheless, it is probable that in the ultimate solution of the problem of human cancer, eugenical measures will play their part.

[1] Cloudman, A. M., *Amer. J. Cancer*, **16**, 568; 1932.
[2] Bittner, J. J., *Amer. J. Cancer*, **15**, 2202; 1931.
[3] Lynch, C. J., *J. Exp. Med.*, **46**, 917; 1927.
[4] Curtis, Dunning and Bullock, *Amer. Nat.*, **67**, 73; 1933.
[5] Murray, W. S., *Science*, **75**, 646; 1932.
[6] Zavadskaia, *J. Genetics*, **27**, 181; 1933.

[From JOURNAL OF GENETICS, Vol. 54, No. 1,
pp. 54–55, January 1956.]
 PRINTED IN GREAT BRITAIN

THE DETECTION OF ANTIGENS WITH AN ABNORMAL GENETIC DETERMINATION

By J. B. S. HALDANE
Department of Biometry, University College, London

Since the pioneer work of Little, it is generally believed that all members of the F_1 between two pure lines of animals possess all the antigens of the parent lines, and no more. This, if true, is explicable on the one gene-one antigen theory of Haldane (1933) provided all the genes concerned are autosomal. This theory has been a useful guide to action, but it seems in danger of becoming a dogma, and I wish to suggest the need for a systematic search for exceptions to it. This search will be easiest in mice. Such a search is made possible by the technique of skin grafts developed by Medawar and his colleagues.

I symbolize pure lines by letters *A*, *B* and so on, the progeny of *A*♀ × *B*♂ by *AB*, and so on. *A*♀ → *BA*♂ means a graft of skin from an *A* female to a male whose mother was *B* and whose father was *A*, and so on.

The failure or success of grafts to grow is most readily detected when the skin colour of donor and host is different. I therefore suggest that F_1 hybrids be made between pure lines in such a way that, as far as possible, the colour of the F_1 differs from that of both parents. If a graft between two stocks fails, there is a presumption that the donor possesses an antigen which is absent in the host. I think that the prospects of success might be considerably increased if one or more of the pure lines tested were derived from a subspecies other than *Mus musculus musculus*.

If the graft *A* → *BA*♂ breaks down, this could be due to the fact that *BA*♂ lacks an antigen determined either by a gene in an X-chromosome from *A* or a cytoplasmic or milk factor from *A*. In the former case the graft *A* → *BA*♀ should take, in the latter it should break down. The converse case, a breakdown of *A*♂ → *BA*♀ but not of *A*♂ → *BA*♂, would suggest a Y-borne antigenic gene in the *A* line. This is most unlikely, as it would lead to the breakdown of *A*♂ → *A*♀ grafts, which has never been observed. Thus a study of *A*♂ → *BA*♂ and *A*♂ → *BA*♀ grafts would detect any of these types of antigenic determination. In any particular case it is easy to predict additional results. Thus if *A* carried an X-linked antigen absent in *B*, not only would *A* → *BA*♂ fail, but *AB* → *BA*♂ and *BA*♀ → *BA*♂ would fail.

Much more interesting is the possibility of the formation of hybrid antigens, that is to say, the possibility that *AB* or *BA* possesses an antigen found in neither *A* nor *B*. Billingham, Brent & Medawar (1953) have shown that by injecting minced tissues of *A* into *B* embryos, the graft *A* → *B* is often made possible. If we call these *B* individuals on which *A* grafts will take *B*(*A*), then if hybrid antigens are formed the graft *AB* → *B*(*A*) or *BA* → *B*(*A*) will probably break down, though *A* → *B*(*A*) does not.

Hybrid antigens have been found in species hybrids (Irwin, 1947) and in *Drosophila melanogaster* by Fox and his colleagues (e.g. Fox & White, 1953). Filitti-Wurmser, Jacquot-Armand, Aubel-Lesure & Wurmser (1954) have found a hybrid protein (so far not known to be antigenic) in *Homo sapiens*. The genes which co-operate to form a hybrid antigen or protein have so far always proved to be approximately allelomorphic, though, as in Chovnick & Fox's (1953) case, they may prove to be pseudo-alleles. Miller (1954) found that one of Irwin's hybrid antigens was produced by the interaction of two apparently allelomorphic genes. It is possible, however, that the relation of the Lewis antigens and the secretor factor in man may show interaction between different loci. It is certainly too early to state as a general principle that the presence of an antigen in a tissue is never determined by the interaction of genes at two different loci. None of the studies on mouse tumours demonstrate the absence of hybrid antigens. They show that AB mice have all the antigens of A and all those of B. They do not show that they have no others in addition.

If n pure lines are available, it is not necessary to make all the $n(n-1)$ possible matings to demonstrate the presence or absence of sex-linked or milk-determined antigens. Such a scheme as $A \times B$, $B \times C$, $C \times D$, $D \times E$, or $A \times B$, $A \times C$, $A \times D$, $A \times E$ would be sufficient. For if A and E differ by a sex-linked gene, then one of the crosses $A \times B$, $B \times C$, $C \times D$ or $D \times E$ will differ by this gene, and so on. However, as many crosses as possible should be made in a search for hybrid antigens.

If any exceptions are found to the 'one-autosomal gene, one-antigen' theory, it is of course entirely possible that they may prove to be due to some other cause than those suggested. Thus a cytoplasmic factor and a milk factor could only be distinguished by fostering experiments, a hybrid antigen could be due to the interaction of a gene and a cytoplasmic or milk factor, and so on.

However, I suggest that a systematic search for exceptions should be undertaken. A negative result would place the generally accepted theory on a much more secure foundation. A positive result would either add to the small stock of sex-linked genes and milk factors known in mice, disclose a new method of determination of antigens, or conceivably a mechanism of graft resistance which did not depend on antigens. Moreover, further work on the nature of a hybrid antigen, were one discovered, would probably be easier with mice than with pigeons.

When I wrote in 1933, the existence of hybrid antigens was doubtful, and some workers believed that the X-chromosome of the mouse carried very few genes. Moreover, the only method for the demonstration of a hybrid antigen in AB was the exhaustion of the serum of an animal immunized against AB cells by a mixture of cells from A and B, and a subsequent test of the exhausted serum on AB cells. This method is practicable with erythrocytes, but much harder with other cells. New prospects of disproving the theory enunciated in 1933, or of giving it additional support, are therefore open.

Unfortunately, no facilities for such work exist here. I suggest that it be undertaken by workers elsewhere.

REFERENCES

BILLINGHAM, R. E., BRENT, L. & MEDAWAR, P. B. (1953). *Nature, Lond.*, **172**, 603.

CHOVNICK, A. & FOX, A. S. (1953). *Proc. Nat. Acad. Sci., Wash.*, **39**, 1035–43.

FILITTI-WURMSER, S., JACQUOT-ARMAND, Y., AUBEL-LESURE, G. & WURMSER, R. (1954). *Ann. Eugen., Lond.*, **18**, 183–202.

FOX, A. S. & WHITE, T. B. (1953). *Genetics*, **38**, 152–67.

HALDANE, J. B. S. (1933). *Nature, Lond.*, **132**, 265.

IRWIN, M. R. (1947). *Adv. Genet.* **1**, 133.

MILLER, W. J. (1954). *Genetics*, **39**, 983–4.

Radiation Genetics

Haldane's main contribution to experimental mammalian radiation genetics was in suggesting methods that would be more efficient than the specific locus method in detecting recessive lethals and sublethals. These suggestions arose out of his earlier interest in linkage. When he was invited by the official British group working on radiation genetics of mammals (first formed in 1947 at the Institute of Animal Genetics in Edinburgh but moved to the Medical Research Council's Radiobiological Research Establishment at Harwell in 1954), Haldane declined, saying that he would be more useful as an external critic.

After the atomic bombing of Hiroshima and Nagasaki in 1945, Haldane (1947) examined the genetic consequences of exposure to ionizing radiation. As can be seen in that paper, his calculations were in substantial agreement with those of H.J. Muller at that time.[1] In his paper on the detection of autosomal lethals in mice, Haldane (1956) applied the "swept radius" concept of Carter and Falconer.[2] It is of interest that he suggested the study of other mutagenic agents, such as food preservatives, drugs, and caffeine. His paper (1957) on the detection of sublethal recessives was an extension of Carter's method for detecting autosomal recessive lethals in mice, using linked autosomal markers.[3] Finally, Haldane's (1960) interpretation of Carter's results presents an interesting discussion of the differences between his and Carter's analyses. Following Haldane's suggestion, Auerbach et al.[4] developed a method for detecting sex-linked mutations in the mouse, using sex-linked marker genes that were available by then.

1. Muller, H.J., The role played by radiative mutation in mankind. *Science*, *93*: 438, 1941.
2. Carter, T.C., and Falconer, D.S., Stocks for detecting linkage in the mouse, and the theory of their design. *J. Genet.*, *50*: 307–323, 1951.
3. Carter, T.C., The use of linked marker genes for detecting recessive autosomal lethals in the mouse. *J.Genet.*, *55*: 585–597, 1957.
4. Auerbach, C., Falconer, D.S., and Isaacson, J.H., Test for sex-linked lethals in irradiated mice. *Genet. Res.*, *3*: 444–447, 1962.

THE DYSGENIC EFFECT OF INDUCED RECESSIVE MUTATIONS

By J. B. S. HALDANE

The particles and radiations of high energy produced by radioactivity and nuclear fission can doubtless produce mutations in man, as in other organisms. Such mutations will generally be harmful, though very rarely desirable. Some will be genes or chromosomal rearrangements with wholly or partly dominant effects. These effects will be apparent within a few generations, and independently of inbreeding. In so far as they lower fitness, such genes will disappear relatively rapidly, their frequencies in successive generations forming a geometric series. Thus, the effects of an atomic bomb explosion, in so far as they are due to dominant genes, will appear at once. The delay will be only a little greater in the case of sex-linked recessive genes. Other mutations will be recessive and produce visible effects only as the result of unions between two heterozygotes. It is the object of this paper to show that the visible effects of such induced mutations will reach their maximum after about four or five generations and remain at about the same level for a very long time.

As a preliminary we consider a gene which is completely neutral as regards selective value and which arises by mutation in a very large population. Any fully recessive autosomal gene is neutral until two heterozygotes mate. If one such gene arises by mutation, we have to calculate the probability that it will occur in x loci after n generations. Since Fisher (1930) first posed this problem and solved it formally the distribution of x may be called the Fisher distribution, though of course it is only one of a number described by Fisher.

Moments and cumulants of the Fisher distribution

Let a_r be the probability that a gene carried by one zygote should be present in r zygotes of the nth generation of a large population, generations being supposed to be separate; and let

$$f(t) = a_0 + a_1 t + a_2 t^2 + \dots .$$

Then $f(1) = 1, f(0) = a_0$, and, since the gene is neutral, then in a stationary population

$$f'(1) = a_1 + 2a_2 + 3a_3 + \dots = 1.$$

Fisher considered the special case $f(t) = e^{t-1}$, which is particularly appropriate if zygotes are counted in each generation at sexual maturity; however, some information can be obtained in a more general case (Haldane, 1939). Let $p_{n,x}$ be the probability that a mutant gene is present in one locus each of x zygotes in the nth generation. Then Fisher showed that, if

$$\phi(n,t) = p_{n,0} + tp_{n,1} + t^2 p_{n,2} + \dots ,$$

then $$\phi(n+1,t) = \phi[n, f(t)].$$

If we are concerned with the progeny of a single mutant gene, $\phi(0,t) = t$; if we start with g genes $\phi(0,t) = t^g$.

The mean value of x is unity if $g = 1$, as we shall assume to be the case for the present. After a number of generations by far the commonest value of x is zero, but the mean of the non-zero values is high. The distribution of the non-zero values will be called the truncated Fisher distribution. Two methods are available for the calculation of their moments. The first is applicable to any admissible function $f(t)$. The nth factorial moment of x about zero is

$$\overline{x^{[n]}} = \left[\left(\frac{d}{dt}\right)^n \phi(n,t)\right]_{(t=1)}.$$

Thus $\bar{x} = \phi'(n,1)$. $\overline{x^2} = \phi''(n,1)+\phi'(n,1)$, $\overline{x^3} = \phi'''(n,1)+3\phi''(n,1)+\phi'(n,1)$, etc.

The coefficients are 'difference quotients of powers of zero'. Now

$$\phi'(n,t) = \frac{d}{dt}\phi[n-1,f(t)]$$
$$= f'(t)\phi'[n-1,f(t)].$$

So
$$\phi'(n,1) = f'(1)\phi'(n-1,1)$$
$$= [f'(1)]^n$$
$$= 1,$$

if $f'(1) = 1$, as we have assumed to be the case, and shall assume in what follows. Also

$$\phi''(n,t) = [f'(t)]^2\phi''[n-1,f(t)]+f''(t)\phi'[n-1,f(t)].$$

So
$$\phi''(n,1) = \phi''(n-1,1)+f''(1)$$
$$= nf''(1),$$

since
$$\phi''(0,1) = 0.$$

Similarly,
$$\phi'''(n,1) = \phi'''(n-1,1)+3f''(1)\phi''(n-1,1)+f'''(1)\phi'(n-1,1)$$
$$= \tfrac{3}{2}n(n-1)[f''(1)]^2+nf'''(1), \quad \text{etc.}$$

By such methods we find

$$\bar{x} = 1,$$
$$\overline{x^2} = nf''(1)+1,$$
$$\overline{x^3} = \tfrac{3}{2}n(n-1)[f''(1)]^2+n[f'''(1)+3f''(1)]+1,$$
$$\overline{x^4} = 3n(n-1)(n-2)[f''(1)]^3+n(n-1)f''(1)[5f'''(1)+\tfrac{3}{2}\{f''(1)\}^2+9f''(1)]$$
$$+n[f^{\text{iv}}(1)+6f'''(1)+7f''(1)]+1, \quad \text{etc.,}$$

whence
$$\left.\begin{aligned}
\kappa_1 &= 1,\\
\kappa_2 &= \mu_2 = nf''(1),\\
\kappa_3 &= \mu_3 = \tfrac{3}{2}n(n-1)[f''(1)]^2+nf'''(1),\\
\mu_4 &= 3n(n-1)(n-2)[f''(1)]^3+n(n-1)f'''(1)[5f''(1)+\tfrac{3}{2}\{f''(1)\}^2+3f''(1)]\\
&\quad +n[f^{\text{iv}}(1)+2f'''(1)+f''(1)],\\
\kappa_4 &= 3n(n-1)(n-2)[f''(1)]^3+n(n-1)f''(1)[5f'''(1)+\tfrac{3}{2}\{f''(1)\}^2]\\
&\quad +n[f^{\text{iv}}(1)+2f'''(1)+f''(1)-3\{f''(1)\}^2].
\end{aligned}\right\} \quad (1)$$

If $f(t) = e^{t-1}$, then $f'(1) = f''(1) = f'''(1)$, etc. $= 1$. In general this is not the case. Where fertility is very variable, the higher derivatives of $f(1)$ will exceed unity. On the other hand, in a community where there were efficient propaganda and incentives both against sterility and against large families, $f''(1)$, etc., might be found to be less than unity.

We now consider the case where $f(t) = e^{t-1}$. The moment-generating function of the Fisher distribution in the nth generation is

$$\begin{aligned} M_n(\theta) &= \phi(n, e^\theta) \\ &= \phi[n-1, f(e^\theta)] \\ &= \phi[0, f^n(e^\theta)] \\ &= f^n(e^\theta), \end{aligned}$$

where the index denotes n-fold iteration of the function f. Thus if $f(t) = e^{t-1}$,

$$M_n(\theta) = f^{n+1}(1+\theta),$$

and $$K_n(\theta) = \log M_n(\theta) = \log f^{n+1}(1+\theta) = f^n(1+\theta) - 1 = M_{n-1}(\theta) - 1,$$

or $$M_n(\theta) = \exp[M_{n-1}(\theta) - 1].$$

That is to say the cumulants of the Fisher distribution for the nth generation are its moments about zero for the $(n-1)$th generation. They can be calculated from this peculiar property. The formulae for moments in terms of cumulants (Kendall, 1943, p. 62) give us the cumulants or the moments of the nth generation in terms of those of the $(n-1)$th. If $\Delta\kappa_r$ is the difference between the rth cumulants in successive generations, we have, since $\kappa_1 = 1$ in each generation,

$$\left.\begin{aligned} \Delta\kappa_2 &= 1, \\ \Delta\kappa_3 &= 3\kappa_2 + 1, \\ \Delta\kappa_4 &= 4\kappa_3 + 3\kappa_2^2 + 6\kappa_2 + 1, \\ \Delta\kappa_5 &= 5\kappa_4 + 10\kappa_3\kappa_2 + 10\kappa_3 + 15\kappa_2^2 + 10\kappa_2 + 1, \\ \Delta\kappa_6 &= 6\kappa_5 + 15\kappa_4\kappa_2 + 15\kappa_4 + 10\kappa_3^2 + 60\kappa_3\kappa_2 + 20\kappa_3 + 15\kappa_2^3 + 45\kappa_2^2 + 15\kappa_2 + 1, \text{ etc.} \end{aligned}\right\} \quad (2)$$

By summing the right-hand sides of these equations, we find, for the cumulants of the nth generation, or the moments about zero of the $(n-1)$th generation,

$$\left.\begin{aligned} \kappa_1 &= 1, \\ \kappa_2 &= n, \\ \kappa_3 &= \tfrac{1}{2}n(3n-1), \\ \kappa_4 &= \tfrac{1}{2}n(2n-1)(3n-1), \\ \kappa_5 &= \tfrac{1}{6}n(45n^3 - 65n^2 + 30n - 4), \\ \kappa_6 &= \tfrac{1}{24}n(540n^4 - 1155n^3 + 890n^2 - 273n + 22). \end{aligned}\right\} \quad (3)$$

Of course equations (1) lead to the same results. Clearly κ_r tends to infinity with n^{r-1}, and γ_r with $n^{\frac{1}{2}r}$. The distribution is bimodal, and does not approximate to any of the Pearsonian types.

The truncated Fisher distribution

Let us consider the distribution of those values of x which are not zero, in other words of the numbers of zygotes which carry a mutant gene. In the nth generation $x = 0$ with frequency $f^n(0)$. Writing $v_n = \dfrac{1}{1-f^n(0)}$, and using x' to denote non-zero values of x, we find $\overline{x'^r} = \overline{x^r}v_n$. Thus from equations (3) which give the values of $\overline{x^r}$ in the $(n-1)$th generation, we find on substituting $n+1$ for n:

$$\overline{x'} = v_n, \quad \overline{x'^2} = (n+1)v_n, \quad \overline{x'^3} = \tfrac{1}{2}(n+1)(3n+2)v_n, \text{ etc.}$$

Fisher (1930) investigated the behaviour of v_n when $f(t) = e^{t-1}$ and found that

$$v_n = \tfrac{1}{2}n + \tfrac{1}{6}\log_e v_n + 1{\cdot}01464{,}8607 - \frac{1}{72v_n} + O(v_n^{-2}),$$

whence $$v_n = \tfrac{1}{2}(n + \tfrac{1}{3}\log n + 1{\cdot}7982515) + O(n^{-1}\log n).$$

Hence we find for the cumulants of the distribution of x',

$$\kappa_1 = v_n,$$
$$\kappa_2 = (n+1)v_n - v_n^2,$$
$$\kappa_3 = \tfrac{1}{2}(n+1)(3n+2)v_n - 3(n+1)v_n^2 + 2v_n^3,$$
$$\kappa_4 = \tfrac{1}{2}(n+1)(2n+1)(3n+2)v_n - (n+1)(9n+7)v_n^2 + 12(n+1)v_n^3 - 6v_n^4, \text{ etc.},$$

or
$$\left.\begin{aligned}\kappa_1 &= \tfrac{1}{2}n + \tfrac{1}{6}\log_e n + 0{\cdot}89913 + O(n^{-1}\log n),\\ \kappa_2 &= \tfrac{1}{4}n(n+2) + \tfrac{1}{6}n\log_e n + O(\log n),\\ \kappa_3 &= \tfrac{1}{4}n^3 + O(n^2),\\ \kappa_4 &= \tfrac{3}{8}n^4 + O(n^3\log n),\end{aligned}\right\} \quad (4)$$

whence $$\gamma_1 = 2 - n^{-1}\log_e n + O(n^{-1}), \quad \gamma_2 = 6 + O(n^{-1}\log n).$$

Thus as n tends to infinity the mean and standard deviation are closely represented by $\tfrac{1}{2}n$, while γ_1 and γ_2 approximate to 2 and 6 respectively. In fact, the distribution approximates to a discontinuous Pearsonian distribution of type III, and as all the reduced cumulants γ_r approximate to finite values, this comparison can be made without reservations. Further, the shape parameters γ_1 and γ_2 approximate to those of the χ^2 distribution for two degrees of freedom, though of course the location and scale parameters are different.

A simple example shows how rapidly the truncated Fisher distribution approximates to the Pearsonian form. If $n = 10$, $v_n = 6{\cdot}323$. Thus ten generations after a group of recessive mutations at different loci, 84·2 % of the mutant genes have disappeared by random extinction. But the number of recessive genes in the population is unaltered; and in the remaining 15·8 % of cases, the mean number of heterozygotes is 6·323, and its standard duration 5·44, while $\gamma_1 = 1{\cdot}86$, $\gamma_2 = 5{\cdot}07$. Thus the distribution is already fairly close to the form to which it approximates when n tends to infinity, with $\gamma_1 = 2$, $\gamma_2 = 6$.

In the more general case, Haldane (1939, equation (3)) showed that if μ_2 and μ_3 are the second and third moments about the mean of the fertility distribution whose generating function is $f(t)$, then

$$v_n = \tfrac{1}{2}\mu_2 n + \left(\tfrac{1}{2}\mu_2 - \frac{\mu_3}{3\mu_2}\right)\log n + c + O(n^{-1}\log n).$$

Thus if μ_2 is somewhat larger than unity, as seems to be the case with man, we should have, since $f''(1) = \mu_2$,

$$\kappa_1 = v_n = \tfrac{1}{2}\mu_2 n + \left(\tfrac{1}{2}\mu_2 - \frac{\mu_3}{3\mu_2}\right)\log n + C,$$
$$\kappa_2 = v_n(n\mu_2 + 1 - v_n) = \tfrac{1}{4}\mu_2^2 n^2 + O(n), \text{ etc.},$$

in place of equations (4).

In an increasing population $f'(1)$ exceeds unity. If successive generations increase by a factor $1+k$, then $1 - f^n(0)$ does not tend to zero, but to $2k - \tfrac{8}{3}k^2 + \tfrac{28}{9}k^3 + \ldots$.

The first cumulants of the Fisher distribution are

$$\kappa_1 = (1+k)^n, \quad \kappa_2 = k^{-1}(1+k)[(1+k)^n - 1],$$

and so on, if $f(t) = e^{k(t-1)}$.

In all cases which are at all likely to occur the distribution of the probabilities of x after n generations consists of a large value for $x = 0$, and a somewhat positively skew distribution over a series of non-zero values. In view of the uncertainty of data on mutation rates, equations (3) will be sufficiently accurate for our purpose.

The appearance of recessives

Suppose that there were x_n heterozygotes **Aa** in the nth generation, we have next to calculate the expected number of recessives. Let α be the mean coefficient of inbreeding, that is to say if q be the frequency of **a** gametes, let the probability that a given **a** gamete unites with another be $\alpha + (1-\alpha)q$. Then Bernstein (1930) showed that α is independent of q, and Haldane & Moshinsky (1939) showed that α is of the order of 10^{-3} for several European populations. Let N be the number of the population.

Then if there are x heterozygotes the expected number of recessives in the next generation of a population of hermaphrodites would be $\frac{1}{2}\alpha x + \frac{(1-\alpha)x^2}{4N}$. However, the human species is bisexual. Assuming a sex ratio of equality, the probability that the x zygotes will consist of y females and $x-y$ males is $\binom{x}{y}2^{-x}$. The term $\frac{1}{2}\alpha x$ must therefore be multiplied by a correction factor of

$$\sum_{y=0}^{x} \frac{4y(x-y)}{x^2}\binom{x}{y}2^{-x}, \quad \text{or} \quad \frac{x-1}{x},$$

so the expected number is $\frac{1}{2}\alpha(x-1) + \frac{(1-\alpha)x^2}{4N}$, provided x exceeds zero. The correction to the term involving x^2 is negligible, since it only becomes relevant when x is of the order of $N^{\frac{1}{2}}$. Thus the expected number of recessives in the $(n+1)$th generation is

$$\begin{aligned} r_{n+1} = \Sigma\left[\frac{\alpha}{2v_n}(x'-1) + \frac{1-\alpha}{4N}x^2\right]p_{n,x} &= \frac{\alpha(v_n-1)}{2v_n} + \frac{(1-\alpha)}{4N}(n+1) \\ &= \frac{\alpha}{2}\left(1 - \frac{2}{n+\frac{1}{3}\log n + c}\right) + \frac{(1-\alpha)(n+1)}{4N} \\ &= \frac{\alpha}{2} + \frac{n}{4N} \text{ approximately.} \end{aligned} \tag{5}$$

The second term is negligible, provided N is of the order of 10^6, for before n reaches a value of the order of 1000, we shall have to correct for the effect of selection.

If the homozygotes have a fitness $1-k$, the number of recessive genes will be reduced by a factor $1-\alpha k$ or approximately $e^{-k\alpha}$ in each generation. Thus in n generations they would be reduced to $e^{-k\alpha n}$. For serious conditions $k > \frac{1}{2}$, so although the process will be slightly speeded up when n reaches the order $N^{\frac{1}{2}}$, i.e. after some thousands of generations, the rate of appearance of homozygotes per mutation will be at first very nearly $\frac{1}{2}\alpha$, later approximating to $\frac{1}{2}\alpha e^{-k\alpha n}$.

However, the process does not begin at once. Apart from the correction for bisexuality, inbreeding does not begin immediately. Incest is negligible, first-cousin marriages account for about 72 % of the total value of α according to Haldane & Moshinsky, marriages of first cousins once removed for another 8 %, and so on. Thus r_n will not effectively equal $\frac{1}{2}\alpha$ for about ten generations, but will reach $0{\cdot}2\alpha$ after four generations.

So far we have only considered single mutations at different loci. Two other cases must be considered. In the first place several mutations may occur simultaneously at the same locus. Secondly one or more mutations may occur giving genes which are already present in the population. Doubtless both events occurred among the survivors of atomic bomb explosions.

THE FISHER DISTRIBUTION WITH SEVERAL INITIAL MUTATIONS

Suppose that the same mutation has occurred in one generation in g different zygotes, so that $\phi(0, t) = t^g$. Then the moment-generating function for the nth generation becomes

$$\begin{aligned} M_n(\theta) &= \phi[0, f^n(e^\theta)] \\ &= [f^n(e^\theta)]^g, \\ K_n(\theta) &= g \log [f^n(e^\theta)] \\ &= g[\{M_{n-1}(\theta)\} g^{-1} - 1] \\ &= g[\exp \{g^{-1} K_{n-1}(\theta)\} - 1]. \end{aligned}$$

To calculate the cumulants of one generation from those of the preceding one we have therefore to multiply each product of r cumulants by g^{1-r}. Thus $\kappa_1 = g$ and equations (2) become

$$\begin{aligned} \Delta\kappa_2 &= g^{-1}\kappa_1^2, \\ \Delta\kappa_3 &= 3g^{-1}\kappa_2 + g^{-2}\kappa^3, \\ \Delta\kappa_4 &= g^{-1}(4\kappa_3\kappa_1 + 3k_2^2) + 6g^{-2}\kappa_1^2\kappa_2 + g^{-3}\kappa_1^4, \\ \Delta\kappa_5 &= 5g^{-1}(\kappa_4\kappa_1 + 2\kappa_3\kappa_2) + 5g^{-2}(2\kappa_3\kappa_1^2 + 3\kappa_2^2\kappa_1) + 10g^{-3}\kappa_2\kappa_1^3 + g^{-4}\kappa_1^5, \\ \Delta\kappa_6 &= g^{-1}(6\kappa_5\kappa_1 + 15\kappa_4\kappa_2 + 10\kappa_3^2) + 15g^{-2}(\kappa_4\kappa_1^2 + 4\kappa_3\kappa_2\kappa_1 + \kappa_2^3) + 5g^{-3}(4\kappa_3\kappa_1^3 + 9\kappa_2^2\kappa_1^2) \\ &\quad + 15g^{-4}\kappa_2\kappa_1^4 + g^{-5}\kappa_1^6. \end{aligned}$$

Hence, in the nth generation,

$$\begin{aligned} \kappa_1 &= g, \\ \kappa_2 &= ng, \\ \kappa_3 &= ng + \tfrac{3}{2}n(n-1), \\ \kappa_4 &= \tfrac{1}{2}ng(2n^2 + 7n - 7) + 2n(n-1)(n-2). \end{aligned}$$

The moments about zero are

$$\begin{aligned} \bar{x} &= g, \\ \overline{x^2} &= g^2 + ng, \\ \overline{x^3} &= g^3 + 3ng^2 + ng + \tfrac{3}{2}n(n+1), \\ \overline{x^4} &= g^4 + 6ng^3 + n(3n+4)g^2 + \tfrac{1}{2}n(2n^2 + 19n - 19)g + 2n(n-1)(n-2), \text{ etc.} \end{aligned}$$

Now the probability that x will be zero in the nth generation is $[f^n(0)]^g = \left(1 - \frac{1}{v_n}\right)^g$. Thus the moments of x' about zero are those of x divided by $1 - \left(1 - \frac{1}{v_n}\right)^g$. If $w_n = \frac{v_n^g}{v_n^g - (v_n - 1)^g}$, then $w_n = \frac{n}{2g} + O(\log n)$, and we have for the cumulants of the distribution of x',

$$\begin{aligned} \kappa_1 &= \tfrac{1}{2}(n+g) + O(\log n), \\ \kappa_2 &= \tfrac{1}{2}n(\tfrac{1}{2}n + g) + \dots, \\ \kappa_3 &= \tfrac{1}{4}n^3\left(\frac{3}{g} - 2\right) + \dots, \\ \kappa_4 &= n^4\left(\frac{7}{8} - \frac{n}{g}\right) + \dots, \end{aligned}$$

The expressions are complicated, but κ_3 is clearly negative for large n:

$$r_{n+1} = \alpha g \frac{(w_n - 1)}{2w_n} + \frac{(1-\alpha)}{N} g(n+g)$$

$$= \frac{\alpha g}{2}\left[1 - \frac{2g}{n} + O(n^{-2})\right] + \frac{g(n+g)}{N} \text{ approximately.}$$

Thus the frequency is, as before, equal to $\frac{1}{2}\alpha$ multiplied by the number of mutant genes over a long period.

The addition of mutants to previously existing recessives

Suppose that the gene frequency of a recessive in a population is q, then the number of recessives expected per generation is $[\alpha q + (1-\alpha)q^2]N$. If q is increased to $q + \delta q$, this number is increased by $[\alpha + 2(1-\alpha)q]\delta q N$, or approximately $(\alpha + 2q)\delta q N$. Now a single mutant gene increases q to $q + 1/2N$ so $\delta q = 1/2N$ and $r_{n+1} = \frac{1}{2}\alpha + q$. It follows that if q is of the order of magnitude of α the dysgenic effect begins immediately, though it rises for a few generations. It is also appreciably larger, that is to say, it is over sooner. This argument depends on the assumption that qN is of such magnitude that it does not fluctuate appreciably as the result of the sampling process by which one generation is derived from another.

Discussion

To sum up, the conclusion is that the rate at which recessive zygotes are to be expected will rise in 200 years or less to a level of $\frac{1}{2}\alpha$ per generation for each mutation produced in a gamete which gives rise to a viable zygote. This will be somewhat exceeded if the recessive gene in question is already frequent in the population. In the long run each harmful recessive mutation will involve the elimination of half a zygote on the average. This elimination may occur in different ways. If the gene is lethal at a very early stage, like yellow in mice, the only effect will be an occasional missed period, and perhaps a lowering of fertility. If it is lethal at later stages it will cause abortions, stillbirths, and infantile or juvenile mortality. Or it may lower the fitness drastically without being completely lethal. Such genes are perhaps the most serious, as the elimination of a single pair involves the production of more than one person destined to chronic invalidism from a condition such as one of the recessive nervous diseases. Finally, it may slightly lower the fitness of a large number of individuals, for example reducing the mean fitness of ten people by 5 % on an average. If an expanding population is irradiated, more than half a life must be sacrificed per harmful mutation, if a diminishing population, less. It must be emphasized that this applies not merely to lethal and sublethal mutations, but to all mutations which appreciably lower the fitness of homozygotes, and are therefore ultimately eliminated.

The rate depends on the coefficient of inbreeding α. The value of this quantity increases with every generation of ancestors considered, and may approach unity if we reckon back to palaeolithic times (Haldane & Moshinsky, 1939). How it will behave in the next ten thousand years depends on unpredictable features of social structure. It may be that 0·001 is a serious underestimate of its effective value. If so the rate of production of homozygotes may rise very gradually for some thousand years.

We have now to consider the probable rate of production of new mutations. Consider an atom bomb explosion in which some 50,000 persons are killed at once or die within a few weeks, while another million are exposed to appreciable doses of γ-radiation. The lethal dose is probably of the order of 500 roentgens, so we may suppose that the million survivors have received a mean dose of between 10 and 50 r., say 20. Those who receive just sublethal doses may be permanently sterilized. Mutations will occur in gametes and in spermatogonia and oogonia. On an average, in a stationary population each individual will produce two gametes which give rise to zygotes. So we have to consider 2×10^6 gametes derived from cells which have received a mean dose of 20 r.

Now the probability that a particular gene will mutate with a dose of 1 r. varies from about $0{\cdot}5 \times 10^{-8}$ to 16×10^{-8} in *Drosophila*, and (if the phenomenon is comparable) in bacteria and viruses (Lea, 1946, p. 144). The median value is about 2×10^{-8}. Thus with a dose of 4×10^7 r. we should expect the same locus to be affected twice in a minority of cases. Human genes cannot be much more sensitive to radiation than those of *Drosophila*, otherwise the rate of spontaneous mutation in man would probably be higher than is the case.

A dose of 1000 r. of X- or γ-rays produces recessive lethal mutations in about 3 % or rather less of the spermatozoa of irradiated *D. melanogaster*. And the number is roughly proportional to the dose (Lea, 1946, p. 151). However, about one-third of these are associated with gross structural changes in chromosomes, and these increase more than proportionally to the dose. So probably a dose of 20 r. would induce lethals in about 4×10^{-4} rather than 6×10^{-4} of the X-chromosomes. However, the total number of genes at risk is about five times the number of sex-linked genes. So about 2×10^{-3} of the irradiated gametes would carry a recessive lethal of some kind. Thus the number of recessive lethal mutations expected in 2×10^6 would be about 4000. This number may well have to be increased by a factor of 10 or 50 if man has more genes per nucleus than *Drosophila*, or if on account of their larger size or some other reason they are more sensitive to radiation. 4000 mutations would involve 2000 deaths in all, spread over very many generations and occurring at a rate of the order of two per generation.

This may be a serious underestimate. No doubt an atomic bomb exploding over a crowded area of a large city might cause considerably more mutations than the number calculated above. But it would also cause more immediate deaths. The relevant quantity is twice the dose in roentgens summed over the number of individuals irradiated but surviving, and weighted downwards in so far as they are wholly or partially sterilized. This has been taken as 4×10^7. It might be ten times as great. But even this would only give about twenty deaths per generation; and many of these might be in early embryonic life, and therefore negligible either from a humanitarian point of view or from the point of view of mere population size.

The effect of dominant and semi-dominant mutations will certainly be more spectacular, as these will all appear and mostly be eliminated in a few generations. If it is possible to discover their approximate frequency from observations on Japanese populations this may lead to a revision of the estimates given above. It should, however, be remembered that many dominants and semi-dominants are due to structural changes, and that these increase approximately with the square of the dose, and are not likely to be very numerous with doses below 100 r.

Muller (1941) has made calculations similar to the above, and which are in substantial agreement with them. However, his work has to the best of my knowledge only appeared in a summary, which is perhaps liable to misinterpretation. He writes of a 'latent period' of 5000 years for the inbreeding effect. If this denotes the mean time before a recessive zygote appears, it is in substantial agreement with my own calculation. However, the frequency of appearance of recessives should approach its maximum in a century or two, so the term 'latent period' may be rather misleading.

It is realized that the calculation of the expected mutation frequency may require drastic revision when, on the one hand, more facts are available concerning atomic bomb explosions and, on the other, the results of at present secret experiments conducted on mice in the U.S.A. are published. There is, however, a very simple reason for comparative optimism regarding the genetic effect of atomic bombs, namely, that the dose of X- or γ-rays which is lethal when given instantaneously is probably not much more than tenfold, and almost certainly not more than a hundredfold, the dose of natural radiation received during a normal lifetime. The situation in *Drosophila* is wholly different. Mitosis is not essential to the life of an imago. An insect imago can therefore survive about twenty times the dose of X- or γ-rays which would kill a man if absorbed in a short period. On the other hand, the mean age of a man at reproduction is about 500 times that of *D. melanogaster*. Thus the ratio of the maximum tolerated dose of radiation to that normally received is about 10,000 times greater in *Drosophila* than in man. Any attempt to argue from one species to the other, which does not include an allowance for this very great difference, is therefore likely to be misleading.

Summary

Expressions are found for the moments and cumulants of the distribution of the probability that a neutral mutant gene originally present in one individual will have x descendants after n generations. Assuming a Poisson distribution for the number of offspring of an individual, it is found that when n is large the gene has disappeared in all but about $2/n$ cases, but in the remainder the numbers of genes give a type III distribution.

The number of recessive homozygotes expected per generation from a single induced recessive mutation is half the mean coefficient of inbreeding of the population concerned. The total number of deaths from recessive mutations to be expected as the result of an atomic bomb explosion is a small fraction of the number immediately killed, and is spread out over thousands of generations.

REFERENCES

F. Bernstein (1930). Fortgesetzte Untersuchungen aus des Theorie der Blutgruppen. *Z. indukt. Abstamm. u. VererbLehre*, **56**, 233.

R. A. Fisher (1930). The distribution of gene ratios for rare mutations. *Proc. Roy. Soc. Edinb.* **50**, 205.

J. B. S. Haldane (1939). The equilibrium between mutation and random extinction. *Ann. Eugen., Lond.*, **9**, 400.

J. B. S. Haldane & P. Moshinsky (1939). Inbreeding in Mendelian populations with special reference to human cousin marriage. *Ann. Eugen., Lond.*, **9**, 321.

M. G. Kendall (1943). *The Advanced Theory of Statistics*. London.

D. E. Lea (1946). *Actions of Radiations on Living Cells*. Cambridge.

H. J. Muller (1941). The role played by radiative mutation in mankind. *Science*, **93**, 438.

[FROM JOURNAL OF GENETICS, VOL. 54, No. 2, pp. 327–342, MAY 1956.]

THE DETECTION OF AUTOSOMAL LETHALS IN MICE INDUCED BY MUTAGENIC AGENTS

BY J. B. S. HALDANE
Department of Biometry, University College London

(With Two Text-figures)

(*Received* 22 *December* 1955)

INTRODUCTION

In view of the increase in the amount of high-frequency radiation to which some human begins are exposed, work has been undertaken to assess the mutagenic effect of such radiation on mammals, of which mice are the most convenient. High doses of such radiation, or of particles such as neutrons which provoke high-energy events in tissues, produce a fair number of more or less dominant mutations, such as translocations giving rise to semisterility, provided they are given within a short time. On the other hand, if the daily dose does not exceed one roentgen, the large majority of mutations should be more or less completely recessive lethals and sublethals. Such have been found by Hertwig (1941). But it appears from Russell's (1954) review that up to June 1952 no systematic search for them had been made which would give any estimate of the frequency with which they arise. I have no reason to believe that it has been made since.

It is probable that most of the undesired effects of high-energy events in human tissues on future generations will be due to recessive (or nearly recessive) lethal genes, including very small deletions and inversions, which may be produced by single events. The undesirability of a human lethal is a function of the time in the life cycle at which it acts. Lethals acting before foetal implantation will slightly reduce fertility, which, according to many writers, is by no means undesirable. Those acting shortly afterwards will cause little more than a missed period. Those leading to death later in foetal life will cause abortions, which are distressing, and not without danger to the mother. Those acting still later will cause stillbirths and neonatal deaths. Even these are less serious than genes causing premature death of children who have received affection and on whose upbringing social effort has been expended. Perhaps the most undesirable of all are lethals such as Duchenne's type of muscular dystrophy which kill round the age of 20. Though it is arguable that a mutation such that a pair of mutant genes is extinguished by a death about this age is preferable to one which is only eliminated by the deaths of several partially fertile individuals who have been chronic invalids. When a hundred or so recessive lethals have been studied in mice it may be possible to extrapolate to man with some confidence. Thus, if it were found that most of these genes killed before implantation, like A^y and t^1, rather than at or soon after birth, like *ch* and *W*, or considerably later, like *gl*, the prognosis for man would be less serious than if they mostly acted in infancy. It is clear that a search on lines similar to those adopted by Hertwig (1941) will lead to the discovery of lethals acting late in development, and thus give a biased picture.

Meanwhile we know nothing as to the mean number of roentgens needed to produce a lethal. In *Drosophila melanogaster* this is known to be very different at different stages of the life cycle, and the same is probably true in mice. Thus the effect of a given dose is nothing absolute. However, speculations as to its possible order of magnitude give some guidance in the planning of experiments. When *Drosophila* sperm is irradiated, about one sex-linked lethal is induced per 35,000 r. (roentgens). The rate for autosomes is four to five times as great. So a lethal is produced for every 6,000 r. or so. There is a much more sensitive stage just before the formation of mature sperm, but spermatogonia are only about half as sensitive (Muller, 1954). So the dose needed per lethal is perhaps on an average 10,000 r. Now a mammalian nucleus contains about thirty times as much DNA as a *Drosophila* nucleus (Vendrely, 1955). If it is equally sensitive we might expect one lethal per 300 r. On the other hand, Russell (1954) obtained fifty-four mutations, as compared with two in an almost equal number of controls, at seven loci in 48,007 mice whose fathers had received 600 r. Only about one-third of these were lethal. However, 'point mutations' at the loci in question are very probably non-lethal. The mean mutation frequency per locus was $2{\cdot}6 \times 10^{-7}$ per r. This is about six* times the mean rate in *Drosophila melanogaster*. So if mouse loci, on an average, contain no more DNA than *Drosophila* loci, mouse DNA must be about six times as sensitive as *Drosophila* DNA. If so, we should expect about one lethal mutation for every 50 r. Other calculations suggest a frequency of the order of one per 1000 r. I shall use the figure 300 r. as a reasonable guess.

Autosomal lethals are detected in *Drosophila melanogaster* by the use of inversions with marker genes. No such inversions are available in mammals; and were they available they would probably cause semisterility. It will therefore be necessary to search for recessive lethals by their effects on the segregation of genes carried by structurally normal chromosomes. It will be seen that this involves the production of such large families that, for the present, research must be restricted to mice. The question then arises, what is the most economical and accurate method of estimating the mean number of autosomal lethals per gamete of a mouse whose ancestors have received known amounts of radiation or particles of high energy.

Outline of the method suggested

I shall first describe the simplest method which seems to be practicable. I shall later discuss improvements on it.

Two stocks of mice are set up, one a multiple autosomal dominant, the other a multiple autosomal recessive. All the genes concerned must give clear segregation in steady ratios, and all the phenotypes occurring in F_2 should be distinguishable. Not more than one gene in the dominant stock might be lethal when homozygous. The complications induced if such a patent lethal is used are discussed later.

The following list of nine markers is tentatively suggested:

Dominant *C, S, A, B, Ln, Se, Je, Re, T.*
Recessive c^{ch}, *s, a, b, ln, se, je, re, t.*

They are all located in different linkage groups. *TT* is lethal. The mutant characters are *chinchilla, piebald, non-agouti, brown, leaden, short-ear, jerker, Rex, Brachyury*. I think

* Russell (1955) gives the factor as fifteen. To avoid overestimating the efficiency of the proposed method, I have adopted a lower figure justified by other work.

that it would also be possible to use *cr* (*crinkled*) if it turns out to be unlinked with the genes mentioned, and a skilled worker might be able to score the simultaneous segregation of *Re* and *wa*-1. The latter is independent of the list suggested. Similarly *Ca* might be substituted for *Re* or *bt* for *s*. Many other possibilities will occur to mouse geneticists, and it is certainly desirable that as many loci as possible should be used, even if only one set is used in a particular laboratory. I return later to the possibility of using linked markers, e.g. *a* and *pa*.

For the sake of simplicity I designate only one locus, at which the allels are G and g. In the experiment suggested in Fig. 1 males of the multiple recessive stock are irradiated during three generations, and unrelated animals are bred together so as to accumulate recessive lethals. But of course females only, or both sexes, could be irradiated, only one parent in P_2 could be irradiated, and so on. Whatever has been done in earlier generations, a multiple recessive mouse (P_1) with irradiated ancestry but not itself irradiated, is crossed to the multiple dominant stock. One pair of their progeny (F_1) both carrying any 'patent lethal' such as T, which may be used, are bred together to produce a large F_2.

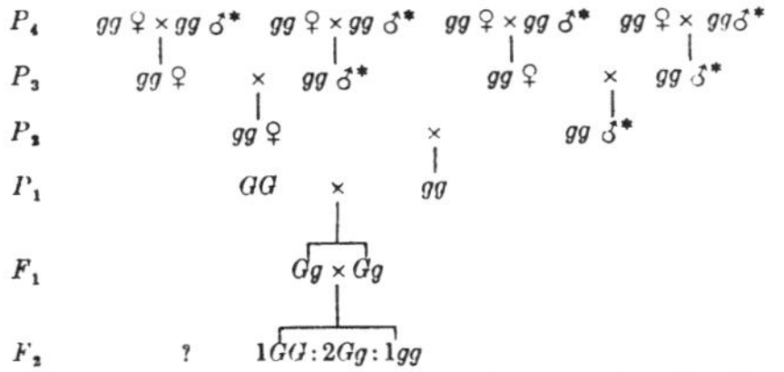

Fig. 1. A possible scheme for experiment. Asterisks denote irradiated animals.

Let us suppose that a recessive lethal l has arisen near a particular recessive locus g, which may be any of the markers in the multiply recessive stock. Then the P_1 recessive parent is gL/gl. So half of the F_1 will be GL/gl, and one-quarter of the F_2's will segregate for l. If, however, both recessive parents in P_2 have been irradiated or their ancestors have been irradiated, as in Fig. 1, then one-quarter of the F_2's test one of the P_1 chromosomes carrying g. Another quarter test the other chromosome so marked. Thus, half the F_2's test for lethals in the neighbourhood of any particular locus. I shall later show how, in the case of one locus, this number can be increased.

The expected frequencies of surviving genotypes in an F_2 from GL/gl♀ × GL/gl♂ are given in Table 1. Here c and c' are the frequencies of recombination between the loci of g and l in the two sexes.

Table 1

GL/GL	$\frac{1}{3}(1-c-c'+cc')$	$\frac{1}{3}(1-cc')$
GL/Gl	$\frac{1}{3}(c+c'-2cc')$	
GL/gL	$\frac{1}{3}(c+c'-2cc')$	$\frac{1}{3}(2-c-c'+2cc')$
GL/gl	$\frac{2}{3}(1-c-c'+cc')$	
Gl/gL	$\frac{2}{3}cc'$	
gL/gL	$\frac{1}{3}cc'$	$\frac{1}{3}(c+c'-cc')$
gL/gl	$\frac{1}{3}(c+c'-2cc')$	

The expected frequency of gg is therefore

$$x=\tfrac{1}{3}(c+c'-cc') \quad (1)$$

if the genotypes GG, Gg, and gg are equally viable. I later consider the effects expected when their viabilities are unequal. If GG is lethal, the expected frequency of gg is

$$x = \frac{c + c' - cc'}{2 + cc'} \tag{2}$$

and this expression can also be used if GG and Gg can be distinguished with certainty. For the present I assume that gg is fully recessive and fully viable. The frequency of gg expected is $\frac{1}{4}$ if there is no lethal linked with g. Otherwise it is x, which is very nearly zero if c and c' are small, and tends to $\frac{1}{4}$ as c and c' tend to $\frac{1}{2}$.

If the F_2 includes sufficiently few recessives at any locus a further search for a lethal is made. If it includes too many, it is discarded. Thus errors of two kinds (cf. Neymann & Pearson, 1933) are inevitable. We can calculate their probabilities if the search for lethals in an F_2 of n members is continued if, *and only if* it includes r or fewer recessives.

Let $P(n, r, x)$ be the probability that, for a given value of x, an F_2 of n includes r or fewer recessives. The probability that there are no recessives is $(1-x)^n$, the probability that there is just one is $nx(1-x)^{n-1}$, and so on. Thus

$$\begin{aligned} P(n, r, x) &= \sum_{i=0}^{r} \binom{n}{i} x^i (1-x)^{n-i} \\ &= (1-x)^n + \binom{n}{1} x(1-x)^{n-1} + \binom{n}{2} x^2 (1-x)^{n-2} \ldots + \binom{n}{r} x^r (1-x)^{n-r}. \end{aligned} \tag{3}$$

This is the fraction of those lethals whose x value is given by their 'map distances' $100c$ and $100c'$, which is expected to be detected in a large number of F_2's. The probability

Table 2

n	20–27	28–34	35–41	43–47	48–53
r	0	1	2	3	4

of an error due to missing a lethal is $1 - P(n, r, x)$. The probability of an error of the other kind, namely suspecting a lethal which is not present, and thus wasting time and labour in trying to locate it, is

$$P(n, r, \tfrac{1}{4}) = 3^{n-r} 4^{-n} \left[3^r + 3^{r-1} n + 3^{r-2} \binom{n}{2} + \ldots 3\binom{n}{r-1} + \binom{n}{r} \right]. \tag{4}$$

It is convenient, when calculating it, to remember that $(\frac{3}{4})^8 = 0{\cdot}100113$.

If, for a given value of n, we increase r, we increase the number of 'false clues', but we also increase the probability of detecting a lethal at any given distance from the marker. Some compromise must be made. I here suggest choosing the values of r so that $P(n, r, \frac{1}{4})$ never exceeds $\frac{1}{300}$ for any locus. Even this is fairly serious. If we were using nine markers, it would lead to false clues in about 3 % of all F_2's. Table 2 gives values of r for given n calculated on this basis. However, the mean value of $P(n, r, \frac{1}{4})$ is well below $\frac{1}{300}$. Thus for $n = 34$, $r = 1$, it is $0{\cdot}000697$, and the mean value for $n = 28$ to 34 is $0{\cdot}001732$, or $1{\cdot}56$ % for nine loci.

It must be emphasized that this set of values is quite arbitrary. In the early stages of a research higher values of r might be acceptable. But if, say, five lethals were detected in the first twenty F_2's, when only one was expected, the values of r might be lowered in future work. Further, the value of r adopted need not be the same for all loci. If no lethals had been detected on one chromosome, it might be desirable to search it more intensively, at the cost of more false clues. All that is needed is that the value of r for a given n should be fixed before a given F_2 is examined, and not, for example, raised because two of the recessive markers were each appearing in rather low numbers, though greater than the number previously chosen for r. For this reason I have not extended Table 2 farther. It might well be desirable to draw up several such tables at different levels of error. It is clear that at the level adopted an F_2 of at least three litters will usually be needed if n is to exceed 20. However, since the dominant and recessive lines will be almost unrelated, large F_2 litters may be expected.

Of course, other mutant types besides recessive lethals linked with markers will be found. The visible mutants will include some lethals acting at birth or later. These must of course be excluded in any estimate of the rate at which lethals are induced. Some translocations will be detected by semisterility. It is also possible that two markers in an F_2 may exhibit significant evidence of coupling. If the F_2 contains a double dominants, b single recessives, and d double recessives, the simplest efficient estimate of linkage is that given by Haldane (1952). If $y=(1-c)(1-c')$, where c and c' are the recombination values of the two genes concerned, then the estimate of y is

Table 3. *The probability P of detection of a lethal as a function of its recombination frequency c with a marker, if n = 40, r = 2.*

c	0	0·0151	0·0305	0·0461	0·0619	0·0780	0·0945	0·1112	0·1282
x	0	0·01	0·02	0·03	0·04	0·05	0·06	0·07	0·08
P	1	0·9925	0·9543	0·8822	0·7855	0·6767	0·5665	0·4624	0·3694
c		0·1450	0·1633	0·2000	0·2384	0·2789	0·3216	0·3675	0·5000
x		0·09	0·10	0·12	0·14	0·16	0·18	0·20	0·25
P		0·2894	0·2228	0·1261	0·06760	0·03448	0·01691	0·006309	0·001016

$$\frac{2(c+1)(2a-b+1)}{4(a+1)(c+1)+(a+c+2)(b+1)}.$$

Its sampling variance is $\frac{2y(1-y)(2+y)}{(1+2y)n}$, or $\frac{9}{16n}$ if $y=\frac{1}{4}$. So the estimate will only exceed $\frac{1}{4}$ by $3/4n^{\frac{1}{2}}$ in 2·275% of all cases in the absence of linkage. If a pair of linked markers were used, evidence of a similar kind would suggest the presence of an inversion. It is at least possible that in this way translocations or inversions might be found which caused little or no semisterility. These would assist greatly in the search for recessive lethals.

The logical basis of this method is essentially that of Carter & Falconer's (1951) systematic search for linkages. They employ five stocks containing twenty-five markers in all, and choose a level of significance corresponding to two standard errors. The probability of a 'false clue', that is to say the probability that a new mutant will appear to be linked with any particular marker, is therefore 0·02275. The probability that at least one of the twenty-five markers will give a false clue, is $1-0{\cdot}97725^{25}$, or 42·7%. However, this large risk is justifiable because if 500 progeny are scored, the probability of discovering a linkage is over 50%.

THE LENGTH OF CHROMOSOME SEARCHED

Given c and c', and hence by equation (1), x, we can readily calculate $P(n, r, x)$, the probability of detecting a lethal at the map distances corresponding to x. Thus for $n = 40$, $r = 2$,

$$P(40, 2, x) = (1-x)^{40} + 40x(1-x)^{39} + 780x^2(1-x)^{38}$$
$$= (1-x)^{38}\,(1+38x+741x^2).$$

Table 3 shows P as a function of x and of c when $c = c'$, and Fig. 2 shows the same figures graphically. When c and c', are unequal, we have

$$x = \tfrac{1}{2}[c + c' - \tfrac{1}{4}(c+c')^2 + \tfrac{1}{4}(c-c')^2],$$

so x is larger than the value corresponding to the mean map distance $50(c+c')$ if c and c' were equal. However, the error in taking c and c' as equal is generally small. Thus for c and p Grüneberg (1936) found $c = 0{\cdot}1610$, $c' = 0{\cdot}1190$. So $x = 0{\cdot}08695$. $\tfrac{1}{2}(c+c') = 0{\cdot}1400$, which would give $x = 0{\cdot}08680$, while the approximation $x = \tfrac{1}{3}(c+c')$ would give $x = 0{\cdot}09333$.

Table 3 shows that the majority of lethals are detected if c is less than 0·1 (10 cM.), while less than 13 % are detected if c exceeds 0·2.

It is not possible to determine the mean radius swept, in Carter & Falconer's (1951) terminology, with any great accuracy, for the following reason. The loci of genes are by no means evenly distributed on the linkage map, even of *Drosophila melanogaster*, where they tend to cluster at the free ends of chromosomes and near the centromeres, still less in organisms such as the Cyprinodont fishes, where chiasmata seem to be sharply localized. This means that if a mutation (e.g. the mutation to *brown*) has occurred at a given locus, another mutation (including a lethal) is more likely to occur at a map distance of 0–5 units than at a map distance of 30–35 units. Hence the mean map distances swept will be overestimated, but the number of lethals found will be more than proportional to the map distance swept. The same criticism applies to Carter & Falconer's calculation. But in their case it is unimportant, as their concept of radius swept is mainly a guide to design, rather than estimation. Their evaluation of this radius could be made more precise by the method here developed, but this is probably not worth doing. Moreover, the linkage maps for mouse genes suggest that bunching may be less marked in the mouse than in *Drosophila melanogaster*. *d* and *se* are the only pair of genes known to me which give under 1 % recombination.

It is possible to determine the radius swept round the locus of each marker on the assumption, which is certainly somewhat incorrect, that mutable loci are evenly distributed over the genetical map. I define the radius swept, or searched, s, as follows. If all the lethals within a map distance of $100s$ cM. on each side of the marker were detected, and none beyond this distance, while the total number of lethals detected was the same as that found, then s is the radius swept. That is to say, if the abscissa in Fig. 2 were map distance instead of recombination frequency, the radius swept would be as shown. The area in the rectangle in this figure is equal to the area below the curve.

If then m is the map distance, reckoned in morgans, not centimorgans,

$$s = \int_0^M P(n, r, x)\,dm, \qquad (5)$$

where M is the maximum attainable value of m. The mean map distance of lethals from the marker is $\int_0^M mP(n, r, x)\, dm \div \int_0^M P(n, r, x)\, dm$. This is usually somewhat less than s. In a preliminary statement as to this work I gave the mean map distance as an estimate of the radius swept. This is not so good an estimate as s, and slightly underestimates the power of the method proposed.

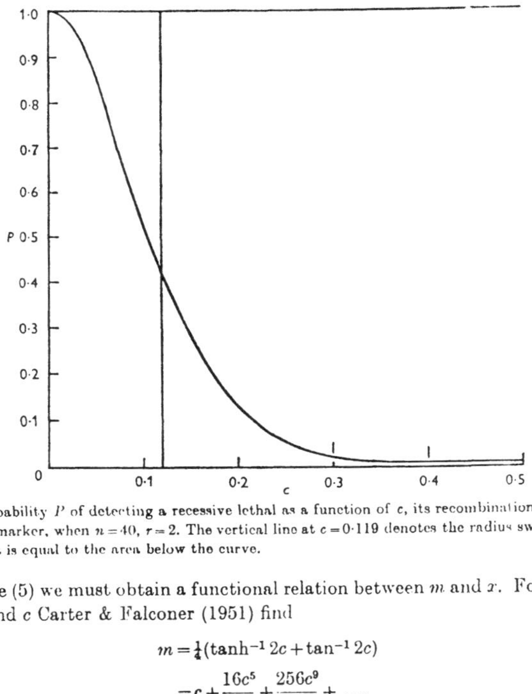

Fig. 2. The probability P of detecting a recessive lethal as a function of c, its recombination frequency with a recessive marker, when $n=40$, $r=2$. The vertical line at $c=0{\cdot}119$ denotes the radius swept. The area to the left of it is equal to the area below the curve.

To evaluate (5) we must obtain a functional relation between m and x. For the relation between m and c Carter & Falconer (1951) find

$$m = \tfrac{1}{4}(\tanh^{-1} 2c + \tan^{-1} 2c)$$
$$= c + \frac{16c^5}{5} + \frac{256c^9}{9} + \dots.$$

This means that the error in taking $m=c$ is less than 0·5 % unless c exceeds 0·2. Other functional relations, such as Kosambi's (1944) give somewhat larger errors, but would not, I think, lead to an increase of 1 % in the value of s unless n exceeded 60. As in what follows I shall be neglecting even the fourth power of c, I take $m=c$, that is to say I neglect double crossing over. I also take $c=c'$, which, as we saw, introduces an error less than 0·2 % in the example here considered. So (5) becomes

$$s = \int_0^{\frac{1}{2}} P(n, r, x)\, dc. \qquad (6)$$

The upper limit of $\frac{1}{3}$ corresponds to a very long map distance. If the marker is near the end of a chromosome a lower limit must be taken. Now from (1)

$$c=1-(1-3x)^{\frac{1}{2}}$$

$$\frac{dc}{dx}=\tfrac{3}{2}(1-3x)^{-\frac{1}{2}}.$$

Hence
$$s=\frac{3}{2}\int_0^{\frac{1}{4}}(1-3x)^{-\frac{1}{2}}P(n,r,x)\,dx. \tag{7}$$

We shall have to deal with several expressions of this type. On expanding $(1-3x)^{-\frac{1}{2}}$ we obtain a series whose terms are of the form $x^kP(n,r,x)\,dx$, multiplied by numerical constants, where k is zero or a positive integer. From (3)

$$\begin{aligned}\int_0^{\frac{1}{4}}x^kP(n,r,x)\,dx&=\sum_{i=0}^{r}\binom{n}{i}\int_0^{\frac{1}{4}}x^{i+k}(1-x)^{n-i}\,dx\\&=\sum_{i=0}^{r}\binom{n}{i}\int_0^{1}x^{i+k}(1-x)^{n-i}\,dx-\sum_{i=0}^{r}\binom{n}{i}\int_{\frac{1}{4}}^{1}x^{i+k}(1-x)^{n-i}\,dx\\&=\sum_{i=0}^{r}\binom{n}{i}\frac{(i+k)!(n-i)!}{(n+k+1)!}-\sum_{i=0}^{r}\binom{n}{i}\int_{\frac{1}{4}}^{1}x^{i+k}(1-x)^{n-i}\,dx\\&=\sum_{i=0}^{r}\frac{(i+1)(i+2)\dots(i+k)}{(n+1)(n+2)\dots(n+k+1)}-\sum_{i=0}^{r}\binom{n}{i}\int_{\frac{1}{4}}^{1}x^{i+k}(1-x)^{n-i}\,dx\\&=\frac{(r+k+1)!\,n!}{(k+1)\,r!\,(n+k+1)!}-\sum_{i=0}^{r}\binom{n}{i}\int_{\frac{1}{4}}^{1}x^{i+k}(1-x)^{n-i}\,dx.\end{aligned}$$

The first term may be written $\dfrac{(r+1)(r+2)\dots(r+k+1)}{(k+1)(n+1)(n+2)\dots(n+k+1)}$. The second term is $-\int_{\frac{1}{4}}^{1}x^kP(n,r,x)\,dx$. Now r has been chosen so that $P(n,r,\frac{1}{4})$ is less than $\frac{1}{300}$, while $P(n,r,0)=1$. Thus for the values of n and r considered, the integral, which is the contribution of the tail of a distribution such as that of Table 3 beyond $x=\frac{1}{4}$ to a moment of x, is negligible. To take numerical examples, with the smallest values of n permitted by Table 2, if $n=20$, $r=0$,

$$\int_0^1(1-x)^n\,dx=\tfrac{1}{21},\quad\int_{\frac{1}{4}}^{1}(1-x)^n\,dx=\tfrac{1}{21}(\tfrac{3}{4})^{21}.$$

Since $(\frac{3}{4})^{21}=0{\cdot}00238$, the error is $0{\cdot}24\%$.

Again with $n=32$, $r=1$,

$$\int_0^1(1-x)^n\,dx=\tfrac{1}{33},\quad\int_{\frac{1}{4}}^{1}(1-x)^n\,dx=\tfrac{1}{33}(\tfrac{3}{4})^{33}=\tfrac{1}{33}\times0{\cdot}75\times10^{-4},$$

$$\int_0^1x(1-x)^{n-1}dx=\frac{1}{32.33},\quad\int_{\frac{1}{4}}^{1}x(1-x)^{n-1}dx=\frac{1}{32.33}\times9\times10^{-4}.$$

Thus the error is less than $0{\cdot}1\%$. We may therefore take

$$\int_0^{\frac{1}{4}}x^kP(n,r,x)\,dx=\frac{(r+k+1)!\,n!}{(k+1)\,r!\,(n+k+1)!} \tag{8}$$

for example,

$$\int_0^{\frac{1}{2}} P(n, r, x)\, dx = \frac{r+1}{n+1},$$

$$\int_0^{\frac{1}{2}} xP(n, r, x)\, dx = \frac{(r+1)\ (r+2)}{2(n+1)\,(n+2)},$$

with negligible error, and in fact take the upper limit of integration in such equations as (7) as unity. (7) may be written

$$s = \frac{3}{2}\int_0^1 (1 + \tfrac{3}{2}x + \tfrac{27}{8}x^2 + \tfrac{135}{16}x^3 + \ldots)\, P(n, r, x)\, dx$$

$$= \frac{3(r+1)}{2(n+1)}\left[1 + \frac{3(r+2)}{4(n+2)} + \frac{9(r+2)\,(r+3)}{8(n+2)\,(n+3)} + \frac{135(r+2)\,(r+3)\,(r+4)}{64(n+2)\,(n+3)\,(n+4)} + \ldots\right]$$

$$= \frac{3(r+1)}{2(n+1)}\left[1 + \frac{3(r+2)}{4n} + \frac{3(r+2)\,(3r+5)}{8n^2} + \frac{3(r+2)\,(45r^2+195r+244)}{64n^3} + \ldots\right]$$

$$= \frac{3(r+1)}{2(n+1)}\left[1 - \frac{3(r+2)}{4n} - \frac{3(r+2)\,(3r+4)}{16n^2} - \frac{3(r+2)\,(18r^2+99r+160)}{64n^3} - \ldots\right]^{-1}.$$

$$= 6(r+1)\left[4n - (3r+2) - \frac{3(r+2)}{4n}\left\{3r+8+\frac{18r^2+111r+176}{4n}+\ldots\right\} + O(n^{-3})\right]^{-1} \quad (9)$$

$$= \frac{6(r+1)}{4n-3r-2}, \text{ nearly.}$$

For example, when $n = 40$, $r = 2$, the four terms given above yield

$$18 \div (160 - 8 - 1{\cdot}05 - 0{\cdot}220),$$

or 0·1194, while the simpler formula gives 0·1184. The error is somewhat greater for smaller values of n. However, an error of even 2% would only become serious compared with the sampling errors when over 1000 lethals had been found! It is of course quite practicable to calculate (6) and (7) with any desired accuracy mechanically for a large range of values of n and r, making allowance for double crossing over if desired.

Assuming that the P_1 recessive is from irradiated ancestry on both sides, then, if the markers are not near the ends of chromosomes, the total map length swept per locus will be $2s$, but it will only be swept in half the F_2's. So if there are k recessive markers, the total length, in centimorgans, swept per F_2 is approximately

$$100s = \frac{600(r+1)\,k}{4n-3r-2} \quad (10)$$

It must, however, be remembered that the values of n and r will not usually be the same for all markers. Some marker genes can be scored at birth, others not, perhaps, till after weaning. Table 4 gives some representative values of $100s$, calculated from (9) for representative values of n and r taken from Table 2. The last two rows give values calculated from (13) and (14).

It will be seen that $100s$ increases roughly with $\frac{1}{3}n$. However it falls while n increases with constant r, the lowest value being 5·7 when $n = 27$, $r = 0$. So since the number of animals used in the search for a lethal always exceeds the number in the F_2, it will always be desirable to continue the breeding of an F_2 during the joint lives of the parents. This will inevitably cause some difficulties, since occasionally a search for a lethal will begin before an F_2 is completed. In such a case the radius swept should, I think, be calculated from the value of n when the search began, and not from its final value.

The mean map distance of genes from the marker is

$$\int_0^M mP(n, r, x)\, dm \div \int_0^M P(n, r, x)\, dm.$$

Making the same approximations as before, it can be shown that this is

$$3(r+2)\left[4n-3r-4-\frac{3(r+3)}{4n}\left\{3r+16+\frac{3(3r^2+33r+80)}{2n}+\dots\right\}\right]^{-1}.$$

This is somewhat less than s if r exceeds zero. For example, for $n=30$, $r=1$, it is 0·080.

Table 4

n	23	30	38	45	51
r	0	1	2	3	4
$100s$	6·9	10·5	12·6	14·3	15·9
$100s'$	11·7	17·9	21·2	23·9	26·2
$100s''$	0·2	0·3	0·3	0·3	0·4

Lengths swept for representative values of n and r.
Third row, autosomal recessive marker.
Fourth row, non-crossover lethals using a and a^t.
Fifth row, crossover lethals using a and a^t.

Allowance for low viability of recessives

I have assumed that recessives can always be distinguished from dominants. They may, however, appear with a frequency different from $\frac{1}{4}$ in control experiments, owing to lowered (or raised) viability. The various genes used may have unexpected reactions on viability or be linked with others which do so. Let us suppose then that the frequency of a recessive in control F_2's is $\frac{1}{4}p$, where p differs significantly from unity.

If so, the probability of a false clue is increased if p is less than unity; for example, for $n=43$, $p=0{\cdot}8$, r must be zero if $P(n, r, 0{\cdot}2)$ is to be less than $\frac{1}{300}$:

$$x=\tfrac{1}{3}p(2c-c^2),\quad \text{so}\quad c=(1-3p^{-1}x)^{\frac{1}{2}},\quad \frac{dc}{dx}=\tfrac{3}{2}p^{-1}(1-3p^{-1}x)^{-\frac{1}{2}}.$$

Hence (7) becomes

$$s=\frac{3}{2p}\int_0^1(1-3p^{-1}x)^{-\frac{1}{2}}P(n, r, x)\, dx$$

$$=\frac{3(r+1)}{2p(n+1)}\left[1+\frac{3(r+2)}{4p(n+2)}+\frac{9(r+2)(r+3)}{8p^2(n+2)(n+3)}+\dots\right]$$

$$=6(r+1)\left[4pn-(3r+6-4p)-\frac{3(r+2)}{4pn}(3r+12-4p+\dots)\right]^{-1}. \qquad (11)$$

It is not worth giving further terms, as the value of p will be uncertain. Roughly speaking, then, for given values of n and r, s is increased by a factor p^{-1}. This does not, on an average, make up for the loss of information due to the lowered value of r. But high values of p, due to relative inviability of a dominant, would be advantageous.

PATENT LETHALS AS MARKERS

I have, for many years, designated a gene such as T (*Brachyury*) or A^y (*Yellow*) as a patent lethal, as opposed to a latent, or fully recessive, lethal such as *ch* (*congenital hydrocephalus*) or *gl* (*grey lethal*). This avoids the ambiguous phrase 'dominant lethal'. From (2) we see that to a first approximation $x = c$, so the radius swept is roughly $(r+1)/n$. This apparent disadvantage is outweighed by the fact that one can use much larger values of r without raising $P(n, r, \frac{1}{3})$ above its critical value. If this value is chosen, as before, at $\frac{1}{300}$, the highest permissible values of r are given in Table 4. It is convenient to remember that $(\frac{2}{3})^{17} = 0{\cdot}0010150$.

TABLE 4

n	15–19	20–25	26–29	30–35	36–38	39–43
r	0	1	2	3	4	5

From (2) $$x = \frac{2c - c^2}{2 + c^2}, \quad \text{so} \quad c = (1+x)^{-1}[1 - (1 - 2x - 2x^2)^{\frac{1}{2}}]$$

$$= x + \tfrac{1}{2}x^2 + x^3 + \tfrac{13}{8}x^4 + \ldots$$

$$\frac{dc}{dx} = 1 + x + 3x^2 + \tfrac{13}{2}x^3 + \ldots.$$

Hence $$s = \int_0^1 (1 + x + 3x^2 + \tfrac{13}{2}x^3 + \ldots)\, P(n, r, x)\, dx$$

$$= \frac{r+1}{n+1}\left[1 + \frac{r+2}{2(n+2)} + \frac{(r+2)(r+3)}{(n+2)(n+3)} + \frac{13(r+2)(r+3)(r+4)}{8(n+2)(n+3)(n+4)} + \ldots\right]$$

$$= 2(r+1)\left[2n - r - \frac{(r+2)}{2n}\left(3r + 8 + \frac{6r^2 + 29r + 36}{2n} + \ldots\right)\right]^{-1}. \quad (12)$$

Thus, if $n = 30$, $r = 3$, $s = 14{\cdot}4$, as compared with $10{\cdot}5$ from (9) if GG is not lethal. But with $n = 35$, $r = 3$, $s = 12{\cdot}2$, as compared with $13{\cdot}8$ when GG is not lethal. Thus a patent lethal perhaps on the whole gives rather more information than an ordinary dominant, though not for all values of n. The advantage may well be offset by the smaller litter size in F_2. The main advantage of a patent lethal is that it makes it easier to detect suspected lethals, and very much easier to keep them once they are found.

THE USE OF MULTIPLE ALLELOMORPHS

If there are two recessive allels at a given locus, there is a slight advantage in using two different recessive stocks, one homozygous for each. Suppose the allels of G are g^1 and g^2, then one quarter of the F_2's will be from $Gg^1 \times Gg^1$, and another quarter from $Gg^2 \times Gg^2$. It should thus be possible to say with a fairly high probability from which parent in P_2 a lethal was derived. However the one locus where a considerable advantage may be gained is the a (non-agouti) locus.

It should be possible to make up two multiple recessive stocks, one being $aa\, c^{ch} c^{ch}\, ss$ ...., and the other $a^t a^t c^{ch} c^{ch}\, ss$ ... and to irradiate each of them. a^t is *black-and-tan*, a is *non-agouti*, or black. The P_1 recessive parent is then aa^t. Half the F_1 are Aa, the other half Aa^t. These genotypes can be distinguished, since the latter has the lighter belly.

Thus all F_1 matings can be $Aa \times Aa$ or $Aa^t \times Aa^t$. Now suppose the P_1 recessive was a^tL/al, then the expected frequencies in F_1 will be:

$$\tfrac{1}{2}(1-c)AL/a^tL, \quad \tfrac{1}{2}cAL/aL, \quad \tfrac{1}{2}cAL/a^tl, \quad \tfrac{1}{2}(1-c)AL/al.$$

So a fraction $(1-c)^2$ of the $Aa \times Aa$ F_1 matings will be $AL/al \times AL/al$, and will segregate for the lethal. Another fraction c^2 will segregate for any lethal linked with a^t. So if a lethal is present in the P_1 recessive a fraction $\tfrac{1}{2}(1-2c+2c^2)$ of all F_2's will segregate for it. This is substantially larger than $\tfrac{1}{4}$.

Consider first the lethals derived from the *aa* stock. The mean distance searched for them is approximately:

$$s = 2\int_0^1 (1-c)^2\, P(n, r, x)\, dc.$$

The factor 2 arises because both sides of the marker locus are searched in all F_2's, instead of only half. $(1-c)^2 = 1-3x$, $\dfrac{dc}{dx} = \tfrac{3}{2}(1-3x)^{-\frac{1}{2}}$. So approximately

$$\begin{aligned} s &= 3\int_0^1 (1-3x)^{\frac{1}{2}}\, P(n, r, x)\, dx \\ &= 3\int_0^1 (1-\tfrac{3}{2}x-\tfrac{9}{8}x^2-\tfrac{27}{16}x^3-\ldots)\, P(n, r, x)\, dx \\ &= \frac{3(r+1)}{n+1}\left[1-\frac{3(r+2)}{4(n+2)}\left\{1+\frac{r+3}{2(n+3)}+\frac{9(r+3)(r+4)}{16(n+3)(n+4)}+\ldots\right\}\right] \\ &= 12(r+1)\left[4n+3r+10+\frac{3(r+2)}{4n}\left(5r+8+\frac{30r^2+91r+80}{4n}+\ldots\right)\right]^{-1}. \end{aligned} \qquad (13)$$

A representative set of values is given in Table 4.

The mean distance searched for lethals derived from the a^ta^t stock, due to two independent crossovers in the gametogenesis of the P_1 recessive parent, is nearly

$$\begin{aligned} s &= 2\int_0^1 c^2\, P(n, r, x)\, dx \\ &= \frac{27}{4}\int_0^1 (x^2+\tfrac{9}{4}x^3+\tfrac{45}{8}x^4+\ldots)\, P(n, r, x)\, dx \\ &= \frac{27}{4}\cdot\frac{(r+1)(r+2)(r+3)}{(n+1)(n+2)(n+3)}\left[\frac{1}{3}+\frac{9(r+4)}{16(n+4)}+\frac{9(r+4)(r+5)}{8(n+4)(n+5)}+\ldots\right] \\ &= 9(r+1)(r+2)(r+3)\,[4n^3-\tfrac{3}{4}(9r+4)\,n^2-\tfrac{1}{16}(135r^2+240r-1376)\,n-\ldots]^{-1}. \end{aligned} \qquad (14)$$

Table 4 shows that s never reaches 1 cM.

If both parents are about equally irradiated, this locus is nearly twice as useful as any other. If, on the other hand, only one grandparent of the F_1 is irradiated, it is more than three times as useful as any other locus, since almost all the chromosomes derived from the irradiated grandparent can be tested, instead of only one quarter of them. It may prove possible to use similar devices at other loci. The advantage of using an incompletely recessive marker is particularly great when only one grandparent is irradiated.

THE CONFIRMATION OF SUSPECTED LETHALS

Supposing a lethal linked with any marker is suspected, the F_2 should be continued as long as possible. This may give decisive evidence. For example, an F_2 of 56 containing only three recessives would only be expected once in 28,000 trials in the absence of a lethal. Meanwile the male parent of the F_2 should be mated to all his other sisters (or all those with the same allel at the a locus if a lethal near it is suspected). Half of the resulting F_2's should segregate for the same lethal. They will also of course yield information about lethals in other chromosomes.

Table 1 shows that of the gg recessives in F_2, all but a fraction $\frac{cc'}{c+c'-2cc'}$, or about $\frac{1}{2}c$, should be heterozygous for the lethal. They can therefore be used to set up new intercrosses, preferably with a stock carrying G and one or more markers linked with it. Among the dominants few of the GG mice will be Ll. But of the Gg mice $\frac{2(1-c-c'+cc')}{2-c-c'+2cc'}$, that is to say a fairly large majority, should be GL/gl. Unless GG and Gg differ phenotypically, the dominants in F_2 should first be tested with gg mates, and those which prove to be Gg mated with their father or with one another. If, after all, the search yields negative results, it would perhaps be reasonable to abandon it when a lethal at a distance of $100s$ cM. would have been detected with about 99% probability. An allowance can then be made for lethals lost in this way. Meanwhile more information (positive or negative) as to lethals in other chromosomes will have been obtained. The computations involved are tedious but not difficult. Thus, if an F_1 male is mated with several sisters, half the F_2's are testing the same chromosome as in the original F_2, with an allowance for crossing over in $1-c$ of all cases. The treatment is similar to that of (13).

A complication will of course arise from the induction of a certain number of genes which are sublethal when recessive. Unless they produce visible effects, most of them will be missed. Suppose, for example, that the viability of a sublethal homozygote is v, then the expected frequency of recessives is raised from x to $\frac{v+3x-3vx}{3+v}$, or $x+\frac{v(1-4x)}{3+v}$. Thus, if $x=0$, $v=\frac{1}{2}$, this frequency is $\frac{1}{7}$, as with a fully lethal gene about 24 cM. from the marker. Such a gene would very seldom be detected.

Again, if the homozygote is fully lethal but the heterozygote somewhat inviable, the lethal gene will tend to disappear in the course of several generations. But it is easier to detect in F_2, since most of the gg mice which are not ll are Ll. It can be seen from Table 1 that the frequency of gg expected in F_2 is

$$\frac{v(c+c'-2cc')+cc'}{1+2v}, \quad \text{or} \quad x-\frac{(1-v)(c+c'-4cc')}{3(1+2v)}.$$

So the map distance searched is somewhat increased. But the increase is by a factor of about $1+\frac{1-v}{3v}$ which will seldom be very large. It may, however, be necessary to allow for it in estimating mutation rates.

Discussion

I do not try to prove that the method here given is the best possible method of searching for lethals. But I think any method must use equation (9) or (12) in some form. It is, however, easy to show that it is better than any method based on disturbances of a 1:1 ratio. Suppose, for example, that the test matings were between the P_1 recessive and its F_1 progeny. Then if both P_2 mice were irradiated or from irradiated stock, all such matings would search for lethals. In the absence of a lethal we should expect $\frac{1}{2}gg$, in presence of a lethal very close to g we should expect $\frac{1}{3}gg$. For example in a backcross family of 30, we should expect $15 \pm 2{\cdot}74gg$, and $10 \pm 2{\cdot}58gg$ on the two hypotheses. Our only hope of detecting such lethals without too many false clues would be to take r about 7 or 8, in which case we should only detect about a third of the lethals. Even with a backcross of 60, detection would be harder than in an F_2 of 20.

A possible method would be the irradiation of mice heterozygous for several patent lethals, such as *Yellow*, *Brachyury*, *Oligosyndactyly* and *Splotch*, and breeding brothers and sisters together. The radius swept is given by (12), but the litter size would be drastically reduced. The same is true if any of the translocations so far discovered were used this way.

An obvious objection to the method here proposed is that the various families of mice from irradiated parents (seven in Fig. 1) are only used for the testing of one set of chromosomes, and that in only half the tests. If two F_2's were bred from different F_1 pairs, then only once in four trials would the same chromosome be tested twice. But if two P_1 recessives were mated to multiple dominants, this would happen less often. The experiment will have to be designed to minimize the number of mice bred per unit of chromosome searched. If an experiment were done in which only the P_2 mice, or one of them, was irradiated, then it would clearly be desirable to test as many of the P_1 mice as possible. All of them would carry different lethals, except when a lethal mutation had occurred early in the germ track and given rise to a number of gametes carrying the same lethal.

Any programme of research is likely to include the study of a group of mice irradiated moderately (say not receiving more than one roentgen per day) for many generations. They would presumably carry few chromosomal rearrangements, and their study would throw more light than that of heavily irradiated mice on human perils. Such a stock should be maximally outbred; but the neighbourhood of the same marker will certainly be searched repeatedly, and special calculations, similar to those of Woolf (1954) will be needed.

Finally some kind of sequential method may well be tried. One might reject any F_2 of 20 which contained four or more recessives at each marked locus. Such a procedure would save material, but it would need supplementary calculations. Unless a plan like that of Table 2 is laid down in advance and rigorously adhered to, accurate work will be impossible.

The tendency of loci to crowd together on the linkage map, noted above, will lead to an overestimate of the mutation rate. For if, as suggested below, 6 % of the linkage map is tested, this is likely to include more than 6 % of the loci. The median of the number of lethals found near different loci may yield a better estimate than their mean. It is also probable that some of the markers used will turn out to be near the ends of chromosomes. A majority of those suggested happen to be terminal in existing linkage maps. This will lead to an underestimate of the mutation rate. But the correction to be made is smaller than in the search for linkage, since the radius swept is much smaller. If each lethal found is located fairly accurately on the chromosome map, it will be possible to find the mean radius swept from the observed location of the lethals found, as a check on the formulae here given. This will, however, entail so much extra work that it may not be considered worth while.

The total autosomal genetical map is about 1824 cM. (Slizynski, 1955) on cytological data and a little less (Carter, 1955) on genetical data, perhaps as a result of the bunching effect. An F_2 of 30 mice segregating for a or a^t, T, and seven other autosomal loci would search $18{\cdot}2+14{\cdot}4+7\times10{\cdot}5$, or 106 cM. This is about 5·8 % of the total map length. Thus, if a P_1 recessive were formed from gametes which between them carried k recessive lethals, an F_2 raised from it would have a probability of about $0{\cdot}029k$ of detecting a lethal. If both parents and all grandparents of the P_1 recessive had received a dose of 400 r., k would be about 5 on the basis of the guess made in the introduction. If so, about one lethal would be detected in seven F_2's, or 210 mice examined, to which must be added perhaps 150 to allow for ancestors and mice used in the determination of the lethal. As was pointed out in the introduction, the value of k might be a good deal larger. Russell detected one visible mutation in every 889 mice examined. Thus it is at least possible that the method suggested would be more economical than Russell's.

If, on the other hand, with the dosage suggested above, only two lethals were detected in 200 F_2's, which would mean scoring about 6000 mice, we should have evidence that a given dosage of radiation produced only about a fifteenth as many lethal mutations in a given weight of mouse DNA as compared with the same weight of *Drosophila* DNA. This would be very reassuring. I conclude then that a test even on as few as 200 F_2's would be of real value.

I have considered the desirability of using linked markers. Dr C. Auerbach has kindly communicated to me a scheme for using them to detect sex-linked lethals, and Dr T. C. Carter has raised the same possibility for autosomal loci. If the conclusions of this paper are accepted, I propose to investigate it. The difficulty is as follows. If we are concerned with two linked markers a and b; we have to base our criterion for search or rejection on three numbers, those of *aa B*, *A bb* and *aabb*. The last gives a powerful test for lethals between the two loci, while the former two must be given more weight in the case of lethals not between them. It is thus hard to find the most efficient criterion. Nevertheless, I think that if *a a pa pa fi fi* and a^t a^t *pa pa fi fi* stocks were irradiated and crossed, and their hybrids crossed to *Ra*/+, one could search about 80 units of chromosome IV, one end in almost all F_2's, the other in somewhat over half. In addition, segments of other chromosomes, for example round the loci of *b* and *s* or *se*, could be searched. The fraction of lethals lost in the different segments would have to be calculated. This would, I think, best be done numerically once a scheme was agreed on. The total length searched would not, I think, greatly if at all exceed that searched by the procedure suggested above.

Finally I would make the following plea. In addition to experiments on the effect of photons and particles of high energy, I believe that experiments should be instituted on the mutagenic effect of substances which are frequently added to human food as preservatives or otherwise, or used as drugs over long periods. An investigation of the mutagenic effect on mice of substances which are mutagens for *Drosophila* would of course be of great interest. But it is clear that a substance mutagenic for one organism may not be so for another. It is entirely possible that 'agene', which was extensively used to bleach flour, and altered the methionine residues of the proteins in bread, may have been responsible for more human mutation than all the radioactive elements so far produced by atomic bombs. The methyl-purines, such as caffeine, may be mutagenic for mammals, as they are for some fungi. In such cases it would be even rasher to extrapolate from Drosophila to mammals than in that of X-rays.

The question of extrapolation from mice to men remains. It is possible that human genetic material is as sensitive as that of mice, or more so. It is equally possible that in long-lived animals selection in favour of genes reducing mutability is much stronger than in shorter-lived ones. Research on long-lived mammals would be very expensive. But it might be possible to compare the mutability, in human and mouse tissue cultures, of genes responsible for the synthesis of particular antigens, which could probably be detected in single cells. It might be difficult to distinguish mutation from somatic crossing over (Pontecorvo, Gloor & Forbes, 1954) but such work should, I believe, form part of any comprehensive programme of research on human mutation.

Summary

A method is proposed for searching for recessive lethals in mice. A multiple recessive stock is irradiated, and members of it are crossed to a multiple dominant stock. Lethal genes are detected by deficiencies of recessives in F_2. The length of chromosome searched is evaluated. It should be possible to search about 6% of the genetical map in each F_2.

I have to thank Dr C. A. B. Smith, Mrs S. Maynard Smith and Dr Sewall Wright for helpful criticism, and Dr T. C. Carter for asking important questions, some of which I have tried to answer

References

CARTER, T. C. (1955). The estimation of total genetical map lengths from linkage test data. *J. Genet.* **53**, 21–8.

CARTER, T. C. & FALCONER, D. S. (1951). Stocks for detecting linkage in the mouse, and the theory of their design. *J. Genet.* **50**, 307–23.

GRÜNEBERG, H. (1936). Further linkage data on the albino chromosome of the house-mouse. *J. Genet.* **33**, 255–65.

HALDANE, J. B. S. (1952). A class of efficient estimates of a parameter. *Bull. Int. Stat. Inst.* **33**, 231–48.

HERTWIG, P. (1941). Erbanderungen bei Maüsen nach Röntgenbestrahlung. *Proc. 7th Int. Gen. Cong. J. Genet.* supplement.

KOSAMBI, D. D. (1944). The estimation of map distances from recombination values. *Ann. Eugen., Lond.*, **12**, 172–5.

MULLER, H. J. (1954). In *Radiation Biology*, vol. **1**, 351–626 (New York).

NEYMANN, J. & PEARSON, E. S. (1933). On the testing of statistical hypotheses in relation to probability *a priori*. *Proc. Camb. Phil. Soc.* **29**, 492.

PONTECORVO, G., GLOOR, E. T. & FORBES, E. (1954). Analysis of mitotic recombination in *Aspergillus nidulans*. *J. Genet.* **52**, 226–37.

RUSSELL, W. L. (1954). Genetic effects of radiation in mammals. *Radiation Biology*, **1**, 825–59 (New York).

RUSSELL, W. L. (1955). Genetic effects of radiation in mice and their bearing on the estimation of human hazards. *Report of Int. Conf. on the peaceful uses of atomic energy.*

SLIZYNSKI, B. M. (1955). Chiasmata in the male mouse. *J. Genet.* **53**, 597–605.

VENDRELY, R. (1955). The deoxyribonucleic acid content of the nucleus. In Chargaff and Davidson's *The Nucleic Acids in Chemistry and Biology.*

WOOLF, B. (1954). Estimation of mutation rates. I. Visible recessive characters detected in inbred lines maintained by single sib-matings. *J. Genet.* **52**, 332–53.

APPENDIX

The Detection of Sublethal Recessives by the use of Linked Marker Genes in the Mouse

By J. B. S. Haldane

Indian Statistical Institute, Calcutta

Carter has shown that by the use of linked marker genes recessive lethal mutations induced by high frequency radiation or otherwise can be detected, and what is more important, their frequency can be estimated. In this note I point out a further advantage of this method. It makes possible the detection of sublethal recessive mutations. These cannot be detected with any very high probability by the method of Haldane (1956) where unlinked markers are used. On the other hand, it does not seem that Carter's method will allow an accurate enumeration of sublethal mutations.

Carter considers the results to be expected if a member of an irradiated $\dfrac{+\ \mathbf{a}\ \mathbf{pa}\ \mathbf{fi}\ +}{+\ \mathbf{a}\ \mathbf{pa}\ \mathbf{fi}\ +}$ stock is crossed with a $\dfrac{\mathbf{Ra}\ +\ +\ +\ \mathbf{Sd}}{+\ +\ +\ +\ +}$ mouse, and the F_1 inbred. The symbols represent the linked recessives *non-agouti*, *pallid*, *fidget*, and the patent lethals *Ragged* and *Danforth's short-tail*. These are 'dominants' lethal when homozygous. It may be remarked that the efficiency of the method will be very considerably increased if one recessive stock containing **a** and one containing $\mathbf{a}^t$ (*tan*) are irradiated, and their F_1 crossed to a dominant. If two $\dfrac{+}{\mathbf{a}}$ mice or two $\dfrac{+}{\mathbf{a}^t}$ mice are mated, this will ensure that at least the **a** locus in each of them is derived from the same irradiated grandparental chromosome. This will double the chance of finding a lethal very close to **a**, and perhaps increase the overall chance by about 50%.

This involves finding a female and a male in the F_1 both of which are $\dfrac{\mathbf{Ra}\ +\ \mathbf{Sd}}{+\ \mathbf{a}\ +}$ or both $\dfrac{\mathbf{Ra}\ +\ \mathbf{Sd}}{+\ \mathbf{a}^t\ +}$. The frequency of **Ra + Sd** gametes is about 0·28, being a little over one-quarter owing to linkage. Those of **+ a +** and **+ $\mathbf{a}^t$ +** gametes are one-half. Assuming a sex ratio of equality the probability that a family of n will contain at least one **Ra Sd** female and at least one **Ra Sd** male is $1-2\times 0{\cdot}86^n+0{\cdot}72^n$. This is 0·5958 when $n=10$, and 0·9035 when $n=20$. Thus an F_1 of 20 should generally suffice.

Similarly the frequency of $\dfrac{\mathbf{Ra}\ +\ \mathbf{Sd}}{+\ \mathbf{a}\ +}$ or $\dfrac{\mathbf{Ra}\ +\ \mathbf{Sd}}{+\ \mathbf{a}^t\ +}$ is 0·14. So the probability of finding at least one female and male is $1-4\times 0{\cdot}86^n+4\times 0{\cdot}79^n-0{\cdot}72^n$. This is 0·4588 when $n=10$, and 0·8396 when $n=20$. Again, an F_1 of 20 should generally suffice.

Carter bases his search for lethals on the enumeration of double recessives, such as $\dfrac{\mathbf{a}\ \mathbf{pa}}{\mathbf{a}\ \mathbf{pa}}$. He proposes, if I understand him correctly, to go on breeding until either the number x of double recessives due to each adjacent pair of loci exceeds x_1, when a lethal is assumed to be absent, or until for one pair at least, the value of x falls below x_2, in which case a lethal is assumed to be present in the segment in question. x_1 and x_2 are calculated from the number of F_2 mice observed and the recombination values so as to render the probabilities of falsely supposing a lethal to be present, or of missing one, both less than 1%. I am not wholly convinced of the validity of Carter's calculations, but they are clearly an approximation to the truth.

'When x lies between x_1 and x_2,' Carter continues, 'the data fail to discriminate between the hypotheses, and the F_2 must be continued.' In fact, if x_1 and x_2 differ considerably, and x lies between them, we should, I think, consider a third hypothesis, namely, that a sublethal gene is present in the segment and there is evidence against lethals in the segments on each side of it.

A concrete example will make the matter clear.

Suppose that an F_2 of twenty-five mice contains four **+**^{Ra} **a**, two **a pa**, three **pa fi**, five **fi +**^{Sd}. Except for the **a pa**, these numbers do not seriously suggest a lethal. For **a pa**, in Carter's terminology $r_1 = 0{\cdot}263$, $r_2 = 0{\cdot}010$. The expected number of **a pa** in absence of a lethal is 6·575, in presence of a lethal in the **a pa** segment 0·25 or less. The probability of finding two or less **a pa** is 0·0234 in absence of a lethal, that of finding two or more is 0·0256 or less in presence of a lethal. If it were not for the figures for the other double recessives, the **a pa** figures could be explained by the presence of a lethal outside the **a pa** segment, but near it. If this were the case the number of double recessives in one of the adjoining segments would almost certainly be less than two. Now if there is a sublethal of which a fraction s of homozygotes survive the expected number of **a pa** is nearly $n[sr_1 + (1-s)r_2]$ or $n(0{\cdot}010 + 0{\cdot}253s)$. This condition is satisfied if $s = 0{\cdot}277$. But even if s were as low as 0·1 the expected numbers of **a pa** could be as high as 0·8, and it would not be surprising to find 2.

Carter's suggested programme of continuing the breeding of an F_2 as long as possible if x lies between x_1 and x_2 is therefore well adapted for the discovery of sublethal mutations. It is unlikely to find any where the survivorship is as high as 50%, and those whose survivorship is as low as 5% are likely to be reported as lethals. So it is not fully quantitative.

One further point which should be made is the following. A physiological disturbance which would be sublethal in the mouse would not necessarily be so in a monotocous species such as man or cattle. In all mouse stocks there is a considerable loss of embryos, and homozygotes for a number of well-known genes have heightened prenatal mortality. A homozygote in which the embryonic growth rate was sufficiently slowed down might be effectively almost lethal in large litters, and harmless in a species where most births were of single individuals. Thus, until the nature of the lethal or sublethal action of a gene in the mouse is discovered, it will not be quite safe to assume that a homologous or analogous mutation in man would have a similar effect, even though this is probably true for all the lethals so far known.

I have to thank Dr Carter for a valuable criticism.

CONCLUSION

Carter's proposed method is well adapted for the discovery of sublethal mutations.

Reprinted from the JOURNAL OF GENETICS Vol. 57, No. 1, June 1960.
Pages 131—136

THE INTERPRETATION OF CARTER'S RESULTS ON INDUCTION OF RECESSIVE LETHALS IN MICE

By J. B. S. HALDANE
Indian Statistical Institute, Calcutta-35

Carter (1959) using a method suggested by Haldane (1956) bred from 158 pairs of irradiated mice and as many controls. He concluded that two recessive lethals had appeared by mutation among the controls, and only one among the irradiated mice. I give reasons why this conclusion seems to me questionable. It can be argued that three of Carter's irradiated pairs showed evidence that each was heterozygous for a recessive lethal. If this is so his further conclusions require considerable modification.

Carter's method was this. A stock of mice homozygous for six recessive markers (counting **d** and **se** as one) was irradiated. The total dose was 600 r to the father and both grandfathers of the mice whose gametes were tested. It is not stated whether X or gamma rays were used, but the dose appears to have been fairly acute, and breeding began after the sterility following it had ceased. The progeny of an irradiated father and two irradiated grandfathers were mated to wild-type mice, and from each mating one F_1 pair was mated. 158 pairs raised four litters each. 11 of these F_2 contained so few of one or other of the six recessives as to "qualify for further investigation". This took two forms. Further F_2 litters were raised, where possible. And the F_1 father was mated to daughters of "wild" phenotype (at the locus under investigation) previously shown to be heterozygous by a test mating. Full details are given in Carter's Tables 3, 4, and 5.

Let us consider pair 126. The first four litters included only 3 **a**/**a** (non-agouti) mice out of 51. A fifth litter of 13 containing no **a**/**a** confirmed the hypothesis of a lethal linked with **a**. The F_1 mother then died. A number (not stated) of "wild-type" i.e. +/+ or +/**a** daughters were tested by mating with **a**/**a** males. Four were found to be heterozygous and mated with their father. They produced 8 **a**/**a** out of 43, 8 out of 48, 13 out of 46, and 6 out of 12. I now quote Carter. "In pair 126 the female died after raising her fifth litter; her great fertility (64 young classified in 5 litters) argues against the presence of a lethal, but if one were present, its recombination with **a** would be estimated to be 7·3 per cent. In that event the expected frequency of **aa** homozygotes, upon back-crossing to the F_1 male his +/**a** daughters, would be 9·8 per cent, or 14·6 among 149 classified young; the observed number, 35, is greatly in excess of this. It must be concluded that there was no linked lethal present."

I believe that this argument is incorrect and misleading for several reasons. First, in such a case it is incorrect to choose, in order to test a hypothesis, the value of an unknown parameter given by a part only of the numerical data.

Let us ask two questions.

(1) What is the frequency with which a pair would give 3 or fewer recessives out of 64 in the absence of a linked lethal, 16 recessives being expected ?

(2) What is the frequency with which one set of matings would give 3 recessives out of 64 and another 35 out of 149 when the same frequency was expected in each ?

The answer to the first question is

$$P = 4^{-64}\times 3^{61}(3^3+3^2\cdot 63+\tfrac{1}{2}\cdot 3\cdot 63\cdot 62+\tfrac{1}{6}\cdot 63\cdot 62\cdot 61)$$
$$= 4^{-64}\times 3^{63}\times 13954$$
$$= 4\cdot 694\times 10^{-5}.$$

The answer to the second is approximately found from the 2×2 table

61	3
114	35

which gives $\chi^2_1=10\cdot 78$, $P=1\cdot 03\times 10^{-3}$.

Thus even if we suppose that all the tested daughters had the same genotype as their mother, it seems that we should be justified in deciding in favour of the less unlikely hypothesis, namely that a linked lethal was present. It can easily be seen that the estimate of the recombination frequency is about 32%. However if Carter's argument were correct, we should be forced to choose between two hypotheses both of which are very improbable.

We have now to consider Carter's second assumption. This is that if we calculate the expected number of recessives in the progeny of a group of families produced by back-crossing to daughters, we can then treat this estimate as if it were obtained on the basis of Mendelian expectation. This is not so. The daughters may be of three different genotypes, and if, as in this case, four daughters are used, there are 81 possible expectations, and it is not a simple matter to calculate the standard error of their weighted mean. To explain the calculations which follow, it will be necessary to repeat some of the argument of Haldane (1956). I assume a recessive marker **a** linked with a recessive lethal **l**, the frequency of recombination being p. I have shown that the differences in recombination frequency between the two sexes may be neglected without serious loss of accuracy. In a F_2 or other family from $\frac{+\ \ +}{\mathbf{a}\ \ \mathbf{l}}\times\frac{+\ \ +}{\mathbf{a}\ \ \mathbf{l}}$, we expect the following frequencies of genotypes:

+ +/+ +	$\frac{1}{3}(1-p)^2$	
+ +/+ **l**	$\frac{2}{3}p(1-p)$	
+ +/**a l**	$\frac{2}{3}(1-p)^2$	} $\frac{2}{3}(1-p+p^2)$
+ +/**a** +	$\frac{2}{3}p(1-p)$	
a +/+ **l**	$\frac{2}{3}p^2$	
a +/**a** +	$\frac{1}{3}p^2$	} $\frac{1}{3}p(2-p)$
a +/**a l**	$\frac{2}{3}p(1-p)$	

The expected frequency of recessives is $x=\frac{1}{3}p(2-p)$. The three genotypes of +/**a** daughters are all detected with equal frequency by matings with **a** +/**a** + males. Their frequencies, among + **a** daughters are:

$$\frac{(1-p)^2}{1-p+p^2}\ +\ +/\mathbf{a}\ \mathbf{l},\quad \frac{p(1-p)}{1-p+p^2}\ +\ +/\mathbf{a}\ +,\ \text{and}\ \frac{p^2}{1-p+p^2}\ \mathbf{a}\ +/+\ \mathbf{l}.$$

Mated with their father, the expected frequencies of recessive offspring are $\frac{1}{3}p(2-p)$, $\frac{1}{4}$, and $\frac{1}{3}(1-p+p^2)$. For example if $p=0{\cdot}25$, which we shall see is a plausible value, we should expect only $\frac{9}{13}$ of the daughters to be + +/**a l** like their mother. And the probability that all four daughters mated to the father were + +/**a l** is only ·2297. Thus Carter's results become a great deal more explicable, since one or two of the tested daughters were probably + +/**a** +.

A rigorous calculation, either of the likelihood of a value of p in a given neighbourhood, or of the probability of getting a worse fit to expectation than the observed, is extremely laborious. For each value of p it would be necessary to compute probabilities for each of the 81 different sets of genotypes to which the four daughters might belong. I shall merely show that some values of p are quite likely, on the evidence given by Carter. This is all that is usually done in a F_2 analysis.

Let $p=\cdot25$, and suppose, first, that one daughter was $\frac{+\ \ +}{\mathbf{a}\ \ +}$ and three were $\frac{+\ \ +}{\mathbf{a}\ \ \mathbf{l}}$. This would occur in 30·6% of all cases. Further suppose that this daughter was the one which produced 6 recessives out of 12. We have the results of Table 1. $\chi^2_5=16{\cdot}66$, $P=\cdot0054$. If however throughout the expectation is one quarter recessives we have the results of Table 2. $\chi^2_5=20{\cdot}93$, $P=\cdot00084$. Let us now suppose that two daughters

TABLE 1

Mother of family			Total	Recessives	Expectation	χ^2
F_1 female			64	3	9·333	5·031
F_2	,,	1	43	8	6·271	0·558
,,	,,	2	48	8	7	0·167
,,	,,	3	46	13	6·708	6·908
,,	,,	4	12	6	3	4·000
Total			213	38	32·312	16·664

χ^2 table for pair 126, assuming $p=\cdot25$, and the daughter $\frac{+\ \ +}{\mathbf{a}\ \ +}$, the other 3 $\frac{+\ \ +}{\mathbf{a}\ \ \mathbf{l}}$.

TABLE 2

Mother of family			Total	Recessives	Expectation	χ^2
F_1 female			64	3	16	14·083
F_2	,,	1	43	8	10·75	0·937
,,	,,	2	48	8	12	1·778
,,	,,	3	46	13	11·5	0·130
,,	,,	4	12	6	3	4·000
Total			213	38	63·25	20·928

χ^2 table for pair 126, assuming no lethal present.

were $\frac{+\ +}{\mathbf{a}\ +}$ and two $\frac{+\ +}{\mathbf{a}\ \mathbf{l}}$. This would be so in 15·3% of all cases. Further suppose that the two $\frac{+\ +}{\mathbf{a}\ +}$ daughters were the mothers of 46 and 12 offspring respectively. In Table 2 we have to substitute 0·130 for 6·908 in the χ^2 column. χ^2_5 is reduced to 9·886. P=·074, which is not significantly low. A similar calculation for p=·20 gives χ^2_5=11·955. These values would be slightly lowered if the mother (4) of the family of 12 were $\frac{\mathbf{a}\ +}{+\ \mathbf{l}}$, in which case χ^2 is reduced by 1·964. I conclude that there is no serious reason to doubt that the members of pair 126 were heterozygous for the same lethal, probably distant 20-25 cM from the locus of **a**.

Similarly let us consider pair 107. The recessive marker with which linkage was suspected is **c**$^{\mathbf{ch}}$. I have used the symbol **c** for convenience. The numbers are unfortunately small. In Table 3 I give the expectations on the hypothesis that p=·25,

TABLE 3

Mother of family			Total	Recessives	Expectation	χ^2
F_1 female			42	3	6·125	1·870
F_2	,,	3	31	10	7·75	0·871
,,	,,	1	38	11	9·5	0·316
,,	,,	4	30	7	4·375	0·820
,,	,,	5	43	7	6·271	0·099
,,	,,	2	38	4	5·542	0·502
Total			222	42	39·563	4·478

χ^2 table for pair 107, assuming p=·25, and daughters 3 and 1 to be $\frac{+\ +}{\mathbf{a}\ +}$, the other three being $\frac{+\ +}{\mathbf{a}\ \mathbf{l}}$.

and 3 daughters were $\frac{+\ +}{\mathbf{c}\ \mathbf{l}}$ while 2 were $\frac{+\ +}{\mathbf{c}\ +}$. This is the most probable distribution, since the frequencies of $\frac{+\ +}{\mathbf{c}\ \mathbf{l}}$, $\frac{+\ +}{\mathbf{c}\ +}$, and $\frac{\mathbf{c}\ +}{+\ \mathbf{l}}$ daughters are $\frac{8}{13}$, $\frac{4}{13}$ and $\frac{1}{13}$. I further assume that daughters 3 and 1 were $\frac{+\ +}{\mathbf{c}\ +}$. χ^2_6=4·478, P=·61. The fit is excellent, Table 4 shows that with p=·5 (no lethal) χ^2_6=12·60, P=·050. No doubt a better fit could be obtained by using a different value of p, and assuming that daughter 3 was $\frac{\mathbf{c}\ +}{+\ \mathbf{l}}$, as she may have been. Moreover the value ·05 is too high, for it would probably be better not to consider daughters 3 and 1. We should then have $\chi^2_4 = 11{\cdot}418$, $P = {\cdot}025$. We cannot come to a very firm conclusion, given the small sizes of the families. But there is no ground for rejecting the hypothesis of a linked lethal, as Carter claims. And as a rule for decision has been laid down, this pair should, I think, be regarded as heterozygous for the same lethal.

The remaining suspected progenies from irradiated ancestries were regarded as false clues because in the fifth and later litters recessives appeared in such numbers as to lead to rejection on the criteria given in Carter's Table 1.

I conclude then, that among 158 pairs from unirradiated ancestors there were two lethals; among 158 from irradiated ancestors, there were two lethals (in pairs 55 and

TABLE 4

Mother of family			Total	Recessives	Expectation	χ^2
F_1 female			42	3	10·5	7·143
F_2	,,	3	31	10	7·75	0·871
,,	,,	1	38	11	9·5	0·316
,,	,,	4	30	7	7·5	0·044
,,	,,	5	43	7	10·75	1·047
,,	,,	2	38	4	9·5	3·184
Total			222	42	55·5	12·605

χ^2 table for pair 107, assuming no lethal present.

126) with very high probability and one more (in pair 107) with a moderately high probability, which must however be taken as present according to the criteria adopted, and therefore the length of chromosome scanned.

The length scanned in the irradiated series is only very slightly less than in the control series (see Carter's Table 6). The number of lethals found according to my argument, namely 3, is of course not significantly greater than 2. It is quite consistent with the expectation calculated by Carter from Russell's data, namely 2·3, the control value being unexpectedly high. On Haldane's (1956) "guess" of one recessive lethal mutation per gamete per 300 r, confirmed by Carter (1957) we should have expected about 14 lethals. This figure is therefore almost certainly too high. But a figure of 1 per 600 r is quite possible.

One of the most surprising features of Carter's work is the discovery of two recessive lethals in the controls. Carter states that his multiple recessive (PCA) stock was maintained with the minimum amount of inbreeding. This may perhaps be undesirable. We must reckon with the possibility that some lethal genes increase fitness in heterozygotes, and will therefore spread in outbred populations.

If it is considered that my criticism of Carter's conclusions is valid, I must accept a fair share of the blame, as I only dealt in a rather cursory manner with the

9

confirmation of suspected lethals. However it is to be noted that Carter did not use the principal method which I suggested, namely the use of the recessive mice appearing in F_2 to build up new stocks heterozygous for the lethal and the marker gene.

I do not know whether research on these lines is being continued at Harwell. According to Sugahara, Tutikawa, and Tanaka (1959) it is being continued at the National Institute of Genetics, Misima, Japan. It is, I think, clear from my discussion that each lethal believed to have been detected should be very thoroughly investigated. This is in any case desirable, since it is important to know at what stage in the life cycle a lethal acts; and if any extrapolation is made to man, this is very important (Haldane 1956).

SUMMARY

An analysis of Carter's data on the induction by X-rays of autosomal recessive genes in mice leads to the conclusion that he almost certainly obtained two, and very probably three such lethals in his irradiated stock, whereas he only claims to have obtained one.

REFERENCES

CARTER, T. C. (1957). Recessive lethal mutation induced in the mouse by chronic gamma radiation. *Proc. Roy. Soc. B*, **147**, 402-411.

CARTER, T. C. (1959). A pilot experiment with mice, using Haldane's method for detecting induced autosomal recessive lethal genes, *J. Genet.*, **56**, 353-362.

HALDANE, J. B. S. (1956). The detection of autosomal lethals in mice induced by mutagenic agents. *J. Genet.*, **54**, 327-342.

RUSSELL, W. L. (1959). Genetic effects of radiation in mammals. Radiation Biology 825-859 (New York).

SUGAHARA, T., TUTIKAWA, K., AND TANAKA, T. (1959). Studies on mutation rates after chronic irradiation in mice. A preliminary report on the sex ratio. *Ann. Rep. Nat. Inst. Genetics, Japan*, **9**, 102-104.

Haldane's Rule

In 1922, Haldane formulated a law that later came to be called "Haldane's Rule." This was based on a large body of data, which he assembled, relating heterogametic sex in the progeny of interspecific crosses with sex-ratio and sterility. With a few rare exceptions this rule has been generally found to be valid in most situations so far studied. It is the only rule or law that is widely known to be associated with Haldane's name.

VOLUME XII OCTOBER, 1922 No. 2

SEX RATIO AND UNISEXUAL STERILITY IN HYBRID ANIMALS.

BY J. B. S. HALDANE, M.A.
Fellow of New College, Oxford.

Many observers have noted that the crossing of different animal species produces an offspring one sex of which is rare or absent, or if present sterile, whilst occasionally the missing sex is represented by intermediate forms. Doncaster(1) concluded that the missing sex was generally the female, but, as will be shown later, this is by no means always the case. I believe, however, that the following rule applies to all cases so far observed, with one certain, and a few doubtful exceptions:—

When in the F_1 offspring of two different animal races one sex is absent, rare, or sterile, that sex is the heterozygous sex.

By the heterozygous sex is meant that sex which is known to be heterozygous for sex factors and sex-linked factors, to contain an odd pair or an odd number of chromosomes, and to produce two different classes of gametes, which normally determine the sex of the offspring. The heterozygous or digametic sex is in most groups the male, but in birds and Lepidoptera the female. Groups in which the male sex is haploid are only extreme cases of the normal type, in that all the chromosomes here behave like the sex-chromosomes of other groups.

Disturbances of sex-ratio and unisexual sterility have been observed as the result of crosses in Lepidoptera, Aves, Diptera, Mammalia, Anoplura, and Cladocera. I have here recorded all cases known to me in which (*a*) the animals were bred in captivity; (*b*) more than 10 offspring were raised, and (*c*) one sex was absent or sterile, or the sex-ratio was more than 2 : 1. In the tables *F* denotes fertility, *S* sterility established by testing several individuals. Of course the fertility is often subnormal.

Table I summarizes the data for Lepidoptera. Goldschmidt's results were each obtained with several different races. In the other crosses there were 24 cases where females were absent or rare, 10 where males were fertile and females sterile, and a number where there was an unstated excess of males; or else the males, though not known to have been fertile, were anatomically normal, whilst the females were clearly sterile.

Of exceptions to the rule there is first the case described by Goldschmidt(20) where crosses between two races of *Lymantria* gave

TABLE I.

Lepidoptera.

Mother	Father	Offspring	Offspring of reciprocal cross	Reference
Cerura erminea ...	*Cerura vinula*	9 ♂, 1 *S* ♀	—	Guillemot (2)
Clostera curtula ...	*Clostera anachoreta* ...	21 *F* ♂, 3 ☿, 2 *S* ♀	Excess *F* ♂'s, *S* ♀'s	Tutt (3)
Deilephila galii ...	*Chaerocampa elpenor* ...	>20 ♂, 8 ♀ [1]	—	Castek (4)
				Grosse (5)
Smerinthus ocellata ...	*Mimas tiliae*	20 ♂, no ♀	—	Standfuss (6)
,, ,, ...	*Calasymbolus astylus* ...	25 ♂, no ♀ [2]	—	Neumögen (7)
Amorpha populi ...	*Smerinthus ocellata* ...	490 ♂, 10 ♀ and ☿ [3]	2 ♂, no ♀	Tutt (8)
				Standfuss (6, 9)
,, ,, ...	,, *atlanticus* ...	9 ♂ : 1 ♀	>20 ♂, no ♀	,, (9)
				Dannenberg (10)
,, *austauti* ...	,, *ocellata* ...	93 ♂ : 7 ♀	—	,, (10)
,, ,, ...	,, *atlanticus* ...	45 ♂, 5 ♀	Excess ♂'s	Standfuss (9)
				Austaut (11)
				Dannenberg (10)
Saturnia spini	*Saturnia pavonia* ...	113 *F* ♂ : 100 *S* ♀	Excess ♂'s, *S* ♀'s	Standfuss (6, 12)
,, *pyri*	,, ,, ...	106 *F* ♂ : 100 *S* ♀	No ♂, 2 ♀	,, (6, 12)
Malacosoma franconica .	*Malacosoma neustria* ...	12 ♂, no ♀ [4]	No ♂, 1 ♀	,, (13)
Nyssia graecaria ...	*Lycia hirtaria*	65 *S* ♂, no ♀	—	Harrison (14)
,, *zonaria* ...	,, ,, ...	208 *S* ♂, no ♀	181 *F* ♂, 279 *S* ♀ [5]	,, (16)
,, ,, ...	*Poecilopsis isabellae* ...	32 ♂, no ♀	—	,, (16)
,, ,, ...	,, *pomonaria* ...	90 ♂, no ♀	44 ♂, 102 ♀	,, (16)
,, ,, ...	,, ,, (inbred)	71 ♂, 7 ♀	—	,, (16)
,, ,, ...	,, *lapponaria* ...	93 ♂, no ♀	Excess ♀'s	,, (16)
,, ,, ...	,, ,, (inbred)	62 ♂, 3 ♀	—	,, (16)
Lycia hirtaria (English)	,, *pomonaria* ...	86 *F* ♂, 75 *S* ♀	98 *F* ♂, 92 *F* ♀	,, (14)
,, (Scottish)	,, ,, ...	190 *F* ♂, 14 *S* ♀	—	,, (14)
Poecilopsis isabellae ...	*Lycia hirtaria*	38 *F* ♂, 32 *S* ♀	—	,, (14)
,, *lapponaria* ...	*Poecilopsis pômonaria* ...	38 *F* ♂, 1 ☿, 39 *S* ♀	—	,, (15)
Oporabia dilutata ...	*Oporabia autumnata* ...	6 ♂, no ♀ [6]	52 *F* ♂, 47 *S* ♀	,, (17)
Tephrosia bistortata ...	*Tephrosia crepuscularia*	378 *F* ♂, 12 *F* ♀	313 *F* ♂, 327 *F* ♀	,, (18)
				Tutt (19)
Lymantria dispar ...	*Lymantria dispar* ...	*F* ♂'s, *S* ♀'s	1 *F* ♂ : 1 *F* ♀	Goldschmidt (20)
,, ,, ...	,, ,, ...	*F* ♂'s, ☿'s	,,	,,
,, ,, ...	,, ,, ...	*F* ♂'s, no ♀	,,	,,
Fumea affinis	*Fumea nitidella* ...	♂'s, no ♀ [7]	♂'s, no ♀ [7]	Standfuss (12)
Basilarchia archippus ...	*Basilarchia arthemis* ...	>9 ♂, no ♀ [8]	—	Field (21)

[1] Grosse obtained 20 ♂, 8 ♀, Castek a number of ♂'s and no ♀'s.

[2] 20 chrysalides wintered over. Their sex was not recorded owing to the author's death, so they may have been the missing ♀'s.

[3] Out of about 500 imagines 98% were ♂'s, the remainder ♀ s, never normally developed, often with ♂ appendages.

[4] "Ein reichliches Dutzend."

[5] I have described the male as fertile, though several males between them only fathered one egg which hatched.

[6] 6 out of 400 pupae, all ♂, survived.

[7] "Eine Anzahl."

[8] These 9 were bred in captivity. All the wild examples were also ♂.

intersexual males, and an excess of males. This took place in two broods only. Goldschmidt's other intersexual males occurred either sporadically or in generations later than F_1, and are therefore not exceptions. It seems just possible that the intersexuality of the two aberrant broods may have been due to disease or other external conditions, or to unsuspected heterozygosis of one parent. His theoretical explanation of them is not convincing, since he ascribes to the race "Fukuoka" on p. 103 (*loc. cit*) a formula which, according to the analysis on p. 66, is entirely inconsistent with its being a "weak" race as stated on p. 12 and borne out by its behaviour in other crosses.

In two of Harrison's reciprocal crosses noted in the table there was a moderate excess of females, though in one of them these females were sterile. Standfuss(6, 12) mentions five cases where a species-cross gave only females. In three of these the numbers of females recorded were two, one, and one, which are insignificant; one (*Drepana falcataria* ♀ × *D. curvatula* ♂) was subsequently shown by him to give both sexes in equal numbers. In the last (*Malacosoma castrensis* ♀ × *neustria* ♂) Bacot(22) found that the males emerged a year after the females, but in only slightly smaller numbers.

Finally Fletcher(23) obtained a brood of 33 females and no males from a *Cymatophora or* ♀, supposed to have been fertilized by a *C. ocularis* ♂, but he was himself dubious of their paternity. There are thus no undoubted exceptions outside *Lymantria*.

The data for Aves are summarized in Table II.

TABLE II.

Aves.

Mother	Father	Offspring	Reference
Turtur orientalis ...	*Columba livia* ...	13 *S* ♂, 1 ♀	Whitman and Riddle (24)
Streptopelia risoria ...	,, ...	38 *F* ♂, no ♀[1]	,, ,, ,,
,, *alba-risoria*[2]	,, ...	11 ♂, no ♀	,, ,, ,,
,, *risoria* ...	*Zenaidura carolinensis*	16 *S* ♂, no ♀	,, ,, ,,
,, *alba-risoria*	*Stigmatopelia senegalensis*	17 *F* ♂, 1 ♂ or ☿, 9 *F* ♀	,, ,, ,,
,, *alba* and hybrids[2]	*Ectopistes migratorius*	10 *S* ♂, no ♀	,, ,, ,,
Gallus domesticus ...	*Phasianus colchicus* ...	>100 *S* ♂, 1 ? ♂	Lewis Jones (in litt.)
Phasianus reevesi ...	,, *torquatus* ,, *versicolor*	161 *S* ♂, 6 *S* ♀	Smith and Haig-Thomas (25)
Tetrao urogallus ...	*Tetrao tetrix*	40 ♂, 8 ♀	Suchetet, cit. Guyer (26)

Besides these crosses many have been made, giving smaller numbers, or less aberrant sex-ratios. They are described by the authorities cited

[1] One male begot a few living young, most were sterile. .

[2] *Alba* and *risoria* yield fertile hybrids with normal sex-ratio. It therefore seems legitimate to include crosses of such hybrids along with crosses of pure species.

7—2

above, and Phillips(27). With regard to unisexual sterility the evidence is not clear. Whitman and Riddle(24) report one case (*Columba livia* ♀ × *Turtur orientalis* ♂) which gave two fertile males and one sterile female with rudimentary ovaries, and four cases where the males were fertile, and the females not known to be so, though not apparently proved sterile. The only possible exception is the cross of *Turtur orientalis* ♀ × *T. turtur* ♂, which gave 7 males and 14 females, all fertile. This may be compared with some of Harrison's cases which gave a moderate excess of females.

In Diptera the male is heterozygous. The data for the only recorded cross are given below, from Sturtevant(28).

Drosophila melanogaster ♀ × *D. simulans* ♂ gave 2 ♂, 3552 ♀, the reciprocal 588 ♂, 171 ♀.

Drosophila melanogaster XXY ♀ × *D. simulans* ♂ gave 59 ♂, 128 ♀.

All these hybrids were sterile. The males produced from XXY ♀'s were shown genetically to contain a *simulans* X like those of the reciprocal cross. These latter all die in some families, but all or almost all survive in others, the difference perhaps depending on the *simulans* parent. Thus, though one cross often gives an excess of males, there is a far greater excess of females in the reciprocal, the two recorded males being perhaps non-disjunctional exceptions.

The data with regard to mammals, where again the male is heterozygous, are given in Table III.

TABLE III.

Mammalia.

Mother		Father		Offspring	Reference
Cavia porcellus	...	*Cavia rufescens*	...	14 *S* ♂, 23 *F* ♀	Detlefsen (29)
Bos indicus	...	*Bibos frontalis*	...	19 *S* ♂, *F* ♀'s	Kuhn[1]
,, ,,	...	,, *sondaicus*	...	1 *S* ♂, *F* ♀'s	,,
,, *taurus*	...	,, *grunniens*	...	*S* ♂'s, *F* ♀'s	,,
,, ,,	...	*Bison americanus*	...	6 *S* ♂, 39 *F* ♀	Boyd (30)
,, ,,	...	,, *bonasus*	...	1 *S* ♂, 3 *F* ♀	Iwanow (31)

Here the males are always sterile, and sometimes rare. This sterility and paucity may persist after one or more generations of back-crossing. Thus in the guinea-pig cross the F_1 females with *porcellus* males gave 31*S* ♂, 52*F* ♀, and it was only in the next generation that a few of the males proved fertile. Similarly 19 yak-cow male hybrids containing $\frac{1}{8}$, $\frac{1}{4}$, $\frac{1}{2}$, $\frac{3}{4}$, and $\frac{7}{8}$ cow "blood" were all sterile, and three out of four males containing $\frac{1}{4}$ bison blood were sterile. Mammalian crosses sometimes give small excesses of males, not exceeding 30 %. Buffon (33)

[1] Quoted by Detlefsen (29) and Ackermann (32).

states that he obtained 7 males and 2 females from *Ovis aries* ♀ × *Capra hircus* ♂, but this has never been confirmed.

In Anoplura the method of sex-determination is unknown. Keilin and Nuttall(34) found that *Pediculus corporis* ♀ × *P. capitis* ♂ gave 310 ♂, 12 ☿, 107 ♀, whilst the reciprocal cross gave 242 ♂, 187 ♀. The normal sex rates for *P. corporis* is 144 ♂ : 100 ♀. The increased excess of males suggests that sex-determination is here perhaps on avian and lepidopteran lines, the female being heterozygous.

In Cladocera there seems to be no obvious cytological difference between the sexes. *Daphnia obtusa* ♀ × *D. pulex* ♂ was found by Agar(35) to give a great excess of sexual broods and males (all sterile) among the descendants by parthenogenesis of the single original female hybrid. As these disturbances did not occur in the first generation they are not really comparable with the other cases cited.

Thus, with the exception of Goldschmidt's intersexual male families the rule always holds as regards sterility, while in the rare cases where an excess of the heterozygous sex is produced the reciprocal cross always gives a greater excess of the homozygotes.

As pointed out by Sturtevant(28) the excess of homozygotes may be due to two distinct processes, a killing-off of the heterozygotes, or their transformation into members of the normally homozygous sex. In *Drosophila* the missing males die as larvae, on the other hand both Goldschmidt and Harrison have shown that in certain moth hybrids partial or complete transformation occurs. If the generalization of this paper is more than a mere coincidence it must be shown how these two effects, and also sterility, may be explained as due to the same cause.

Goldschmidt and Harrison have shown that many of their results can be explained by difference of intensity of the sex factors carried by the Z or X chromosomes in the two parental species. In *Drosophila* at least the other chromosomes play a part as well. In the pure races these factors are balanced by the cytoplasm or W chromosome, but in the hybrids there is a lack of balance. This will be most serious in the heterozygous sex, since in the homozygotes the effect of the two Z or X chromosomes will be the average of the parental values. The heterozygotes will tend to be pushed either towards the homozygous sex or towards an exaggeration of their own sex. Either of these effects in moderation may be expected to cause sterility, as pointed out by Harrison. The former may cause gynandromorphism, sex-reversal, or death when pushed further, the latter only death. Thus where both reciprocal crosses yield males only, as in *Fumea*, we may suppose that in one case some of the males are transformed females as in *Lymantria*, whilst in the other the zygotes with an exaggerated tendency to maleness have died. This hypothesis may be compared with the demonstration by Bridges(36) that in *Drosophila melanogaster* both supermales with one *X* chromosome and 3 sets of autosomes and superfemales with 3 *X*'s and 2 sets of autosomes are sterile and not very viable.

But since in some cases the heterozygotes are transformed, in others killed off, alteration of sex-potential must have different effects in different animals. That this should be so is intelligible when we consider the great difference between the effects of castration or parabiosis in different groups. In Lepidoptera these conditions have little or no effect on somatic development, in mammals a great deal. The case here is by no means parallel, since the somatic cells are affected directly and not through an internal secretion, but the analogy shows that we need not expect the same effect from the same cause in different groups.

Although the explanation in terms of sex factors is attractive we have no satisfactory evidence of their existence. If sex is due simply to a double dose of a factor in the *X* chromosome (or sex-linked factor group) we should expect this factor occasionally to mutate like its neighbours. This would lead, if the factor were lost in mammals or Diptera, to the production of males with two *X* chromosomes and two sets of sex-linked factors, which would now exhibit partial and not complete sex-linkage. But such a condition has never been observed.

Moreover, upsets of the sex-ratio similar to those found in species crosses have been recorded in which factors which are certainly not sex factors are involved. Examples from Drosophila are given in Table IV.

The missing males are not transformed, but die as embryos. The characters concerned are all sex-linked recessives to the normal, "glazed" and "rugose" being multiple allelomorphs. They appear in the normal

TABLE IV.

Mother	Father	Offspring	Offspring of reciprocal cross	Observer
Fused *melanogaster*	Normal *melanogaster*	No ♂, 823 *F* ♀	1 ♂ : 1 ♀	Lynch (37)
Fused *XXY melanogaster* ...	,, ,,	9 ♂, 744 *F* ♀	—	,,
Rudimentary ,, ...	,, ,,	10 ♂, 923 *F* ♀	1 ♂ : 1 ♀	Lynch (37) and Bridges (38)
Rudimentary *XXY melanogaster*	,, ,,	93 ♂, 647 *F* ♀	—	Lynch (37)
Rugose *virilis*	Glazed *virilis* ...	No ♂, *S* ♀'s	Nil	Metz and Bridges (39)

sex-ratio when the mother is a wild type heterozygote, but in each case the recessive female is almost wholly sterile. However "rudimentary" females have given 7 ♀ and 13 ♂ offspring with rudimentary males, so the upset of the sex-ratio is conditioned by crossing. The analogy with species crosses is striking, and may throw light on them. Two autosomal recessives in *melanogaster*, "morula" and "dwarf," behave similarly, except that with morula and dwarf males the recessive females have given 2 ♀ and 7 ♀ respectively, with no males. Finally according to Doncaster(40) colour-blind men have an excess of daughters by normal women. Although the data here are not so satisfactory, there is no sterility in the recessives.

Entia non sunt multiplicanda praeter necessitatem, and if ordinary factors, either sex-linked, like "rudimentary," or autosomal like "morula," can cause the disappearance of the heterozygous sex in crosses, we have no right to postulate sex factors for this purpose. A possible explanation of the phenomena under discussion is then as follows. In the course of the evolution of a species factorial differences arise between it and its parent species. They are perpetuated, probably by natural selection. Some of these factors, like "rudimentary," cause the death (or transformation) of the heterozygous sex when the new form is crossed with the ancestral. How this happens is quite obscure, but such factors do exist, whereas sex factors, though an attractive hypothesis, are nothing more. Moreover Bridges' (36) work on triploidy shows that sex may be determined by other groups of factors than those which normally determine it. It seems possible then, that sex is normally determined, not by a specific factor, but by the simultaneous activity of a fairly large group of factors, each of which has, or may have, other effects. The loss of any one member of this group will not cause a change of sex, though it may cause partial sterility. If sex were determined by a single factor it is very difficult to see what advantage there could be in its being linked with other factors. If on the other hand a number of factors determine it, it is essential that they should be linked. If in any animals sex is determined by one factor, there is probably no sex-linkage or chromosome difference between the sexes. As soon as another factor becomes necessary, complete linkage between the two must appear in the heterozygous sex, and the same mechanism which prevents them from crossing over may be expected to hinder or prevent crossing over of all factors in that sex.

I shall not attempt here to discuss the phenomena observed in the F_2 of the crosses considered. Their variability is partly explained by the fact that the fertile F_1 may either be all homozygotes, or in part transformed heterozygotes, partly by failures in reduction.

It is worth noticing that other disturbing influences do not affect the heterozygous sex more than the homozygous. Thus late fertilization turns XX frog zygotes into males, and the blood of their brothers converts XX mammalian embryos into freemartins. On the other hand the distinction between homozygous and heterozygous sex is more fundamental than that between male and female in determining the intensity of partial linkage between factors. Obviously sex-linked factors must be completely linked in the heterozygous sex, but linkage between autosomal factors is also always stronger in that sex. In *Drosophila melanogaster*, *simulans* and *virilis* linkage is always complete in the heterozygous male, in Bombyx, as shown by Tanaka(41), in the heterozygous female. Nabours(42) in *Apotettix* and Haldane(43) in *Paratettix* found linkage much stronger in the heterozygous male. And Dunn(44) showed that in the rat and mouse linkage is slightly stronger in the heterozygous male. If these facts are anything more than a coincidence they may be due to a greater difficulty of fusion of chromosome pairs in the heterozygous sex, and this in turn may be a contributory cause of its sterility. A possible evolutionary explanation of this stronger linkage has been suggested above.

I wish to record my thanks to the Rev. E. Lewis Jones for his information concerning pheasant-poultry hybrids.

Summary.

When in the F_1 offspring of a cross between two animal species or races one sex is absent, rare, or sterile, that sex is always the heterozygous sex.

REFERENCES.

1. DONCASTER. *The Determination of Sex*, p. 87.
2. GUILLEMOT. *Ann. Soc. Entom.* France, 1856, p. 29.
3. TUTT. *British Lepidoptera*, Vol. IV. pp. 1—38.
4. CASTEK. *Int. Ent. Zeit.* Vol. IV. p. 181, 1910.
5. GROSSE. *Int. Ent. Zeit.* Vol. V. p. 327, 1912.
6. STANDFUSS. *Proc.* VII. *Int. Zool. Congress*, pp. 113—115, 1907.
7. NEUMÖGEN. *Entom. News*, Vol. V. p. 326, 1894.
8. TUTT. *British Lepidoptera*, Vol. III. pp. 395, 448—459, 495.
9. STANDFUSS. *Bull. Soc. Entom.* France, 1901, pp. 87—89.
10. DANNENBERG. *Zeit. Wiss. Insektenbiol.* Vol. VIII. p. 27, 1912, Vol. IX. p. 294, 1913.

11. AUSTAUT. *Le Naturaliste.* Vol. XIV. p. 236.
12. STANDFUSS. *Handbuch der Palaearktische Grossschmetterlinge*, pp. 54—117.
13. ——. *Stett. Ent. Zeit.* Vol. XLV. p. 193, 1895.
14. HARRISON. *Journal of Genetics*, Vol. VI. p. 95, 1916.
15. ——. *Journal of Genetics*, Vol. VI. p. 269, 1917.
16. ——. *Journal of Genetics*, Vol. IX. p. 1, 1919.
17. ——. *Journal of Genetics*, Vol. IX. p. 195, 1920.
18. ——. *Journal of Genetics*, Vol. X. p. 61, 1920.
19. TUTT. *British Lepidoptera*, Vol. V. p. 31.
20. GOLDSCHMIDT. *Zeitsch. Ind. Abst. u. Ver.* Vol. XXIII. p. 1, 1920.
21. FIELD. *Psyche*, Vol. 21, p. 115, 1914.
22. BACOT. *Ent. Record*, Vol. XIV. p. 106, 1902, Vol. XV. p. 134, 1903.
23. FLETCHER. *Ent. Record*, Vol. IV. p. 304, 1893.
24. WHITMAN and RIDDLE. *Carn. Inst. Wash. Pub.* 257, Vol. II. 1919.
25. SMITH and HAIG-THOMAS. *Journal of Genetics*, Vol. III. p. 39, 1913.
26. GUYER. *Biol. Bull.* Vol. XVI. p. 193, 1909.
27. PHILLIPS. *Journ. Exp. Zool.* Vol. XVI. p. 143, 1914.
28. STURTEVANT. *Genetics*, Vol. V. p. 488, 1920, Vol. VI. p. 179, 1921.
29. DETLEFSEN. *Carn. Inst. Wash. Pub.* 205, 1914.
30. BOYD. *Journal of Heredity*, Vol. V. p. 189, 1914.
31. IWANOW and PHILIPTCHENKO. *Zeit. Ind. Abst. u. Ver.* Vol. XVI. p. 1, 1916.
32. ACKERMANN. *Thierbastarde.*
33. BUFFON. *Histoire Naturelle*, Oeuvres Complètes. Quadrupèdes, VI. 1787, p. 378.
34. KEILIN and NUTTALL, *Parasitology*, Vol. II. p. 279.
35. AGAR. *Journal of Genetics*, Vol. X. p. 303, 1920.
36. BRIDGES. *Am. Nat.* Vol. LVI. p. 51, 1922.
37. LYNCH. *Genetics*, Vol. IV. p. 501, 1919.
38. BRIDGES and MORGAN. *Carn. Inst. Wash. Publ.* 278, p. 231, 1919.
39. METZ and BRIDGES. *Proc. Nat. Ac. Sci.* Vol. III. p. 673, 1917; Vol. VI. p. 421, 1920.
40. DONCASTER. *The Determination of Sex*, p. 48.
41. TANAKA. *Trans. Sapporo Nat. Hist. Soc.* Vol. V. 1914.
42. NABOURS. *Am. Nat.* Vol. LIII. p. 131, 1919.
43. HALDANE. *Journal of Genetics*, Vol. X. p. 47, 1920.
44. DUNN. *Genetics*, Vol. V. p. 325, 1919.

Origins of Life

Throughout his life, Haldane was greatly interested in finding an adequate explanation to account for the origin of life on earth. In a series of papers he put forward novel ideas and hypotheses and preferred to use the plural "origins" to suggest the possibility of the independent appearance of systems with a quasi-vital degree of complexity. Haldane and A.I. Oparin independently suggested a plausible mechanism for the origin of life in an anaerobic prebiotic world. A summary of Haldane's ideas first appeared in *Nature*.[1] Both N.W. Pirie and A.I. Oparin have recognized the place that Haldane's ideas occupy in studies of the origin of life.[2]

1. News and Views. *Nature, 122*: 933–934, 1928.
2. See Dronamraju, K.R.: (Ed.) *Haldane and Modern Biology*. Baltimore: Johns Hopkins University Press, 1968; pp. 251–264.

1929

THE ORIGIN OF LIFE

UNTIL 1668 it was generally believed that living beings were constantly arising out of dead matter. Maggots were supposed to be generated spontaneously in decaying meat. In that year Redi showed that this did not happen provided insects were carefully excluded. And in 1860 Pasteur extended the proof to the bacteria which he had shown were the cause of putrefaction. It seemed fairly clear that all the living beings known to us originate from other living beings. At the same time Darwin gave a new emotional interest to the problem. It had appeared unimportant that a few worms should originate from mud. But if man was descended from worms such spontaneous generation acquired a new significance. The origin of life on the earth would have been as casual an affair as the evolution of monkeys into man. Even if the latter stages of man's history were due to natural causes, pride clung to a supernatural, or at least surprising, mode of origin for his ultimate ancestors. So it was with a sigh of relief that a good many men, whom Darwin's arguments had convinced, accepted the conclusion of Pasteur that life can originate only from life. It was possible either to suppose that life had been supernaturally created on earth some millions of years ago, or that it had been brought to earth by a meteorite or by micro-organisms floating through interstellar space. But a large number, perhaps the majority, of biologists believed, in spite of Pasteur, that at some time in the remote past life had originated on earth from dead matter as the result of natural processes.

The more ardent materialists tried to fill in the details of this process, but without complete success. Oddly enough, the few scientific men who professed idealism agreed with them. For if one can find evidence of mind (in religious terminology the finger of God) in the most ordinary events, even those which go on in the chemical laboratory, one can without too much difficulty believe in the origin of life from such processes. Pasteur's work therefore appealed most strongly to those who desired to stress the contrast between mind and matter. For a variety of obscure historical reasons, the Christian Churches have taken this latter point of view. But it should never be forgotten that the early Christians held many views which are now regarded as materialistic. They believed in the resurrection of the body, not the immortality of the soul. St Paul seems to have attributed consciousness and will to the body. He used a phrase translated in the revised version as 'the mind of the flesh', and credited the flesh with a capacity for hatred, wrath, and other mental functions. Many modern physiologists hold similar beliefs. But, perhaps fortunately for Christianity, the Church was captured by a group of very inferior Greek philosophers in the third and fourth centuries AD. Since that date views as to the relation between mind and body which St Paul, at least, did not hold have been regarded as part of Christianity, and have retarded the progress of science.

It is hard to believe that any lapse of time will dim the glory of Pasteur's positive achievements. He published singularly few experimental results. It has even been suggested by a cynic that his entire work would not gain a Doctorate of Philosophy today! But every experiment was final. I have never heard of anyone who has repeated any experiment of Pasteur's with a result different from that of the master. Yet his deductions from these experiments were sometimes too sweeping. It is perhaps not quite irrelevant that he worked in his later years with half a brain. His right cerebral hemisphere had been extensively wrecked when he was only forty-five years old; and the united brain power of the microbiologists who succeeded him has barely compensated for that accident. Even during his lifetime some of the conclusions which he had drawn from his experimental work were disproved. He had said that alcoholic fermentation was impossible without life. Buchner obtained it with a cell-free and dead extract of yeast. And since his death the gap between life and matter has been greatly narrowed.

When Darwin deduced the animal origin of man a search began for a 'missing link' between ourselves and the apes. When Dubois found the bones of Pithecanthropus some comparative anatomists at once proclaimed that they were of animal origin, while others were equally convinced that they were parts of a human skeleton. It is now generally recognized that either party was right, according to the definition of humanity adopted. Pithecanthropus was a creature which might legitimately be described either as a man or an ape, and its existence showed that the distinction between the two was not absolute.

Now the recent study of ultramicroscopic beings has brought up at least one parallel case, that of the bacteriophage, discovered by d'Herelle, who had been to some extent anticipated by Twort. This is the cause of a disease or, at any rate, abnormality of bacteria. Before the size of the atom was known there was no reason to doubt that

> *Big fleas have little fleas*
> *Upon their backs to bite 'em;*
> *The little ones have lesser ones,*
> *And so* ad infinitum.

But we now know that this is impossible. Roughly speaking, from the point of view of size, the bacillus is the flea's flea, the bacteriophage the bacillus' flea; but the bacteriophage's flea would be of the dimensions of an atom, and atoms do not behave like fleas. In other words, there are only about as many atoms in a cell as cells in a man. The link between living and dead matter is therefore somewhere between a cell and an atom.

D'Herelle found that certain cultures of bacteria began to swell up and burst until all had disappeared. If such cultures were passed through a filter fine enough to keep out all bacteria, the filtrate could infect fresh bacteria, and so on indefinitely. Though the infective agents cannot be seen with a microscope, they can be counted as follows. If an active filtrate containing bacteriophage be poured over a colony of bacteria on a jelly, the bacteria will all, or almost all, disappear. If it be diluted many thousand times, a few islands of living bacteria survive for some time. If it be diluted about ten million fold, the bacteria are destroyed round only a few isolated spots, each representing a single particle of bacteriophage.

Since the bacteriophage multiplies, d'Herelle believes it to be a living organism. Bordet and others have taken an opposite view. It will survive heating and other insults which kill the large majority of organisms, and will multiply only in presence of living bacteria, though it can break up dead ones. Except perhaps in presence of bacteria, it does not use oxygen or display any other signs of life. Bordet and his school therefore regard it as a ferment which breaks up bacteria as our own digestive ferments break up our food, at the same time inducing the disintegrating bacteria to produce more of the same ferment. This is not as fantastic as it sounds, for most cells while dying liberate or activate ferments which digest themselves. But these ferments are certainly feeble when compared with the bacteriophage.

Clearly we are in doubt as to the proper criterion of life. D'Herelle says that the bacteriophage is alive, because, like the flea or the tiger, it can multiply indefinitely at the cost of living beings. His opponents say that it can multiply only as long as its food is alive, whereas the tiger certainly, and the flea probably, can live on dead products of life. They suggest that the bacteriophage is like a book or a work of art which is constantly being copied by living beings, and is therefore only metaphorically alive, its real life being in its copiers.

The American geneticist Müller has, however, suggested an intermediate view. He compares the bacteriophage to a gene—that is to say, one of the units concerned in heredity. A fully coloured and a spotted dog differ because the latter has in each of its cells one or two of a certain gene, which we know is too small for the microscope to see. Before a cell of a dog divides, this gene divides also, so that each of the daughter cells has one, two, or none according with the number in the parent cell. The ordinary spotted dog is healthy, but a gene common among German dogs causes a roan colour when one is present, while two make the dog nearly white, wall-eyed, and generally deaf, blind, or both. Most of such dogs die young, and the analogy to the bacteriophage is fairly close. The main difference between such a lethal gene, of which many are known, and the bacteriophage is that the one is only known inside the cell, the other outside. In the present state of our ignorance we may regard the gene either as a tiny organism which can divide in the environment provided by the rest of the cell, or as a bit of machinery which the 'living' cell copies at each division. The truth is probably somewhere in between these two hypotheses.

Unless a living creature is a piece of dead matter plus a soul (a view which finds little support in modern biology), something of the following kind must be true. A simple organism must consists of parts A, B, C, D, and so on, each of which can multiply only in presence of all, or almost all, of the others. Among these parts are genes, and the bacteriophage is such a part which has got loose. This hypothesis becomes more plausible if we believe in the work of Handuroy, who finds that the ultramicroscopic particles into which the bacteria have been broken up, and which pass through filters that can stop the bacteria, occasionally grow up again into bacteria after a lapse of several months. He brings evidence to show that such fragments of bacteria may cause disease, and d'Herelle and Peyre claim to have found the ultramicroscopic form of a common staphylococcus, along with bacteriophage, in cancers, and suspects that this combination may be the cause of that disease.

On this view the bacteriophage is a cog, as it were, in the wheel of a life cycle of many bacteria. The same bacteriophage can act on different species, and is thus, so to say, a spare part which can be fitted into a number of different machines, just as a human diabetic can remain in health when provided with insulin manufactured by a pig. A great many kinds of molecule have been got from cells, and many of them are very efficient when removed from it. One can separate from yeast one of the many tools which it uses in alcoholic fermentation, an enzyme called invertase, and this will break up six times its weight of cane sugar per second for an indefinite time without wearing out. As it does not form alcohol from the sugar, but only a sticky mixture of other sugars, its use is permitted in the US in the manufacture of confectionery and cake-icing. But such fragments do not reproduce themselves, though they take part in the assimilation of food by the living cell. No one supposes that they are alive. The bacteriophage is a step beyond the enzyme on the road to life, but it is perhaps an exaggeration to call it fully alive. At about the same stage on the road are the viruses which cause such diseases as smallpox, herpes, and hydrophobia. They can multiply only in living tissue, and pass through filters which stop bacteria.

With these facts in mind we may, I think, legitimately speculate on the origin of life on this planet. Within a few thousand years from its origin it probably cooled down so far as to develop a fairly permanent solid crust. For a long time, however, this crust must have been above the boiling point of water, which condensed only gradually. The primitive atmosphere probably contained little or no oxygen, for our present supply of that gas is only about enough to burn all the coal and other organic remains found below and on the earth's surface. On the other hand, almost all the carbon now combined in chalk, limestone, and dolomite were in the atmosphere as carbon dioxide. Probably a good deal of the nitrogen now in the air was combined with metals as nitride in the earth's crust, so that ammonia was constantly being formed by the action of water. The sun was perhaps slightly brighter than it is now, and as there was no oxygen in the atmosphere, the chemically active ultra-violet rays from the sun were not, as they now are, mainly stopped by ozone (a modified form of oxygen) in the upper atmosphere, and oxygen itself lower down. They penetrated to the surface of the land and sea, or at least to the clouds.

Now, when ultra-violet light acts on a mixture of water, carbon dioxide, and ammonia, a vast variety of organic substances are made, including sugars and apparently some of the materials from which proteins are built up. This fact has been demonstrated in the laboratory by Baly of Liverpool and his colleagues. In this present world such substances, if left about, decay—that is to say, they are destroyed by micro-organisms. But before the origin of life they must have accumulated till the primitive oceans reached the consistency of hot dilute soup. Today an organism must trust to luck, skill, or strength to obtain its food. The first precursors of life found food available in considerable quantities, and had no competitors in the struggle for existence. As the primitive atmosphere contained little or no oxygen, they must have obtained the energy which they needed for growth by some other process than oxidation—in fact, by fermentation. For, as Pasteur put it, fermentation is life without oxygen. If this was so, we should expect that high organisms like ourselves would start life as anaerobic beings, just as we start as single cells. This is the case. Embryo chicks for the first two or three days after fertilization use very little oxygen, but obtain the energy which they need for growth by fermenting sugar into lactic acid, like the bacteria which turns milk sour. So do various embryo mammals, and in all probability you and I lived mainly by fermentation during the first week of our pre-natal life. The cancer cell behaves in the same way. Warburg has shown that with its embryonic habit of unrestricted growth there goes an embryonic habit of fermentation.

The first living or half-living things were probably large molecules synthesized under the influence of the sun's radiation, and only capable of reproduction in the particularly favourable medium in which they originated. Each presumably required a variety of highly specialized molecules before it could reproduce itself, and it depended on chance for a supply of them. This is the case today with most viruses, including the bacteriophage, which can grow only in presence of the complicated assortment of molecules found in a living cell.

The unicellular organisms, including bacteria, which were the simplest living things known a generation ago, are far more complicated. They are organisms—that is to say, systems whose parts co-operate. Each part is specialized to a particular chemical function, and prepares chemical molecules suitable for the growth of the other parts. In consequence, the cell as a whole can usually subsist on a few types of molecule, which are transformed within it into the more complex substances needed for the growth of the parts.

The cell consists of numerous half-living chemical molecules suspended in water and enclosed in an oily film. When the whole sea was a vast chemical laboratory the conditions for the formation of such films must have been relatively favourable; but for all that life may have remained in the virus stage for many millions of years before a suitable assemblage of elementary units was brought together in the first cell. There must have been many failures, but the first successful cell had plenty of food, and an immense advantage over its competitors.

It is probable that all organisms now alive are descended from one ancestor, for the following reason. Most of our structural molecules are asymmetrical, as shown by the fact that they rotate the plane of polarized light, and often form asymmetrical crystals. But of the two possible types of any such molecule, related to one another like a right and left boot, only one is found throughout living nature. The apparent exceptions to this rule are all small molecules which are not used in the building of the large structures which display the phenomena of life. There is nothing, so far as we can see, in the nature of things to prevent the existence of looking-glass organisms built from molecules which are, so to say, the mirror images in our own bodies. Many of the requisite molecules have already been made in the laboratory. If life had originated independently on several occasions, such organisms would probably exist. As they do not, this event probably occurred only once or, more probably, the descendants of the first living organism rapidly evolved far enough to overwhelm any later competitors when these arrived on the scene.

As the primitive organisms used up the foodstuffs available in the sea, some of them began to perform in their own bodies the synthesis formerly performed at haphazard by the sunlight, thus ensuring a liberal supply of food. The first plants thus came into existence, living near the surface of the ocean, and making food with the aid of sunlight as do their descendants today. It is thought by many biologists that we animals are descended from them. Among the molecules in our own bodies are a number whose structure resembles that of chlorophyll, the green pigment with which the plants have harnessed the sunlight to their needs. We use them for other purposes than the plants—for example, for carrying oxygen—and we do not, of course, know whether they are, so to speak, descendants of chlorophyll or merely cousins. But since the oxygen liberated by the first plants must have killed off most of the other organisms, the former view is the more plausible.

The above conclusions are speculative. They will remain so until living creatures have been synthesized in the biochemical laboratory. We are a long way from that goal. It was in 1928 that Pictel for the first time made cane sugar artificially. It is doubtful whether any enzyme has been obtained quite pure. Nevertheless I hope to live to see one made artificially. I do not think I shall behold the synthesis of anything so nearly alive as a bacteriophage or a virus, and I do not suppose that a self-contained organism will be made for centuries. Until that is done the origin of life will remain a subject for speculation. But such speculation is not idle, because it is susceptible of experimental proof or disproof.

Some people will consider it a sufficient refutation of the above theories to say that they are materialistic, and that materialism can be refuted on philosophical grounds. They are no doubt compatible with materialism, but also with other philosophical tenets. The facts are, after all, fairly plain. Just as we know of sight only in connection with a particular kind of material system called the eye, so we know only of life in connection with certain arrangements of matter, of which the biochemist can give a good, but far from complete, account. The question at issue is: 'How did the first such system on this planet originate?' This is a historical problem to which I have given a very tentative answer on the not unreasonable hypothesis that a thousand million years ago matter obeyed the same laws that it does today.

This answer is compatible with, for example, the view that pre-existent mind or spirit can associate itself with certain kinds of matter. If so, we are left with the mystery as to why mind has so marked a preference for a particular type of colloidal organic substances. Personally I regard all attempts to describe the relation of mind to matter as rather clumsy metaphors. The biochemist knows no more, and no less, about this question than anyone else. His ignorance disqualifies him no more than the historian or the geologist from attempting to solve a historical problem.

Systems of Predication

Haldane was greatly interested in systems of logic and predication, which can be widely applied to scientific results and their interpretation. In India, he explored both Hindu and Jaina philosophies—especially those aspects that seemed to him to offer systems of logic that can be applied to the classification and interpretation of scientific results. This is, of course, as relevant to genetic analyses as any other branch of science. The following paper is concerned with the logical system of Bhadrabahu, a Jaina philosopher of fourth century B.C.

Reprinted from Sankhyā: The Indian Journal of Statistics, Vol. 18, Parts 1 & 2, 1957.

THE SYĀDVĀDA SYSTEM OF PREDICATION

By J. B. S. HALDANE

University College, London

The search for truth by the scientific method does not lead to complete certainty. Still less does it lead to complete uncertainty. Hence any logical system which allows of conclusions intermediate between certainty and uncertainty should interest scientists. The earliest such system known to me is the *Syādvāda* system of the Jaina philosopher Bhadrabahu (?433-357 B.C.). Mahalanobis (1954) has commented on it. A central feature of this system is the *saptabhangīnaya* or list of seven types of predication. These are as follows.

(1) *syādasti.*	May be it is.
(2) *syātnāsti.*	May be it is not.
(3) *syādasti nāsti ca.*	May be it is and is not.
(4) *syādavaktavyah.*	May be it is indeterminate.
(5) *syādasti ca avaktavyaśca.*	May be it is and is indeterminate.
(6) *syātnāsti ca avaktavyaśca.*	May be it is not and is indeterminate.
(7) *syādasti nasti ca avaktavyaśca.*	May be it is, is not, and is indeterminate.

Mahalanobis illustrated this from the throw of a coin, and held that it could serve as a foundation for statistics. However I wish to show that it arises naturally in simpler cases, including simple cases where the affirmative predication *asti* would be "This is hot", or "This is a man".

In any such case an uncertain judgement is usually somewhat quantitative, as in "I think this is a man, though it may be a statue." I therefore begin with a very abstract field, that of algebra. Here we may be certain of our answer. If $x+2 = 3$, then $x = 1$. But if $x^2-3x+2=0$, then $x = 1$ or 2. We cannot say that the probability that $x = 1$ is greater than, less than, or equal to the probability that $x = 2$. Further data may lead to either of these judgements. Five hundred years ago one might perhaps have spoken of indeterminate solutions of equations. Thus if $x^3-x^2+x-1 = 0$, $x = 1$ or $\pm\sqrt{-1}$. The last two solutions were *avakta* (incapable of being spoken) until the invention of complex numbers. Today we can find better examples in the field of finite arithmetic.

Consider the finite arithmetic *modulo* m. The only admissible values of a variable are the m residues $0, 1, 2, \ldots m-2, m-1$, that is to say the possible remainders after division by m. For example *modulo* 5, $4+3 = 7 = 5+2$, so we write $4+3 \equiv 2$. And $4\times 3 = 12 = 2\times 5+2$, so we write $4\times 3 \equiv 2$. Let us consider the theory of functions *modulo* m. We can define any function $f(x)$ by a table of the values which it assumes for the different admissible values of x. Thus the function $3x$ (*mod*.5) can be defined by the table 0, 3, 1, 4, 2. For example if $x = 4$, $3x \equiv 2$. Of course many other functions are identical with it. For example $3x^5 \equiv x^9+2x^5 \equiv 3x$. A function which assumes all the admissible values unequivocally is called biunivocal[1], and it is easy to show that there are $m!$ biunivocal functions. However some functions are univocal, but their inverses are not. In this case some residues do not occur in the table, while others occur more than once. For example the table of $3x^2+1$ (*mod.*5) is 1, 4, 3, 3, 4. The number of univocal functions is m^m, since each place in the table can be filled in m ways.

If a function is not univocal, but its inverse is univocal, we obtain a table such as that for $x^{\frac{1}{2}}$, namely 0, 1 or 4, अ. अ. 1 or 4. Here I introduce the symbol अ, for *avakta*, for an undefined number. There is no number whose square (*mod.* 5) is 2 or 3. अ may occur in a table as an alternative to a number. For example the function e^x is never integral when x is a residue other than zero. Nor is it integral for most values of x which are *avakta*, such as $\sqrt{2}$. But it is integral for such numbers as log 2. Hence the table of e^x is 1; अ; अ; अ; अ: and 0, 1, 2, 3, 4, or अ. The last place in the table corresponds to $x =$ अ. Similarly if we consider the function y defined by $y^3-y^2 = x^2$, then we find the table

0 or 1, अ, 2 or अ, 2 or अ, अ, 3 or 4 or अ.

For when $x = 2$ or 3, $y^3-y^2-4 \equiv 0$, so $y = 2$ or $2 \pm \sqrt{2}$, the latter two roots being congruent with $\frac{1}{2}(-1 \pm \sqrt{-7})$. These quantities are inexpressible (*avakta*) *modulo* 5. And when $x =$ अ, $x^2 = 2, 3$, or अ, so y may be 3 or 4, as well as अ.

Thus for a full enumeration of functions *modulo* m we need a table with $m+1$ places corresponding to the residues $0, 1, 2, \ldots, m-1$, and अ. In each place we can set one, or any number, of these symbols, but we must set at least one. So each place can be filled in $2^{m+1}-1$ ways, for each of the $m+1$ symbols can be present or absent, except that all cannot be absent. Thus the total number of functions *modulo* m is $(2^{m+1}-1)^{m+1}$, for example 62, 523, 502, 209 if $m = 5$, as compared with only 120 biunivocal functions, and 3125 univocal.

Now consider the simplest of the finite arithmetics, namely arithmetic *modulo* 2. There are only two elements, 0 and 1. Electronic calculators are based on this arithmetic. These machines are so designed that each unit, as the result of any instruction, will be active (1) or inactive (0) at any given moment. And it is possible, in principle, to predict whether it will be active or inactive. That is to say ambiguity is avoided, and the machine is designed to operate in terms of univocal functions. Nevertheless it is possible to provide such a machine with an instruction to which it cannot give a definite answer. It is said that some such machines, when given an instruction equivalent to one of the paradoxes of Principia Mathematica, come to no conclusion, but print 101010...indefinitely. Clearly a machine could be designed to print अ in such a case. It is obviously possible to design a machine which would print "0 or 1" in response to the instruction $x^2-x = 0$. A machine with the further refinement suggested above would respond "0, 1, or अ" to the instruction "$(x^2-x)\cos x \equiv 0 \pmod 2$". Such a machine could give any of 7 responses, namely :

0, 1, अ, 0 or 1, 0 or अ, 1 or अ, 0 or 1 or अ.

These are the *saptabhanghīnaya* with the ommission of the syllable *syād*.

[1] I have deliberately chosen a word with the same root (Latin *vox* = Sanskrit *vak*) as *avakta*.

I now pass to an example where the *saptabhanghīnaya* is actually applied in scientific research, and which I suspect is not far from what was in Bhadrabahu's mind. In the study of the physiology of the sense organs it is important to determine a threshold. For example a light cannot be seen below a certain intensity, or a solution of a substance which is tasted as bitter when concentrated cannot be distinguished from water when it is diluted. Some experimenters order their subjects to answer "yes" or "no" to the question "Is this illuminated ?", or "Is this bitter ? ". If the experimenter is interested in the psychology of perception he will permit the subject also to answer "It is uncertain", or some equivalent phrase. The objection to this is that some subjects may do so over a wide range of intensities.

Now consider a subject who is shown a series of illuminated patches, some above his threshold of perception, some below it, and others very close to it, in a randomised series. We will suppose that he is in a steady state of sensory adaptation, that he replies in Sanskrit, and that he is aware that his answers will sometimes be incorrect. At any given trial he will answer "*syādasti*", "*syādavaktavyah*", or "*syātnāsti*". After the second trial of a light of an intensity near the threshold he may have given two of these answers, for example "*syātnāsti ca avaktavyaśca*". After the third he may have given all three, though this is not very probable. The possibilities may be schematised as follows:

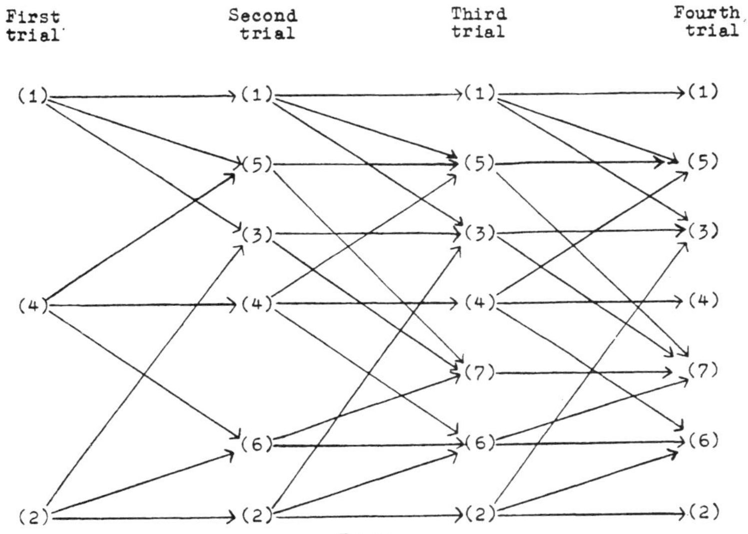

(Fig. 1)

Diagram showing the possible sequences of predications. After the third trial no new possibilities arise.

It is clear that the seven possibilities are exhaustive. My only possible criticism of Bhadrabahu is this. If the subject has given two different answers he may be aware that there is a possibility that he will later give the third. Once he has given all three, no further possibility is open. It might therefore be argued that the seventh type of predication should be "*asti nāsti ca avaktavyaśca*".

On the hypothesis that the subject is in a steady physiological and psychological state, the probabilities of each of the three answers to any given stimulus are constant. Let the probabilities of answering *syādasti*, *syādavaktavyah* and *syātnāsti* be p, q, and r, where $p+q+r = 1$. If, after n trials, the probabilities of the 7 types of predication are $P_{1,n}$, $P_{2,n}$, etc. where $P_{1,n}$ is the probability of *syādasti*, etc., then the vector $[P_{1,n}; P_{2,n}; P_{3,n}; P_{4,n}; P_{5,n}; P_{6,n}; P_{7,n}]$ is transformed into the vector $[P_{1,n+1}; P_{2,n+1}; \ldots$ etc.$]$ by multiplication by the matrix

$$\begin{pmatrix} p & 0 & 0 & 0 & 0 & 0 & 0 \\ 0 & r & 0 & 0 & 0 & 0 & 0 \\ r & p & p+r & 0 & 0 & 0 & 0 \\ 0 & 0 & 0 & q & 0 & 0 & 0 \\ q & 0 & 0 & p & p+q & 0 & 0 \\ 0 & q & 0 & r & 0 & q+r & 0 \\ 0 & 0 & q & 0 & r & p & 1 \end{pmatrix}$$

Evidently this could be made a little more symmetrical by transposing row and column (3) and (4).

The latent roots of this matrix are :

$$1,\ p+q,\ q+r,\ p+r,\ p,\ q,\ r.$$

So

$$P_{1n} = p^n$$
$$P_{2n} = r^n$$
$$P_{3n} = (p+r)^n - p^n - r^n$$
$$P_{4n} = q^n$$
$$P_{5n} = (p+q)^n - p^n - q^n$$
$$P_{6n} = (q+r)^n - q^n - r^n$$
$$P_{7n} = 1 - (q+r)^n - (r+p)^n - (q+r)^n + p^n + q^n + r^n.$$

Thus unless one of p, q, or r is zero the final predication will be *syādasti nāsti ca avaktavyaśca*. In many cases when the stimulus is far from the threshold, p or r will be unity. The subject will always, or never, say "this is bitter", or "this is illuminated". It is unlikely that q will ever be unity. So in this case *syādavaktavyah* will almost always be at best a provisional predication. It is however possible that p or r (say r) should be small, but not zero. If so $P_{5,n}$ will reach a maximum for some value of n and then decline. For example if $p = .6$, $q = .3$, $r = .1$, P_5 reaches its maximum value of .5184 when $n = 4$.

I have dealt with a case which arises when the question asked is as simple as possible. Human judgements are generally more complicated. We may attend to the data of several different senses, and of our memories. Thus we arrive at one conclusion from one set of data, and another from another set. We say that wood is hard when compared with clay, soft when compared with iron, indeterminate when compared with similar wood.

The close analysis of vision with a dark adapted eye shows that in this case at least, Mahalanobis was correct in regarding the *saptabhangīnaya* as foreshadowing modern statistical theory. It appears that when dark adaptation is complete, about five quanta of radiation must arrive within a short time in a small area of the retina before light is reported. Whether they will do so with a given intensity of illumination can only be stated as a probability. It is probable, though not by any means certain, that more complicated judgements depend on similar probabilities of events within the central nervous system.

Whatever philosophers of other schools may think, a Jaina can hardly object to regarding human predication as a special kind of animal behaviour. In this he agrees with followers of Darwin, such as myself. Attempts at a logical classification of animal behaviours frequently lead to a separation of 2^n-1 types, where however n may exceed 3. Thus Haldane (1953) classified the possible results of learning in an animal as follows. In any situation an animal will, or will not, give a certain response R, say eating a particular type of food within a minute of its presentation, or lifting its leg within ten seconds after an auditory signal is given.

If we compare the set of possible situations in which an animal may be placed before and after an experience E, they fall into four categories, $r\,r$, rR, $R\,r$, and RR. A situation $r\,r$ is one in which the response is not given before or after the experience. A situation $r\,R$ is one which it is given after E, but not before E, and so on. All situations may be $r\,r$. For example no-one has taught a dog to write. Some may be $r\,r$ and some rR. For example a dog which did not previously bring objects from the water to his master can learn to do so on command. In Pavlov's experiments a dog which previously only salivated (R) when given food will do so when certain auditory or other stimuli are given. Thus for such a dog all situations fall into the classes $r\,r$, RR, and rR. It can easily be seen that the effect of any experience on an animal can be classified according as the situations in which it can be placed fall into one, two, three, or all four of these classes. There are thus 2^4-1, or 15 qualitatively different results of an experiment in which an attempt is made to alter an animal's behaviours. In this classification the animal is assumed never to give an indeterminate response. If it can do so, both before and after, there are, as I pointed out, 2^9-1, or 511 possible results. The same principles may be applied to the comparison of the behaviour of two different animals, or two different races or species.

It is foolish to pretend that ancient philosophers anticipated all modern intellectual developments. And I believe that we, today, can do more honour to their memories by thinking for ourselves, as they did, than by devoting our lives to commentaries on them. But if we do so it is our duty to point out cases where it turns out that our own thought has run parallel to theirs. I was unaware of Bhadrabahu's existence when I wrote the paper to which I refer. The fact that I reached a conclusion so like his own suggests that we may both have seen the same facet of many-splendoured truth.

No doubt we reached it by very different methods, Bhadrabahu by meditation, I by thinking about the results of concrete experiments on animals. Such methods will often lead to different conclusions. This was the view of Warren Hastings in his introduction to Wilkins' translation of the Bhagavad Gita.

"But if we are told that there have been men who were successively, for ages past, in the daily habit of abstracted contemplation, begun in the earliest period of youth, and continued in many to the maturity of age, each adding some portion of knowledge to the store accumulated by his predecessors, it is not assuming too much to conclude, that as the mind ever gathers strength, like the body, with exercise, so in such exercise it may in each have acquired the faculty to which they aspired, and that their collective studies have led them to the discovery of new tracks and combinations of sentiment, totally different from the doctrines with which the learned of other nations are acquainted: doctrines, which however speculative and subtle, still, as they possess the advantage of being derived from a source so free from every adventitious mixture, may be equally founded on truth with the most simple of our own".

If, on the other hand, the contemplation of one's own mind, and that of the minds of animals, lead to similar results, such results are, perhaps, worthy of serious consideration.

REFERENCES

MAHALANOBIS, P. C. (1954): The foundations of statistics. *Dialectica*, **8**, 95-111.

HALDANE, J. B. S. (1954): A logical analysis of learning, conditioning, and related processes. *Behaviour*, **6**, 256-270.

Paper received : November, 1956.

Science Citation Index 1988

HALDANE JB

32 CAUSE EVOLUTION					
OTTAVIAN E	THEOR A GEN		76	601	88

HALDANE JBS

12 J PHYSIOL-LONDON 45 12					
VONRESTO W	AVIAT SP EN		59	929	88
12 J PHYSIOL-LONDON 45 22					
MELINYSH MJ	AM J PHYSL		255	H 77	88
STERN FB	AM J EPIDEM		128	1276	88
15 J GENET 5 133					
MULLER G	EMBO J		7	2723	88
19 J GENET 8 229					
GOLDGAR DE	AM J HU GEN		43	38	88
19 J GENET 8 291					
SINGH NK	THEOR A GEN		75	642	88
19 J GENET 8 299					
BLANK RD	CURR T MICR	R	137	25	88
CROW JF	GENETICS	E	118	1	88
GRUNDY P	NATURE		336	374	88
LEE C	THEOR A GEN		75	362	88
NARUSE K	ZOOL SCI	N	5	489	88
WATKINS PC	BIOTECHNIQU	R	6	310	88
22 J GENET 12 101					
ERICKSON RP	DEVELOPMENT		101	25	87
GOSALVEZ J	GENOME		30	656	88
HENDRIKS A	ENT EXP APP		48	213	88
SCHMUTZ SM	J HEREDITY		78	388	87
STASIAK RH	EXPERIENTIA	N	44	262	88
TEGELSTR H	BIOCHEM GEN		26	223	88
WISHART WD	CAN J ZOOL		66	1664	88
ZOUROS E	EVOLUTION		42	1321	88
24 P CAMB PHIL SOC BIOL 158					
CUGUEN J	HEREDITY		60	91	88
24 P ROY SOC BIOL 96 1					
HOFF SD	J PARENT EN		12	414	88
OSTER JR	LIFE SCI		42	811	88
24 T CAMBRIDGE PHILOS S 23 19					
SEE SSCI FOR 1 ADDITIONAL CITATION					
HARRIS AC	J RS NZ		18	333	88
27 P CAMBRIDGE PHILOS S 23 607					
ABUGOV R	J THEOR BIO		132	437	88
27 P CAMB PHIL SOC 23 838					
HASTINGS A	GENETICS		118	543	88
LANGLEY CH	"		119	619	88
MIYASHIT N	"		120	199	88
POGSON GH	CAN J ZOOL		66	1139	88
SCHAEFFE SW	MOL BIOL EV		5	30	88
28 J PHYSIOL-LONDON 68 1068					
PIANTADO CA	J APP PHYSL		65	878	88
29 RATIONALIST ANN 3					
KAMMINGA H	ORIGIN LIFE		18	1	88
29 RATIONALIST ANN 148					
WACHTERS G	MICROBIOL R	R	52	452	88
29 RATIONALIST ANN 148 3					
CAVALIER T	COLD S HARB		52	805	87
ESCHENMO A	ANGEW CHEM	R	27	5	88
30 ENZYMES					
GAUTAN N	J BIOL CHEM		263	5400	88
GOEDDERT JG	J ENV ENG		114	1063	88
HERMES JD	COLD S HARB		52	597	87
JARDETZK TS	BIOCHEM		27	6758	88
KRAUT J	SCIENCE		242	533	88
MAZRAJI E	BIOSYSTEMS		22	11	88
"	J THEOR BIO		129	163	87
30 ENZYMES 83					
VERHAMME IM	EUR J BIOCH		172	615	88
30 ENZYMES 84					
KUHL PW	BIO CHEM HS	M	369	1204	88
30 ENZYMES 182					
FERSHT AR	BIOCHEM		26	8031	87
SHOHAM G	P NAS US		85	684	88
30 J GENETICS 22 359					
SOLTIS DE	HEREDITY		60	375	88
30 P CAMBRIDGE PHILOS S 26 220					
TREXLER JC	EVOLUTION		42	1006	88
31 CYTOLOGIA TOKYO 3 54					
UKAI Y	JPN J GENET	N	63	258	88
31 GENETICS 16 357					
BURR B	GENETICS		118	519	88
CECI JD	GENE		59	171	87
COWEN NM	THEOR A GEN		75	857	88
MORTON NE	ANN HUM GEN		52	309	88
NOSHIRO M	BIOCHEM		27	6434	88
SKOW LC	BIOCHEM GEN		26	557	88
SNAPE JW	THEOR A GEN		76	125	88
WHITEHEA AS	IMMUNOGENET		28	388	88
32 ALLGEMEINE CHEM ENZY					
MUNOZ J	PLANTA		175	460	88
32 CAUSES EVOLUTION					
SEE SSCI FOR 2 ADDITIONAL CITATIONS					
CHRISTIA FB	PHI T ROY B		319	587	88
CURY P	CAN J FISH		45	1080	88
FUTUYMA DJ	EVOLUTION		42	217	88
HARPENDI H	YEAR PH ANT		30	127	87
KELLER L	ANIM BEHAV		36	159	88
POGSON GH	CAN J ZOOL		66	1139	88
SNOW AA	EVOLUTION		42	1085	88
WRIGHT S	AM NATURAL	N	131	115	88
32 CAUSES EVOLUTION 131					
PAUL DB	J HIST BIOL		21	411	88
33 NATURE 132 265					
SHREFFLE DC	J IMMUNOL	R	141	1791	88
35 J GENETICS 31 317					
BARDONI B	HUM GENET	N	79	86	88
BOBROW M	ARCH NEUROL	N	45	85	88
DAVIDSON BL	J CLIN INV	N	82	2164	88
GITSCHIE J	AM J HU GEN		43	274	88
GRIMM T	AM J MED G	L	29	445	88
JEANPIER M	J MED GENET		25	863	88
KANE WH	BLOOD	R	71	539	88
KNOERS N	HUM GENET		80	31	88
LANE RJM	LANCET	L	2	971	88
MULLEY JC	AUST PAEDIA		24	92	88
PELET A	ANN BIOL CL		46	456	88
ROMEO G	EUR J PED		147	412	88
ROSES AD	ARCH NEUROL		45	84	88
SIGURET V	BR J HAEM		70	411	88
STOUT JT	TRENDS GEN	R	4	175	88
WOOD S	HUM GENET		78	282	88
YANG TP	SOM CELL M		14	293	88
YOUSSOUF H	AM J HU GEN		42	718	88
"	"		42	867	88
"	HUM GENET		80	143	88
35 RESPIRATION					

HALDANE JBS

			VOL	PG	YR
VONRESTO W	AVIAT SP EN		59	925	88
36 ANN EUGEN LOND 7 28					
GOODFELL PJ	DEVELOPMENT		[illegible]	[illegible]	87
36 J GENETICS 32 393					
MORGAN MT	EVOLUTION		42	496	88
37 ADVENTURES BIOL 151					
PAUL DB	J HIST BIOL		21	411	88
37 AM NAT 71 337					
BERNSTEI H	ADV GENETIC	R	24	323	87
GRAFEN A	J THEOR BIO		131	163	88
HOPF FA	THEOR POP B		33	243	88
KONDRASH AS	GENETICS		120	853	88
REDFIELD RJ	"		119	213	88
UYENOYAM MK	AM NATURAL		131	700	88
37 BIOMETRIKA 29 133					
HABERMAN SJ	J AM STAT A		83	555	88
MIELKE PW	BIOMETRIKA	N	75	790	88
38 ANN EUGENICS 14 33					
ROGATKO A	AM J HU GEN		42	889	88
39 ANN EUGEN LOND 9 400					
CROW JF	EVOLUTION		42	482	88
39 ENZYMES					
HUTCHINS DH	APPL MICR B		29	599	88
39 J GENET 37 365					
STEWART AJA	BIOL J LINN		34	57	88
39 J HYGIENE 39 289					
HAAS CN	APPL ENVIR		54	2996	88
40 BIOMETRIKA 31 346					
BERRY KJ	PSYCHOL B		103	256	88
MIELKE PW	BIOMETRIKA	N	75	790	88
41 J GENETICS 41 149					
RIDLEY RM	J MED GENET		25	589	88
41 NEW PATHS GENETICS					
SEE SSCI FOR 1 ADDITIONAL CITATION					
LIBERTIN G	J THEOR BIO		132	145	88
PENZLIN H	BIOL ZBL	I	107	617	88
42 ANN EUGENICS 11 179					
RAFTERY AE	BIOMETRIKA		75	223	88
42 NEW PATHS GENETICS					
NESSE RM	EXP GERONT		23	445	88
45 BIOMETRIKA 33 222					
BEAL SL	BIOMETRICS		43	941	87
45 NATURE 73 375					
PENZLIN H	BIOL ZBL	I	107	617	88
46 ANN EUGEN LONDON 13 197					
BECKER HC	PLANT BREED	R	101	1	88
KHOURY MJ	AM J HU GEN		42	89	88
46 ANN EUGENICS 13 262					
YOUSSOUF H	AM J HU GEN		42	867	88
46 P ANN S EUGEN SOC 13 262					
YOUSSOUF H	HUM GENET		80	143	88
47 ANN EUGEN LONDON 14 10					
AMAR A	ISR J MED S		24	28	88
47 ANN EUGEN LONDON 14 117					
BONNEY GE	BIOMETRICS		43	951	87
DEBRAEKE M	CAN J NEUR		15	139	88
HARDING AE	J MED GENET		25	528	88
MALAMA IM	BR J PSYCHI		152	482	88
47 EUGENICS 13 197					
BAKER RJ	CAN J PLANT		68	405	88
48 J GENET 49 104					
KLEIN J	METH ENZYM	R	150	163	87
48 P ROY SOC B 135 147					
MCKUSICK VA	MEDICINE	R	67	1	88
49 ANN EUGEN 15 15					
HOLSINGE KE	ACT OEC-PLA		9	95	88
"	EVOLUTION		42	1235	88
49 EVOLUTION 3 51					
HUNTER RST	MICROPALEON		34	181	88
MACFADDE BJ	BIOL J LINN		35	37	88
"	EVOLUT BIOL	R	22	131	88
"	NATURE		336	466	88
49 RIC SCI 19 1					
NADEAU JH	GENETICS		118	131	88
49 RICERCA SCIENTIFIC S 19 68					
(ANON)	LANCET	E	2	608	88
BARRETT JA	PHI T ROY B		319	473	88
GIBBS A	J CELL SCI			319	87
PARKER MA	EVOLUTION		42	239	88
PRICE PW	AM NATURAL		131	544	88
SEGER J	PHI T ROY B		319	541	88
TRAGER W	ANN TROP M	R	81	511	87
WEATHERA DJ	PHI T ROY B		321	327	88
49 8 P INT C GEN HER S 35 367					
WEATHERA DJ	ANN TROP M		81	539	87
51 ANN EUGENICS 16 359					
FRODA S	J AM GER SO	L	36	179	88
HUFF FJ	"	L	36	180	88
54 AMER BIOL 58 89					
HOYLE CHV	COMP BIOC C		90	113	88
54 BR J ANIM BEHAV 2 1					
54 BEHAVIOUR 6 256					
CLONINGE CR	J PSYCH RES		21	457	87
54 CARYOLOGIA S 480					
ULIZZI L	HUMAN HERED		38	129	88
54 EVOLUTION PROCESS 109					
BARRETT JA	PHI T ROY B		319	473	88
54 J GENET 52 631					
LOUIS EJ	BIOMETRICS		43	805	87
54 NEW BIOL 16 12					
CHMELIK J	CHEM LISTY	R	82	24	88
54 9TH P INT C GEN CA S 480					
LEVIN DA	AM J BOTANY		75	1632	88
54 9 P INT C GEN 1 480					
CHARLESW B	EVOLUTION		42	1129	88
SCHLUTER D	"		42	849	88
55 ANN HUM GENET 19 251					
WOODROW JC	J RHEUMATOL	E	15	197	88
55 ANN HUMAN GENETICS 20 309					
BONATI M	EUR J PED		147	468	88
COOPER DN	HUM GENET	R	78	299	88
DEBRUIN TWA	BR MED J		296	1292	88
DEMAINE AG	IMMUNOGENET		27	19	88
DEMOOR P	BR J HAEM		69	225	88
KLEMP P	TISSUE ANTI		32	12	88
LINET MS	"		31	71	88
MAT MC	INT J DERM		27	246	88
PEVNITSK LA	VA MED NAUK			48	88
REYNOLDS KM	PHYTOPATHOL		78	240	88
ROWE JR	HUMAN IMMUN		22	51	88
55 EVOLUTION 9 484					
CHAMBERS RC	CAN J FISH	R	44	1936	87
"	MAR ECOL-PR		47	1	88
55 NEW BIOL 19 7					
ROPER JA	CANC SURV	I	7	229	88
55 P R SOC B 144 217					
ALLEN JA	PHI T ROY B		319	485	88
ANDRIYAS MA	GENETIKA	R	23	2085	87
55 11 ACT C INT ORN 454					
HOTKER H	J ANIM ECOL		57	109	88
LUBOYA K	ACT OEC-GEN		9	293	88
SAETHER BE	NATURE		331	616	88
56 ANN HUM GENET 20 209					
MITCHELL RJ	HUMAN HERED		38	117	88
"	"		38	144	88
56 ANN HUMAN GENET 20 309					
CAMARGOS PA	INT J EPID		17	193	88
COX RA	J INFEC DIS		158	1302	88
GAMMON WR	J INVES DER		91	228	88
JOHNSON N	BR J OBST G		95	877	88
KAMPGEN E	ARCH DERMAT		124	1372	88
PURRMANN J	J RHEUMATOL		15	1658	88
"	Z GASTROENT		26	658	88
ZERBE TR	AM J CARD	N	61	1359	88
56 ANN HUMAN GENETICS 20 344					
WORTON RG	INT R NEURO	R	29	1	88
56 BIOMETRIKA 43 96					
AKOPYAN MV	NUCL INST A		272	855	88
56 J GENET 45 294					
CLARK AG	GENETICS		118	471	88
56 J GENETICS 54 294					
INNES DJ	EVOLUTION		42	1024	88
TUCIC N	HEREDITY		60	55	88
56 P ROYAL SOC B 145 306					
ELLIOTT JM	J ANIM ECOL		57	49	88
57 ACTA GENET STAT MED 6 321					
GOUTEUX JP	ANN PARASIT		63	315	88
57 J GENET 55 511					
ANDRIYAS MA	GENETIKA	R	23	2085	87
KIMURA M	JPN J GENET		63	1	88
OTTAVIAN E	THEOR A GEN		76	601	88
WALLACE B	PERSP BIOL		31	201	88
57 NATURE 179 832					
ANDREASE NC	SCHIZO BULL		14	471	88
BOUNAUD JY	EUR J CAN C		24	461	88
CLARK ER	J STEROID B		29	375	88
JENSEN JD	P SOC EXP M		189	28	88
JORDAN VC	CRC C R LAB	R	26	97	88
MILLER DJ	J DAIRY SCI		71	239	88
REUL JMHM	NEUROBIOL A		9	253	88
57 SANKHYA A 18 195					
BARTHOLO DJ	J ROY STA A		151	137	88
60 J BOMBAY NAT HIST SO 57 243					
GOPAL B	CURRENT SCI	N	57	348	88
60 J GENET 57 351					
WALLACE B	PERSP BIOL		31	201	88
60 NATURE 185 87					
MASON SF	BIOCH PHARM		37	1	88
60 NATURE 187 879					
BANERJEE K	I J MED RES		87	134	88
IKAL MA	T RS TROP M		82	628	88
63 BIOMETRIKA 50 89					
LEADBETT MR	ANN PROBAB	R	16	431	88
63 J GENET 58 237					
CHARLESW B	J THEOR BIO		130	191	88
GROSBERG RK	EVOLUTION		42	900	88
HEDRICK AV	AM NATURAL		132	267	88
PAMILO P	ANN ZOO FEN		25	99	88
63 J GENET 58 318					
TUCKER GM	HEREDITY		60	329	88
64 PERSPECT BIOL MED 1 343					
CASWELL H	ECOL MODEL		43	33	88
64 PERSPECT BIOL MED 7 343					

HALDANE JBS

			VOL	PG	YR
WALLACE B	PERSP BIOL		[illegible]	[illegible]	88
65 ENZYME					
SATO [illegible]	WATER RES		[illegible]	[illegible]	88
65 ENZYMES					
PLUCKTHUN A	COLD S HARB		52	[illegible]	87
PROFY AT	PROG NUCL A	R	35	[illegible]	88
SINGHAL N	CHEM ENG J		39	B37	88
SUIDAN MT	J ENV ENG		114	1259	88
ZVELEBIL MJ	PROTEIN ENG			[illegible]	88
65 ORIGIN PREBIOLOGICAL 11					
ALLEN G	ORIGIN LIFE		[illegible]	289	88
CAVALIER T	COLD S HARB		52	805	87
LAZCANO A	J MOL EVOL		[illegible]	283	88
65 11TH P INT C GEN 2 R 91					
WALLACE B	PERSP BIOL		31	201	88
67 ORIGIN LIFE 242					
DANCHIN A	RECHERCHE		19	[illegible]	88
69 CORRECTION 31 220					
MIELKE PW	BIOMETRIKA	N	[illegible]	[illegible]	88
82 RACIONALIST ANN 48					
ALBARRAN G	RADIAT PH C		[illegible]	82	88
85 BEING RIGHT SIZE OTH					
MASON J	J CHEM EDUC		65	[illegible]	88

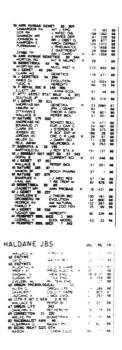

Bibliography

Books reviewed by Haldane in the *Journal of Genetics* (1959–64)

1 Lea DE 1956 *Actions of Radiations on Living Cells*. Cambridge University Press, London

2 Barlow N (ed) 1958 *The Autobiography of Charles Darwin*. Collins, London

3 Wolstenholme GEW, O'Connor CM (eds) *Biochemistry of Human Genetics*. Churchill, London

4 Poehlman JM 1959 *Breeding Field Crops*. Holt, New York

5 Hayashi T (ed) 1959 *Subcellular Particles*. The Ronald Press, New York

6 Rudnick D (ed) 1959 *Developmental Cytology*. The Ronald Press, New York

7 Avery AG, Satina S, Rietsema J 1959 *Blakeslee: The Genus Datura*. The Ronald Press, New York

8 Dittrich M 1959 *Getreide-Umwandlung und Artproblem. Eine Historische Orientierung*. Gustav Fischer, Jena

9 Harris H 1959 *Human Biochemical Genetics*. Cambridge University Press, London

10 OEEC, ENEA and the Danish Atomic Energy Commission 1959 *Health Physics in Nuclear Installations*. OEEC, Paris

11 Bell PR (ed) 1959 *Darwin's Biological Work: Some Aspects Reconsidered*. Cambridge University Press, London

12 1959 *Genetics and Cancer*. University of Texas Press, Austin

13 Hsia DY 1959 *Inborn Errors of Metabolism*. Yearbook Publishers, Chicago

14 Rudnick D (ed) 1960 *Developing Cell Systems and Their Control*. The Ronald Press, New York

15 Bartlett MS 1960 *Stochastic Population Models*. Methuen, London

16 Roberts F 1960 *An Introduction to Human Blood Groups*. Heinemann, London

17 The National Spastics Society 1960 *A Proposed Standard of Nomenclature of Human Mitotic Chromosomes: Human Chromosomes Study Group Suppl. to Cerebral Palsy Bull.*, vol 2. The National Spastics Society, London

18 Prywes M (ed) 1960 *Medical and Biological Research in Israel*. R. Mass, Jerusalem

19 Falconer DS 1960 *Introduction to Quantitative Genetics*. Oliver and Boyd, Edinburgh

20 Le Roy HL 1960 *Statistiche Methoden der Populationsgenetik*. Birkhauser, Basel

21 Strehler BL *et al* (eds) 1960 *The Biology of Aging*. American Institute of Biological Sciences, Washington DC

22 Lasker GW (ed) 1960 *The Process of Ongoing Evolution*. Wayne State University Press, Detroit

23 Parkes AS 1960 *Marshall's Physiology of Reproduction*, 3rd edn. Longmans Green, London

24 Adelberg EA (ed) 1960 *Papers on Bacterial Genetics*. Little, Brown, Boston

25 Stent GS (ed) 1960 *Papers on Bacterial Viruses*. Little, Brown, Boston

26 Muntzing A 1961 *Genetic Research*. LT Forlag, Stockholm

27 British Council 1961 Human genetics. *British Medical Bulletin* 17(3)

28 Banton M (ed) 1961 *Darwinism and the Study of Society*. Quadrangle Books, Chicago

29 Jones FA (ed) 1961 *Clinical Aspects of Genetics*. Pitman Medical Publishing, London

30 1961 *Selected Papers of AH Sturtevant*. WH Freeman, San Francisco

31 Neyman J (ed) 1961 *Proc. of 4th Berkeley Symp. on Mathematical Statistics and Probability*, vol. 4: *Biology and Problems of Medicine*. University of California Press, Berkeley

32 Dept of Commerce 1961 *Fundamental Aspects of Radiosensitivity, Brookhaven Symposia in Biology 14*. Department of Commerce, Washington, DC

33 MacLeod AM, Cobley LS (eds) 1961 *Contemporary Botanical Thought*. Oliver and Boyd, Edinburgh

34 Lasker GW 1961 *The Evolution of Man*. Holt, Rinehart and Winston, New York

35 Potter EL 1961 *Pathology of the Fetus and Infant*. Yearbook Publishers, Chicago
36 Galton F 1962 *Hereditary Genius*. Collins, London
37 Edds MV (ed) 1962 *Macromolecular Complexes*. The Ronald Press, New York
38 Bonner DM (ed) 1962 *Control Mechanisms in Cellular Processes*. The Ronald Press, New York
39 Auerbach C 1962 *The Science of Genetics*. Hutchinson, London
40 Auerbach C 1962 *Mutation: An Introduction to Research on Mutagenesis*. Part 1: *Methods*. Oliver and Boyd, Edinburgh
41 Schull WJ (ed) 1962 *Mutations*. University of Michigan Press, Ann Arbor
42 Good R 1962 *Features of Evolution in the Flowering Plants*. Longmans, Green, London
43 Dawson GWP 1962 *An Introduction to Cytogenetics of Polyploids*. Blackwell, Oxford
44 1962 *The Molecular Basis of Neoplasia*. The university of Texas Press, Austin
45 King RC 1962 *Genetics*. Oxford University Press, Oxford
46 1962 *Life Sciences*, vol 1. Pergamon Press, Oxford
47 CIBA Foundation Study Group 1962 *Resistance of Bacteria to the Penicillins*. Churchill, London
48 CIBA Foundation Study Group 1962 *CIBA Foundation Symposium on Transplantation*. Churchill, London
49 Robinson HP (ed) 1962 *Papers on Quantitative Genetics and Related Topics*. North Carolina State College, Raleigh
50 Spiess EB (ed) 1962 *Papers on Animal Population Genetics*. Little, Brown, Boston
51 Hamerton JL (ed) 1962 *Chromosomes in Medicine*. Heinemann, London
52 Ministere de L'education 1962 *Problemes Actuels de Paleontologie (Evolution des Vertebres)*. CNRS, Paris
53 1962 *Approaches to Genetic Analysis of Mammalian Cells*. University of Michigan Press, Ann Arbor
54 Dreyfus JC, Schapira G 1962 *Biochemistry of Hereditary Myopathies*. CC Thomas, Springfield
55 Burdette WJ (ed) 1962 *Methodology in Human Genetics*. Holden-Day, San Francisco
56 Case RAM *et al* 1962 *The Chester Beatty Research Institute Life Tables*. Chester Beatty Research Institute and Royal Cancer Hospital, London
57 Muller HJ 1962 *Studies in Genetics*. Indiana University Press, Bloomington
58 Sturtevant AH, Beadle GW 1962 *An Introduction to Genetics*. Dover Publications
59 Mayr E 1963 *Animal Species and Evolution*. Belknap Press, Harvard, Cambridge
60 Kerkut GA (ed) 1963 *Problems in Biology*, vol 1. Pergamon Press, Oxford
61 Neel JV 1963 *Changing Perspectives in the Genetic Effects of Radiation*. CC Thomas, Springfield
62 Schull WJ (ed) 1963 *Genetic Selection in Man*. University of Michigan Press, Ann Arbor
63 Huxley JS (ed) 1963 *Evolution: The Modern Synthesis*. Allen and Unwin, London
64 Weyl N, Possony ST 1963 *The Geography of Intellect*. Henry Regnery, Chicago
65 Feibleman JR 1963 *Mankind Behaving: Human Needs and Material Culture*. CC Thomas, Springfield
66 Wagner RP, Mitchell HK 1964 *Genetics and Metabolism*. John Wiley, New York
67 Tazima Y 1964 *The Genetics of the Silkworm*. Academic Press, New York
68 Ford EB 1964 *Ecological Genetics*. Methuen, London
69 Campbell DH *et al* 1964 *Methods in Immunology*. Benjamin, New York

The Scientific Publications of JBS Haldane

Haldane JBS 1912 The dissociation of oxyhaemoglobin in human blood during partial CO poisoning. *J. Physiol.* 45: 22

Haldane JBS, Douglas CG, Haldane JS 1912 The Laws of combination of haemoglobin with CO and oxygen. *J. Physiol.* 44: 275

Haldane JBS, Sprunt AD, Haldane NM 1915 Reduplication in mice. *J. Genet.* 5: 133

Haldane JBS 1919a The probable errors of calculated linkage values, and the most accurate method of determining gametic from certain zygotic series. *J. Genet.* 8: 291
Haldane JBS 1919b The combination of linkage values, and the calculation of distances between loci of linked factors. *J. Genet.* 8: 299

Haldane JBS 1920a Note on a case of linkage in Paratettix. *J. Genet.* 10: 47
Haldane JBS 1920b Some recent work on heredity. *Trans. Oxford Univ. Jr. Sci. Club* 1(3): 3
Haldane JBS, Davies HW, Kennaway EL 1920 Experiments on the regulation of the blood's alkalinity, I. *J. Physiol.* 54: 32

Haldane JBS 1921a Experiments on the regulation of the blood's alkalinity, II. *J. Physiol.* 55: 265
Haldane JBS 1921b Linkage in poultry. *Science* 54: 663
Haldane JBS, Bazett HC 1921 Some effects of hot baths on man. *J. Physiol.* 55: 4

Haldane JBS 1922 Sex-ratio and unisexual sterility in hybrid animals. *J. Genet.* 12: 101
Haldane JBS, Baird MM 1922 Salt and water excretion in man. *J. Physiol.* 56: 259
Haldane JBS, Davies HW, Peskett GL 1922 The excretion of chlorides and bicarbonates by the human kidney. *J. Physiol.* 56: 269

Haldane JBS 1923 *Daedalus, or Science and the Future.* Kegan Paul, Trench, Trubner, London (EP Dutton, New York 1924)
Haldane JBS, Baird MM, Douglas CG, Priestley JG 1923 Ammonium chloride acidosis. *J. Physiol.* 57: xli
Haldane JBS, Hill R, Luck JM 1923 Calcium chloride acidosis. *J. Physiol.* 57: 301

Haldane JBS 1924a A mathematical theory of natural and artificial selection, pt 1. *Trans. Camb. Phil. Soc.* 23: 19–41
Haldane JBS 1924b A mathematical theory of natural and artificial selection, pt 2. The influence of partial self-fertilization, inbreeding, assortative mating, and selective fertilization on the composition of Mendelian populations, and on natural selection. *Proc. Camb. Phil. Soc.* 1: 158
Haldane JBS 1924c Uber Halluzinationen infolge von Anderungen des Kohlen-sauredrucks. *Psychologische Forschung* 5: 356
Haldane JBS 1924d The possible existence of a growth regulating substance in termites. *Nature, London* 113: 676
Haldane JBS, Quastel JH 1924 The changes in alveolar carbon dioxide pressure after violent exercise. *J. Physiol.* 59: 138
Haldane JBS, Kay HD, Smith W 1924 The effect of insulin on blood volume. *J. Physiol.* 59: 193
Haldane JBS, Stewart CP 1924 Experimental alterations in the calcium content of human serum and urine. *Biochem. J.* 28: 855
Haldane JBS, Wigglesworth VB, Woodrow CE 1924a Effect of reaction changes on human inorganic metabolism. *Proc. Roy. Soc. B* 96: 1
Haldane JBS, Wigglesworth VB, Woodrow CE 1924b The effect of reaction changes on human carbohydrate and oxygen metabolism. *Proc. Roy. Soc. B* 96: 15

Haldane JBS 1925a The production of acidosis by ingestion of magnesium chloride and strontium chloride. *Biochem. J.* 29: 249
Haldane JBS 1925b On the origin of the potential differences between the interior and exterior of cells. *Proc. Camb. Phil. Soc. (Biol. Sci.)* 1: 243
Haldane JBS 1925c *Callinicus: A Defence of Chemical Warfare.* Kegan Paul, Trench, Trubner, London
Haldane JBS, Bourguignon G 1925 Electricite physiologique-evolution de la chronaxie au cours de la crise de tetanie experimentale par hyperpnee volontaire chez l'homme. *C. R. Acad. Sci. Paris* 180: 231
Haldane JBS, Briggs GE 1925 Note on the kinetics of enzyme action. *Biochem. J.* 29: 338
Haldane JBS, Crew FAE 1925 Change of linkage in poultry with age. *Nature, London* 115: 641

Haldane JBS 1926 A mathematical theory of natural and artificial selection, pt 3. *Proc. Camb. Phil. Soc.* 23: 363

Haldane JBS 1927a A mathematical theory of natural and artificial selection, pt 4. *Proc. Camb. Phil. Soc.* 23: 607
Haldane JBS 1927b A mathematical theory of natural and artificial selection, pt 5. Selection and mutation. *Proc. Camb. Phil. Soc.* 23: 838
Haldane JBS 1927c The comparative genetics of colour in rodents and carnivora. *Biol. Rev.* 11: 199
Haldane JBS 1927d Carbon monoxide as a tissue poison. *Biochem. J.* 21: 1068
Haldane JBS 1927e Carbon monoxide poisoning in the absence of haemoglobin. *Nature, London* 119: 352
Haldane JBS 1927f Biological fact and theory. *Nature, London* 119: 456
Haldane JBS 1927g *Possible Worlds and Other Essays*. Chatto and Windus, London
Haldane JBS, Huxley JS 1927 *Animal Biology*. Clarendon Press, Oxford

Haldane JBS 1928a Pituitrin and the chloride concentrating power of the kidneys. *J. Physiol.* 66: 10
Haldane JBS 1928b The affinity of different types of enzyme for their substrates. *Nature, London* 121: 207
Haldane JBS 1928c The universe and irreversibility. *Nature, London* 122: 808
Haldane JBS, Linder GC, Hilton R, Fraser FR 1928 The arterial blood in ammonium chloride acidosis. *J. Physiol.* 65: 412

Haldane JBS 1929a Natural selection. *Nature, London* 124: 444
Haldane JBS 1929b The species problem in the light of genetics. *Nature, London* 124: 514
Haldane JBS 1929c The scientific point of view. *The Realist* 1(4): 10
Haldane JBS 1929d The place of science in Western civilization. *The Realsist* 2: 149
Haldane JBS 1929e Genetics of polyploid plants. *Conference on Polyploidy*. John Innes Horticultural Institute, p 9
Haldane JBS 1929f The origin of life. *Rationalist Annual*, p 3
Haldane JBS, Gairdner AE 1929 A case of balanced lethal factors in *Antirrhinum majus*. *J. Genet.* 21: 315

Haldane JBS 1930a *Enzymes*. Longmans, Green, London
Haldane JBS 1930b A note on Fisher's theory of the origin of dominance and on a correlation between dominance and linkage. *American Naturalist* 64: 87
Haldane JBS 1930c La cinétique des actions diastasiques. *J. Chim. Phys.* 27: 277
Haldane JBS 1930d A mathematical theory of natural and artificial selection, pt 6. Isolation. *Proc. Camb. Phil. Soc.* 26: 220
Haldane JBS 1930e Theoretical genetics of autopolyploids. *J. Genet.* 22: 359
Haldane JBS 1930f Genetics of some autopolyploid plants. *Rep. Proc. 5th Int. Bot. Congr.* Cambridge, p 232
Haldane JBS 1930g The principles of plant breeding, illustrated by the Chinese Primrose. *Proc. Roy. Inst.* 26: 199
Haldane JBS 1930h Origin of asymmetry in gastropods. *Nature, London* 126: 10
Haldane JBS 1930i Natural selection intensity as a function of mortality rate. *Nature, London* 126: 883

Haldane JBS 1931a A mathematical theory of natural and artificial selection, pt 7. Selection intensity as a function of mortality rate. *Proc. Camb. Phil. Soc.* 27: 131
Haldane JBS 1931b A mathematical theory of natural selection, pt 8. Metastable populations. *Proc. Camb. Phil. Soc.* 27: 137
Haldane JBS 1931c Embryology and evolution. *Nature, London* 126: 956; 127: 274
Haldane JBS 1931d Oxidation by living cells. *Nature, London* 128: 175
Haldane JBS 1931e The molecular statistics of an enzyme action. *Proc. Roy. Soc. B* 108: 559
Haldane JBS 1931f Prehistory in the light of genetics. *Proc. Roy. Inst.* 26: 355
Haldane JBS 1931g The cytological basis of genetical interference. *Cytologia* 3: 54
Haldane JBS, De Winton D 1931 Linkage in the tetraploid *Primula sinensis*. *J. Genet.* 24: 121
Haldane JBS, Waddington CH 1931 Inbreeding and linkage. *Genetics* 16: 357
Haldane JBS, Cook RP, Mapson LW 1931 The relationship between the respiratory catalysts of *B. coli*. *Biochem. J.* 25: 534

Haldane JBS, Cook RP 1931 The respiration of *B. coli communis*. *Biochem. J.* 25: 880

Haldane JBS 1932a A note on inverse probability. *Proc. Camb. Phil. Soc.* 28: 55
Haldane JBS 1932b On the non-linear difference equation. *Proc. Camb. Phil. Soc.* 28: 234
Haldane JBS 1932c A mathematical theory of natural and artificial selection, pt 9. Rapid selection. *Proc. Camb. Phil Soc.* 28: 244
Haldane JBS 1932d Discussion on recent advances in the study of enzymes and their action. *Proc. Roy. Soc. B* 111: 280
Haldane JBS 1932e The time of action of genes, and its bearing on some evolutionary problems. *American Naturalist* 66: 5
Haldane JBS 1932f Note on a fallacious method of avoiding selection. *American Naturalist* 66: 479.
Haldane JBS 1932g A method for investigating recessive characters in man. *J. Genet.* 25: 251
Haldane JBS 1932h Genetical evidence for a cytological abnormality in man. *J. Genet.* 26: 341
Haldane JBS 1932i Determinism. *Nature, London* 129: 315
Haldane JBS 1932j The hereditary transmission of acquired characters. *Nature, London* 129: 817, 856
Haldane JBS 1932k Eland-ox hybrid. *Nature, London* 129: 906
Haldane JBS 1932l The inheritance of acquired characters. *Nature, London* 130: 20, 204
Haldane JBS 1932m Chain reactions in enzymatic catalyses. *Nature, London* 130: 61
Haldane JBS 1932n *The Inequality of Man and Other Essays*. Chatto and Windus, London
Haldane JBS 1932o *The Causes of Evolution*. Longmans, Green, London

Haldane JBS 1933a The part played by recurrent mutation in evolution. *American Naturalist* 67: 5
Haldane JBS 1933b Two new allelomorphs for heterostylism in *Primula*. *American Naturalist* 67: 559
Haldane JBS 1933c The genetics of cancer. *Nature, London* 132: 265
Haldane JBS 1933d The biologist and society. In: Adams M (ed) 1933 *Science in the Changing World*. Allen and Unwin, London
Haldane JBS, De Winton D 1933 The genetics of *Primula sinensis*, II. Segregation and interaction of factors in the diploid. *J. Genet.* 27: 1
Haldane JBS, Gairdner AE 1933 A case of balanced lethal factors in *Antirrhinum majus*., ii *J. Genet.* 27: 287

Haldane JBS 1934a Quantum mechanics as a basis for philosophy. *Phil. Sci.* 1: 78
Haldane JBS 1934b A contribution to the theory of price fluctuations. *Rev. Econ. Stud.* 1: 186
Haldane JBS 1934c Anthropology and human biology. *Man* 34: 142
Haldane JBS 1934d Anthropology and human biology. *Man* 34: 163
Haldane JBS 1934e A mathematical theory of natural and artificial selection, pt 10. Some theorems on artificial selection. *Genetics* 19: 412
Haldane JBS 1934f The attitude of the German government towards science. *Nature, London* 132: 726
Haldane JBS 1934g Science and politics. *Nature, London* 133: 65
Haldane JBS 1934h Science at the universities. *Nature, London* 134: 571
Haldane JBS 1934i Methods for the detection of autosomal linkage in man. *Ann. Eugen.* 6: 26
Haldane JBS 1934j Human biology and politics. *The British Science Guild: 10th Norman Lockyer lecture*, p 3
Haldane JBS 1934k Race and culture. *Proc. Royal Anthroplogical Institute and the Institute of Sociology*. Le Play House Press, London, p 8
Haldane JBS 1934l The relative efficiency of two methods of measuring human linkage. *American Naturalist* 68: 286
Haldane JBS 1934m Genetika i sovremennye sotsyalyie teorie. *Usp. Sovrem Biol.* 3: 426
Haldane JBS 1934n *Fact and Faith*. Watts, London
Haldane JBS, Bartlett MS 1934 The theory of inbreeding in autotetraploids. *J. Genet.* 29: 175
Haldane JBS, Baker JR 1934 *Biology in Everyday Life*. George Allen and Unwin, London
Haldane JBS, Darlington CD, Koller PC 1934 Possibility of incomplete sex linkage in mammals. *Nature, London* 133: 417

Haldane JBS 1935a Genetics since 1910. *Nature, London* 135: 726
Haldane JBS 1935b Blood group inheritance. *Nature, London* 136: 432
Haldane JBS 1935c Human genetics and human ideals. *Nature, London* 136: 894
Haldane JBS 1935d The rate of spontaneous mutation of a human gene. *J. Genet.* 31: 317
Haldane JBS 1935e *Contribution de la génétique a la solution de quelques problèmes physiologiques.* Réunion Plenière de la Societé de Biologie, Paris
Haldane JBS 1935f Some problems of mathematical biology. *J. Math. Phys.* 14: 125
Haldane JBS 1935g *The Outlook of Science.* Kegan Paul, Trench, Trubner, London
Haldane JBS 1935h *Science and Well-being.* Kegan Paul, Trench, Trubner, London
Haldane JBS, Penrose LS 1935 Mutation rates in man. *Nature, London* 135: 907
Haldane JBS, De Winton D 1935 The genetics of *Primula sinensis* III. Linkage in the diploid. *J. Genet.* 31: 67
Haldane JBS, Bartlett MS 1935 The theory of inbreeding with forced heterozygosis. *J. Genet.* 31: 327.
Haldane JBS, Lunn A 1935 *Science and the Supernatural.* Eyre and Spottiswoode, London

Haldane JBS 1936a A provisional map of a human chromosome. *Nature, London* 137: 397
Haldane JBS 1936b Carbon dioxide content of atmospheric air. *Nature, London* 137: 575
Haldane JBS 1936c Natural selection. *Nature, London* 138: 1053
Haldane JBS 1936d Linkage in *Primula sinensis*: A correction. *J. Genet.* 32: 373
Haldane JBS 1936e The amount of heterozygosis to be expected in an approximately pure line. *J. Genet.* 32: 375
Haldane JBS 1936f Some natural populations of *Lythrum salicaria*. *J. Genet.* 32: 393
Haldane JBS 1936g Some principles of causal analysis in genetics. *Erkenntnis* 6: 346
Haldane JBS 1936h A search for incomplete sex-linkage in man. *Ann. Eugen.* 7: 28
Haldane JBS 1936i Is space-time simply connected? *The Observatory* 59: 228
Haldane JBS 1936j A discussion on the present state of the theory of natural selection. Primary and secondary effects of natural selection. *Proc. Roy. Soc. B* 121: 67
Haldane JBS, Bell J 1936 Linkage in man. *Nature, London* 138: 759
Haldane JBS, Ashby E, Crew FAE, Darlington CD, Ford EB, Salisbury EJ, Turrill WB, Waddington CH 1936 Genetics in the universities. *Nature, London* 138: 972

Haldane JBS 1937a Physical science and philosophy. *Nature, London* 139: 1003
Haldane JBS 1937b Genetics in Madrid. *Nature, London* 140: 331
Haldane JBS 1937c The position of genetics. *Nature, London* 140: 428
Haldane JBS 1937d The exact value of the moments of the distribution of χ^2 used as a test of goodness of fit, when expectations are small. *Biometrika* 29: 133
Haldane JBS 1937e Some theoretical results of continued brother-sister mating. *J. Genet.* 34: 265
Haldane JBS 1937f The effect of variation on fitness. *American Naturalist* 71: 337
Haldane JBS 1937g A probable new sex-linked dominant in man. *J. Hered.* 28: 58
Haldane JBS 1937h L'analyse génétique des populations naturelles. *Réunion internat. de Physique-Chimique-Biologie. Congrès du Palais de la découverte, Paris* 8: 517
Haldane JBS 1937i Science and future warfare. *J. Roy. United Services Inst.* 82: 713
Haldane JBS 1937j Dialectical account of evolution. *Science and Society* 1: 473
Haldane JBS 1937k Biochemistry of the individual. In: Needham J, Green DE (eds) 1937 *Perspectives in Biochemistry.* Cambridge University Press, Cambridge
Haldane JBS, Gruneberg H 1937 Tests of goodness of fit applied to records of Mendelian segregation in mice. *Biometrika* 29: 144
Haldane JBS, Bell J 1937 The linkage between the genes for colour-blindness and haemophilia in man. *Proc. Roy. Soc. B* 123: 119

Haldane JBS 1938a The first six moments of χ^2 for an n-fold table with n degrees of freedom when some expectations are small. *Biometrika* 29: 389
Haldane JBS 1938b The approximate normalization of a class of frequency distributions. *Biometrika* 29: 392
Haldane JBS 1938c Heterostylism in natural populations of the primrose. *Biometrika* 30: 196
Haldane JBS 1938d Social relations of science. *Nature, Lond.* 141: 730
Haldane JBS 1938e Mathematics of air raid protection. *Nature, Lond.* 142: 791

Haldane JBS 1938f The estimation of the frequencies of recessive conditions in man. *Ann. Eug.* 8: 255
Haldane JBS 1938g A hitherto unexpected complication in the genetics of human recessives. *Ann. Eug.* 8: 263
Haldane JBS 1938h The location of the gene for haemophilia. *Genetica* 20: 423
Haldane JBS 1938i Indirect evidence for the mating system in natural populations. *J. Genet.* 36: 213
Haldane JBS 1938j The nature of interspecific differences. *Evolution*. p 79.
Haldane JBS 1938k Blood royal. A study of haemophilia in the royal families of Europe. *The Modern Quarterly* 1: 129
Haldane JBS 1938l Congenital disease. *Lancet* ii: 1449
Haldane JBS 1938m *The Chemistry of the Individual. 38th Robert Boyle Lec.* Oxford University Press, Oxford
Haldane JBS 1938n Forty years of genetics. In: Needham J, Pagel W (eds) 1938 *Background to Modern Science*. Cambridge University Press, Cambridge, p 225
Haldane JBS 1938o *ARP*. Victor Gollancz, London
Haldane JBS 1938p *Heredity and Politics*. George Allen and Unwin, London
Haldane JBS, Bedichek S 1938 A search for autosomal recessive lethals in man. *Ann. Eugen* 8: 245
Haldane JBS 1939a The theory of the evolution of dominance. *J. Genet.* 37: 365.
Haldane JBS 1939b Speculative biology. *The Modern Quarterly* 2: 1
Haldane JBS 1939c Protoplasm. *The Modern Quarterly* 2: 128
Haldane JBS 1939d The spread of harmful autosomal recessive genes in human populations. *Ann. Eug.* 9: 232
Haldane JBS 1939e The equilibrium between mutation and random extinction. *Ann. Eug.* 9: 400
Haldane JBS 1939f Note on the preceding analysis of Mendelian segregations. *Biometrika* 31: 67
Haldane JBS 1939g Corrections to formulae in papers on the moments of χ^2. *Biometrika* 31: 220
Haldane JBS 1939h Sampling errors in the determination of bacterial or virus density by the dilution method. *J. Hyg.* 39: 289
Haldane JBS, Moshinsky P 1939 Inbreeding in Mendelian populations with special reference to human cousin marriage. *Ann. Eug.* 9: 321
Haldane JBS, Phillip U 1939a The daughters and sisters of haemophilics. *J. Genet.* 33: 193
Haldane JBS, Phillip U 1939b Relative sexuality in unicellular algae. *Nature, Lond.* 143: 334
Haldane JBS, Alexander W, Duff P, Ives G, Renton D 1939 After-effects of exposure of men to carbon dioxide. *Lancet* ii: 419

Haldane JBS 1940a The mean and variance of χ^2, when used as a test of homogeneity, when expectations are small. *Biometrika* 31: 346
Haldane JBS 1940b The cumulants and moments of the binomial distribution, and the cumulants of χ^2 for a $(n \times 2)$ fold table. *Biometrika* 31: 392
Haldane JBS 1940c Blood groups of anthropoids. *Nature, Lond.* 146: 562
Haldane JBS 1940d The conflict between selection and mutation of harmful recessive genes. *Ann. Eug.* 10: 417
Haldane JBS 1940e The estimation of recessive gene frequencies by inbreeding. *Proc. Ind. Acd. Sci.* 12: 109
Haldane JBS 1940f The blood-group frequencies of European peoples and racial origins. *Human Biology* 12: 457
Haldane JBS 1940g Preface and notes. In: Dutt C (ed) 1940 *Dialectics of Nature*. Lawrence and Wishart, London
Haldane JBS 1940h *Science in Peace and War*. Lawrence and Wishart, London
Haldane JBS 1940i *Science in Everyday Life*. Macmillan, New York
Haldane JBS 1940j *Keeping Cool and Other Essays*. Chatto and Windus, London
Haldane JBS, Gruneberg H 1940 Congenital hyperglycaemia in mice. *Nature, Lond.* 145: 704

Haldane JBS 1941a The partial sex-linkage of recessive spastic paraplegia. *J. Genet.* 41: 141

Haldane JBS 1941b The relative importance of principal and modifying genes in determining some human diseases. *J. Genet.* 41: 149
Haldane JBS 1941c Can science be independent? *Nature, Lond.* 147: 416
Haldane JBS 1941d The relation between science and ethics. *Nature, Lond.* 148: 342
Haldane JBS 1941e Human life and death at high pressures. *Nature, Lond.* 148: 458
Haldane JBS 1941f Science in the USSR. *Nature, Lond.* 148: 598
Haldane JBS 1941g Number of primes and probability considerations. *Nature, Lond.* 148: 694
Haldane JBS 1941h Physiological properties of some common gases at high pressures. *Chemical Products* 4: 83
Haldane JBS 1941i The faking of genetical results. *Eureka* 6: 8
Haldane JBS 1941j The fitting of binomial distributions. *Ann. Eug.* 11: 179
Haldane JBS 1941k How to write a popular scientific article. *The Scientific Worker* 13: 122
Haldane JBS 1941l The cumulants of the distribution of the square of a variate. *Biometrika* 32: 199
Haldane JBS 1941m The laws of Nature. *Rationalist Annual* p. 35
Haldane JBS 1941n *New Paths in Genetics.* George Allen and Unwin, London
Haldane JBS, Case EM 1941a Tastes of oxygen and nitrogen at high pressures. *Nature, Lond.* 148: 84
Haldane JBS, Case EM 1941b Human physiology under high pressure. I. Effects of nitrogen, carbon dioxide and cold. *J. Hyg.* 41: 225

Haldane JBS 1942a Moments of the distributions of powers and products of normal variates. *Biometrika* 32: 226
Haldane JBS 1942b The mode and median of a nearly normal distribution with given cumulants. *Biometrika* 32: 294
Haldane JBS 1942c Selection against heterozygosis in man. *Ann. Eug.* 11: 333
Haldane JBS 1942d The selective elimination of silver foxes in Eastern Canada. *J. Genet.* 44: 296
Haldane JBS 1942e Civil defence against war gases. *Nature, Lond.* 150: 769
Haldane JBS, Poole R 1942 A new pedigree of recurrent bullouse eruption of the feet. *J. Hered.* 33: 17

Haldane JBS 1943a Statistics of occupational mortality. *Camb. Univ. Medical Soc. Mag.* 20: 38
Haldane JBS 1943b James Prescott Joule and the unit of energy. *Nature, Lond.* 152: 479
Haldane JBS, Rendel JM 1943 Variation in the weights of hatched and unhatched ducks. *Biometrika* 33: 56

Haldane JBS 1944a Mutation and the Rhesus reaction. *Nature, Lond.* 153: 106
Haldane JBS 1944b Radioactivity and the origin of life in Milne's cosmology. *Nature, Lond.* 153: 555
Haldane JBS 1944c Heredity, development and genetics. *Nature, Lond.* 154: 429
Haldane JBS 1944d New deep-sea diving method: the case for helium. *Fairplay* 163: 740
Haldane JBS 1944e Reshaping plants and animals. In: Huxley JS (ed) 1944 *Reshaping Man's Heritage.* Allen and Unwin, London
Haldane JBS, Whitehouse HLK 1944 Symmetrical and asymmetrical post-reduction in Ascomycetes. *Nature, Lond.* 154: 704
Haldane JBS, Phillip U, Rendel JM, Spurway H 1944 Genetics and karyology of *Drosophila subobscura. Nature, Lond.* 154: 260

Haldane JBS 1945a A labour saving method of sampling. *Nature, Lond.* 155: 49
Haldane JBS 1945b A quantum theory of the origin of the solar system. *Nature, Lond.* 155: 133
Haldane JBS 1945c Inverse statistical variates. *Nature, Lond.* 155: 453
Haldane JBS 1945d Cosmic rays and kinematical relativity. *Nature, Lond.* 156: 266
Haldane JBS 1944e On a method of estimating frequencies. *Biometrika* 33: 222
Haldane JBS 1944f Moments of r and χ^2 for a fourfold table in the absence of association. *Biometrika* 33: 231

Haldane JBS 1945g Use of χ^2 as a test of homogeneity in a ($n \times 2$)-fold table when expectations are small. *Biometrika* 33: 234

Haldane JBS 1945h A new theory of the past. *Amer. Scientist* 33: 129

Haldane JBS 1945i Cnance effects and the Gaussian distribution. *Phil. Mag.* (7): 36, 184

Haldane JBS 1946a The cumulants of the distribution of Fisher's 'u_{11}' and 'u_{11}' scores used in the detection and estimation of linkage in man. *Ann. Eug.* 13: 122

Haldane JBS 1946b The interaction of nature and nurture. *Ann. Eug.* 13: 197

Haldane JBS 1946c Auld Hornie, FRS. *Modern Quarterly* p 32

Haldane JBS 1946d *A Banned Broadcast and Other Essays*. Chatto and Windus, London

Haldane JBS, Gilchrist BM 1946 Sex-linkage in *Culex molestus*. *Experientia* 11: 372

Haldane JBS, Whitehouse HLK 1946 Symmetrical and asymmetrical reduction in Ascomycetes. *J. Genet.* 47: 208

Haldane JBS 1947a The mutation rate of the gene for haemophilia, and its segregation ratios in males and females. *Ann. Eug.* 13: 262

Haldane JBS 1947b The dysgenic effect of induced recessive mutations. *Ann. Eug.* 14: 35

Haldane JBS 1947c Effect of nuclear explosions. *Ann. Eug.* 14: 35

Haldane JBS 1947d *Science Advances*. George Allen and Unwin, London

Haldane JBS 1947e *What is life?* Boni and Gaer, New York

Haldene JBS, Gilchrist BM 1947 Sex-linkage and sex determination in a mosquito *Culex molestus*. *Hereditas*. 33: 175

Haldane JBS, Lea DE 1947 A mathematical theory of chromosomal rearrangements. *J. Genet.* 48: 1

Haldane JBS, Smith CAB 1947 A new estimate of the linkage between the genes for colour-blindness and haemophilia in man. *Ann. Eug.* 14: 10

Haldane JBS 1948a The precision of observed values of small frequencies. *Biometrika* 35: 297

Haldane JBS 1948b A note on the median of a multivariate distribution. *Biometrika* 35: 414

Haldane JBS 1948c The theory of a cline. *J. Genet.* 48: 277

Haldane JBS 1948d The number of genotypes which can be formed with a given number of genes. *J. Genet.* 49: 117

Haldane JBS 1948e Differences. *Mind* 57 (NS): 227

Haldane JBS 1948f The formal genetics of man. *Proc. Roy. Soc. B* 135: 147

Haldane JBS, Smith CAB 1948 A simple exact test for birth order effect. *Ann. Eug.* 14: 117

Haldane JBS, Snell GD 1948 Methods for histocompatibility of genes. *J. Genet.* 49: 104

Haldane JBS 1949a Parental and fraternal correlations for fitness. *Ann. Eug.* 14: 288

Haldane JBS 1949b A test for homogeneity of records of familial abnormalities. *Ann. Eug.* 14: 339

Haldane JBS 1949c The association of characters as a result of inbreeding and linkage. *Ann. Eug.* 15: 15

Haldane JBS 1949d Suggestions as to quantitative measurement of rates of evolution. *Evolution*, 3: 51

Haldane JBS 1949e Some statistical problems arising in genetics. *J. Roy. Stat. Soc. B* 11: 14

Haldane JBS 1949f The rate of mutation of human genes. *Proc. 8th International Congress of Genetics. Hereditas Suppl.* p. 267

Haldane JBS 1949g A note on non-normal correlation. *Biometrika* 34: 467

Haldane JBS 1949h In defence of genetics. *Modern Quarterly* (NS) 4: 194

Haldane JBS 1949i Human evolution: Past and future. In: Jepsen GL, Mayr E, Simpson GG (eds) 1949 *Evolution*. Princeton University Press, Princeton p. 405

Haldane JBS 1949j Disease and evolution. *La ricerca scientifica Suppl.* 19: 68

Haldane JBS, Dewar D, Davies CM 1949 *Is Evolution a Myth? A Debate*. London: C. A. Watts and Co and The Paternoster Press

Haldane JBS 1951a La methode dans la génétique. *C.R. 10th Cong. Internat. Phil. Sci.* 6: 34

Haldane JBS 1951b La narcose par les gaz indifférents. *Mecanisme de la Narcose*. CNRS, Paris, p 47

Haldane JBS 1951c The rate of evolution. *Rat. Ann.* p 7

Haldane JBS 1951d The mathematics of biology. *Sci. J. Roy. Coll. Sci.* 22: 11

Haldane JBS 1951e A class of efficient estimates of a parameter. *Bull. Internat. Stat. Inst.* 32: 231
Haldane JBS 1951f The extraction of square roots. *Math. Gaz.* 35: 89
Haldane JBS 1951g *Everything has a History*. George Allen and Unwin, London

Haldane JBS 1952a The mechanical chess player. *Brit. J. Phil. Sci.* 3: 189
Haldane JBS 1952b Variation. *New Biology* 12: 9
Haldane JBS 1952c Simple tests for bimodality and bitangentiality. *Ann. Eug.* 16: 359
Haldane JBS 1952d Relations between biology and other sciences. *Sci. Culture*, 17: 407
Haldane JBS 1952e The origin of language. *Rat. Ann.* p 38

Haldane JBS 1953a The gentics of some biochemical abnormalities. *Lectures on the Scientific Basis of Medicine* 3: 41
Haldane JBS 1953b Animal ritual and human language. *Diogenes* (UNESCO) 4: 61
Haldane JBS 1953c Foreword. 'Evolution' *Symp. Soc. Expt. Biol.* 7: 9
Haldane JBS 1953d The estimation of two parameters from a sample. *Sankhya* 12: 313
Haldane JBS 1953e Animal populations and their regulation. *New biology* 15: 9
Haldane JBS 1953f On some statistical formulae. *Sci. Culture* 18: 598
Haldane JBS 1953g Some animal life-tables. *J. Inst. Actuaries*. 79: 53
Haldane JBS 1953h Closing address. *IUBS Symp. on Genetics of Population*, p 139
Haldane JBS, Spurway H 1953 The comparative ethology of vertebrate breathing. I. Breathing in newts with a general survey. *Behaviour* 6: 8

Haldane JBS 1954a A logical analysis of learning, conditioning and related processes. *Behaviour* 6: 4
Haldane JBS 1954b The measurement of natural selection. *Caryologia* (Turin). Suppl. 6: 480
Haldane JBS 1954c Introducing Douglas Spalding. *Brit. J. Anim. Behaviour* 2: 1
Haldane JBS 1954d The genetical determination of behaviour. *Brit. J. Anim. Behaviour* 2: 118
Haldane JBS 1954e A rationalist with a halo. *Rationalist Annual* p 14
Haldane JBS 1954f The origins of life. *New Biology* 16: 12
Haldane JBS 1954g La signalisation animale. *L'Annee Biologique* 30: 89
Haldane JBS 1954h Substitutes for χ^2. *Biometrika* 42: 265
Haldane JBS 1954i An exact test for randomness of mating. *J. Genet.* 52: 631
Haldane JBS 1954j The statistics of evolution. In: Huxley JS, Hardy AC, Ford EB (eds) 1954 Allen and Unwin, London p 109
Haldane JBS 1954k *The Biochemistry of Genetics*. George Allen and Unwin, London
Haldane JBS, Spurway H 1954a A statistical analysis of communication in *Apis mellifera* and a comparison with communication in other animals. *Insectes Soc.* 1: 247
Haldane JBS, Spurway H 1954b A statistical analysis of some data on infra-red communication. *Brit. J. Anim. Behaviour* 2: 38
Haldane JBS, Capildeo R 1954 The mathematics of bird population growth and decline. *J. Anim. ecol.* 23: 215

Haldane JBS 1955a Genetical effects of radiation from products of nuclear explosions. *Nature, Lond.* 176: 115
Haldane JBS 1955b Origin of man. *Nature, Lond.* 176: 169
Haldane JBS 1955c Educational problems of the colonial territories. *Nature, Lond.* 176: 750
Haldane JBS 1955d Population genetics. *New Biology* 18: 34
Haldane JBS 1955e Some alternatives to sex. *New Biology* 19: 7
Haldane JBS 1955f A problem in the significance of small numbers. *Biometrika* 42: 266
Haldane JBS 1955g The rapid calculation of χ^2 as a test of homogeneity from a $2 \times n$ table. *Biometrika* 42: 519
Haldane JBS 1955h Biometry. *Sankhya* 16: 207
Haldane JBS 1955i A logical basis for genetics? *Brit. J. Phil. Science* 6: 245
Haldane JBS 1955j Natural selection. *Trans. Bose. Res. Inst. Calcutta* 10: 17
Haldane JBS 1955k The genetic effects of atomic bomb explosions. *Current Science* 24: 399
Haldane JBS 1955l The prospects of eugenics. *The Roy. Inst. of Gt. Brit.* 36: 290
Haldane JBS 1955m Targets. *Math. Gaz.* 39: 1

Haldane JBS 1955n The complete matrices for brother–sister and alternate parent–offspring mating involving one locus. *J. Genet.* 53: 315

Haldane JBS 1955o Aristotle's account of bees' dances. *J. Hellenic Studies* 75: 24

Haldane JBS 1955p On the biochemistry of heterosis, and the stabilization of polymorphism. *Proc. Roy. Soc. B* 144: 217

Haldane JBS 1955q Animal communication and the origin of human language. *Sci. Progr.* 171: 385

Haldane JBS 1955r The biochemistry of human genetics. *Society of Biological Chemists, India, Silver Jubilee. Souvenir*, p 21

Haldane JBS 1955s Suggestions for evolutionary studies in India. *Nat. Inst. of Sci. Ind. Bulletin No. 7, Symposium on Organic Evolution*, p 25

Haldane JBS 1955t The calculation of mortality rates from ringing data. *Acta Congr. Int. Orn.* p 454

Haldane JBS 1955u Introduction p 14 and, Critique de la méthode statistique utilisée pour l'etude de la *pars stridens* alair de *Locusta migratoria*. In: Busnel RG (ed) 1955 *Colloque sur l'acoustique des Orthoptères*. Publ. Inst. Nat. Rech. Agronom. Paris, p 102

Haldane JBS 1955v Remaniement du patrimoine héréditaire humain, and Mecanismes biochimiques d'action des gènes. In: Turpin R (ed) 1955 *La Progénèse*. Masson et Cie, Paris, pp 389, 397

Haldane JBS, Spurway H 1955 The respiratory behaviour of the Indian climbing perch in various environments. *Brit. J. Anim. Behaviour* 3: 74

Haldane JBS 1956a The detection of antigens with an abnormal genetic determination. *J. Genet.* 54: 54

Haldane JBS 1956b The conflict between inbreeding and selection. 1. Self-fertilization. *J. Genet.* 54: 56

Haldane JBS 1956c The estimation of viabilities. *J. Genet.* 54: 294

Haldane JBS 1956d The detection of autosomal lethals in mice induced by mutagenic agents. *J. Genet.* 54: 327

Haldane JBS 1956e Almost unbiased estimates of functions of frequencies. *Sankhya* 17: 201

Haldane JBS 1956f The estimation and significance of the logarithm of a ratio of frequencies. *Ann. Human Gen.* 20: 309

Haldane JBS 1956g Mutation in the sex linked recessive type of muscular dystrophy. A possible sex difference. *Ann. Human Gen.* 20: 344

Haldane JBS 1956h The theory of selection for melanism in *Lepidoptera*. *Proc. Roy. Soc. B* 145: 303

Haldane JBS 1956i The relation between density regulation and natural selection. *Proc. Roy. Soc. B* 145: 306

Haldane JBS 1956j Some reflections on non-violence. *Mankind* 1: 1

Haldane JBS 1956k The sources of some ethological notions. *Brit. J. Anim. Behaviour* 4: 162

Haldane JBS 1956l Die Bedeutung der Makromolekule fur Evolution und Differenzierung. In 'Vergleichend Biochemische Fragen'. *Colloquium Ges. Physiol. Chemie* 6: 165

Haldane JBS 1956m Natural selection in man. *Acta. Genet.* 6: 321

Haldane JBS 1956n The estimation of mutation rates produced by high energy events in mammals. *Current Sci.* 25: 75

Haldane JBS 1956o The argument from animals to men. An examination of its validity for anthropology. *J. Roy. Anthropol. Inst.* 86: 1

Haldane JBS 1956p Time in biology. *Sci. Progr.* 175: 385

Haldane JBS 1956q The biometrical analysis of fossil populations. *Journal of the Paleontological Society of India* (Lucknow) 1: 54

Haldane JBS 1956r Les aspects physico-chimiques des instincts. *L'Instinct dans le comportement des animaux et del l'homme*. Masson et Cie, Paris, p 547

Haldane JBS 1956s Can a species concept be justified? In: Sylvester-Bradley PC (ed) 1956 The species concept in paleontology. *Syst. Assoc. Publ.* 2: 95

Haldane JBS 1956t Radiation hazards. *Lancet* i: 1066.

Haldane JBS, Smith SM 1956 The sampling distribution of a maximum likelihood estimate. *Biometrika* 43: 96

Haldane JBS, Spurway H 1956a Abnormal breathing behaviour in a fish. *Brit. J. Anim. Behavior* 4: 37
Haldane JBS, Spurway H 1956b Imprinting and the evolution of instincts. *Nature, Lond.* 178: 85

Haldane JBS 1957a The conditions for coadaptation in polymorphism for inversions. *J. Genet.* 55: 218
Haldane JBS 1957b The cost of natural selection. *J. Genet.* 55: 511
Haldane JBS 1957c The prospects of eugenics. *New Biology* 22: 7
Haldane JBS 1957d Karl Pearson, 1857–1957. *Biometrika* 44: 303 (Also published in *New Biology* 25: 7)
Haldane JBS 1957e The elementary theory of population growth. *J. Mad. Univ. B* 27: 237
Haldane JBS 1957f Graphical methods in enzyme chemistry. *Nature, Lond.* 179: 832
Haldane JBS 1957g Methods for the detection and enumeration of mutations produced by irradiation in mice. *Proc. Int. Genetics Symp.* (Cytologia supplement)
Haldane JBS 1957h Genesis of life. In: Bates DR (ed) 1957 *The Planet Earth*. Pergamon Press, London p 287
Haldane JBS, Carter TC 1957 The use of linked marker genes for detecting recessive autosomal lethals in the mouse. *J. Genet.* 55: 596

Haldane JBS 1958a Syadvada system of predication. *Sankhya* 18: 195
Haldane JBS 1958b The scope of biological statistics. *Sankhya* 20: 195
Haldane JBS 1958c Parthenogenesis. *Triangle* (Basle) 3: 142
Haldane JBS 1958d Sex determination in Metazoa. *Proc. Zool. Soc. Calcutta, Mukherjee Memorial* 4: 13
Haldane JBS 1958e Mathematics and jute breeding. *Jute and Gunny Review* 10: 3
Haldane JBS 1958f The present position of Darwinism. *J. Sci. Ind. Res.* (India) 17a: 97
Haldane JBS 1958g The statistical study of animal behaviour. *Trans. Bose Research Institute* 22: 201
Haldane JBS 1958h The genetic effects of quanta and particles of high energy. *Sci. Culture* 24: 16
Haldane JBS 1958i The theory of evolution before and after Bateson. *J. Genet.* 56: 11
Haldane JBS 1958j *The Unity and Diversity of Life*. Publications Division, Government of India
Haldane JBS, Roy SK 1958 A research project for some Indian schools. *Vigyan Shikshak* 2: 35
Haldane JBS, Spurway H 1958 The quantitative study of animal behaviour in an approximately steady state. *Memoriam Methodi Popov, Bulgarian Academy of Sciences*, p. 89

Haldane JBS 1959a The scope of biological statistics. *Sankhya* 20: 195
Haldane JBS 1959b The analysis of heterogeneity. *Sankhya* 21: 209
Haldane JBS 1959c An Indian perspective of Darwin. *Centenn. Rev. Arts Sci. Mich. St. Univ.* 3: 357.
Haldane JBS 1959d Suggestions for research on coconuts. *Ind. Coconut J.* 12: 1
Haldane JBS 1959e The non-violent scientific study of birds. *J. Bombay Nat. Hist. Soc.* 56: 375
Haldane JBS 1959f Parthenogenese *Naturwissenschaftliche Rundschau* 12: 453
Haldane JBS 1959g Natural selection. In: Bell PR (ed) 1959 *Darwin's Biological Work*. Cambridge University Press, Cambridge, p 101

Haldane JBS 1960a The theory of natural selection today. In: Purchon RD (ed) 1960 *Proc. Cent. Bicent. Cong. Biol.* University Malaya Press, Singapore, p 1 (Also *Nature, Lond.* 183: 710)
Haldane JBS 1960b Pasteur and cosmic asymmetry. *Nature, Lond.* 185: 87
Haldane JBS 1960c The scientific work of JS Haldane. *Nature, Lond.* 187: 102
Haldane JBS 1960*d 'Dex' or 'order of magnitude'? Nature, Lond.* 187: 879
Haldane JBS 1960e The interpretation of Carter's results on induction of recessive lethals in mice. *J. Genet.* 57: 131
Haldane JBS 1960f More precise expressions for the cost of natural selection. *J. Genet.* 57: 351

Haldane JBS 1960g Physiological problems at high pressure. *Aero Med. Soc. J. (New Delhi)* 5: 1
Haldane JBS 1960h Genetics in relation to medicine. *Proc. Acad. Med. Sci. (Andhra Pradesh)* 1: 216
Haldane JBS 1960i Suggestions for research on human physiology in India. *The Medico (Gandhi Medical College, Hyderabad)* 4: 2
Haldane JBS 1960j On expecting the unexpected. *Rationalist Annual*, p 5
Haldane JBS 1960k The addition of random vectors. *Sankhya*, 22: 213
Haldane JBS 1960l Blood grouping and human trisomy. *Current Sci.* 29: 375
Haldane JBS 1960m Mind in evolution. *Zool. Jahrb. Abt. Syst.* 88: 117
Haldane JBS 1960n Physiological variation and evolution. *Maharajah Sayajirao Memorial Lecture*, p 1

Haldane JBS 1961a Some simple systems of artificial selection. *J. Genet.* 57: 345
Haldane JBS 1961b Natural selection in man. *Prog. Med. Genet.* 1: 27
Haldane JBS 1961c The scientific work of JS Haldane. *Penguin Science Survey* (2), p 11
Haldane JBS 1961d Simple approximations to the probability integral and $P(\chi^2, 1)$ when both are small. *Sankhya* 23: 9
Haldane JBS 1961e Evolution as a test for ethics. *Current Sci.* 30: 214
Haldane JBS 1961f Conditions for stable polymorphism at an autosomal locus. *Nature, Lond.* 193: 1108
Haldane JBS, Jayakar SD 1961 A statistical analysis of some data on ant and wasp behavior. *Att. IV Congresso UIEIS—Pavia, Symposia Genetica et Biol. Ital.* 12: 221

Haldane JBS 1962a Human needs. In: Mitchison N (ed) 1962 *What the Human Race is Up To.* Gollancz, London, p 395
Haldane JBS 1962b Evidence for heterosis in woodlice. *J. Genet.* 58: 39
Haldane JBS 1962c Natural selection in a population with annual breeding but overlapping generations. *J. Genet.* 58: 122
Haldane JBS 1962d The selection of double heterozygotes. *J. Genet.* 58: 125
Haldane JBS, Dronamraju KR 1962 Inheritance of hairy pinnae. *Amer. J. Hum. Genet.* 14: 102
Haldane JBS, Jayakar SD 1962 An enumeration of some human relationships. *J. Genet.* 58: 81

Haldane JBS 1963a Tests for sex-linked inheritance on population samples. *Ann. Hum. Genet.* 27: 107
Haldane JBS 1963b The design of experiments on mutation rates. *J. Genet.* 58: 232
Haldane JBS 1963c Life and mind as physical realities. *Penguin Science Survey* (2), p. 224
Haldane JBS 1963d The concentration of rare recessive genes in the past and in modern times. In: Goldschmidt E (ed.) 1963 *The Genetics of Migrant and Isolate Populations.* Williams and Wilkins, Baltimore, p. 243
Haldane JBS 1963e Some lies about science. *Rationalist Annual*, p. 32
Haldane JBS 1963f Biological possibilities for the human species in the next ten thousand years. In: Wolstenholme GEW (ed) 1963 J and A Churchill, London, p 337
Haldane JBS 1963g A possible development of JS Haldane's views on the relation between quantum mechanics and biology. In: Cunningham DJC, Lloyd BB (eds) 1963 *The Regulation of Human Respiration.* Blackwell, Oxford, p 103
Haldane JBS, Spurway H 1963 The regulation of breathing in a fish, *Anabas testudineus.* In: *The Regulation of Human Respiration.* Cunningham DJC, Lloyd BB (eds) 1963 Blackwell, Oxford, p. 431
Haldane JBS, Jayakar SD 1963a The distribution of extremal and nearly extremal values in samples from a normal distribution. *Biometrika* 50: 89
Haldane JBS, Jayakar SD 1963b Polymorphism due to selection of varying direction. *J. Genet.* 58: 237
Haldanes JBS, Jayakar SD 1963c The elimination of double dominants in large random mating populations. *J. Genet.* 58: 243
Haldane JBS, Jayakar SD 1963d The solution of some equations occurring in population genetics. *J. Genet.* 58: 291

Haldane JBS, Jayakar SD 1963e Polymorphism due to selection depending on the composition of a population. *J. Genet.* 58: 318
Haldane JBS, Jayakar SD 1963f A new test of significance in sampling from finite populations, with application to human inbreeding. *J. Genet.* 58: 402

Haldane JBS 1964a A defence of beanbag genetics. *Perspectives in Biology and Medicine*, 7: 343
Haldane JBS 1964b The origin of lactation. *Rationalist Annual*, p. 19
Haldane JBS 1964c The implications of genetics for human society. *Proc. 11th Inter. Congr. Genet.* xci.
Haldane JBS 1964d The proper social application of the knowledge of human genetics. In: Goldsmith M, Mackay A (ed) 1964 Souvenir Press and Penguin Books, London, p 150
Haldane JBS, Jayakar SD 1964 Equilibria under natural selection at a sex-linked locus. *J. Genet.* 59: 29

Haldane JBS 1965a On being finite. *Rationalist Annual*, p. 3
Haldane JBS 1965b The possible evolution of lactation. *Zool. Jahr. Syst. Bd.* 92: 41
Haldane JBS 1965c Data needed for a blueprint of the first organism. In: Fox S W (ed) 1965 *The Origins of Prebiological Systems*. Academic Press, New York, p 11
Haldane JBS 1965d Biological research in developing countries. In: Wolstenholme GEW, O'Connor M (eds) 1965 *Man and Africa*. CIBA Foundation Symposium. J and A Churchill, London, p 222
Haldane JBS 1965e *Science and Indian Culture*. New Age Publishers Private, Calcutta
Haldane JBS, Jayakar SD 1965a The nature of human genetic loads. *J. Genet.* 59: 53
Haldane JBS, Jayakar SD 1965b Selection for a single pair of allelomorphs with complete replacement. *J. Genet.* 59: 81
Haldane JBS, Ray AK 1965 The genetics of a common Indian digital anomaly. *Proc. Nat. Acad. Sci. Wash.* 53: 1050

Haldane JBS 1966 An autobiography in brief. *Persp. Biol. Med.* 9: 476

Haldane JBS 1969 *Science and Life*. Pemberton Publishing, London

Haldane JBS 1971 The comparison of coefficients of inbreeding. *J. Genet.* 60: 250

Haldane JBS, Jayakar SD 1972 The equilibrium between mutation and selection in bisexual diploids. *J. Genet.* 61: 1

Haldane JBS 1973 *Reader of Popular Scientific Essays*. (Feldman GE, Meshkov OD eds) Nauka, Moscow

Haldane JBS 1976 *The Man with Two Memories*. Merlin Press, London